Medical Terminology Systems

Systems

A Body Systems Approach

8TH EDITION

Medical Terminology Systems

A Body Systems Approach

8TH EDITION

Barbara A. Gylys, MEd, CMA-A (AAMA)
Professor Emerita
University of Toledo
Toledo, OH

Mary Ellen Wedding, MEd, MT(ASCP), CMA (AAMA), CPC (AAPC)
Professor Emerita
University of Toledo
Toledo, OH

F.A. Davis Company • Philadelphia

F. A. Davis Company
1915 Arch Street
Philadelphia, PA 19103
www.fadavis.com

Copyright © 2017 by F. A. Davis Company

Printed in the United States of America

Last digit indicates print number: 10 9 8 7 6 5 4 3

Publisher: T. Quincy McDonald
Director of Content Development: George W. Lang
Developmental Editor: Brenna Mayer
Art and Design Manager: Carolyn O'Brien

As new scientific information becomes available through basic and clinical research, recommended treatments and drug therapies undergo changes. The author(s) and publisher have done everything possible to make this book accurate, up to date, and in accord with accepted standards at the time of publication. The author(s), editors, and publisher are not responsible for errors or omissions or for consequences from application of the book, and make no warranty, expressed or implied, in regard to the contents of the book. Any practice described in this book should be applied by the reader in accordance with professional standards of care used in regard to the unique circumstances that may apply in each situation. The reader is advised always to check product information (package inserts) for changes and new information regarding dose and contraindications before administering any drug. Caution is especially urged when using new or infrequently ordered drugs.

Library of Congress Cataloging-in-Publication Data

Names: Gylys, Barbara A., author. | Wedding, Mary Ellen, author.
Title: Medical terminology systems : a body systems approach / Barbara A.
   Gylys, Mary Ellen Wedding.
Description: Eighth edition. | Philadelphia : F.A. Davis Company, [2017] |
   Includes bibliographical references and indexes.
Identifiers: LCCN 2016054225| ISBN 9780803658677 (pbk.) | ISBN 0803658672
   (pbk.)
Subjects: | MESH: Terminology as Topic | Problems and Exercises
Classification: LCC R123 | NLM W 15 | DDC 610.1/4—dc23
LC record available at https://lccn.loc.gov/2016054225

This Book Is Dedicated with Love

To my best friend, colleague, and husband, Dr. Julius A. Gylys, and to my children, Regina Maria and Dr. Julius Anthony, and to my grandchildren, Andrew Masters, Dr. Julia Halm, Caitlin Masters, Anthony Bishop-Gylys, Matthew Bishop-Gylys, and the little ones, Liam, Harrison, and Emmett Halm

B.A.G.

To my loving grandchildren, Andrew Arthur Kurtz, Katherine Louise Kurtz, Daniel Keith Wedding II, Carol Ann Estelle Wedding, Jonathan Michael Kurtz, Donald Keith Wedding III, Emily Michelle Wedding, Katelyn Christine Wedding, and David Michael Wedding

M.E.W.

Acknowledgments

The authors would like to acknowledge the valuable contributions of F. A. Davis's editorial and production team who were responsible for this project:

- **Quincy McDonald, Publisher,** who provided the overall design and layout for the eighth edition. His vision and guidance focused the authors at the onset of the project, and his support throughout this endeavor provided cohesiveness.
- **Brenna H. Mayer, Developmental Editor,** whose careful and conscientious edits and suggestions for the manuscript are evident throughout the entire work. Her enthusiasm and untiring assistance and support during this project are deeply appreciated, and the authors extend their sincerest gratitude.
- **George W. Lang, Director of Content Development,** who meticulously guided the manuscript through the developmental and production phases of the textbook.
- **Margaret Biblis, Editor-in-Chief,** once again provided her support and efforts for the quality of the finished product.

In addition, we wish to acknowledge the many exceptionally dedicated publishing partners who helped in this publication:

- Nichole Liccio, Editorial Associate
- Elizabeth Bales, Developmental Editor and Digital Products Manager
- Kate Margeson, Illustrations Coordinator
- Bob Butler, Production Manager
- Carolyn O'Brien, Art and Design Manager
- Cynthia Breuninger, Managing Editor
- Kirk Pedrick, Director, Digital Solutions
- Julie Chase, Content Product Manager

We also extend our sincerest appreciation to Neil Kelly, Executive Director of Sales, and his staff of sales representatives whose continued efforts have undoubtedly contributed to the success of this textbook.

Preface

Building on the success of previous editions, *Medical Terminology Systems,* 8th edition, continues its well-established record of presenting medical word building principles based on competency-based curricula. Because of the pedagogical success of previous editions, the 8th edition continues its structural design as a textbook–workbook that complements all teaching formats, including traditional lecture, distance learning, and independent or self-paced study. The 8th edition continues to present eponyms without showing the possessive form, such as *Bowman capsule, Cushing syndrome,* and *Parkinson disease.* Medical dictionaries as well as the American Association for Medical Transcription and the American Medical Association support these changes.

The popular basic features of the previous edition have been enhanced and expanded. The updated body systems chapters include diseases and conditions, current medical and diagnostic procedures, treatments, and pharmaceutical agents. The textbook continues to present authentic medical records with activities designed to enhance application of medical terminology to the "real world of medicine." This approach provides the essential tools students of various learning levels need to communicate effectively in today's health-care settings.

As in earlier editions, illustrations that clearly and accurately enhance textual material are integrated throughout the textbook. *Medical Terminology Systems,* 8th edition, includes over 36 new illustrations specifically designed to portray real-life medical conditions, procedures, and treatments. The illustrations supplement course content in new and interesting ways and help make difficult concepts clear. Unique to this edition are innovative illustrations created for Chapters 1 through 3 to help students understand the various applications of suffixes and prefixes in word building. Also new to the 8th edition are Documenting Health-Care Activities sections in each body systems chapter. These sections emphasize the role of the electronic medical record (EMR) in today's health-care industry.

Documenting Health-Care Activities are first introduced in Chapter 4, Body Structure. The introduction provides information related to the transition of the medical record from a paper medical chart to a digital version. Reinforcement of this introduction continues throughout each body systems chapter so that students fully understand how today's digital medical record allows practitioners to electronically monitor and track the history of a patient's medical treatment.

Although the fundamental characteristics of the 8th edition remain the same as those in previous editions, this edition offers significant updates and enhancements to aid in the learning process and improve retention of medical terms. To achieve this goal, each illustration in the textbook presents clinically accurate and aesthetically pleasing representations of anatomical structures, disease conditions, and medical procedures. In addition, ICD-10-PCS replacement terms for discontinued eponyms are summarized in Appendix H. As in previous editions, we continue to incorporate the excellent suggestions offered by instructors and students and appreciate all of their contributions. Undoubtedly, the recommendations have helped make *Medical Terminology Systems: A Body Systems Approach* a leading textbook in educational institutions and one that continues to be well received by instructors and students. Here is a brief summary of chapter content:

- **Chapter 1** explains the techniques of medical word building using basic word elements.
- **Chapter 2** categorizes major surgical, diagnostic, symptomatic, and grammatical suffixes.
- **Chapter 3** presents major prefixes of position, number and measurement, direction, and other parameters.
- **Chapter 4** introduces anatomical, physiological, and pathological terms. It also presents combining forms denoting cellular and body structures, body position and direction, and regions of the body, in addition to combining forms related to diagnostic methods and pathology. General diagnostic and therapeutic terms are described and provide a solid foundation for specific terms addressed in the body systems chapters that follow.
- **Chapters 5 through 16** are organized according to specific body systems and may be taught in any sequence. These chapters include key anatomical and physiological terms, basic anatomy and physiology, a body systems connections table, and a comprehensive table of word elements, including combining forms, suffixes, and prefixes. The remaining chapter material consists of a disease focus section, followed by tables that include updated diseases and conditions; diagnostic, surgical, and therapeutic procedures; pharmacology; and abbreviations. Each body systems chapter concludes with several learning activities that assess comprehension of material and medical record activities that

illustrate various clinical applications and reinforce medical record documentation.

- **Appendix A: Answer Key** contains answers to each learning activity to validate proficiency and provide immediate feedback for student assessment. Although the answer key for the terminology section of each Documenting Health-Care Activity is not included in this appendix, it is available to adopters in the Instructor's Guide.
- **Appendix B: Common Abbreviations and Symbols** includes an updated, comprehensive list of medical abbreviations and their meanings and an updated summary of common symbols.
- **Appendix C: Glossary of Medical Word Elements** contains alphabetical lists of medical word elements and their meanings. This appendix presents two methods for word-element indexing—first by medical word element, then by English term.
- **Appendix D: Index of Genetic Disorders** lists genetic disorders presented in the textbook.
- **Appendix E: Index of Clinical, Laboratory, and Imaging Procedures** lists radiographic and other diagnostic imaging procedures presented in the textbook.
- **Appendix F: Index of Pharmacology** lists drug classifications presented in the textbook.
- **Appendix G: Index of Oncological Terms** lists oncological diseases presented in the textbook.
- **Appendix H: Index of Discontinued Abbreviations and Eponyms** summarizes abbreviations discontinued in medical charts. It also contains discontinued eponyms along with their replacement terms for coding purposes.

Medical Language Lab (MLL)

Included in every new copy of *Medical Terminology Systems: A Body Systems Approach*, 8th edition, is access to the ultimate online medical terminology resource for students. The MLL is a rich learning environment utilizing proven language development methods to help students become effective users of medical language. To access the MLL, students simply go to *http://www.medicallanguagelab.com* and redeem the access code provided in their new copies of *Medical Terminology Systems: A Body Systems Approach*, 8th edition.

Each lesson in the MLL teaches students how to listen critically for important terms, respond to terms using medical terminology, and generate their own terminology-rich writing and speaking skills. By following the activities in each lesson, students graduate from simple memorization to becoming stronger users of medical language.

In addition, the MLL provides students with a wide variety of practice activities that help them to solidify their recall of key terms from the chapter. It also contains an audio glossary in which students can hear words pronounced and used properly in context.

Designed to work seamlessly with *Medical Terminology Systems: A Body Systems Approach*, 8th edition, each activity in the MLL has been crafted with content specific to the textbook. Every chapter in *Medical Terminology Systems: A Body Systems Approach*, 8th edition, contains a corresponding lesson in the MLL that is relevant and useful in helping students develop medical terminology skills.

Instructors benefit from an instructor's page that is powerful yet easy to understand and allows them to decide which chapters and activities will be available to their students. Instructors also control how the MLL reports student scores, either through the native MLL grade book or to their own BlackBoard, Angel, Moodle, or SCORM-compliant course management solution.

Davis*Plus* Online Resource Center

Although the study of medical terminology demands hard work and discipline, various self-paced activities offer interest and variety to the learning process. Many activities and resources are available to adopters of the textbook at the Davis*Plus* Instructor and Student Online Resource Center. The Online Resource Center is designed to help teachers teach and students learn medical terminology in an exciting, challenging, effective fashion. Visit *http://davisplus.fadavis.com* for the Instructor and Student Online Resource Center to explore the various ancillaries available for instructors and students.

Instructor Online Resource Center

The Davis*Plus* Instructor Online Resource Center provides many updated, innovative instructional activities. These activities make teaching medical terminology easier and more effective. Teachers can use the supplemental activities in various educational settings—traditional classroom, distance learning, or independent or self-paced studies. The many ancillaries help instructors maximize the benefits of the textbook and include the following:

- Electronic test bank with *ExamView Pro* test-generating software
- PowerPoint presentations for each chapter

- Searchable image bank
- Printable Instructor's Guide
- Resources in Blackboard, Angel, Moodle, and SCORM formats

Electronic Test Bank

This edition offers a powerful updated *ExamView Pro* test-generating program that allows instructors to create custom-made or randomly generated tests in a printable or online format from a test bank of more than 2,500 test items.

PowerPoint Lecture Notes

The lecture notes provide a unique and reinforcing dimension to the learning process.

Over 1,400 slides are carefully designed to supplement and augment the material covered in the textbook. The PowerPoint presentations suggest various teaching techniques to make learning and teaching profoundly effective. Notes at the bottom of various slides offer faculty suggestions to tailor or expand the presentations to suit their individual academic needs.

Each chapter has an outline-based presentation, consisting of a chapter overview, main functions of the body system, and selected pathology, vocabulary, and procedures. Included are interactive clinically related exercises that highlight real-life situations. Full-color illustrations reinforce many of the clinically related exercises.

Image Bank

The image bank contains all illustrations from the textbook. It is fully searchable and allows users to zoom in and out and display a JPG image of an illustration that can be copied into a Microsoft Word document or PowerPoint presentation.

Instructor's Guide

The printable Instructor's Guide is a resource full of instructional activities that have been updated to meet today's instructional needs. It is available in PDF format on the Instructor's Online Resource Center and includes the following elements:

- *Suggested Course Outlines.* Course outlines of various lengths, provide effective methods of covering material presented in the textbook. A course outline is also provided for Term*Plus,* the interactive software that is available separately from F. A. Davis Co. The outline makes it easy to correlate the instructional software with the textbook chapters.

- *Student- and Instructor-Directed Activities.* These comprehensive teaching aids are updated and extended for this edition. They offer an assortment of activities for each body systems chapter that are easily incorporated as course requirements, supplemental activities, or collaborative projects. Included are peer evaluation forms and community and Internet resources. This section provides an updated list of resources, including technical journals, community organizations, and Internet sites to complement course content.

- *Supplemental Documenting Health-Care Activities.* The supplemental medical record activities have been updated to parallel the new Documenting Health-Care Activities sections presented in each of the body systems chapters. As in the textbook, these activities use actual medical records to show how medical terminology is used to document patient care. Terminology and analysis exercises reinforce the medical vocabulary in the report to help students develop critical thinking skills. Instructors can use the answer key for grading purposes or give it to the students for self-evaluation. In addition, they can use these medical records for various activities, including oral reports, medical coding, medical transcribing, or individual assignments.

- *Pronunciations and Answer Keys.* Answer keys are provided in the IG for the activities in the Medical Word Elements tables and Documenting Health-Care Activities Terminology tables in the textbook. These keys should prove helpful for grading or for class presentations.

Student Online Resource Center

The Davis*Plus* Student Online Resource Center includes many user-friendly activities to reinforce material covered in the textbook. At the same time, it is structured to make learning medical terminology an exciting, challenging activity. Resources include medical record activities, audio tutorials, and animations.

Reinforcement of Medical Record Activities

Health-care providers in hospitals, medical centers, and private practice facilities dictate various types of medical reports that become part of the electronic medical record. Included are chart notes, history and physical examinations, progress notes, consultation reports, operative reports, discharge summaries, and diagnostic studies. Samples of these types of reports are included in the Documenting Health-Care Activities found in the body systems chapters (Chapters 5–16). To reinforce these activities, the Student Online Resource Center includes a medical records activities section in which the key terms in each report are underlined. As students click the underlined terms, they hear the correct pronunciation of each term. All reports are styled following the guidelines established by the American Association of Medical Transcription (AAMT). This formatting provides an opportunity for students to learn the correct styling of various types for medical reports.

Audio Tutorials

The audio tutorials are developed from the Medical Word Elements sections of the body systems chapters (Chapters 5–16). They are designed to strengthen word building, spelling, pronunciation, and understanding of selected medical terms. These tutorials are also useful for students in beginning transcription and medical secretarial courses. Students can develop transcription skills by typing each word as it is pronounced. After typing the words, the student can correct spelling by referring to the textbook or a medical dictionary.

Animations

Several animations are included to help students better visualize complex concepts. For example, one animation explores the pathology of gastroesophageal reflux disease (GERD). Another shows the various stages of pregnancy and delivery. These innovative tools help students better understand important processes and procedures as they learn the associated medical terminology.

Term*Plus*

Term*Plus* continues to be a powerful, interactive CD-ROM program that is available for purchase separately from F. A. Davis Co. Term*Plus* is a competency-based, self-paced, multimedia program that includes graphics, audio, and a dictionary culled from *Taber's Cyclopedic Medical Dictionary*, 22nd edition. Help menus provide navigational support. The software comes with numerous interactive learning activities, including the following:

• Anatomy Focus
• Tag the Elements (drag-and-drop)
• Spotlight the Elements
• Concentration
• Build Medical Words
• Programmed Learning
• Medical Vocabulary
• Chart Notes
• Spelling
• Crossword Puzzles
• Word Scramble
• Terminology Teaser

All activities can be graded, and the results can be printed or e-mailed to the instructor. This feature makes Term*Plus* especially valuable as a distance-learning tool because it provides evidence of student drill-and-practice completion in various learning activities.

Taber's Cyclopedic Medical Dictionary

The world-famous *Taber's Cyclopedic Medical Dictionary* is the recommended companion reference for this book. Virtually all terms in *Systems* may be found in *Taber's*. In addition, *Taber's* contains etymologies for nearly all main entries presented in this textbook.

Discontinued Eponyms with ICD-10-PCS Replacement Terms

ICD-10-CM contains the use of eponyms when assigning certain codes for diagnoses and procedures. However, all surgical eponyms have been removed from ICD-10-PCS. In their place are root terms that describe the objective of the procedure and other parameters to assign the proper code(s). The ICD-10-PCS procedural codes are more specific, more clinically accurate, and use a more logical structure than the previous coding systems. There are still some diagnostic eponyms in ICD-10-PCS, but most have been replaced by a constructed term that identifies the disease or condition. A summary of eponyms found in this textbook along with the ICD-10-PCS 2015 term(s) that replace the eponym are summarized in Appendix H of this textbook.

We hope you enjoy this new edition as much as we enjoyed preparing it. We think you will find this the best edition ever.

Barbara A. Gylys
Mary Ellen Wedding

Reviewers

The authors extend a special thanks to the clinical reviewers who read and edited the manuscript and provided detailed evaluations and ideas for improving the textbook.

Algie LaKesa Bond, MHA, RHIA, PMP
Clinical Assistant Professor
Health Information Management Program
Temple University
Philadelphia, Pennsylvania

Lori Jo Bork, PhD, RN, CCRN
Professor of Nursing
Dakota Wesleyan University
Mitchell, South Dakota

Margaret J. Bower, BS, AMA
Adjunct Instructor
Allied Health Division
Central Pennsylvania College
Summerdale, Pennsylvania

Angela Carmichael, MBA, RHIA, CCS, CCS-P
Director of HIM Compliance
AHIM Approved ICD-10-CM/PCS Instructor
J.A. Thomas and Associates
Atlanta, Georgia

Jean M. Chenu
Associate Professor
Office Technology
Genesee Community College
Batavia, New York

Mary Ellen Hethcox, PharmD, RPh
Assistant Professor of Pharmacy Practice
Director of Drug and Health Information Services
Raabe College of Pharmacy
Ohio Northern University
Ada, Ohio

Gloria Madison, MS, RHIA, CHTS-IM
Health Information Technology Program Director/Faculty
Health Sciences
Moraine Park Technical College
West Bend, Wisconsin

Rich Patterson, MS, LAT, ATC
Clinical Education Coordinator
Department of Athletic Training
Barton College
Wilson, North Carolina

Kim O'Connell-Brock, MS, ATC/L
Assistant Director, Athletic Training Program
Human Performance, Dance and Recreation
New Mexico State University
Las Cruces, New Mexico

Donna Pritchard, RHIT, LPN
Instructor
Allied Health, Health Information Technology Program
Ozarks Technical Community College
Springfield, Missouri

Donna Sue M. Shellman, EdS, CPC
Program Coordinator, Medical Office Administration
Office Systems Technology
Gaston College
Dallas, North Carolina

Staci Waldrep, MS, RHIT
Associate Professor and Program Director of Health Information Technology
Allied Health and Sciences
Lamar Institute of Technology
Beaumont, Texas

Gail Winkler, MHIIM, RHIA
Director Health Information Technology Program
Health Information Technology
Walters State Community College
Morristown, Tennessee

Contents at a Glance

Contents

CHAPTER **5**   **Integumentary System**   *81*

CHAPTER **6**   **Digestive System**   *127*

Basic Elements of a Medical Word

Chapter Outline

Objectives

Upon completion of this chapter, you will be able to:

- Identify the four word elements used to build medical words.
- Divide medical words into their component parts.
- Apply the basic rules to define and build medical words.
- Locate the pronunciation guidelines chart and interpret pronunciation marks.
- Pronounce medical terms presented in this chapter.
- Demonstrate your knowledge of this chapter by completing the learning activities.

Medical Word Elements

The language of medicine is a specialized vocabulary used by health-care providers. Many current medical word elements originated as early as the 4th century B.C. when Hippocrates practiced medicine. With technological and scientific advancements in medicine, new terms have evolved to reflect these innovations. For example, radiographic terms, such as magnetic resonance imaging (MRI) and ultrasound (US), are now commonly used to describe current diagnostic procedures.

A medical word consists of some or all of the following elements:

• word root
• combining form
• suffix
• prefix.

How these elements are combined and whether all or some of them are present in a medical term determines the meaning of a word. To understand the meaning of medical words, it is important to learn how to divide them into their basic elements. The purpose of this chapter is to cover the basic principles of medical word building and learn how to pronounce the terms correctly. Thus, pronunciations of medical terms are provided throughout the textbook. In addition, pronunciation guidelines are located on the inside back cover of this book. They can be used as a convenient reference to help pronounce terms correctly.

Word Roots

A **word root** is the foundation of a medical term and contains its primary meaning. All medical terms have at least one word root. Most word roots are derived from the Greek or Latin language; thus, two different roots may have the same meaning. For example, the Greek word *dermatos* and the Latin word *cutane* both refer to the skin. As a general rule, Greek roots describe a disease, condition, treatment, or diagnosis. Latin roots describe anatomical structures. Consequently, the Greek root *dermat* describes a disease, condition, treatment, or diagnosis of the skin; the Latin root *cutane* describes an anatomical structure. (See Table 1-1.)

Table 1-1   Examples of Word Roots

This table lists examples of English terms with their Greek and Latin origins as well as word analyses of corresponding medical terms. Phonetic pronunciations are provided to help you practice pronouncing the medical terms.

English Term	Greek or Latin Term*	Word Root	Word Analysis
skin	dermatos (Gr)	dermat	**dermat**/itis (dĕr-mă-TĪ-tĭs): inflammation of the skin
			Dermatitis *is a general term used to describe an inflammatory condition of the skin.*
	cutis (L)	cutane	**cutane**/ous (kū-TĀ-nē-ŭs): pertaining to the skin
			Cutaneous *is a term that identifies an anatomical structure.*
kidney	nephros (Gr)	nephr	**nephr**/oma (nĕ-FRŌ-mă): tumor of the kidney
			Nephroma *is a tumor (benign or malignant) of kidney tissue.*
	renes (L)	ren	**ren**/al (RĒ-năl): pertains to the kidney
			Renal *is a term that identifies an anatomical structure.*

Table I-I	Examples of Word Roots—cont'd		
English Term	**Greek or Latin Term***	**Word Root**	**Word Analysis**
mouth	stomatos (Gr)	stomat	**stomat**/itis (stō-mă-TĪ-tĭs): inflammation of the mouth
			The word root stomat is commonly confused with the English term stomach. However, stomat is derived from the Greek word for mouth. The word root for the stomach is gastr, derived from the Greek word gastros.
	oris (L)	or	or/al (OR-ăl): pertaining to the mouth
			Oral is a term that identifies an anatomical structure.

*It is not important to know the origin of a medical word. This information is provided here to clarify and illustrate that there may be two different word roots for a single term.

Combining Forms

A **combining form** is created when a word root is combined with a vowel. The vowel, known as a **combining vowel,** is usually an *o* but is sometimes an *i*. The combining vowel has no meaning of its own but enables the connection of two or more word elements. Like a word root, a combining form is the basic foundation to which other word elements are added to build a complete medical word. In this text, a combining form will be listed as *word root/vowel* (such as *gastr/o*), as illustrated in Table 1-2.

Table I-2	Examples of Combining Forms				
*This table illustrates how word roots and vowels create combining forms. Learning combining forms rather than word roots makes pronunciations easier because of the terminal vowel. For example, in this table, the word roots **gastr** and **nephr** are difficult to pronounce, whereas their combining forms **gastr/o** and **nephr/o** are easier to pronounce.*					
Word Root	**+**	**Vowel**	**=**	**Combining Form**	**Meaning**
erythr/	+	o	=	erythr/o	red
gastr/	+	o	=	gastr/o	stomach
hepat/	+	o	=	hepat/o	liver
immun/	+	o	=	immun/o	immune, immunity, safe
nephr/	+	o	=	nephr/o	kidney
oste/	+	o	=	oste/o	bone

Suffixes

A **suffix** is a word element placed at the end of a word that alters its meaning. All medical terms have a suffix. In the terms *pancreat/itis* (inflammation of the pancreas) and *pancreat/o/pathy* (disease of the pancreas), the suffixes are *-itis* (inflammation) and *-pathy* (disease). In medical terminology, a suffix usually describes a pathology (disease or abnormality), symptom, surgical or diagnostic procedure, or part of speech.

To link a suffix that begins with a vowel, use a word root. To link a suffix that begins with a consonant, use a combining form. Review Table 1-3, which illustrates this principle.

Table 1-3	**Examples of Suffixes**

This table lists examples of pathological suffixes linked with a word root (WR) and a combining form (CF). Phonetic pronunciations are provided to help you practice pronouncing the medical terms.

Suffix	=	Medical Word	Meaning	Rationale
-itis (inflammation)	=	gastr/**itis** găs-TRĪ-tĭs	inflammation of the stomach*	The suffix *-itis* begins with a vowel and requires a WR.
-megaly (enlargement)	=	gastr/o/**megaly** găs-trō-MĔG-ă-lē	enlargement of the stomach	The suffix *-megaly* begins with a consonant and requires a CF.
-oma (tumor)	=	hepat/**oma** hĕp-ă-TŌ-mă	tumor of the liver	The suffix *-oma* begins with a vowel and requires a WR.
-cyte (cell)	=	hepat/o/**cytes** HĔP-ă-tō-sīts	cells in the liver	The suffix *-cytes* begins with a consonant and requires a CF.

*To define a medical term, first define the suffix and then the first part of the word.

Prefixes

A **prefix** is a word element attached to the beginning of a word or word root. However, not all medical terms have a prefix. Adding or changing a prefix changes the meaning of the word. Prefixes usually indicate a number, time, position, direction, or negation. Many of the same prefixes used in medical terminology are also used in the English language. Review Table 1-4 to reinforce the principles of linking a prefix to other word elements.

Table 1-4	**Examples of Prefixes**

This table lists examples of prefixes linked to a word root and a suffix. Note that the suffixes begin with a vowel and are linked to a word root. Phonetic pronunciations of the constructed medical words are provided to help you practice pronouncing the medical terms.

Prefix	+	Word Root	+	Suffix	=	Medical Word	Meaning
an- (without, not)	+	esthes (feeling)	+	-ia (condition)	=	an/esthes/ia ăn-ĕs-THĒ-zē-ă	condition of not feeling
hyper- (excessive, above normal)	+	therm (heat)	+	-ia (condition)	=	hyper/therm/ia hī-pĕr-THĔR-mē-ă	condition of excessive heat
intra- (in, within)	+	muscul (muscle)	+	-ar (pertaining to)	=	intra/muscul/ar ĭn-tră-MŬS-kū-lăr	pertaining to within the muscle
para- (near, beside; beyond)	+	nas (nose)	+	-al (pertaining to)	=	para/nas/al păr-ă-NĀ-săl	pertaining to (area) near the nose
poly (many, much)	+	ur (urine)	+	-ia (condition)	=	poly/ur/ia pŏl-ē-Ū-rē-ă	condition of much urine
pre- (before)	+	nat (birth)	+	-al (pertaining to)	=	pre/nat/al prē-NĀ-tăl	pertaining to before birth

Basic Guidelines

Defining and building medical words are crucial skills in understanding the meaning of a medical word. Following the basic guidelines will help you develop these skills.

Defining Medical Words

Here are three steps for defining medical words using *gastr/o/enter/itis* as an example.

- **Step 1.** Define the **suffix,** or last part of the word. In this case, the suffix *-itis* means *inflammation.*
- **Step 2.** Define the **first part of the word** (which may be a word root, combining form, or prefix). In this case, the combining form *gastr/o* means *stomach.*
- **Step 3.** Define the **middle parts of the word.** In this case, the word root *enter* means *intestine.*

When you analyze *gastr/o/enter/itis* following the three steps, the meaning is:

1. inflammation (of)
2. stomach (and)
3. intestine.

Thus, the meaning of **gastr/o/enter/itis** is *inflammation (of) stomach (and) intestine.* Table 1-5 further illustrates this process.

Table 1-5 Defining Gastroenteritis		
This table illustrates the three steps of defining a medical word using the example gastroenteritis.		
Combining Form	**Middle**	**Suffix**
gastr/o	enter/	-itis
stomach	intestine	inflammation
(step 2)	(step 3)	(step 1)

Building Medical Words

There are three basic rules for building medical words.

Rule 1

A word root links a suffix that begins with a vowel.

Word Root	+	Suffix	=	Medical Word	Meaning
hepat (liver)	+	-itis (inflammation)	=	hepatitis hĕp-ă-TĪ-tĭs	inflammation of the liver

Rule 2

A combining form (root + o) links a suffix that begins with a consonant.

Combining Form	+	Suffix	=	Medical Word	Meaning
hepat/o (liver)	+	-cyte (cell)	=	hepatocyte HĔP-ă-tō-sīt	liver cell

Rule 3

A combining form links one root to another root to form a compound word. This rule holds true even if the second root begins with a vowel, as in **oste/o/arthr/itis**. Keep in mind that the rules for linking multiple roots to each other are slightly different from the rules for linking roots and combining forms to suffixes.

Combining Form	+	Word Root	+	Suffix	=	Medical Word	Meaning
oste/o (bone)	+	chondr (cartilage)	+	-itis (inflammation)	=	osteochondritis ŏs-tē-ō-kŏn-DRĪ-tĭs	inflammation of bone and cartilage
	+	arthr (joint)	+	-itis (inflammation)	=	osteoarthritis ŏs-tē-ō-ăr-THRĪ-tĭs	inflammation of bone and joint

It is time to review medical word elements by completing Learning Activities 1–1 and 1–2 on pages 8–9.

Pronunciation Guidelines

Although pronunciation of medical words usually follows the same rules that govern pronunciations of English words, some medical words may be difficult to pronounce when first encountered. Therefore, selected terms in this book include the phonetic pronunciation. Also, pronunciation guidelines can be found on the inside back cover of this book and at the end of selected tables. Use them whenever you need help with pronunciation of medical words.

It is time to review pronunciations, analysis of word elements, and defining medical terms by completing Learning Activities 1–3, 1–4, and 1–5 on pages 10–12.

Medical Word Building Summary

The illustration that follows demonstrates medical word building. Building a medical word that means *enlargement of the stomach* requires knowledge of the word element for *stomach* (**gastr** or **gastr/o**) and the suffix for *enlargement* (**-megaly**). The medical word for *enlargement of the stomach* is **gastromegaly.** To develop medical word building skills, study the combinations of word building elements in the digestive system illustration that follows.

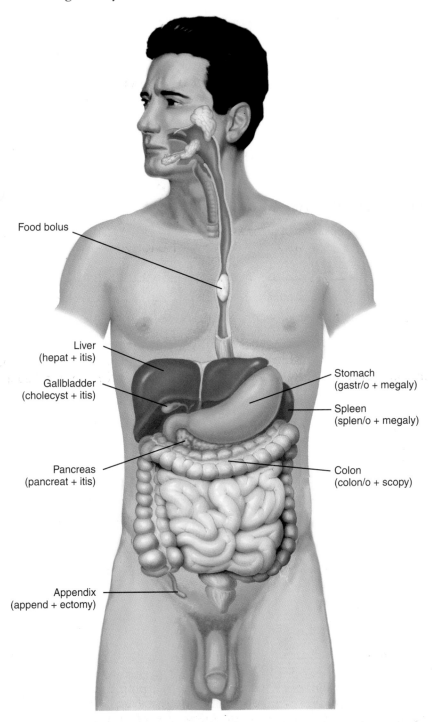

Food bolus

Liver
(hepat + itis)

Gallbladder
(cholecyst + itis)

Pancreas
(pancreat + itis)

Appendix
(append + ectomy)

Stomach
(gastr/o + megaly)

Spleen
(splen/o + megaly)

Colon
(colon/o + scopy)

 It is time to practice building medical words by completing Learning Activity 1–6 on page 14.

LEARNING ACTIVITIES

The learning activities that follow provide a review of the basic medical word elements introduced in this chapter. Complete each activity and review your answers to evaluate your understanding of this chapter.

Learning Activity I-I

Understanding Medical Word Elements

Fill in the blanks to complete the sentences correctly.

1. The four elements used to form words are ___word root, combining form, suffix, prefix___

2. A root is the main part or foundation of a word. In the words *arthritis*, *arthrectomy*, and *arthroscope*, the root is ___arth___.

Identify the statements as true or false. If false, rewrite the statement correctly on the line provided.

3. A combining vowel is usually an e.   True   (False)
   ___it's usually an "o" sometimes an "i"___

4. A word root links a suffix that begins with a consonant.   True   (False)
   ___root links a suffix that begins with a vowel___

5. A combining form links multiple roots to each other.   (True)   False

6. A combining form links a suffix that begins with a consonant.   (True)   False

7. To define a medical word, first define the prefix.   True   (False)
   ___To define a medical word, first define the suffix___

8. In the term *intramuscular*, *intra* is the prefix.   (True)   False

Underline the word root in each of the combining forms.

9. splen/o (spleen)

10. hyster/o (uterus)

11. enter/o (intestine)

12. neur/o (nerve)

13. ot/o (ear)

14. dermat/o (skin)

15. hydr/o (water)

✓ *Check your answers in Appendix A. Review material that you did not answer correctly.*

Correct Answers _____ X 6.67 = _____ % Score

Learning Activity 1-2

Identifying Word Roots and Combining Forms

Underline the word roots in the medical words that follow.

Medical Word	Meaning
1. <u>nephr</u>itis	inflammation of the kidney
2. <u>arthr</u>odesis	fixation of a joint
3. <u>dermat</u>itis	inflammation of the skin
4. <u>dent</u>ist	specialist in teeth
5. <u>gastr</u>ectomy	excision of the stomach
6. <u>chondr</u>itis	inflammation of cartilage
7. hepat/oma	tumor of the liver
8. muscul/ar	pertaining to muscle
9. gastr/ic	pertaining to the stomach
10. oste/oma	tumor of the bone

Underline the combining forms.

11. <u>nephr</u>	kidney
12. <u>hepat/o</u>	liver
13. arthr	joint
14. <u>oste/o</u>/arthr	bone, joint
15. <u>cholangi/o</u>	bile vessel

 Check your answers in Appendix A. Review material that you did not answer correctly.

Correct Answers _____ X 6.67 = _____ % Score

Learning Activity 1-3

Understanding Pronunciations

Review the pronunciation guidelines (located on the inside back cover of this book) and then underline the correct answer in each of the statements.

1. The diacritical mark ⁻ is called a (breve, ⟨macron⟩).

2. The diacritical mark ˘ is called a (⟨breve⟩, macron).

3. The ⁻ indicates the (short, ⟨long⟩) sound of vowels.

4. The ˘ indicates the (⟨short⟩, long) sound of vowels.

5. The combination *ch* is sometimes pronounced like (⟨k⟩, chiy). Examples are *cholesterol, cholemia.*

6. When *pn* is at the beginning of a word, it is pronounced only with the sound of (p, ⟨n⟩). Examples are *pneumonia, pneumotoxin.*

7. When *pn* is in the middle of a word, the *p* (⟨is⟩, is not) pronounced. Examples are *orthopnea, hyperpnea.*

8. When *i* is at the end of a word, it is pronounced like (⟨eye⟩, ee). Examples are *bronchi, fungi, nuclei.*

9. For *ae* and *oe*, only the (first, ⟨second⟩) vowel is pronounced. Examples are *bursae, pleurae.*

10. When *e* and *es* form the final letter or letters of a word, they are commonly pronounced as (combined, ⟨separate⟩) syllables. Examples are *syncope, systole, nares.*

✓ *Check your answers in Appendix A. Review material that you did not answer correctly.*

Correct Answers _____ X 10 = _____ % Score

Learning Activity 1-4

Identifying Suffixes and Prefixes

Pronounce the medical terms that follow. Then analyze each term and write the suffix in the right-hand column. The first suffix is completed for you.

Term	Suffix
1. thoracotomy thōr-ă-KŎT-ō-mē	*-tomy*
2. gastroscope GĂS-trō-skōp	scope
3. tonsillitis tŏn-sĭl-Ī-tĭs	itis
4. gastric GĂS-trĭk	ic
5. tonsillectomy tŏn-sĭl-ĔK-tō-mē	ectomy

Pronunciation Help	Long Sound Short Sound	ā — rate ă — apple	ē — rebirth ĕ — ever	ī — isle ĭ — it	ō — over ŏ — not	ū — unite ŭ — cut

Pronounce the medical terms that follow. Then analyze each term and write the element that is a prefix in the right-hand column. The first prefix is completed for you.

Term	Prefix
6. anesthesia ăn-ĕs-THĒ-zē-ă	*an-*
7. hyperthermia hī-pĕr-THĔR-mē-ă	hyper
8. intramuscular ĭn-tră-MŬS-kū-lăr	intra
9. paranasal păr-ă-NĀ-săl	para
10. polyuria pŏl-ē-Ū-rē-ă	poly

✔ *Check your answers in Appendix A. Review material that you did not answer correctly.*

Correct Answers _____ X 10 = _____ % Score

Learning Activity I-5

Defining Medical Words

The three steps for defining medical words are:

1. Define the last part of the word, or suffix.
2. Define the first part of the word, or prefix, word root, or combining form.
3. Define the middle of the word.

First, pronounce the term aloud. Then apply the three steps to define the terms in the table that follows. If you are not certain of a definition, refer to Appendix C, Part 1, of this textbook, which provides an alphabetical list of word elements and their meanings.

Term	Definition
1. gastritis găs-TRĪ-tĭs	inflammation of the stomach
2. nephritis nĕf-RĪ-tĭs	inflammation of the liver
3. gastrectomy găs-TRĔK-tō-mē	excision of the stomach
4. osteoma ŏs-tē-Ō-mă	tumor of the bone
5. hepatoma hĕp-ă-TŌ-mă	tumor of the liver
6. hepatitis hĕp-ă-TĪ-tĭs	inflammation of the liver

Refer to the section "Building Medical Words" on pages 5–6 to complete this activity. Write the number for the rule that applies to each listed term and give a short summary of the rule. Use the abbreviation WR to designate *word root*, and use CF to designate *combining form*. The first one is completed for you.

Term	Rule	Summary of the Rule
7. arthr/itis ăr-THRĪ-tĭs	I	*A WR links a suffix that begins with a vowel.*
8. scler/osis sklĕ-RŌ-sĭs	1	A WR links a suffix that begins with a vowel
9. arthr/o/centesis ăr-thrō-sĕn-TĒ-sĭs	2	CF links a suffix begins with a consonant
10. colon/o/scope kō-LŎN-ō-skōp	2	CF links a suffix begins with a consonant
11. chondr/itis kŏn-DRĪ-tĭs	1	WR links a suffix that begins with a vowel
12. chondr/oma kŏn-DRŌ-mă	1	WR links a suffix that begins with a vowel

13. oste/o/chondr/itis   3, 1   CF links multiple roots to each other
    ŏs-tē-ō-kŏn-DRĪ-tĭs

14. muscul/ar   1   WR links suffix that begins w/ a vowel
    MŬS-kū-lăr

15. oste/o/arthr/itis   3, 1   CF links multiple roots to each other
    ŏs-tē-ō-ăr-THRĪ-tĭs

✓ *Check your answers in Appendix A. Review material that you did not answer correctly.*

Correct Answers _____ X 6.67 = _____ % Score

Learning Activity 1-6

Building Medical Words

Refer to the figure on page 7 to complete this activity.
Use -ectomy (excision) to build medical words that mean *excision of the:*

1. spleen: _Splenectomy_
2. appendix: _appendectomy_
3. pancreas: _Pancreatectomy_
4. gallbladder: _cholecystectomy_
5. colon: _colectomy_
6. stomach: _gastrectomy_

Use -itis (inflammation) to build medical words that mean *inflammation of the:*

7. spleen: _splenitis_
8. liver: _hepatitis_
9. pancreas: _pancreatitis_
10. gallbladder: _cholecystitis_
11. colon: _colitis_
12. stomach: _gastritis_

Use -megaly (enlargement) to build medical words that mean *enlargement of the:*

13. liver: _hepetomegaly_
14. spleen: _splenomegaly_
15. stomach: _gastromegaly_

✔ *Check your answers in Appendix A. Review material that you did not answer correctly.*

Correct Answers _____ X 6.67 = _____ % Score

Suffixes

Chapter Outline

Objectives

Upon completion of this chapter, you will be able to:

- Identify examples of surgical, diagnostic, pathological, and related suffixes.
- Link combining forms and word roots to suffixes.
- Define and provide surgical, diagnostic, pathological, and related suffixes.
- Define and provide adjective, noun, and diminutive suffixes.
- Locate and apply guidelines for pluralizing terms.
- Pronounce medical terms presented in this chapter.
- Demonstrate your knowledge of the chapter by completing the learning activities.

Suffix Linking

In medical words, a suffix is added to the end of a word root or combining form to change its meaning. Recall Rule 1 and Rule 2 on pages 5–6 for linking suffixes. When a suffix begins with a vowel, use the root word for linking the two word elements. When the suffix begins with a consonant, use the combining form for linking the two word elements. For example, the word root **hemat** means *blood*. The suffix -**emesis** means *vomiting*, and -**logy** means *study of*. Hemat/**emesis** means *vomiting blood*; hemat/o/**logy** is the *study of blood*. Review Table 2-1, which illustrates examples of word roots linked with suffixes that begin with a vowel and combining forms linked with suffixes that begin with consonant.

Table 2-1	**Word Roots and Combining Forms With Suffixes**

This table provides examples of word roots linking a suffix that begins with a vowel. It also provides examples of combining forms (root + o) linking a suffix that begins with a consonant.

Element	+	Suffix	=	Medical Word	Meaning
Word Roots					
hemat (blood)	+	-emesis (vomiting)	=	hemat/emesis hĕm-ăt-ĔM-ĕ-sĭs	vomiting blood
arthr (joint)	+	-itis (inflammation)	=	arthr/itis ăr-THRĪ-tĭs	inflammation of a joint
oste (bone)	+	-oma (tumor)	=	oste/oma ŏs-tē-Ō-mă	tumor of bone
Combining Forms					
hemat/o (blood)	+	-logy (study of)	=	hemat/o/logy hē-mă-TŎL-ō-jē	study of blood
arthr/o (joint)	+	-centesis (surgical puncture)	=	arthr/o/centesis ăr-thrō-sĕn-TĒ-sĭs	surgical puncture of a joint
oste/o (bone)	+	-dynia (pain)	=	oste/o/dynia ŏs-tē-ō-DĬN-ē-ă	pain in bone

Words that contain more than one word root are known as **compound words.** Multiple roots within a compound word are joined together with a vowel, regardless of whether the second root begins with a vowel or a consonant. Notice that a vowel is used in Table 2-2 between *oste* and *arthr,* even though the second root, *arthr,* begins with a vowel.

Table 2-2	**Compound Words With Suffixes**

This table provides examples of medical terms with more than one word root, also known as compound words. The table lists suffixes linked with roots when the suffix begins with a vowel, and it lists combining forms when the suffix begins with a consonant.

Combining Form	+	Word Root	+	Suffix	=	Medical Word	Meaning
oste/o (bone)	+	arthr (joint)	+	-itis (inflammation)	=	oste/o/arthr/itis ŏs-tē-ō-ăr-THRĪ-tĭs	inflammation of the bone and joint
encephal/o (brain)	+	mening (meninges)	+	-itis (inflammation)	=	encephal/o/mening/itis ĕn-sĕf-ă-lō-mĕn-ĭn-JĪ-tĭs	inflammation of the brain and meninges
oste/o (bone)	+	arthr/o (joint)	+	-pathy (disease)	=	oste/o/arthr/o/pathy ŏs-tē-ō-ăr-THRŎP-ă-thē	disease of the bone and joint
encephal/o (brain)	+	mening/o (meninges)	+	-pathy (disease)	=	encephal/o/mening/o/pathy ĕn-sĕf-ă-lō-mĕn-ĭn-GŎP-ă-thē	disease of the brain and meninges

Keep in mind that the rule for linking multiple roots is slightly different from the rules for linking roots to suffixes. To reinforce your understanding of building compound words, refer to Rule 3 on page 6 of this textbook. Use the steps when in doubt about building a medical word.

Suffix Types

An effective method in mastering medical terminology is to learn the major types of suffixes in categories. Grouping the surgical, diagnostic, pathological, related, and grammatical suffixes makes them easier to remember.

Surgical, Diagnostic, Pathological, and Related Suffixes

Surgical suffixes describe a type of invasive procedure performed on a body part. (See Table 2-3.) Diagnostic suffixes describe a procedure performed to identify the cause and nature of an illness. Pathological suffixes describe an abnormal condition or disease. (See Table 2-4.)

Table 2-3	**Surgical Suffixes**	
This table lists commonly used surgical suffixes along with their meanings and word analyses.		
Suffix	**Meaning**	**Word Analysis**
-centesis	surgical puncture	arthr/o/**centesis** (ăr-thrō-sĕn-TĒ-sĭs): surgical puncture of a joint
		arthr/o: joint
		Arthrocentesis is a surgical puncture to remove fluid in a joint by using a needle inserted into the joint space. It may also help to obtain samples of synovial fluid for diagnostic purposes and to instill medications. (See Fig. 2-1.)

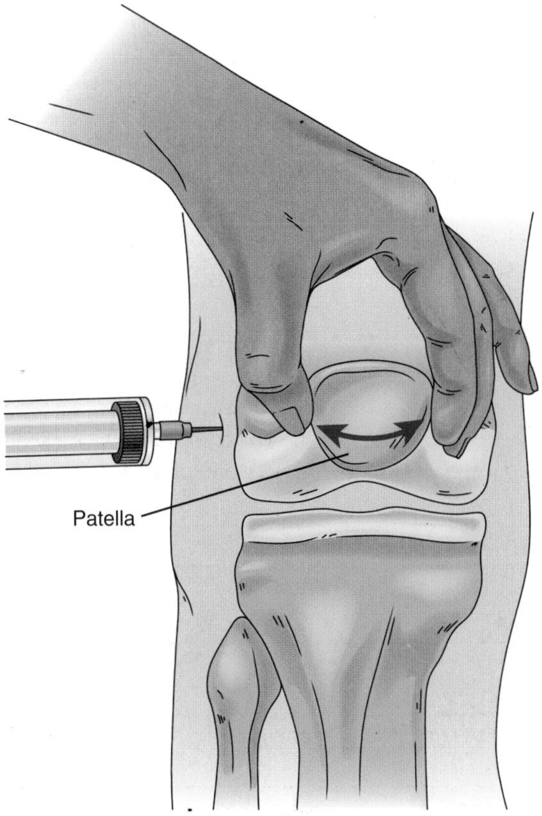

Patella

Figure 2-1 Arthrocentesis of the knee.

Table 2-3	Surgical Suffixes—cont'd	

Suffix	Meaning	Word Analysis
-clasis	to break; surgical fracture	oste/o/**clasis** (ŏs-tē-ŎK-lă-sĭs): surgical fracture of a bone *oste/o*: bone *Osteoclasis is performed to correct a deformity of a bone.*
-desis	binding, fixation (of a bone or joint)	arthr/o/**desis** (ăr-thrō-DĒ-sĭs): binding or fixation of a joint *arthr/o*: joint *Arthrodesis fuses bones across the joint space in a degenerated, unstable joint.*
-ectomy	excision, removal	append/**ectomy** (ăp-ĕn-DĔK-tō-mē): excision of the appendix *append*: appendix
-lysis	separation; destruction; loosening	thromb/o/**lysis** (thrŏm-BŎL-ĭ-sĭs): destruction or separation of a blood clot *thromb/o*: blood clot *Drug therapy is usually used to dissolve a blood clot.*
-pexy	fixation (of an organ)	mast/o/**pexy** (MĂS-tō-pĕks-ē): fixation of the breast(s) *mast/o*: breast *Mastopexy, an elective surgery, affixes sagging breasts in a more elevated position, commonly improving their shape.*
-plasty	surgical repair	rhin/o/**plasty** (RĪ-nō-plăs-tē): surgical repair of the nose *rhin/o*: nose *Rhinoplasty is a type of surgery that changes the size or shape of the nose.*
-rrhaphy	suture	my/o/**rrhaphy** (mī-OR-ă-fē): suture of a muscle *my/o*: muscle
-stomy	forming an opening (mouth)	trache/o/**stomy** (tră-kē-ŎS-tō-mē): forming an opening (mouth) into the trachea *trache/o*: trachea (windpipe) *A tracheostomy is an artificial opening created to bypass an obstructed upper airway.*
-tome	instrument to cut	oste/o/**tome** (ŎS-tē-ō-tōm): instrument to cut bone *oste/o*: bone *An osteotome is a surgical chisel used to cut through bone.*
-tomy	incision	trache/o/**tomy** (tră-kē-ŎT-ō-mē): incision of the trachea *trache/o*: trachea (windpipe) *Tracheotomy opens a direct airway through the neck and into the trachea (the windpipe).*
-tripsy	crushing	lith/o/**tripsy** (LĬTH-ō-trĭp-sē): crushing a stone *lith/o*: stone, calculus *Lithotripsy is a surgical procedure to remove a stone or calculus in the kidney, ureter, bladder, or gallbladder.*

It is time to review surgical suffixes by completing Learning Activities 2-1, 2-2, and 2-3.

Table 2-4	Diagnostic, Pathological, and Related Suffixes

This table lists commonly used diagnostic, pathological, and related suffixes, along with their meanings and word analyses.

Suffix	Meaning	Word Analysis
Diagnostic		
-gram	record, writing	electr/o/cardi/o/**gram** (ē-lĕk-trō-KĂR-dē-ō-grăm): record of electrical activity of the heart *electr/o:* electricity *cardi/o:* heart
-graph	instrument for recording	electr/o/cardi/o/**graph** (ē-lĕk-trō-KĂR-dē-ō-grăf): instrument for recording electrical activity of the heart *electr/o:* electricity *cardi/o:* heart
-graphy	process of recording	electr/o/cardi/o/**graphy** (ē-lĕk-trō-kăr-dē-ŎG-ră-fē): process of recording electrical activity of the heart (see Fig. 2-2.) *electr/o:* electricity *cardi/o:* heart

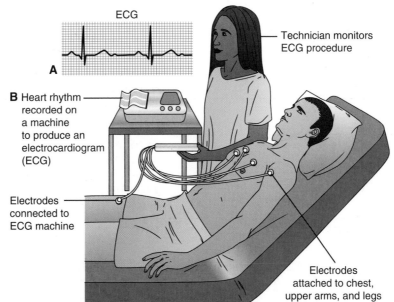

Figure 2-2 Electrocardio**graphy** (ECG) is the ***process of recording*** electrical activity of heart muscle. (A) An electrocardio**gram** is *a record* taken during the procedure that shows as a line tracing on a scrolling graph paper. The dips and peaks of the tracing are labeled with the letters P, Q, R. S, and T, which correspond to events of the cardiac cycle. (B) An electrocardio**graph** is the ***instrument for recording*** the electrical impulses of the heart.

Suffix	Meaning	Word Analysis
-scope	instrument for examining	endo/**scope** (ĔN-dō-skōp): instrument for examining within *endo-:* in, within *An endoscope is a flexible or rigid instrument consisting of a tube and optical system for observing the inside of a hollow organ or cavity.*
-scopy	visual examination	endo/**scopy** (ĕn-DŎS-kō-pē): visual examination within *endo-:* in, within *Endoscopy is performed to visualize a body cavity or canal using a specialized lighted instrument called an endoscope.*

(continued)

Table 2-4   Diagnostic, Pathological, and Related Suffixes—cont'd

Suffix	Meaning	Word Analysis
Pathological and Related		
-algia	pain	neur/**algia** (nū-RĂL-jē-ă): pain of a nerve *neur*: nerve *Neuralgic pain usually occurs along the path of a nerve.*
-dynia		ot/o/**dynia** (ō-tō-DĬN-ē-ă): pain in the ear *ot/o*: ear *Otodynia, also called otalgia, is commonly known as an earache.*
-cele	hernia, swelling	hepat/o/**cele** (hĕ-PĂT-ō-sēl): hernia or swelling of the liver *hepat/o*: liver
-ectasis	dilation, expansion	bronchi/**ectasis** (brŏng-kē-ĔK-tă-sĭs): dilation or expansion of the bronchi *bronchi*: bronchus (plural, *bronchi*)
-emesis	vomiting	hyper/**emesis** (hī-pĕr-ĔM-ĕ-sĭs): excessive vomiting *hyper-*: excessive, above normal
-emia	blood condition	leuk/**emia** (ă-NĒ-mē-ă): white blood *an-*: without, not *Leukemia is a cancer of the white blood cells (leukocytes).*
-gen	forming, producing, origin	carcin/o/**gen** (kăr-SĬN-ō-jĕn): forming, producing, or origin of cancer *carcin/o*: cancer *A carcinogen is a substance or agent, such as a cigarette, that causes the development or increases the incidence of cancer.*
-genesis		carcin/o/**genesis** (kăr-sĭ-nō-JĔN-ĕ-sĭs): forming, producing, or origin of cancer *carcin/o*: cancer *Carcinogenesis is the transformation of normal cells into cancer cells, commonly as a result of chemical, viral, or radioactive damage to genes.*
-itis	inflammation	gastr/**itis** (găs-TRĪ-tĭs): inflammation of the stomach *gastr*: stomach
-malacia	softening	chondr/o/**malacia** (kŏn-drō-măl-Ā-shē-ă): softening of cartilage *chondr/o*: cartilage
-megaly	enlargement	cardi/o/**megaly** (kăr-dē-ō-MĔG-ă-lē): enlargement of the heart *cardi/o*: heart
-oma	tumor	neur/**oma** (nū-RŌ-mă): tumor of a nerve *neur*: nerve *A neuroma is a benign tumor composed of nerve tissue.*
-osis	abnormal condition; increase (used primarily with blood cells)	cyan/**osis** (sī-ă-NŌ-sĭs): dark blue or purple discoloration of the skin and mucous membrane *cyan*: blue *Cyanosis is a bluish discoloration of the skin that indicates a deficiency of oxygen in the blood.*
-pathy	disease	my/o/**pathy** (mī-ŎP-ă-thē): disease of muscle *my/o*: muscle

Table 2-4	Diagnostic, Pathological, and Related Suffixes—cont'd	

Suffix	Meaning	Word Analysis
-penia	decrease, deficiency	oste/o/**penia** (ŏs-tē-ō-PĒ-nē-ă): decrease in bone mass *oste/o:* bone *Osteopenia is characterized by bone loss that is not as severe as that in osteoporosis.*
-phobia	fear	hem/o/**phobia** (hē-mō-FŌ-bē-ă): fear of blood *hem/o:* blood *Hemophobia is an abnormal aversion to the sight of blood.*
-plegia	paralysis	quadri/**plegia** (kwŏd-rĭ-PLĒ-jē-ă): paralysis of four *quadri:* four *Quadriplegia is a paralysis of four extremities, both arms and legs. (See Fig. 2-3.)*

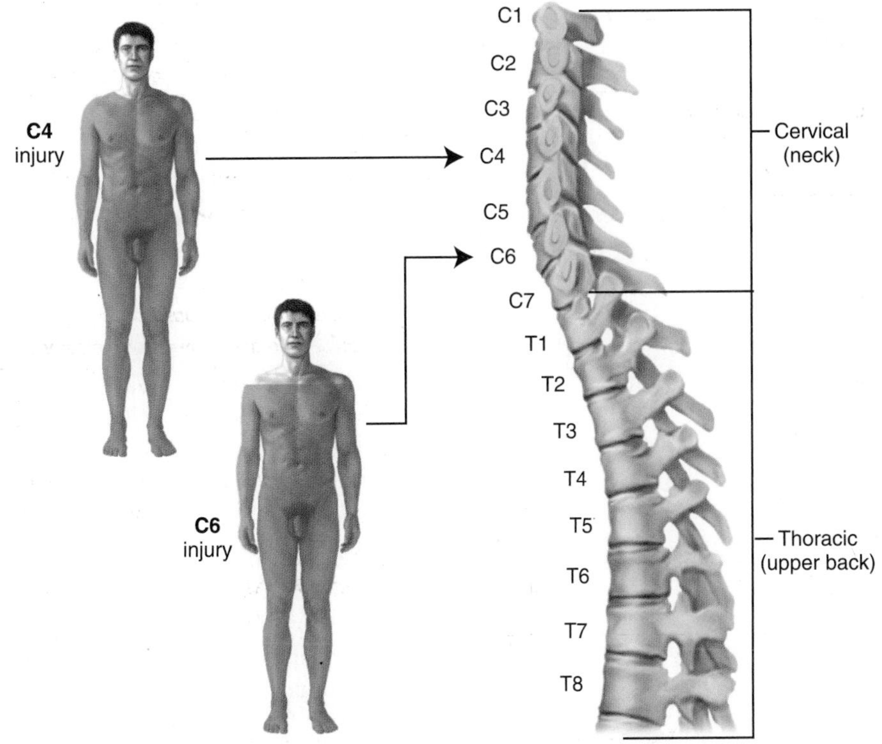

Figure 2-3 Quadriplegia as a result of cervical injuries.

Suffix	Meaning	Word Analysis
-ptosis	prolapse, downward displacement	blephar/o/**ptosis** (blĕf-ă-rō-TŌ-sĭs): prolapse or downward displacement of the eyelid *blephar/o:* eyelid *Blepharoptosis is a drooping of the upper eyelid(s).*
-rrhea	discharge, flow	dia/**rrhea** (dī-ă-RĒ-ă): discharge or flow through *dia-:* through, across *Diarrhea is an abnormally frequent discharge or flow of fluid fecal matter from the bowel.*
-rrhexis	rupture	arteri/o/**rrhexis** (ăr-tē-rē-ō-RĔK-sĭs): rupture of an artery *arteri/o:* artery
-sclerosis	abnormal condition of hardening	arteri/o/**sclerosis** (ăr-tē-rē-ō-sklĕ-RŌ-sĭs): abnormal condition of hardening of an artery *arteri/o:* artery

(continued)

Table 2-4	Diagnostic, Pathological, and Related Suffixes—cont'd	
Suffix	**Meaning**	**Word Analysis**
-spasm	involuntary contraction, twitching	blephar/o/**spasm** (BLĔF-ă-rō-spăsm): involuntary contraction or twitching of the eyelid *blephar/o:* eyelid
-stenosis	narrowing, stricture	arteri/o/**stenosis** (ăr-tē-rē-ō-stĕ-NŌ-sĭs): abnormal narrowing or stricture of an artery *arteri/o:* artery
-toxic	poison	hepat/o/**toxic** (HĔP-ă-tō-tŏk-sĭk): pertaining to poison in the liver *hepat/o:* liver *Alcohol and drugs are examples of agents that have destructive effects on the liver.*

 It is time to review diagnostic, pathological, and related suffixes by completing Learning Activities 2–4 and 2–5.

Grammatical Suffixes

Short grammatical suffixes are attached to word roots to form parts of speech, such as adjectives and nouns. Many of these same suffixes are used in the English language. (See Table 2-5.)

Table 2-5	Adjective and Noun Suffixes	
This table lists adjective and noun suffixes that are attached to word roots in a medical term, along with their meanings and word analyses.		
Suffix	**Meaning**	**Word Analysis**
Adjective		
-ac	pertaining to	cardi/**ac** (KĂR-dē-ăk): pertaining to the heart *cardi:* heart
-al		neur/**al** (NŪ-răl): pertaining to a nerve *neur:* nerve
-ar		muscul/**ar** (MŬS-kū-lăr): pertaining to muscle *muscul:* muscle
-ary		pulmon/**ary** (PŬL-mō-nĕr-ē): pertaining to the lungs *pulmon:* lung
-eal		esophag/**eal** (ē-sŏf-ă-JĒ-ăl): pertaining to the esophagus *esophag:* esophagus
-ic		thorac/**ic** (thō-RĂS-ĭk): pertaining to the chest *thorac:* chest
-ior		poster/**ior** (pŏs-TĒ-rē-or): pertaining to the back (of the body) *poster:* back (of body), behind, posterior
-ous		cutane/**ous** (kū-TĀ-nē-ŭs): pertaining to the skin *cutane:* skin
-tic		acous/**tic** (ă-KOOS-tĭk): pertaining to hearing *acous:* hearing

Table 2-5	Adjective and Noun Suffixes—cont'd	
Suffix	**Meaning**	**Word Analysis**
Noun		
-ia	condition	pneumon/ia (nū-MŌ-nē-ǎ): condition of the lung(s) *pneumon:* air; lung *Pneumonia is an infection of the lung, usually caused by bacteria, viruses, or diseases.*
-ism		thyroid/ism (THĪ-royd-ĭzm): condition of the thyroid gland *thyroid:* thyroid gland *Thyroidism is a condition caused by overactivity of the thyroid gland.*
-iatry	medicine; treatment	psych/iatry (sī-KĪ-ǎ-trē): treatment of the mind *psych/o:* mind *Psychiatry is the medical specialty concerned with treatment of mental illness, emotional disturbance, and abnormal behavior.*

-ist		hemat/o/log/ist (hē-mǎ-TŎL-ō-jĭst): specialist in the study of blood
		    hemat/o: blood
		    log: study of

-y	condition; process	neur/o/path/y (nū-RŎP-ǎ-thē): condition of nerve diseases
		    neur/o: nerve
		    path: disease
		Neuropathy is the study of disorders of the nerves.

Diminutive		
-icle	small, minute	ventr/icle (VĔN-trĭ-kl): small cavity, as of the brain or heart *ventr:* belly, belly side
-ole		arteri/ole (ǎr-TĒ-rē-ōl): small or minute artery *arteri:* artery *Arteries narrow to form arterioles (minute arteries), which branch into capillaries (microscopic blood vessels).*
-ule		ven/ule (VĔN-ūl): small or minute vein *ven:* vein *A venule is a small vein that is continuous with a capillary.*

 It is time to review grammatical suffixes by completing Learning Activity 2-6.

Plural Suffixes

Suffixes are also used to denote singular and plural forms of a word. English endings have also been adopted for commonly used medical terms. When a word changes from a singular to a plural form, the suffix of the word is the part that changes. A summary of the rules for changing a singular word into its plural form is located on the inside back cover of this textbook. Use it to complete Learning Activity 2-7 and whenever you need help forming plural words.

 It is time to review the rules for forming plural words by completing Learning Activity 2-7.

LEARNING ACTIVITIES

These activities provide review of the suffixes introduced in this chapter. Complete each activity and review your answers to evaluate your understanding of the chapter.

Learning Activity 2-1

Building Surgical Words

Use the meanings in the right column to complete the surgical words in the left column. The first one is completed for you. *Note:* The word roots are underlined in the left column.

Incomplete Word	Meaning
1. episi/o/ t o m y	incision of the perineum
2. col e c t o m y	excision (of all or part)* of the colon
3. arthr/o/ c e n t e s i s	surgical puncture of a joint (to remove fluid)
4. splen e c t o m y	excision of the spleen
5. col/o/ s t o m y	forming an opening (mouth) into the colon
6. oste/o/ t o m e	instrument to cut bone
7. tympan/o/ t o m y	incision of the tympanic membrane
8. trache/o/ s t o m y	forming an opening (mouth) into the trachea
9. mast e c t o m y	excision of a breast
10. lith/o/ t o m y	incision to remove a stone or calculus
11. hemorrhoid e c t o m y	excision of hemorrhoids

Build a surgical word that means:

12. forming an opening (mouth) into the colon: colostomy
13. excision of the colon: colectomy
14. instrument to cut bone: osteotome
15. surgical puncture of a joint: arthrocentasis
16. incision to remove a stone: lithotomy
17. excision of a breast: mastectomy
18. incision of the tympanic membrane: typanotomy
19. forming an opening (mouth) into the trachea: tracheostomy
20. excision of the spleen: splectomy

✓ *Check your answers in Appendix A. Review any material that you did not answer correctly.*

Correct Answers _____ X 5 = _____ % Score

*Information in parentheses is used to clarify the meaning of the word but not to build the medical term.

Learning Activity 2-2

Building More Surgical Words

Use the meanings in the right column to complete the surgical words in the left column. The word roots are underlined in the left column.

Incomplete Word	Meaning
1. arthr/o/desis	fixation or binding of a joint
2. rhin/o/plasty	surgical repair of the nose
3. ten/o/plasty	surgical repair of tendons
4. my/o/rrhaphy	suture of a muscle
5. mast/o/pexy	fixation of a (pendulous)* breast
6. cyst/o/rrhaphy	suture of the bladder
7. oste/o/clasis	surgical fracture of a bone
8. lith/o/tripsy	crushing of a stone
9. enter/o/lysis	separation of intestinal (adhesions)
10. neur/o/tripsy	crushing a nerve

Build a surgical word that means:

11. surgical repair of the nose: __rhinoplasty__
12. fixation of a joint: __athrodess__
13. suture of a muscle: __myorrhaphy__
14. fixation of a (pendulous) breast: __mastopexy__
15. suture of the bladder: __cystorrhaphy__
16. surgical repair of tendons: __tenoplasty__
17. surgical fracture of a bone: __osteoclasis__
18. crushing stones: __lithrotripsy__
19. separation of intestinal (adhesions): __enterolysis__
20. crushing a nerve: __neurotripsy__

✓ *Check your answers in Appendix A. Review any material that you did not answer correctly.*

Correct Answers _____ X 5 = _____ % Score

---

*Information in parentheses is used to clarify the meaning of the word but not to build the medical term.

Learning Activity 2-3
Selecting a Surgical Suffix

Use the list of suffixes to build surgical words in the right column that reflect the meanings in the left column. You may use the same suffix more than one time.

-centesis	-ectomy	-plasty	-tome
-clasis	-lysis	-rrhaphy	-tomy
-desis	-pexy	-stomy	-tripsy

1. crushing of a stone: lith/o _tripsy_
2. puncture of a joint (to remove fluid):*   arthr/o/ _centesis_
3. excision of the spleen: splen/ _splenectomy_
4. forming an opening (mouth) into the colon: col/o/ _colostomy_
5. instrument to cut skin: derma/ _dermatome_
6. forming an opening (mouth) into the trachea: trache/o/ _tracheostomy_
7. incision to remove a stone or calculus: lith/ _o_ / _tomy_
8. excision of a breast: mast/ _ectomy_
9. excision of hemorrhoids: hemorrhoid/ _ectomy_
10. incision of the trachea: trache/ _o_ / _tomy_
11. fixation of a breast: mast/ _o_ / _pexy_
12. excision of the colon: col/ _ectomy_
13. suture of the stomach (wall):   gastr/ _o_ / _rraphy_
14. fixation of the uterus: hyster/ _o_ / _pexy_
15. surgical repair of the nose: rhin/ _o_ / _plasty_
16. fixation or binding of a joint: arthr/ _o_ / _desis_
17. to break or surgically fracture a bone: oste/ _o_ / _clasis_
18. loosening of nerve (tissue):   neur/ _o_ / _lysis_
19. suture of muscle: my/o/ _rraphy_
20. incision of the tympanic membrane: tympan/ _o_ / _tomy_

✓ *Check your answers in Appendix A. Review any material that you did not answer correctly.*

Correct Answers _____ X 5 = _____ % Score

_____

*Information in parentheses is used to clarify the meaning of the word but not to build the medical term.

Learning Activity 2-4

Selecting Diagnostic, Pathological, and Related Suffixes

Use the suffixes in this list to build diagnostic, pathological, and related words in the right column that reflect the meanings in the left column.

-algia	-graph	-osis	-rrhea
-cele	-malacia	-pathy	-rrhexis
-ectasis	-megaly	-penia	-spasm
-emia	-oma	-plegia	

1. tumor of the liver: hepat/ _hepatoma_
2. pain (along the course) of a nerve: neur/ _neuralgia_
3. dilation of a bronchus: bronchi/ _bronchiectasis_
4. abnormal condition of the skin: dermat/ _dermatosis_
5. enlargement of the kidney: nephr/o/ _nephromegaly_
6. discharge or flow from the ear: ot/ _o_ / _rrhea_
7. rupture of the uterus: hyster/ _o_ / _rrhexis_
8. twitching of the eyelid: blephar/ _o_ / _spasm_
9. herniation of the bladder: cyst/ _o_ / _cele_
10. paralysis of four extremities: quadri/ _quadriplegia_
11. disease of muscle (tissue):   my/ _o_ / _pathy_
12. softening of the bones: oste/ _o_ / _malacia_
13. white blood condition: leuk/ _leukemia_
14. decrease in bone (mineral density):   oste/ _o_ / _penia_
15. instrument for recording (electrical activity) of the heart: cardi/o/ _cardiograph_

✓ *Check your answers in Appendix A. Review any material that you did not answer correctly.*

Correct Answers _____ X 6.67 = _____ % Score

Learning Activity 2-5

Building Pathological and Related Words

Use the meanings in the right column to complete the pathological and related words in the left column.

Incomplete Word	Meaning
1. bronchi/ _ectasis_	dilation of a bronchus
2. chole/ _lith_	gallstone
3. carcin/o/ _genesis_	forming or producing cancer
4. oste/ _o_ / _malacia_	softening of bone
5. hepat/ _o_ / _megaly_	enlargement of the liver
6. neur/ _o_ / _ma_	tumor composed of nervous tissue
7. hepat/ _o_ / _cele_	herniation of the liver
8. neur/o/ _pathy_	disease of the nerves
9. dermat/ _osis_	abnormal condition of the skin
10. quadri/ _plegia_	paralysis of four extremities
11. blephar/ _o_ / _ptosis_	prolapse or downward displacement of the eyelid
12. arteri/o/ _sclerosis_	abnormal condition of arterial hardening
13. cephal/o/ _dynia_	pain in the head; headache
14. blephar/ _o_ / _spasm_	twitching of the eyelid
15. hem/ _o_ / _phobia_	fear of blood

✓ *Check your answers in Appendix A. Review any material that you did not answer correctly.*

Correct Answers _____ X 6.67 = _____ % Score

Learning Activity 2-6

Selecting Adjective, Noun, and Diminutive Suffixes

Use the adjective suffixes in the list to create medical terms. The first one is completed for you.
Note: When in doubt about the validity of a word, refer to a medical dictionary.

-ac	-ary	-ic	-tic
-al	-eal	-ous	-tix

	Element	Medical Term	Meaning
1.	gastr/	*gastric*	pertaining to the stomach
2.	bacteri/	bacterial	pertaining to bacteria
3.	aqua/	aquatic	pertaining to water
4.	axill/	axillary	pertaining to the armpit
5.	cardi/	cardiac	pertaining to the heart
6.	spin/	spinal	pertaining to the spine
7.	membran/	membranous	pertaining to a membrane

Use the noun suffixes in the list to create medical terms.

-er	-is	-ole
-ia	-ism	-ule
-iatry	-ist	-y

	Element	Medical Term	Meaning
8.	intern/	internist	specialist in internal medicine
9.	arteri/	arteriole	minute artery
10.	sigmoid/o/scop/	sigmoidoscopy	visual examination of the sigmoid colon
11.	alcohol/	alcoholism	condition of (excessive) alcohol
12.	allerg/	allergist	specialist in treating allergic disorders
13.	man/	mania	condition of madness
14.	arteri/	arteriole	minute artery
15.	ven/	venule	small vein

 Check your answers in Appendix A. Review any material that you did not answer correctly.

Correct Answers _____ X 6.67 = _____ % Score

Learning Activity 2-7

Forming Plural Words

Review the guidelines for plural suffixes (located on the inside back cover of this book). Then write the plural form for each of the singular terms and briefly state the rule that applies. The first one is completed for you.

Singular	Plural	Rule
1. diagnosis	*diagnoses*	*Drop the is and add es.*
2. fornix	fornices	Drop ix, add ices
3. vertebra	vertebrae	keep "a", add "e"
4. keratosis	keratoses	drop the is add es
5. bronchus	bronchi	drop the us add "i"
6. spermatozoon	spermatozoa	drop the suffix add the zoa
7. septum	septa	drop the um add a
8. coccus	cocci	drop the i add i
9. ganglion	ganglia	drop the i add i
10. prognosis	prognoses	drop the is, add es
11. thrombus	thrombi	drop us add i
12. appendix	appendices	add es drop ix
13. bacterium	bacteria	add ia drop ium
14. testis	testes	drop is add es
15. nevus	nevi	drop us add i

✓ *Check your answers in Appendix A. Review any material that you did not answer correctly.*

Correct Answers _____ X 6.67 = _____ % Score

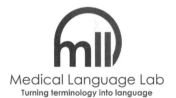

Medical Language Lab
Turning terminology into language

Visit the Medical Language Lab at the website *medicallanguagelab.com*. Use it to enhance your study and reinforcement of suffixes with the flash-card activity related to suffixes. We recommend that you complete the flash-card activity before moving on to Chapter 3.

Prefixes

Chapter Outline

Objectives

Upon completion of this chapter, you will be able to:

- Define common prefixes used in medical terminology.
- Describe how a prefix changes the meaning of a medical word.
- Recognize and define prefixes of position, number and measurement, and direction.
- Pronounce medical terms presented in this chapter.
- Demonstrate your knowledge of this chapter by completing the learning activities.

Prefix Linking

Most medical words contain a root or combining form with a suffix. Some of them also contain prefixes. A prefix is a word element located at the beginning of a word. Substituting one prefix for another alters the meaning of the word. For example, in the term **macro/cyte**, *macro-* is a prefix meaning *large; -cyte* is a suffix meaning *cell*. A **macr/o/cyte** is a *large cell*. Changing the prefix **macro-** (large) to **micro-** (small) changes the meaning of the word. A **micr/o/cyte** is a *small cell*. See Table 3-1 for other examples of how a prefix changes the meaning of a word.

Table 3-1	Changing Prefixes and Meanings

In this table, each word has the same root, nat *(birth), and suffix,* -al *(pertaining to). By substituting different prefixes, new words with different meanings are formed.*

Prefix	+	Word Root	+	Suffix	=	Medical Word	Meaning
pre- (before)	+	nat (birth)	+	-al (pertaining to)	=	pre/nat/al prē-NĀ-tăl	pertaining to (the period) before birth
peri- (around)	+	nat (birth)	+	-al (pertaining to)		peri/nat/al pĕr-ĭ-NĀ-tăl	pertaining to (the period) around birth
post- (after)	+	nat (birth)	+	-al (pertaining to)		post/nat/al pōst-NĀ-tăl	pertaining to (the period) after birth

Prefix Types

Learning the major types of prefixes, such as prefixes of position, number and measurement, and direction, as well as some others, will help you master medical terminology.

Prefixes of Position, Number, Measurement, and Direction

Prefixes used in medical terms denote position, number and measurement, and direction. Prefixes of position describe a place or location. (See Table 3-2.) Prefixes of number and measurement describe an amount, size, or degree of involvement. (See Table 3-3.) Prefixes of direction indicate a pathway or route. (See Table 3-4.)

Table 3-2	Prefixes of Position

This table lists commonly used prefixes of position, along with their meanings and word analyses.

Prefix	Meaning	Word Analysis
endo-	in, within	**endo**/crine (ĔN-dō-krĭn): secrete within -crine: secrete *Endocrine describes a gland that secretes directly into the bloodstream.*

intra-		**intra**/muscul/ar (ĭn-tră-MŬS-kū-lăr): within the muscle
		  muscul: muscle
		  -ar: pertaining to

epi-	above, upon	**epi**/derm/is (ĕp-ĭ-DĔR-mĭs): upon the skin
		  derm: skin
		  -is: noun ending
		The epidermis is the outer layer of the skin.

Table 3-2	Prefixes of Position—cont'd	

Prefix	Meaning	Word Analysis

hypo-	under, below; deficient	hypo/derm/ic (hī-pō-DĔR-mĭk): pertaining to under the skin
		  derm: skin
		  -ic: pertaining to
		Hypodermic needles are used for subcutaneous injections and to take fluid samples from the body, for example, taking blood from a vein in venipuncture. (See Fig. 3-1.)

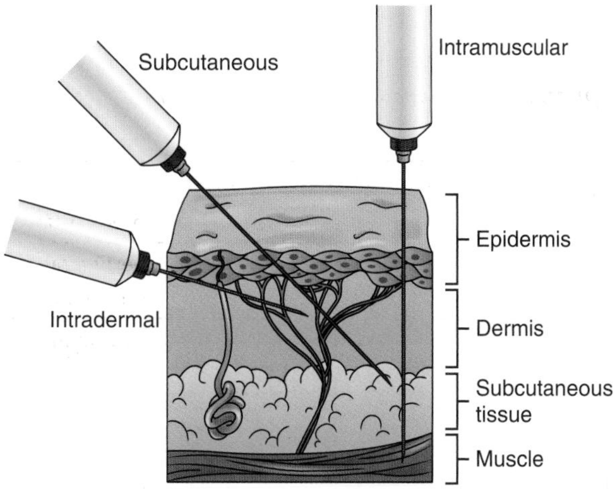

Figure 3-1 **Hypo**dermic needles inserted within the skin (**intra**dermal), under the skin (**sub**cutaneous), or in between the muscular layer (**intra**muscular).

Prefix	Meaning	Word Analysis

infra-	under, below	infra/cost/al (ĭn-fră-KŎS-tăl): below the ribs
		  cost: ribs
		  -al: pertaining to

sub-		sub/cutane/ous (sŭb-kū-TĀ-nē-ŭs): pertaining to under the skin
		  cutane: skin
		  -ous: pertaining to
		The subcutaneous tissue is the lowest layer of skin. It binds the dermis to underlying structures.

inter-	between	inter/cost/al (ĭn-tĕr-KŎS-tăl): between the ribs
		  cost: ribs
		  -al: pertaining to

retro-	backward, behind	retro/version (rĕt-rō-VĔR-shŭn): turning backward *-version:* turning **Retroversion** *refers to tipping backward of an organ (such as the uterus) from its normal position.*

Table 3-3	Prefixes of Number and Measurement

This table lists commonly used prefixes of number and measurement, along with their meanings and word analyses.

Prefix	Meaning	Word Analysis
bi-	two	**bi**/later/al (bī-LĂT-ĕr-ăl): pertaining to two sides *later:* side *-al:* pertaining to
dipl-	double	**dipl**/opia (dĭp-LŌ-pē-ă): double vision *-opia:* vision
diplo-		**diplo**/bacteri/al (dĭp-lō-băk-TĒR-ē-ăl): bacteria linked together in pairs *bacteri:* bacteria *-al:* pertaining to *Diplobacteria reproduce in such a manner that they are joined together in pairs.*
hemi-	one-half	**hemi**/plegia (hĕm-ē-PLĒ-jē-ă): paralysis of one half *-plegia:* paralysis *Hemiplegia is a paralysis of one-half of the body, either the right side or the left side.*
hyper-	excessive, above normal	**hyper**/calc/emia (hī-pĕr-kăl-SĒ-mē-ă): excessive calcium in the blood *calc:* calcium *-emia:* blood condition
macro-	large	**macro**/cyte (MĂK-rō-sīt): large cell *-cyte:* cell
micro-	small	**micro**/scope (MĪ-krō-skōp): instrument for examining small (objects) *-scope:* instrument for examining *A microscope is an optical instrument that greatly magnifies minute objects.*
mono-	one	**mono**/therapy (MŎN-ō-thĕr-ă-pē): one treatment *-therapy:* treatment *An example of monotherapy is treatment using only a single drug or a single treatment modality.*
uni-		**uni**/nucle/ar (ū-nĭ-NŪ-klē-ăr): pertaining to one nucleus *nucle:* nucleus *-ar:* pertaining to
multi-	many, much	**multi**/gravida (mŭl-tĭ-GRĂV-ĭ-dă): woman who has been pregnant more than once *-gravida:* pregnant woman
poly		**poly**/phobia (pŏl-ē-FŌ-bē-ă): fear of many things *-phobia:* fear
quadri-	four	**quadri**/plegia (kwŏd-rĭ-PLĒ-jē-ă): paralysis of four *-plegia:* paralysis *Quadriplegia is a paralysis of all four extremities, usually caused by an injury to or disease of the cervical spinal cord.*
tri-	three	**tri**/ceps (TRĪ-cĕps): three heads *-ceps:* head *Triceps describes a muscle having three heads or points of origin.*

Table 3-4	Prefixes of Direction

This table lists commonly used prefixes of direction as well as their meanings and word analyses.

Prefix	Meaning	Word Analysis
ab-	from, away from	**ab**/duction (ăb-DŬK-shŭn): movement of a limb away from (the body)
		-duction: act of leading, bringing, conducting
		Abduction is a body movement away from the midline or axis of the body. (See Fig. 3-2.)
ad-	toward	**ad**/duction (ăb-DŬK-shŭn): movement of a limb toward (the body)
		-duction: act of leading, bringing, conducting
		Adduction is a body movement toward to the midline or axis of the body. (See Fig. 3-2.)

A **Ad**duction   **B** **Ab**duction

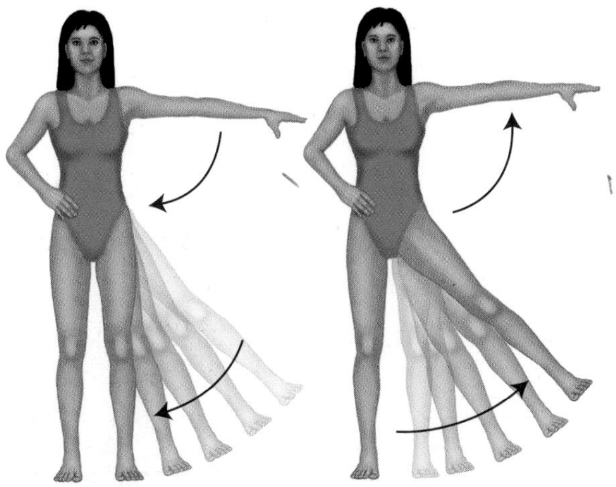

Figure 3-2 Adduction and **Ab**duction.

Prefix	Meaning	Word Analysis
circum-	around	**circum**/ren/al (sĕr-kŭm-RĒ-năl): pertaining to around the kidney
		ren: kidney
		-al: pertaining to
peri-		**peri**/odont/al (pĕr-ē-ō-DŎN-tăl): pertaining to around a tooth
		odont: teeth
		-al: pertaining to
dia-	through, across	**dia**/rrhea (dī-ă-RĒ-ă): flow through
		-rrhea: discharge, flow
		Diarrhea is a condition of abnormally frequent discharge or flow of fluid fecal matter through the bowel.
trans-		**trans**/vagin/al (trăns-VĂJ-ĭn-ăl): pertaining to across or through the vagina
		vagin: vagina
		-al: pertaining to
ecto-	outside, outward	**ecto**/gen/ous (ĕk-TŎJ-ĕ-nŭs): forming outside (the body or structure)
		gen: forming, producing, origin
		-ous: pertaining to
		An ectogenous infection is one that originates outside of the body.
exo-		**exo**/tropia (ĕks-ō-TRŌ-pē-ă): turning outward
		-tropia: turning
		Exotropia refers to the turning outward of the eyes.
extra-		**extra**/crani/al (ĕks-tră-KRĀ-nē-ăl): pertaining to outside the skull
		crani: cranium (skull)
		-al: pertaining to

(continued)

Table 3-4	**Prefixes of Direction—cont'd**	
Prefix	**Meaning**	**Word Analysis**
para-*	near, beside; beyond	**para**/nas/al (păr-ă-NĀ-săl): beside the nose *nas:* nose *-al:* pertaining to
super-	upper, above	**super**/ior (soo-PĒ-rē-or): pertaining to above or the upper part of a structure *-ior:* pertaining to
supra-	above; excessive; superior	**supra**/ren/al (soo-pră-RĒ-năl): pertaining to above the kidney *ren:* kidney *-al:* pertaining to
ultra-	excess, beyond	**ultra**/son/ic (ŭl-tră-SŎN-ĭk): pertaining to sound beyond (that which can be heard by the human ear) *son:* sound *-ic:* pertaining to

*Para- may also be used as a suffix meaning to bear (offspring).

Other Common Prefixes

Many other common prefixes may also change the meaning of a word. See Table 3-5 for a list of other common prefixes.

Table 3-5	**Other Common Prefixes**	
This table lists other commonly used prefixes, along with their meanings and word analyses.		
Prefix	**Meaning**	**Word Analysis**
a-*	without, not	**a**/mast/ia (ă-MĂS-tē-ă): without a breast *mast:* breast *-ia:* condition *Amastia may be the result of a congenital defect, an endocrine disorder, or mastectomy.*
an-**		**an**/esthesia (ăn-ĕs-THĒ-zē-ă): without feeling *-esthesia:* feeling *Anesthesia may be a partial or complete loss of sensation with or without loss of consciousness.*
anti-	against	**anti**/bacteri/al (ăn-tĭ-băk-TĒR-ē-ăl): against bacteria *bacteri:* bacteria *-al:* pertaining to *Antibacterials are substances that kill bacteria or inhibit their growth or replication.*
contra-		**contra**/ception (kŏn-tră-SĔP-shŭn): against conceiving *-ception:* conceiving *Contraceptive techniques prevent pregnancy by means of medication, a device, or a method that blocks or alters one or more of the processes of reproduction.*

*The prefix a- is usually used before a consonant.

** The prefix an- is usually used before a vowel.

| Table 3-5 | **Other Common Prefixes—cont'd** |

Prefix	Meaning	Word Analysis
auto-	self, own	**auto**/graft (AW-tō-grăft); transplantation to self *-graft:* transplantation *An autograft is tissue transplanted from one site and grafted to another site of the same person. (See Fig. 3-3.)*

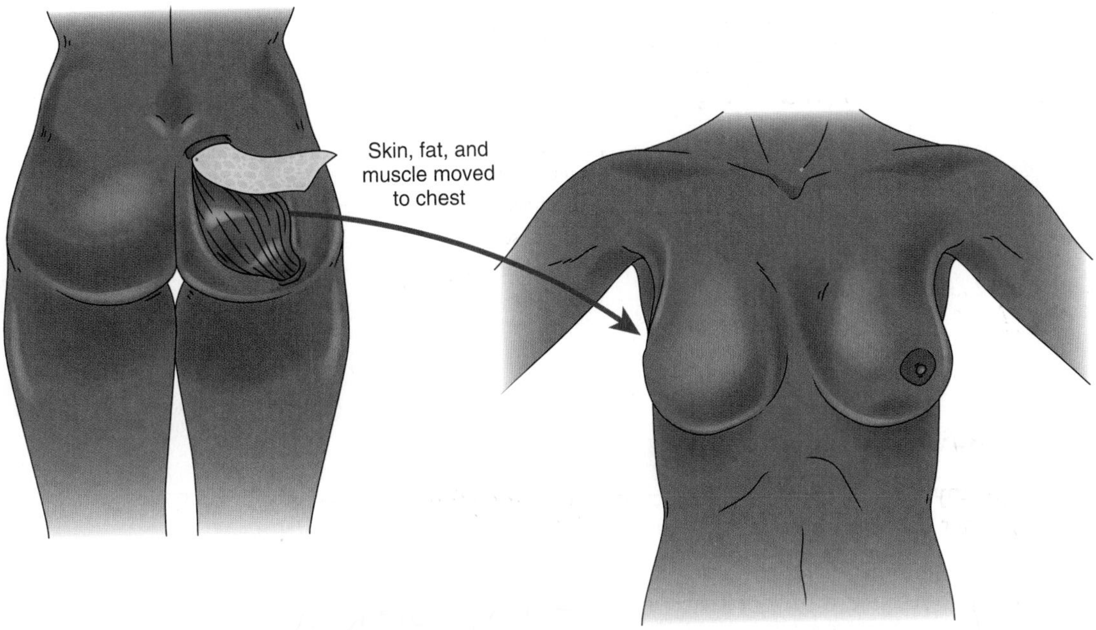

Skin, fat, and muscle moved to chest

Figure 3-3 **Auto**graft in which tissue from the patient's buttocks is transplanted to her breast.

Prefix	Meaning	Word Analysis
brady-	slow	**brady**/cardia (brăd-ē-KĂR-dē-ă): slow heart rate *-cardia:* heart
dys-	bad; painful; difficult	**dys**/tocia (dĭs-TŌ-sē-ă): difficult childbirth *-tocia:* childbirth, labor
eu-	good, normal	**eu**/pnea (ūp-NĒ-ă): normal breathing *-pnea:* breathing

(continued)

Table 3-5	**Other Common Prefixes—cont'd**	

Prefix	Meaning	Word Analysis
hetero-	different	**hetero**/graft (HĔT-ĕ-rō-grăft): different transplantation; also called *xenograft*
		-graft: transplantation
		A heterograft is a transplant from one species to another. (See Fig. 3-4.)

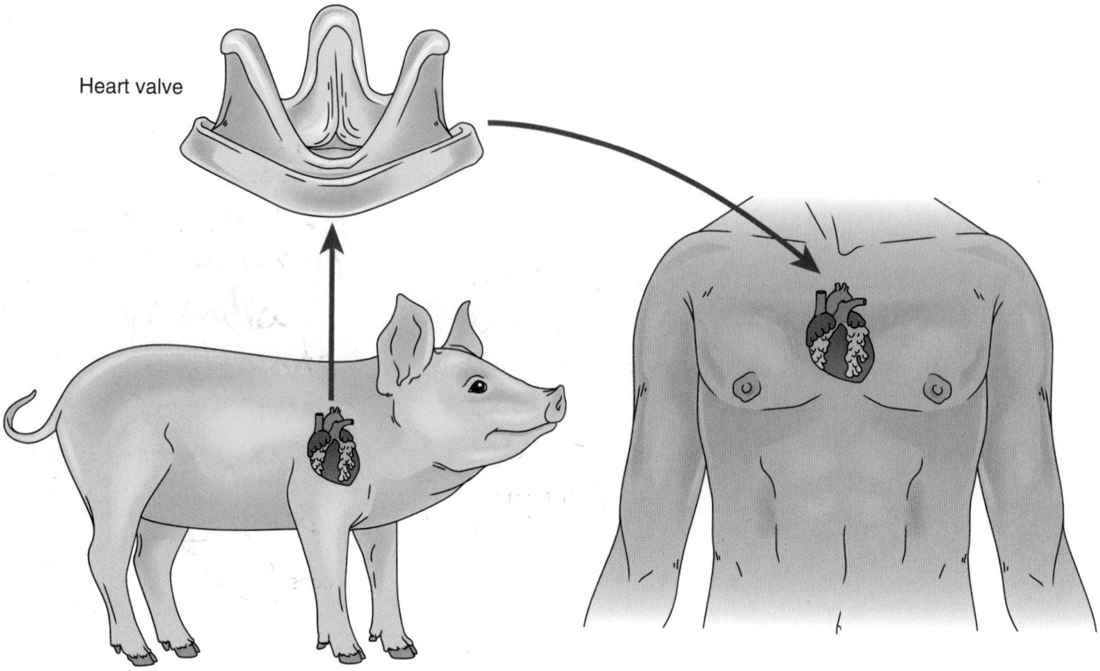

Heart valve

Figure 3-4 Heterograft in which tissue (heart valve) from one species (pig) is transplanted to another species (human).

Prefix	Meaning	Word Analysis
homo-	same	**homo/graft** (HŌ-mō-grăft): same transplantation *-graft:* transplantation *A homograft, also called an allograft, is a graft of tissue or an organ taken from a donor of the same species as the recipient. Commonly transplanted organs include the kidneys, lungs, and heart. (See Fig. 3-5.)*
homeo-		**homeo/plasia** (hō-mē-ō-PLĀ-zē-ă): formation or growth of same (or similar tissue) *-plasia:* formation, growth

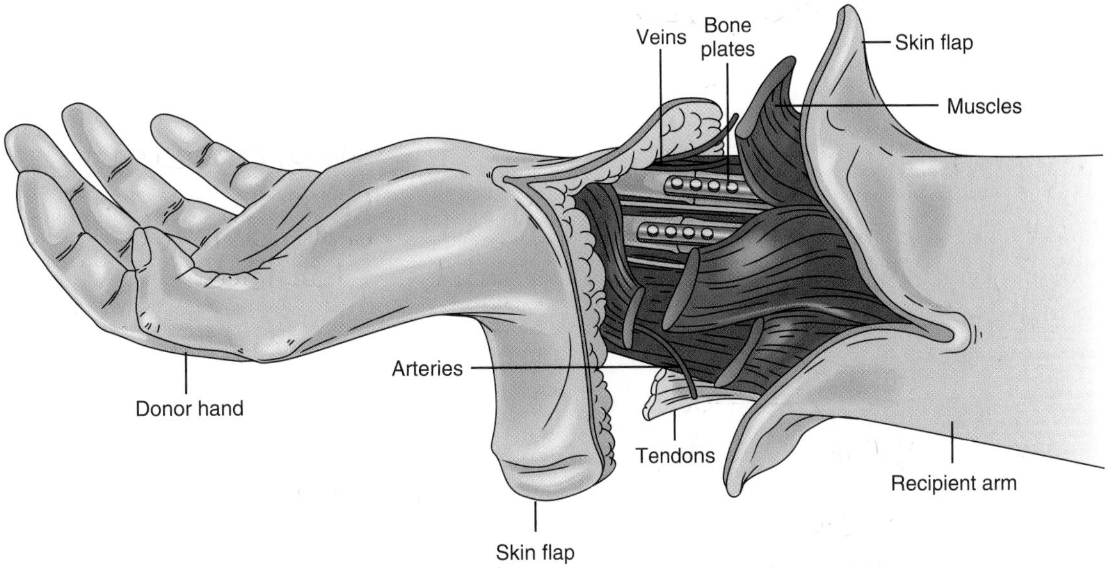

Table 3-5 ## Other Common Prefixes—cont'd

Veins Bone plates Skin flap Muscles

Arteries

Donor hand

Tendons

Recipient arm

Skin flap

Figure 3-5 Homograft of an arm taken from a human donor and transplanted to another human.

tachy-	rapid	**tachy/pnea** (tăk-ĭp-NĒ-ă): rapid breathing *-pnea:* breathing

 It is time to review prefixes by completing Learning Activities 3-1, 3-2, and 3-3.

LEARNING ACTIVITIES

The activities that follow provide review of the prefixes introduced in this chapter. Complete each activity and review your answers to evaluate your understanding of the chapter.

Learning Activity 3-1

Identifying and Defining Prefixes

Place a slash after each of the prefixes and then define the prefix. The first one is completed for you.

Word	Definition of Prefix
1. inter/dental	*between*
2. hypo/dermic	under, below, deficient
3. epi/dermis	above upon
4. retro/version	backward, behind
5. sub/lingual	under, below
6. quadr/iplegia	four
7. micro/scope	small
8. tri/ceps	three
9. an/esthesia	with
10. intra/muscular	in, within
11. supra/pelvic	above, excessive, superior
12. bi/lateral	two
13. peri/odontal	around
14. brady/cardia	slow
15. tachy/pnea	rapid
16. dyst/ocia	bad, painful, difficult
17. eu/pnea	good, normal
18. hetero/graft	diffrent
19. post/natal	after
20. circum/renal	around

✔ *Check your answers in Appendix A. Review any material that you did not answer correctly.*

Correct Answers _____ X 5 = _____ % Score

Learning Activity 3-2

Matching Prefixes of Position, Number and Measurement, and Direction

Match the terms with the definitions in the numbered list.

bradypnea	intercostal	postoperative
diarrhea	macrocyte	quadriplegia
epigastric	monotherapy	retroversion
hemiplegia	periodontal	subnasal
hypodermic	polyphobia	suprarenal

1. _retroversion_ tipping back of an organ
2. _hypodermic_ pertaining to under the skin
3. _bradypnea_ slow breathing
4. _subnasal_ pertaining to under the nose
5. _postoperative_ after surgery
6. _intercostal_ pertaining to between the ribs
7. _epigastric_ pertaining to (the area) above the stomach
8. _periodontal_ pertaining to around the teeth
9. _diarrhea_ flow through (watery bowel movement)
10. _monotherapy_ one treatment
11. _suprarenal_ above the kidney
12. _hemiplegia_ paralysis of one-half (of the body)
13. _quadriplegia_ paralysis of four (limbs)
14. _macrocyte_ (abnormally) large blood cell
15. _polyphobia_ many fears

✓ *Check your answers in Appendix A. Review any material that you did not answer correctly.*

Correct Answers _____ X 6.67 = _____ % Score

Learning Activity 3-3

Matching Other Prefixes

Match the terms with the definitions in the numbered list.

amastia	bradypnea	heterograft
anesthesia	contraception	homeoplasia
antibacterial	dyspepsia	homograft
anticonvulsant	dystocia	tachyphasia
bradycardia	eupnea	tachycardia

1. _____dyspepsia_____ difficult digestion
2. _____heterograft_____ tissue transplant from a different species
3. _____bradypnea_____ slow breathing
4. _____antibacterial_____ against bacteria
5. _____tachycardia_____ slow heartbeat
6. _____anticonvulsant_____ prevents or relieves convulsions
7. _____amastia_____ without a breast
8. _____anesthesia_____ without sensation
9. _____eupnea_____ good or normal breathing
10. _____tachyphasia_____ rapid speech
11. _____tachycardia_____ rapid heartbeat
12. _____contraception_____ against conceiving
13. _____homograft_____ tissue transplant from the same species
14. _____dystocia_____ difficult childbirth
15. _____homephasia_____ formation of the same tissue

✓ *Check your answers in Appendix A. Review any material that you did not answer correctly.*

Correct Answers _____ X 6.67 = _____ % Score

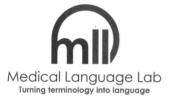

Medical Language Lab
Turning terminology into language

Visit the Medical Language Lab at the website *medicallanguagelab.com*. Use it to enhance your study and reinforcement of prefixes with the flash-card activity related to prefixes. We recommend that you complete the flash-card activity before moving on to Chapter 4.

Body Structure

Chapter Outline

Objectives

Upon completion of this chapter, you will be able to:

- List the levels of organization of the body.
- Define and identify three planes of the body.
- Identify the cavities, quadrants, and regions of the body.
- List and identify terms related to direction, position, and planes of the body.
- Recognize, pronounce, spell, and build words related to body structure.
- Describe diseases, conditions, and procedures related to body structure.
- Demonstrate your knowledge of this chapter by completing the learning and documenting health-care activities.

Introduction

This chapter provides an orientation to the body as a whole and contains general terms that are relevant to all body systems. Learning these terms and how they are used to locate and describe structures within the body helps to master the material presented in subsequent chapters of this book. Included are terms associated with diseases, abnormal conditions, and diagnostic and medical procedures used in the clinical setting. Also, case studies provide prototypes for documenting health-care services in a patient's electronic medical record.

Body Structure Key Terms

This section introduces important terms associated with body structure, along with their definitions and pronunciations. The key terms are highlighted in color throughout the introduction. Word analyses are also provided for selected terms.

Term	Definition
chromatin KRŌ-mă-tĭn ☐	Structural component of the nucleus, composed of nucleic acids and proteins *Chromatin condenses to form chromosomes during cell division.*
chromosome KRŌ-mō-sōm ☐	Threadlike structures within the nucleus composed of deoxyribonucleic acid (DNA) that carries hereditary information encoded in genes *Each sperm or egg has 23 unpaired chromosomes. After fertilization, each cell of the embryo then has 46 chromosomes (23 pairs). In each pair of chromosomes, one chromosome is provided by the father and the other by the mother.*
deoxyribonucleic acid (DNA) dē-ŏk-sē-rī-bō-noo-KLĀ-ĭk ĂS-ĭd ☐	Molecule that holds genetic information capable of replicating and producing an exact copy whenever the cell divides
metabolism mĕ-TĂB-ō-lĭzm ☐	Sum of all physical and chemical changes that take place in a cell or an organism *Metabolism includes the building up (anabolism) and breaking down (catabolism) of body constituents.*
organelle or-găn-ĔL ☐	Cellular structure that provides a specialized function, such as the nucleus (reproduction), ribosomes (protein synthesis), Golgi apparatus (removal of material from the cell), and lysosomes (digestion) *The membranes of many organelles act as sites of chemical reactions.*

Pronunciation Help	Long Sound	ā — rate	ē — rebirth	ī — isle	ō — over	ū — unite
	Short Sound	ă — apple	ĕ — ever	ĭ — it	ŏ — not	ŭ — cut

Levels of Organization

The human body contains several levels of structure and function. Each of these levels builds on the previous level and contributes to the structure and function of the entire organism. Five levels of organization are relevant to understanding anatomy, physiology, and pathology: the cells, tissues, organs, systems, and organism. (See Fig. 4-1.)

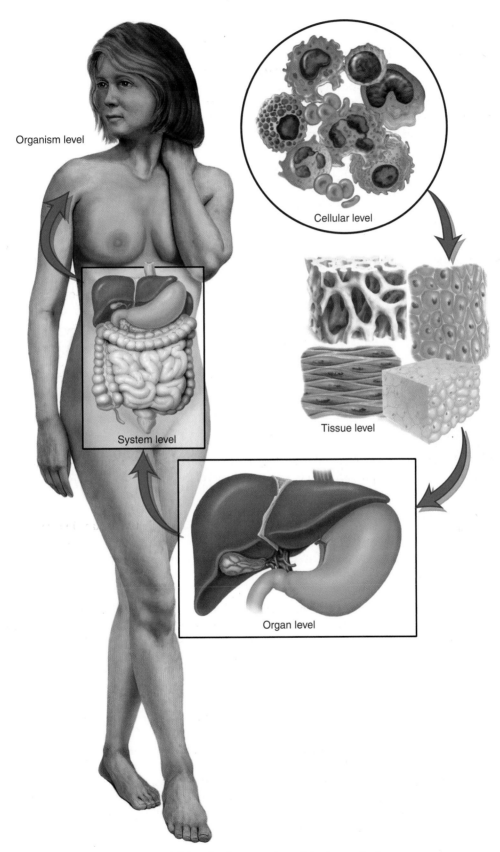

Organism level

Cellular level

Tissue level

System level

Organ level

Figure 4-1 Levels of organization of the human body.

Cells

The cell is the smallest structural and functional unit of life. Body cells perform all activities associated with life, including utilizing food, facilitating reproduction, and eliminating waste products. Cells have many shapes and sizes, but they share three main structures: **cell membrane, cytoplasm,** and **nucleus.** The study of the body at the cellular level is called **cytology.**

Cell Membrane and Cytoplasm

The cell membrane acts as a barrier that supports and protects the intracellular contents. Within the cell membrane is a jellylike matrix of proteins, salts, water, dissolved gases, and nutrients called **cytoplasm.** Inside the cytoplasm are specialized structures called **organelles.** These organelles perform specific functions of the cell, such as reproduction and digestion. The largest cell organelle is the nucleus, which directs the cell's activities and contains **chromosomes.**

Nucleus

The nucleus is responsible for **metabolism,** growth, and reproduction. It also carries the genetic blueprint of the organism. This blueprint is found in a complex molecule called **deoxyribonucleic acid (DNA)** that is organized into a threadlike structure called **chromatin.** When the cell is ready to divide, chromatin forms **chromosomes,** which carry thousands of genes that make up our genetic blueprint. Each body cell, with the exception of the female ovum and the male spermatozoa, contains 23 pairs of chromosomes that determine its genetic makeup. In each of the 23 pairs, one of the chromosomes was inherited from the mother and the other from the father. About 20,000–25,000 genes in the body determine unique human characteristics. Genes pass biological information from one generation to the next. This biological information includes such traits as hair color, body structure, and metabolic activity.

Tissues

Tissue is composed of similar cells that perform specialized or common functions. The study of tissues is called **histology.** Between the cells that make up tissues are varying amounts and types of nonliving, intercellular substances that provide pathways for cellular interaction. The body contains four types of tissues:

- **Epithelial tissue** covers surfaces of organs, lines cavities and canals, forms tubes and ducts, provides the secreting portions of glands, and makes up the outer layer **(epidermis)** of the skin. It is composed of cells arranged in a continuous sheet consisting of one or more layers.
- **Connective tissue** supports and connects other body tissues. There are various types of connective tissue, including cartilage, adipose (fat), bone, elastic fiber, and even blood.
- **Muscle tissue** provides the contractile tissue of the body, which is responsible for movement.
- **Nervous tissue** transmits electrical impulses as it relays information throughout the entire body.

Organs

Organs are body structures that perform specialized functions. They are composed of two or more tissue types. For example, the stomach is made up of connective tissue, muscle tissue, epithelial tissue, and nervous tissue. Muscle and connective tissue form the wall of the stomach. Epithelial and connective tissue cover the inner and outer surfaces of the stomach. Nervous tissue penetrates the epithelial lining of the stomach and its muscular wall to stimulate the release of chemicals for digestion.

Systems

A body system is composed of varying numbers of organs and accessory structures that have similar or related functions. For example, organs of the gastrointestinal system include the esophagus, stomach, small intestine, and colon. Some of its accessory structures include the liver, gallbladder, and pancreas. The main function of the digestive system is to digest food, remove and absorb its nutrients, and expel waste products.

Organism

The highest level of organization is the organism. An organism is a complete living entity capable of independent existence. All complex organisms, including humans, are made up of several body systems that work together to sustain life.

Anatomical Position

Anatomical position is a body posture used among anatomists and clinicians as a position of reference to ensure uniformity and consistency in locating anatomical parts or divisions of the human body. In the anatomical position, the person stands erect, facing forward, and the arms are at the sides of the body, with the palms of the hands turned forward and the feet parallel to each another. No matter how the body is actually positioned—standing or lying down, facing forward or backward—or how the limbs are actually placed, the positions and relationships of a structure are always described as if the body were in the anatomical position.

Body Planes

A **plane** is an imaginary flat surface that divides the body into two sections. When the body is in anatomical position, the planes serve as points of reference to identify the different sections of the body. The most commonly used planes are coronal (frontal), transverse (horizontal), and midsagittal (median). The section is named for the plane along which it is cut. A **coronal (frontal) plane** divides the body into an anterior and posterior section; a **transverse (horizontal) plane** divides the body into top and bottom sections. The **midsagittal plane** runs through the center of the body, dividing the body into right and left halves. (See Fig. 4-2.)

Before the development of modern imaging techniques, standard x-ray images showed only a single plane, and many body abnormalities were difficult, if not impossible, to see. Current

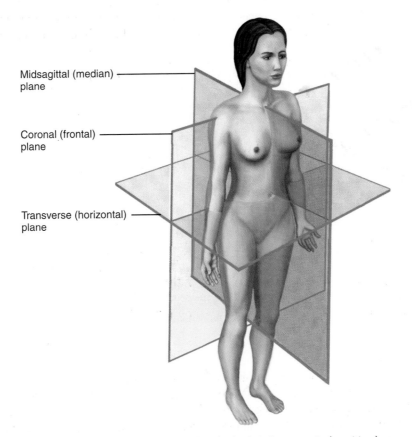

Midsagittal (median) plane

Coronal (frontal) plane

Transverse (horizontal) plane

Figure 4-2 Body planes. (Note that the body is in anatomical position.)

imaging procedures, such as magnetic resonance imaging (MRI) and computed tomography (CT), produce three-dimensional images on more than one plane. Thus, structural abnormalities and body masses that were previously not found using a standard single plane x-ray are now detected with scanning devices that show images taken in several body planes.

Directional Terms

Directional terms help indicate the position of structures, surfaces, and regions of the body. These terms are always identified relative to the anatomical position. For example, the knee is *superior* to the ankle; the legs are *inferior* to the trunk. Refer to Figure 4-3 to locate the directional terms *superior* and *inferior*. Physicians commonly use directional terms in medical reports and in communications with other health-care providers and patients. Directional terms identify the location of diseases, injuries, and surgical sites. In a clinical setting, health-care providers may describe the location of a heart attack to the patient as occurring in the front, or *anterior*, part of the heart. A tumor on the back of the kidney may be described as being located on the *posterior* surface of the kidney. (See Table 4-1.)

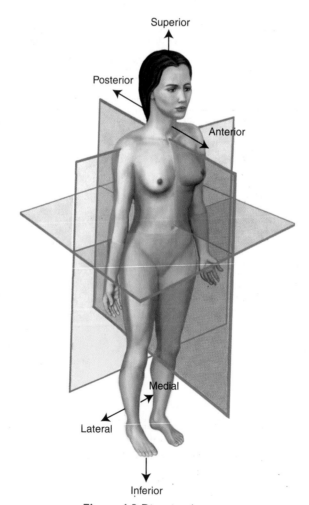

Figure 4-3 Directional terms.

Table 4-1	**Directional Terms**

This table provides a comprehensive summary of directional terms, along with their definitions. Opposing terms are presented consecutively to aid memorization.

Term	Definition
Abduction	Movement away from the midsagittal (median) plane of the body or one of its parts
Adduction	Movement toward the midsagittal (median) plane of the body
Medial	Pertaining to the midline of the body or structure
Lateral	Pertaining to a side
Superior (cephalad)	Toward the head or upper portion of a structure
Inferior (caudal)	Away from the head, or toward the tail or lower part of a structure
Proximal	Nearer to the center (trunk of the body) or to the point of attachment to the body
Distal	Further from the center (trunk of the body) or from the point of attachment to the body
Anterior (ventral)	Front of the body
Posterior (dorsal)	Back of the body
Parietal	Pertaining to the outer wall of the body cavity
Visceral	Pertaining to the viscera, or internal organs, especially the abdominal organs
Prone	Lying on the abdomen, face down
Supine	Lying horizontally on the back, face up
Inversion	Turning inward or inside out
Eversion	Turning outward
Palmar	Pertaining to the palm of the hand
Plantar	Pertaining to the sole of the foot
Superficial	Toward the surface of the body (external)
Deep	Away from the surface of the body (internal)

Body Cavities

Body cavities are spaces within the body that hold, protect, separate, and support internal organs. Clinicians refer to these cavities to locate internal organs and identify abnormalities within the cavities. The body has two main cavities: the **dorsal cavity,** located on the back of the body **(posterior),** and the **ventral cavity,** located on the front of the body **(anterior).** (See Fig. 4-4.)

Dorsal Cavity

The **dorsal cavity** is divided into the *cranial cavity* and the *spinal cavity.* The **cranial cavity,** formed by the skull, contains the brain; the **spinal cavity,** formed by the backbone (spine), contains the spinal cord. The **meninges** are the membranes that line these cavities and also cover the brain and spinal cord. The dorsal cavity is continuous; no wall or structure separates the cranial cavity from the spinal cavity.

Ventral Cavity

The **ventral cavity** is divided into the *thoracic cavity* and *abdominopelvic cavity.* The thoracic cavity is separated from the abdominopelvic cavity by a muscular wall called the **diaphragm.** The **thoracic cavity** contains the lungs and heart. The **abdominal pelvic cavity** is further divided into the *abdominal cavity* and *pelvic cavity.* The **abdominal cavity** contains the liver, stomach, intestines, and kidneys. The **pelvic cavity,** positioned inferior to the abdominal cavity, contains the urinary bladder and reproductive organs, such as the uterus in women and the prostate gland in men. Examine the divisions of the ventral cavity in Figure 4-4.

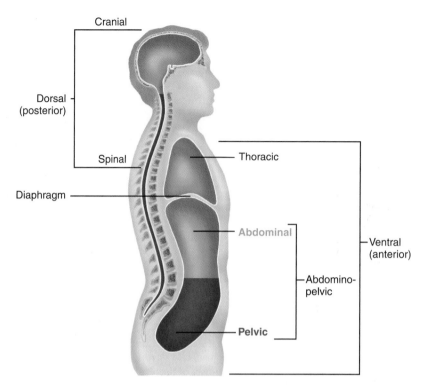

Figure 4-4 Body cavities.

Abdominopelvic Quadrants and Regions

To describe the location of the many abdominal and pelvic organs more easily, anatomists and clinicians use two methods of dividing the abdominopelvic cavity into smaller areas. These two divisions are known as **quadrants** and **regions.**

Quadrants

The abdominopelvic cavity is divided into four **quadrants** with two imaginary lines that form a cross in the midsection of the lower torso. The quadrants provide a means of locating specific sites of the abdomen for descriptive and diagnostic purposes. (See Table 4-2.) They also provide a point of reference in clinical examinations and medical reports. Clinicians will commonly describe pain, lesions, abrasions, punctures, and burns as located in a specific quadrant. They will also identify incision sites by using body quadrants. (See Fig. 4-5.)

Table 4-2	Abdominopelvic Quadrants	
Quadrant	**Abbreviation**	**Major Structures**
Right upper	RUQ	Right lobe of the liver, the gallbladder, part of the pancreas, and part of the small and large intestines
Left upper	LUQ	Left lobe of the liver, the stomach, the spleen, part of the pancreas, and part of the small and large intestines
Right lower	RLQ	Part of the small and large intestines, the appendix, the right ovary, the right fallopian tube, and the right ureter
Left lower	LLQ	Part of the small and large intestines, the left ovary, the left fallopian tube, and the left ureter

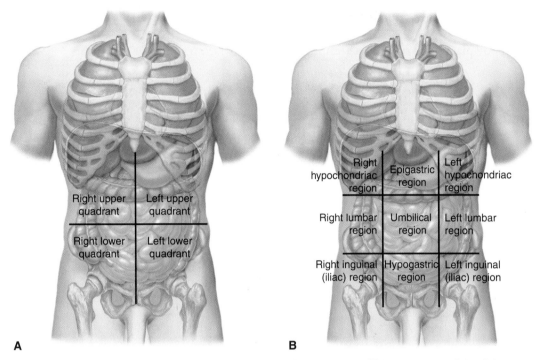

Figure 4-5 Quadrants and regions. (A) Four quadrants of the abdomen. (B) Nine regions of the abdomen.

Regions

Anatomists and clinicians divide the abdominopelvic cavity into nine **abdominopelvic regions.** They use these regions primarily to identify the location of underlying body structures and visceral organs. (See Table 4-3.) For example, the stomach is located in the left hypochondriac and epigastric region; the appendix is located in the right inguinal region.

Table 4-3	**Abdominopelvic Regions**
Region	**Location**
Right hypochondriac	Upper right lateral region beneath the ribs
Epigastric	Upper middle region
Left hypochondriac	Upper left lateral region beneath the ribs
Right lumbar	Middle right lateral region
Umbilical	Region of the navel
Left lumbar	Middle left lateral region
Right inguinal (iliac)	Lower right lateral region
Hypogastric	Lower middle region
Left inguinal (iliac)	Lower left lateral region

Anatomy Review: Body Planes

To review the body planes and directional terms, label the illustration using the terms that follow.

anterior   *lateral*   *posterior*

coronal (frontal) plane   *medial*   *superior*

inferior   *midsagittal (median) plane*   *transverse (horizontal) plane*

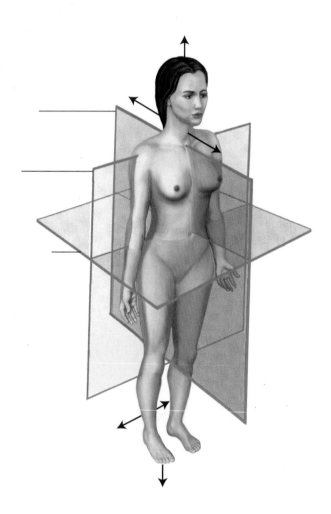

 Check your answers by referring to Figure 4-2 on page 47. Review material that you did not answer correctly.

Anatomy Review: Quadrants and Regions

To review quadrants and regions, label the quadrants in Figure A and the regions in Figure B using the terms that follow.

epigastric region

hypogastric region

left hypochondriac region

left iliac region

left lower quadrant

left lumbar region

left upper quadrant

right hypochondriac region

right iliac region

right lower quadrant

right lumbar region

right upper quadrant

umbilical region

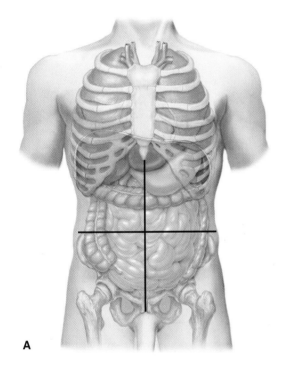

A

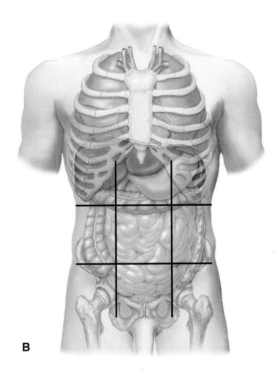

B

Check your answers by referring to Figures 4-5A and 4-5B on page 51. Review material that you did not answer correctly.

Spine

The spine (**vertebral column** or **backbone**) is composed of a series of bones that extend from the base of the skull to the pelvis. It is formed from 26 irregular bones (**vertebrae,** singular: **vertebra**) and connective tissue in such a way that a flexible, curved structure results. The spine is divided into sections corresponding to the vertebrae located in the spinal column. These divisions are as follows:

- Cervical (neck)
- Thoracic (chest)
- Lumbar (loin)
- Sacral (lower back)
- Coccyx (tailbone)

⊕ *It is time to review body cavities, the spine, and directional terms by completing Learning Activity 4-1.*

Medical Word Elements

This section introduces combining forms, suffixes, and prefixes related to body structure. Word analyses are also provided. From the information provided, complete the meaning of the medical words in the right-hand column. The first one is completed for you.

Element	Meaning	Word Analysis and Meaning
Combining Forms		
Cellular Structure		
cyt/o	cell	**cyt/o**/logist (sī-TŎL-ō-jĭst): *specialist in the study of cells* *-logist:* specialist in the study of *Cytologists study the formation, structure, and function of cells.*
hist/o	tissue	**hist/o**/logy (hĭs-TŎL-ō-jē): _____ *-logy:* study of *Histology is the branch of science that investigates the microscopic structures and functions of tissues.*
kary/o	nucleus	kary/o/lysis (kăr-ē-ŎL-ĭ-sĭs): _____ *-lysis:* separation; destruction; loosening *Karyolysis results in death of the cell.*
nucle/o		nucle/ar (NŪ-klē-ăr): _____ *-ar:* pertaining to
Position and Direction		
anter/o	anterior, front	**anter**/ior (ăn-TĒR-ē-or): _____ *-ior:* pertaining to
caud/o	tail	**caud**/ad (KAW-dăd): _____ *-ad:* toward

Medical Word Elements—cont'd

Element	Meaning	Word Analysis and Meaning
cephal/o	head	**cephal**/ad: _____ -*ad:* toward
dist/o	far, farthest	**dist**/al (DĬS-tăl): _____ -*al:* pertaining to
dors/o	back (of body)	**dors**/al (DOR-săl): _____ -*al:* pertaining to
infer/o	lower, below	**infer**/ior (ĭn-FĔR-rē-or): _____ -*ior:* pertaining to
later/o	side, to one side	**later**/al (LĂT-ĕr-ăl): _____ -*al:* pertaining to
medi/o	middle	**medi**/ad (MĒ-dē-ăd): _____ -*ad:* toward
poster/o	back (of body), behind, posterior	**poster**/ior (pōs-TĔR-ē-or): _____ -*ior:* pertaining to
proxim/o	near, nearest	**proxim**/al (PRŎK-sĭm-ăl): _____
ventr/o	belly, belly side	**ventr**/al (VĔN-trăl): _____ -*al:* pertaining to
Color		
albin/o	white	**albin**/ism (ĂL-bĭn-ĭzm): _____ -*ism:* condition *Albinism is characterized by a partial or total lack of pigment in the skin, hair, and eyes.*
leuk/o		**leuk**/o/cyte (LOO-kō-sīt): _____ -*cyte:* cell *A leukocyte is a white blood cell.*
chrom/o	color	hetero/**chrom**/ic (hĕt-ĕr-ō-KRŌ-mĭk): _____ *hetero-:* different -*ic:* pertaining to *Heterochromia is associated with the iris or sections of the iris of the eyes. Thus, the individual with heterochromia may have one brown iris and one blue iris.*

(continued)

Medical Word Elements—cont'd

Element	Meaning	Word Analysis and Meaning
cirrh/o	yellow	**cirrh**/osis (sĭr-RŌ-sĭs): _____ *-osis:* abnormal condition; increase (used primarily with blood cells) *In cirrhosis, the skin, sclera of the eyes, and mucous membranes take on a yellow color.*
jaund/o		**jaund**/ice (JAWN-dĭs): _____ *-ice:* noun ending *Jaundice is the yellowing of the skin, mucous membranes, and sclera caused by excessive bilirubin in the blood.*
xanth/o		**xanth**/oma (ZĂN-thō-sĭs): _____ *-oma:* tumor *A xanthoma is a nodule or patch composed of lipoid material commonly associated with disturbances in lipid metabolism.*
cyan/o	blue	**cyan/o**/tic (sī-ăn-ŎT-ĭk): _____ *-tic:* pertaining to *Cyanosis is associated with lack of oxygen in the blood and a bluish discoloration of the skin.*
erythr/o	red	**erythr/o**/cyte (ĕ-RĬTH-rō-sīt): _____ *-cyte:* cell *An erythrocyte is a red blood cell.*
melan/o	black	**melan**/oma (mĕl-ă-NŌ-mă): _____ *-oma:* tumor *Melanoma is a malignancy that arises from melanocytes.*
poli/o	gray; gray matter (of the brain or spinal cord)	**poli/o**/myel/itis (pō-lē-ō-mī-ĕ-LĪ-tĭs): _____ *myel:* bone marrow; spinal cord *-itis:* inflammation
Other		
radi/o	radiation, x-ray; radius (lower arm bone on thumb side)	**radi/o**/logist (rā-dē-ŎL-ŏ-jĭst): _____ *-logist:* specialist in the study of *Radiologists are physicians who employ imaging techniques to help medical doctors diagnose and treat diseases.*
tom/o	to cut	**tom/o**/graphy (tō-MŎG-ră-fē): _____ *-graphy:* process of recording *Tomography is an imaging procedure that employs a computer to produce images that appear as cuts (or slices) of an organ or structure.*
viscer/o	internal organs	**viscer**/al (VĬS-ĕr-ăl): _____ *-al:* pertaining to

Medical Word Elements—cont'd

Element	Meaning	Word Analysis and Meaning
Suffixes		
-ar	pertaining to	lumb/**ar** (LŬM-băr): _____ _lumb/o:_ loins (lower back)
-ic	pertaining to	gastr/**ic** (ĕp-ĭ-GĂS-trĭk): _____ _epi:_ above, upon _-ic:_ pertaining to
-graphy	process of recording	son/o/**graphy** (sō-NŎG-ră-fĕ): _____ _son/o:_ sound _**Sonography is a diagnostic imaging procedure using sound in the inaudible range (ultrasound) to visualize internal structures.**_
Prefixes		
infra-	below, under	**infra**/cost/al (ĭn-fră-KŎS-tăl): _____ _cost:_ ribs _-al:_ pertaining to
peri-	around	**peri**/umbilic/al (pĕr-ē-ŭm-BĬL-ĭ-kăl): _____ _umbilic:_ umbilicus, navel _-al:_ pertaining to
super-	upper, above	**super**/ior (soo-PĒ-rē-or): _____ _-ior:_ pertaining to _Superior is a directional term meaning toward the head or upper portion of a structure._
ultra-	excess, beyond	**ultra**/son/ic (ŭl-tră-SŎN-ĭk): _____ _son:_ sound _-ic:_ pertaining to _Ultrasound includes sound frequencies too high to be perceived by the human ear._

⊕ *It is time to review medical word elements by completing Learning Activities 4-2 and 4-3.*

Disease Focus

All body cells require oxygen and nutrients for survival. They also need a stable internal environment **(homeostasis)** that provides a narrow range of temperature, water, acidity, and salt concentration. When homeostasis is disrupted and cells, tissues, organs, or systems are unable to function effectively, the condition is called **disease.** From a clinical point of view, disease is a **pathological,** or **morbid,** condition that presents a group of signs, symptoms, and clinical findings. **Signs** are objective indicators that are observable. A rash, tissue redness, and swelling are examples of signs. In Figure 4-6, the rash is a sign of rubella (German measles), which is an acute infectious disease. A **symptom (Sx)** is a subjective indicator of disease. As such, only the patient can experience it. Dizziness, pain, and nausea are examples of symptoms. Clinical findings are the results of radiological, laboratory, and other medical procedures performed on the patient or the patient's specimens. (See Fig. 4-6.)

Establishing a **diagnosis (Dx),** the cause and nature of a disease, helps in the selection of a **treatment (Tx).** A **prognosis** is the prediction of the course of a disease and its probable outcome. An **idiopathic disease** is one whose cause is unknown or exists without any connection with a known cause. Some diseases, injuries, or treatments cause complications. For example, a head injury may cause paralysis, and treatment with a toxic drug may cause deafness.

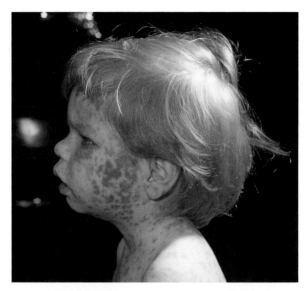

Figure 4-6 Skin rash (a sign of disease).

A variety of diagnostic and therapeutic procedures can help identify and treat diseases. These procedures are categorized as clinical, surgical, endoscopic, laboratory, and imaging procedures. Many diagnostic and therapeutic procedures include more than one testing modality. For example, many surgical procedures are undertaken using radiological methods to guide the surgeon during the procedure.

Each of the various types of imaging modalities produces a unique type of image. Physicians select the type of imaging procedure that provides the information that is relevant to a particular diagnosis or treatment. (See Fig. 4-7.)

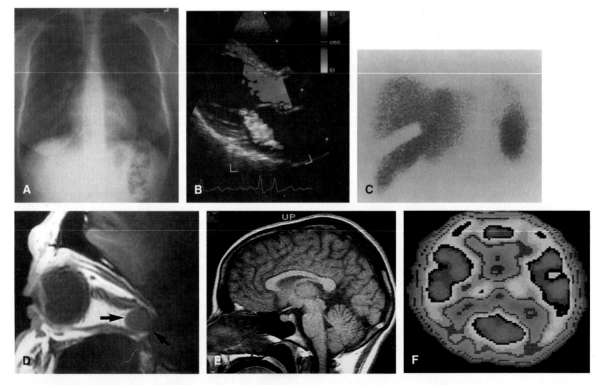

Figure 4-7 Medical imaging. (A) Chest radiograph of the mediastinum. (B) Ultrasonography of blood flow with colors indicating direction. (C) Nuclear scan of the liver and spleen. (D) Computed tomography (CT) scan of the eye in lateral view showing a tumor (arrows). (E) Magnetic resonance imaging (MRI) scan of the midsagittal section of the head. (F) Positron emission tomography (PET) scan of the brain in transverse section (frontal lobes at top).

Diseases and Conditions

This section introduces diseases and conditions, along with their meanings and their pronunciations. These terms are applicable to the body system chapters that follow. Word analyses for selected terms are also provided.

Term	Definition
adhesion ăd-HĒ-zhŭn	Abnormal fibrous band that holds or binds together tissues that are normally separated *Adhesions may occur within body cavities as a result of surgery. (See Fig. 4-8.)*

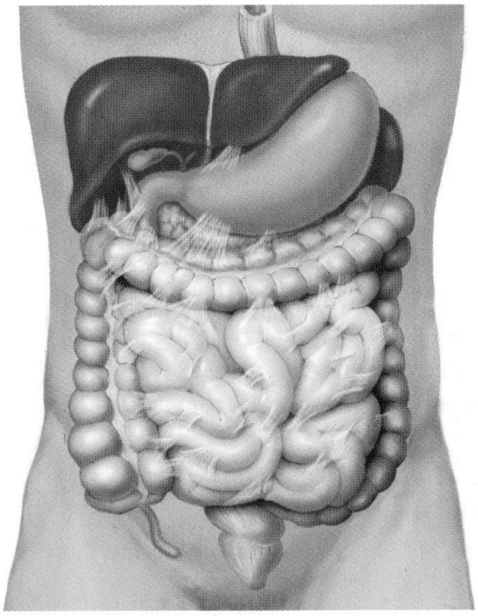

Figure 4-8 Abdominal adhesions.

edema ě-DĒ-mă	Abnormal accumulation of fluid within tissue spaces as a result of systemic disease or failure of the lymphatic system to drain tissue fluid from the site *After applying pressure to a small area, if the indentation persists after the release of pressure, the condition is known as pitting edema. (See Figure 4-9.)*

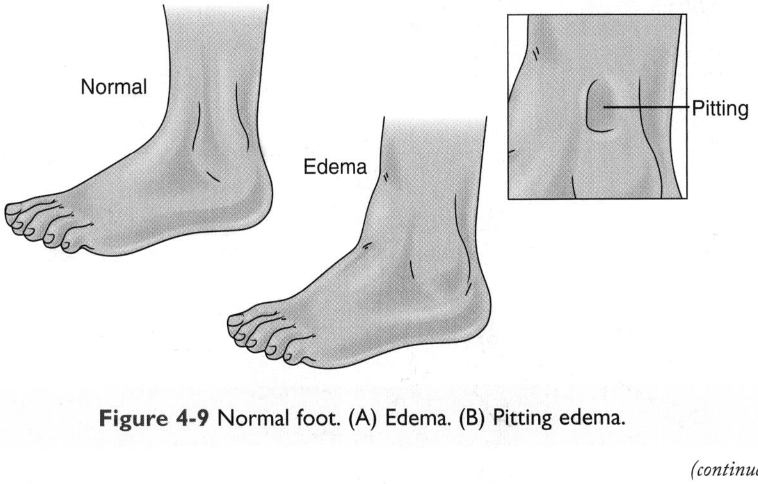

Figure 4-9 Normal foot. (A) Edema. (B) Pitting edema.

(continued)

Diseases and Conditions—cont'd

Term	Definition
febrile FĔ-brĭl	Having or showing symptoms of a fever
gangrene GĂNG-grēn	Death and decay of soft tissue, usually caused by circulatory obstruction or infection *Risk of developing gangrene of the extremities is associated with diabetes and atherosclerosis as a result of poor circulation.*
hernia HĔR-nē-ă	Protrusion of any organ through the structure that normally contains it
inflammation ĭn-flă-MĀ-shŭn	Body defense against injury, infection, or allergy marked by redness, swelling, heat, and pain, sometimes with loss of function *Inflammation is a mechanism used by the body to protect against invasion by foreign organisms and to repair injured tissue.*
mycosis mī-KŌ-sĭs *myc:* fungus (plural, *fungi*) *-osis:* abnormal condition; increase (used primarily with blood cells)	Any fungal infection in or on the body *Mycotic infections can be superficial, affecting the skin, or deep seated, affecting structures beneath the skin, especially the brain, bone marrow, or other internal organs.*
perforation pĕr-fō-RĀ-shŭn	Hole that completely penetrates a structure *A perforation in the gastrointestinal tract is a medical emergency because gastrointestinal contents may flow into the abdominal cavity and infect the peritoneum.*
peritonitis pĕr-ĭ-tō-NĪ-tĭs *periton:* peritoneum *-itis:* inflammation	Inflammation of the peritoneum, the serous membrane that surrounds the abdominal cavity and covers its organs, usually caused by bacteria or fungi *Peritonitis requires prompt medical attention to fight the infection and, if necessary, to treat any underlying medical conditions.*
rupture RŬP-chūr	Sudden breaking or bursting of a structure or organ
septicemia sĕp-tĭ-SĒ-mē-ă	Severe bacterial infection of the tissues that spreads to the blood; also called *sepsis* or *blood poisoning* *In septicemia, bacteria and their endotoxins cause severe systemic symptoms.*
suppuration sŭp-ū-RĀ-shŭn	Process of forming pus *Suppuration occurs when the agent that provoked the inflammation is difficult to eliminate.*

It is time to review diseases and conditions by completing Learning Activity 4-4.

Diagnostic and Surgical Procedures

This section introduces surgical and diagnostic procedures that are applicable in the body systems chapters. Descriptions are provided, along with pronunciations and word analyses for selected terms.

Procedure	Description
Diagnostic	

Clinical

assessment techniques	Sequence of procedures designed to evaluate the health status of a patient
auscultation aws-kŭl-TĀ-shŭn	Listening to the heart, bowel, and lungs with or without a stethoscope to assess the presence and quality of sounds
inspection	General observation of the patient as a whole, progressing to specific body areas
palpation păl-PĀ-shŭn	Gentle application of the hands to a specific structure or body area to determine size, consistency, texture, symmetry, and tenderness of underlying structures
percussion pĕr-KŬSH-ŭn	Tapping a body structure with the hand or fingers to assess consistency and the presence or absence of fluids within the underlying structure *Percussion is especially helpful in assessing the thorax and abdomen.*

Endoscopic

endoscopy ĕn-DŎS-kō-pē *endo-:* in, within *-scopy:* visual examination	Visual examination of a body cavity or canal using a specialized lighted instrument called an endoscope *Endoscopy is used for biopsy, surgery, aspiration of fluids, and coagulation of bleeding areas. The endoscope is usually named for the organ, cavity, or canal being examined, such as gastroscope and sigmoidoscope. (See Fig. 4–10.) A camera and video recorder are commonly used during the procedure to provide a permanent record.*

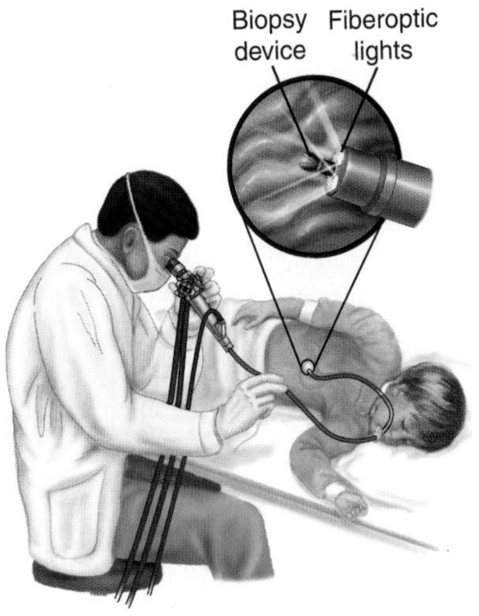

Biopsy device   Fiberoptic lights

Figure 4-10 Endoscopy (gastroscopy).

(continued)

Diagnostic and Surgical Procedures—cont'd

Procedure	Description
Laboratory	
blood chemistry analysis ă-NĂL-ĭ-sĭs	Laboratory test, usually performed on serum, to determine biochemical imbalances, abnormalities, and nutritional conditions *An example of a blood chemistry analysis is the cholesterol test. The results will identify the patient's cholesterol value and where it falls in the normal or abnormal range.*
complete blood count (CBC)	Broad screening test used to evaluate red blood cells, white blood cells, and platelets to determine anemias, infections, and other diseases *The CBC is usually included as part of routine physical examinations to determine general health status.*
Imaging	
computed tomography (CT) kŏm-PŪ-tĕd tō-MŎG-ră-fē *tom/o:* to cut *-graphy:* process of recording	Imaging technique that rotates an x-ray emitter around the area to be evaluated and measures the intensity of transmitted rays from different angles *In a CT scan, the computer generates a detailed cross-sectional image that appears as a slice. (See Fig. 4–7D.) It may detect tumor masses, bone displacement, and fluid accumulation. This technique may be used with or without a contrast medium. (See Fig. 4–11.)*

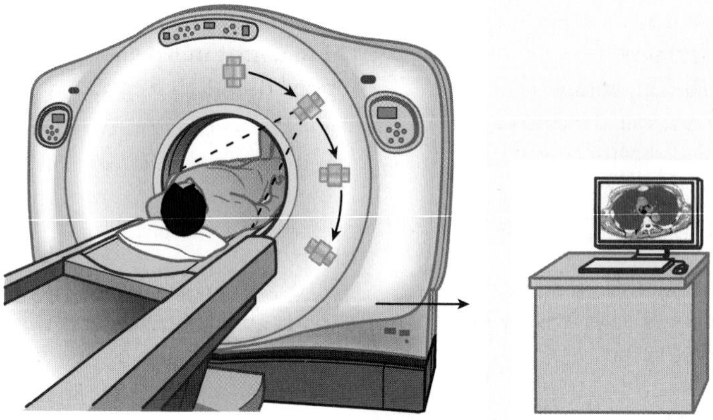

A   B

Figure 4-11 Computed tomography (CT) scan with motorized table (A) and computer (B).

fluoroscopy floo-or-ŎS-kō-pē *fluor/o:* luminous, fluorescent *-scopy:* visual examination	Technique in which x-rays are directed through the body to a fluorescent screen that displays internal structures in continuous motion *Fluoroscopy helps to view the motion of organs and follow the movement of contrast dye during a cardiac catheterization, an angiography, or an upper gastrointestinal series (barium swallow) and to aid in the placement of catheters or other devices.*

Diagnostic and Surgical Procedures—cont'd

Procedure	Description
magnetic resonance imaging (MRI) RĔZ-ĕn-ăns ĬM-ăj-ĭng	Technique that uses radio waves and a strong magnetic field, rather than an x-ray beam, to produce highly detailed, multiplanar, cross-sectional views of soft tissues (See Fig. 4-7E.) *MRI helps diagnose a growing number of diseases because it provides superior soft tissue contrast. It commonly proves superior to CT scan for most central nervous system images, musculoskeletal images, and images of the pelvic areas. The procedure usually does not require a contrast medium.*
nuclear scan NŪ-klē-ăr	Technique in which a radioactive material (radiopharmaceutical) called a tracer is introduced into the body (inhaled, ingested, or injected), and a specialized camera (gamma camera) produces images of organs and structures (See Fig. 4-7C.) *A nuclear scan is the reverse of a conventional radiograph. Rather than being directed into the body, radiation comes from inside the body and is then detected by a specialized camera to produce an image.*
positron emission tomography (PET) PŎZ-ĭ-trŏn ē-MĬSH-ŭn tō-MŎG-ră-fē	Computed tomography records the positrons (positively charged particles) emitted from a radiopharmaceutical to produce a cross-sectional image of the metabolic activity of body tissues to determine the presence of disease (See Fig. 4-7F.) *PET is particularly useful in scanning the brain and nervous system to diagnose disorders that involve abnormal tissue metabolism, such as schizophrenia, brain tumors, epilepsy, stroke, and Alzheimer disease, and pulmonary disorders.*
radiography rā-dē-ŎG-ră-fē *radi/o:* radiation, x-ray; radius (lower arm bone on thumb side) *-graphy:* process of recording	Technique in which x-rays are passed through the body or area and captured on a film to generate an image; also called x-ray (See Fig. 4-7A.) *Radiography of soft tissue usually requires the use of a contrast medium to enhance images. Commonly used x-ray contrast media are barium and iodine compounds.*
single-photon emission computed tomography (SPECT) FŌ-tŏn ē-MĬ-shŭn tō-MŎG-ră-fē *tom/o:* to cut *-graphy:* process of recording	Radiological technique that integrates computed tomography (CT) and a radioactive material (tracer) injected into the bloodstream to visualize blood flow to tissues and organs *SPECT differs from a PET scan in that the tracer remains in the bloodstream rather than being absorbed by surrounding tissue. It is especially useful to visualize blood flow through arteries and veins in the brain.*
ultrasonography (US) ŭl-tră-sōn-ŎG-ră-fē *ultra-:* excess, beyond *son/o:* sound *-graphy:* process of recording	High-frequency sound waves (ultrasound) are directed at soft tissue and reflected as "echoes" to produce an image on a monitor of an internal body structure; also called *ultrasound, sonography,* and *echo* (See Fig. 4-7B.) *US, unlike most other imaging methods, creates real-time moving images, allowing the visualization of organs and functions of organs in motion. A computer analyzes the reflected echoes and converts them into an image on a video monitor. Because this procedure does not utilize ionizing radiation (x-ray), it is used during pregnancy to observe fetal growth and also to study other internal organs for possible pathologies or lesions.*

(continued)

Diagnostic and Surgical Procedures—cont'd

Procedure	Description
Surgical	
biopsy (bx) BĪ-ŏp-sē	Removal of a representative tissue sample from a body site for microscopic examination, usually to establish a diagnosis
excisional ĕk-SĬ-zhŭn-ăl	Biopsy in which the entire lesion is removed
incisional ĭn-SĬZH-ŭn-ăl	Biopsy in which only a small sample of the lesion is removed
Surgical	
ablation ăb-LĀ-shŭn	Removal of a body part, pathway, or function by surgery, chemical destruction, electrocautery, freezing, or radio frequency (RF) *Ablation procedures are common for treating atrial fibrillation and varicose veins and destroying abnormal tissues found in various organs, including the lungs, liver, kidneys, and uterus.*
anastomosis ă-năs-tō-MŌ-sĭs	Surgical joining of two ducts, vessels, or bowel segments to allow flow from one to another (See Fig. 4-12.)

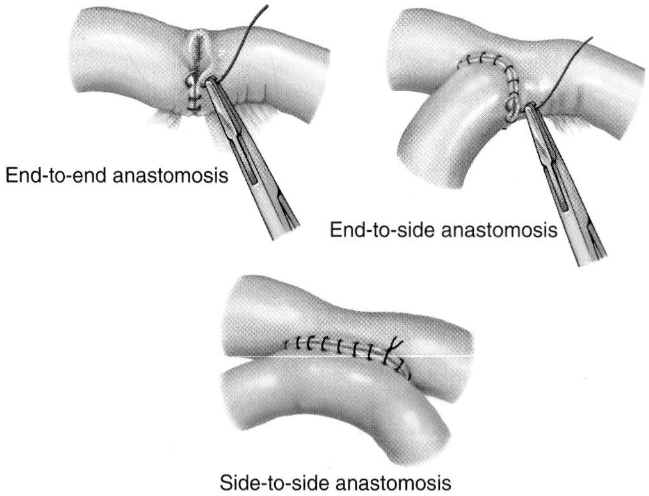

End-to-end anastomosis

End-to-side anastomosis

Side-to-side anastomosis

Figure 4-12 Anastomoses.

Procedure	Description
curettage kū-rĕ-TĂZH	Scraping of a body cavity with a spoon-shaped instrument called a *curette* (curet)
electrocauterization ē-lĕk-trō-KAW-tĕr-ĭ-ZĀ-shŭn *electr/o:* electricity *cauter:* heat, burn *-ization:* process (of)	Use of an electrically activated instrument to burn and destroy diseased tissue *Electrocauterization is common for removing tumors (particularly in the brain) and warts and treating chronic nosebleeds.*
incision and drainage (I&D) ĭn-SĬZH-ŭn, DRĀN-ĭj	Incision made to allow the free flow of fluids and pus from a wound, abscess, or body cavity

Diagnostic and Surgical Procedures—cont'd

Procedure	Description
laser surgery LĀ-zĕr SŬR-jĕr-ē	Use of a high-intensity laser light beam to remove diseased tissues, to stop bleeding, or for cosmetic purposes *Laser surgery is used in a wide variety of noninvasive and minimally invasive procedures, including removal of lesions, scars, tattoos, wrinkles, sunspots, or birthmarks.*
revision	Surgical procedure used to replace or compensate for a previously implanted device or correct an undesirable result or effect of a previous surgery

Abbreviations

This section introduces body structure abbreviations and their meanings.

Abbreviation	Meaning	Abbreviation	Meaning
AP	anteroposterior	MRI	magnetic resonance imaging
Bx, bx	biopsy	PET	positron emission tomography
CBC	complete blood count	RF	rheumatoid factor; radio frequency
CT	computed tomography	RLQ	right lower quadrant
DNA	deoxyribonucleic acid	RUQ	right upper quadrant
Dx	diagnosis	SPECT	single-photon emission computed tomography
I&D	incision and drainage	Sx	symptom
LAT, lat	lateral	Tx	treatment
LLQ	left lower quadrant	U&L, U/L	upper and lower
LUQ	left upper quadrant	US	ultrasound, ultrasonography

It is time to review procedures and abbreviations by completing Learning Activity 4-5.

LEARNING ACTIVITIES

The activities that follow provide review of the body structure terms introduced in this chapter. Complete each activity and review your answers to evaluate your understanding of the chapter.

Learning Activity 4-1

Body Structures and Directional Terms

Match each term on the left with its meaning on the right.

1. _____ abdominopelvic   a. pertaining to the sole of the foot
2. _____ adduction   b. tailbone
3. _____ cervical   c. ventral cavity that contains the heart, lungs, and associated structures
4. _____ coccyx   d. toward the surface of the body (external)
5. _____ deep   e. lying horizontal with face downward
6. _____ eversion   f. turning outward
7. _____ inferior (caudal)   g. nearer to the center (trunk of the body)
8. _____ inversion   h. ventral cavity that contains digestive, reproductive, and excretory structures
9. _____ lumbar   i. turning inward or inside out
10. _____ plantar   j. part of the spine known as the *neck*
11. _____ posterior (dorsal)   k. movement toward the median plane
12. _____ prone   l. away from the head; toward the tail or lower part of a structure
13. _____ proximal   m. away from the surface of the body (internal)
14. _____ superficial   n. part of the spine known as the *loin*
15. _____ thoracic   o. near the back of the body

✓ *Check your answers in Appendix A. Review any material that you did not answer correctly.*

Correct Answers _____ X 6.67 = _____ % Score

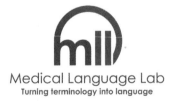

Medical Language Lab
Turning terminology into language

Visit the Medical Language Lab at the website *medicallanguagelab.com*. Use it to enhance your study and reinforcement of this chapter with the flash-card activity. We recommend that you complete the flash-card activity before starting Learning Activities 4-2 and 4-3.

Basic Word Elements

Select the word element that matches the definition in the numbered list.

Combining Forms		Suffixes	Prefixes
anter/o	later/o	-ia	peri-
caud/o	leuk/o	-ar	super-
cyt/o	melan/o		ultra-
cyan/o	medi/o		
dist/o	proxim/o		
dors/o	ventr/o		
erythr/o	xanth/o		
hist/o			

1. black _____
2. far, farthest _____
3. cell _____
4. anterior, front _____
5. white _____
6. blue _____
7. yellow _____
8. back (of body) _____
9. pertaining to _____
10. around _____
11. side, to one side _____
12. tail _____
13. condition _____
14. excess, beyond _____
15. belly, belly side _____
16. upper, above _____
17. tissue _____
18. near, nearest _____
19. middle _____
20. red _____

Check your answers in Appendix A. Review any material that you did not answer correctly.

Correct Answers _____ X 5 = _____ % Score

Learning Activity 4-3

Building Basic Terms

Read the definition in the numbered list. Then select two elements from the table to build a medical word. You may use the elements more than once. The first one is completed for you.

Combining Forms	Suffixes	Prefixes
anter/o	-ad	epi-
cephal/o	-al	hypo-
cirrh/o	-cyte	
dors/o	-ic	
erythr/o	-ior	
gastr/o	-logist	
melan/o	-oma	
radi/o	-osis	
ventr/o		

  1. pertaining to the front (of the body) <u>anterior</u> _____

  2. toward the head _____

  3. pertaining to the back (of the body) _____

  4. pertaining to the belly side (front of the body) _____

  5. abnormal condition of yellow (ing) _____

  6. cell that is red _____

  7. tumor that is black _____

  8. specialist in the study of radiation or x-rays _____

  9. pertaining to above the (area of the) stomach _____

10. pertaining to under or below the (area of the) stomach _____

✓ *Check your answers in Appendix A. Review any material that you did not answer correctly.*

Correct Answers _____ X 10 = _____ % Score

Learning Activity 4-4
Building Medical Words

Use *cyt/o* to build words that mean

1. specialist in the study of cells _____
2. study of cells _____

Use *-cyte* (cells) to build words that mean

3. red cell _____
4. white cell _____
5. black cell _____

Use *-al* (pertaining to) to build words that mean *pertaining to the*

6. belly or belly side _____
7. nearest (point of attachment) _____
8. middle _____
9. farthest (point of attachment) _____
10. side, to one side _____

Check your answers in Appendix A. Review any material that you did not answer correctly.

Correct Answers _____ X 10 = _____ % Score

Learning Activity 4-5
Diseases and Conditions

Match the terms with the definitions in the numbered list.

adhesion	hernia	prognosis
diagnosis	inflammation	rupture
edema	mycosis	septicemia
febrile	perforation	suppuration
gangrene	peritonitis	symptom

1. characterized by an elevated body temperature _____
2. establishing the cause and nature of a disease _____
3. fibrous band that binds together tissues that are normally separated _____
4. death and decay of soft tissue _____
5. protrusion of any organ through the structure that normally contains it _____
6. inflammation of the serous membrane that surrounds the abdominal cavity _____
7. severe bacterial infection of the tissues that spreads to the blood _____
8. producing or forming pus _____
9. prediction of the course of a disease and its probable outcome _____
10. body defense against injury, infection, or allergy, marked by redness, heat, pain, and swelling _____
11. sudden breaking or bursting of a structure or organ _____
12. subjective indicator of a disease _____
13. abnormal accumulation of fluid in tissue spaces _____
14. fungal infection in or on the body _____
15. hole that forms through a structure or a body part _____

✓ *Check your answers in Appendix A. Review any material that you did not answer correctly.*

Correct Answers _____ X 6.67 = _____ % Score

Learning Activity 4-6
Procedures and Abbreviations

Match the terms with the definitions in the numbered list.

ablation	*Dx*	*MRI*
anastomosis	*endoscopy*	*nuclear scan*
electrocautery	*curettage*	*palpation*
CBC	*fluoroscopy*	*percussion*
computed tomography	*I&D*	*revision*

1. assessment technique that involves the gentle tapping of a structure _____

2. scraping of a body cavity with a spoon-shaped instrument _____

3. panel of blood tests used as a broad screening test for anemias, infections, and other diseases _____

4. removal of a part, pathway, or function by surgery, chemical destruction, or other techniques _____

5. visual examination of a cavity or canal using a special lighted instrument _____

6. imaging technique that directs x-rays to a fluorescent screen and displays "live" images on a monitor _____

7. establishing the nature and cause of a disease _____

8. use of an electrically activated instrument to burn and destroy diseased tissue _____

9. surgery to compensate for or correct a previously performed surgery _____

10. imaging procedure that uses radio waves and a strong magnetic field to produce images _____

11. surgical joining of two ducts, vessels, or bowel segments _____

12. imaging procedure that uses a radioactive material introduced into the body to produce an image _____

13. gentle application of hands to evaluate a specific structure of the body _____

14. incision that allows a free flow of fluids or pus from a wound _____

15. imaging procedure that generates detailed cross-sectional images that appear as a slice _____

✓ *Check your answers in Appendix A. Review any material that you did not answer correctly.*

Correct Answers _____ X 6.67 = _____ % Score

DOCUMENTING HEALTH-CARE

The electronic medical record (EMR) is a systematic collection in digital format of a patient's health history. In other words, it is an electronic version of a paper medical chart. The EMR contains a history of the patient's medical care, including diagnoses, treatments, and other vital health information. The digital version allows practitioners to electronically monitor and track the health status, preventive health services, treatments, and care planning of patients and serves as a more efficient method of documenting patient care. The electronic connection provides a platform to share medical documents between providers who are caring for the same patient so that there is continuity of treatment without duplication of effort.

Besides ease of access, this method of documentation decreases errors associated with poor penmanship, lost pages, and misfiled records. It also provides documentation of health-care information that will be needed if legal issues arise. In addition, it is the basis for reimbursement of medical services. Thus, it is important that all information entered into the medical record be complete, current, correct, and maintained in confidentiality.

Currently, increasing numbers of physician offices, clinics, hospitals, and other medical settings are providing patients with access to their individual EMRs. In this way, the EMR is available instantly and securely for patients and other authorized users. The Documenting Health-Care Activities in this chapter and throughout the book are designed to familiarize you to the appearance and terminology of various medical records and to develop the critical thinking skills necessary to interpret these records in a medical setting.

DOCUMENTING HEALTH-CARE ACTIVITIES

This section provides practical application activities in the form of exercises to help students develop skills in documenting patient care. First, read the medical report. Then complete the activities and exercises that follow.

Documenting Health-Care Activity 4-1

Radiology Consultation Letter: Cervical and Lumbar Spine

Physician Center

2422 Rodeo Drive ■ ■ **Sun City, USA 12345** ■ ■ **(555) 333–2427**

May 3, 20xx

John Roberts, MD
1115 Forest Ave
Sun City, USA 12345

Dear Doctor Roberts:

Thank you for referring Chester Bowen to our office. Mr. Bowen presents with neck and lower back pain of more than 2 years' duration. Radiographic examination of June 14, 20xx, reveals the following: AP, lateral, and odontoid views of the cervical spine demonstrate some reversal of normal cervical curvature, as seen on lateral projection. There is some right lateral scoliosis of the cervical spine. The vertebral bodies, however, appear to be well maintained in height; the intervertebral spaces are well maintained. The odontoid is visualized and appears to be intact. The atlantoaxial joint appears symmetrical.

Impression: Films of the cervical spine demonstrate some reversal of normal cervical curvature and a minimal scoliosis, possibly secondary to muscle spasm, without evidence of recent bony disease or injury. AP and lateral films of the lumbar spine, with spots of the lumbosacral junction, demonstrate an apparent minimal spina bifida occulta of the first sacral segment. The vertebral bodies, however, are well maintained in height; the intervertebral spaces appear well maintained.

Pathological Diagnosis: Right lateral scoliosis with some reversal of normal cervical curvature

If you have any further questions, please feel free to contact me.

Sincerely yours,

Adrian Jones, MD
Adrian Jones, MD

aj:bg

Terminology

The terms listed in the table that follows are taken from *Radiology Consultation Letter: Cervical and Lumbar Spine*. Use a medical dictionary such as *Taber's Cyclopedic Medical Dictionary*, the appendices of this book, or other resources to define each term. Then review the pronunciations for each term and practice by reading the medical record aloud.

Term	Definition
atlantoaxial ăt-lăn-tō-ĂK-sē-ăl	
cervical SĔR-vĭ-kăl	
lumbosacral junction lŭm-bō-SĀ-krăl	
odontoid ō-DŎN-toyd	
sacral SĀ-krăl	
scoliosis skō-lē-Ō-sĭs	
spina bifida occulta SPĪ-nă BĬF-ĭ-dă ŏ-KŬL-tă	
vertebral bodies VĔR-tĕ-brăl	

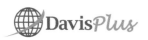 Visit the *Medical Terminology Systems* online resource center at Davis*Plus* to practice pronunciation and reinforce the meanings of the terms in this medical report.

Critical Thinking

Review *Radiology Consultation Letter: Cervical and Lumbar Spine* to answer the questions.

1. What was the presenting problem?

_____

_____

_____

_____

2. What were the three views of the radiological examination of June 14, 20xx?

_____

_____

_____

_____

3. Was there evidence of recent bony disease or injury?

_____

_____

_____

_____

4. Which cervical vertebrae form the atlantoaxial joint?

_____

_____

_____

_____

5. Was the odontoid fractured?

_____

_____

_____

_____

6. What did the AP and lateral films of the lumbar spine demonstrate?

_____

_____

_____

_____

Radiology Report: Injury of Left Wrist, Elbow, and Humerus

General Hospital

1511 Ninth Avenue ■ ■ Sun City, USA 12345 ■ ■ (555) 802–1887

RADIOLOGY REPORT

Date:	June 5, 20xx	Patient:	Hill, Joan
Physician:	Adrian Jones, MD	DOB:	5/25/19xx
Examination:	Left wrist, left elbow, and left humerus	x-ray No.:	43201

Left Wrist: Images obtained with the patient's arm taped to an arm board. There are fractures through the distal shafts of the radius and ulna. The radial fracture fragments show approximately 8-mm overlap with dorsal displacement of the distal radial fracture fragment. The distal ulnar shaft fracture shows ventral-lateral angulation at the fracture apex. There is no overriding at this fracture. No additional fracture is seen. Soft tissue deformity is present, correlating with the fracture sites.

Left Elbow and Left Humerus: Single view of the left elbow was obtained in the lateral projection. AP view of the humerus was obtained to include a portion of the elbow. A third radiograph was obtained but is not currently available for review. There is lucency through the distal humerus on the AP view along its medial aspect. It would be difficult to exclude fracture just above the medial epicondyle. On the lateral view, there is elevation of the anterior and posterior fat pad. These findings are of some concern. Repeat elbow study is recommended.

Jason Skinner, MD
Jason Skinner, MD

JS: bg

D: 6–05–20xx
T: 6–05–20xx

Terminology

The terms listed in the table that follows are taken from *Radiology Report: Injury of Left Wrist, Elbow, and Humerus*. Use a medical dictionary such as *Taber's Cyclopedic Medical Dictionary*, the appendices of this book, or other resources to define each term. Then review the pronunciations for each term and practice by reading the medical record aloud.

Term	Definition
AP	
anterior ăn-TĬR-ē-or	
distal DĬS-tăl	
dorsal DOR-săl	
epicondyle ĕp-ĭ-KŎN-dĭl	
humerus HŪ-mĕr-ŭs	
lucency LOO-sĕnt-sē	
medial MĔ-dē-ăl	
mm	
posterior	
radius RĀ-dē-ŭs	
ulna ŬL-nă	
ventral-lateral VĔN-trăl-LĂT-ĕr-ăl	

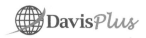 **DavisPlus**   Visit the *Medical Terminology Systems* online resource center at Davis*Plus* to practice pronunciation and reinforce the meanings of the terms in this medical report.

Critical Thinking

Review *Radiology Report: Injury of Left Wrist, Elbow, and Humerus* to answer the questions.

1. Where are the fractures located?

_____

_____

_____

_____

2. What caused the soft tissue deformity?

_____

_____

_____

_____

3. Did the radiologist take any side views of the left elbow?

_____

_____

_____

_____

4. In the AP view of the humerus, what structure was also visualized?

_____

_____

_____

_____

5. What findings are causes of concern for the radiologist?

_____

_____

_____

_____

Integumentary System

Chapter Outline

Objectives

Upon completion of this chapter, you will be able to:

• Locate the major organs of the integumentary system and describe their structure and function.

• Describe the functional relationship between the integumentary system and other body systems.

• Pronounce, spell, and build words related to the integumentary system.

• Describe diseases, conditions, and procedures related to the integumentary system.

• Explain pharmacology associated with the treatment of skin disorders.

• Demonstrate your knowledge of this chapter by completing the learning and documenting health-care activities.

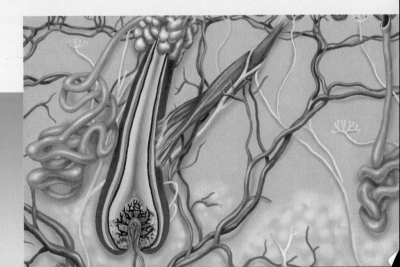

Anatomy and Physiology

The skin, also called the **integument,** is the largest organ in the body. Together with its accessory organs (hair, nails, and glands), the skin makes up the **integumentary system.** This elaborate system of distinct tissues includes glands that produce several types of secretions, nerves that transmit impulses, and blood vessels that help regulate body temperature. The skin covers and protects all outer surfaces of the body and performs many vital functions, including the sense of touch.

Anatomy and Physiology Key Terms

This section introduces important terms, along with their definitions and pronunciations. The key terms are highlighted in color in the Anatomy and Physiology section. Word analyses for selected terms are also provided. Pronounce the term, and place a check mark in the box after you do so.

Term	Definition
androgen ĂN-drō-jĕn ☐	Generic term for an agent (usually a hormone, such as testosterone or androsterone) that stimulates development of male characteristics *Androgens also regulate the production of sebum.*
ductule DŬK-tūl ☐ *duct:* to lead; carry *-ule:* small, minute	Very small duct
homeostasis hō-mē-ō-STĀ-sĭs ☐ *homeo-:* same, alike *-stasis:* standing still	State of equilibrium of the internal environment of the body despite changes in the external environment *Homeostasis encompasses the regulatory mechanisms of the body that control temperature, acidity, and the concentration of salt, food, and waste products.*
synthesize SĬN-thĕ-sīz ☐	Forming a complex substance by the union of simpler compounds or elements *Skin synthesizes vitamin D (needed by bones for calcium absorption).*

Pronunciation Help	Long Sound	ā — rate	ē — rebirth	ī — isle	ō — over	ū — unite
	Short Sound	ă — apple	ĕ — ever	ĭ — it	ŏ — not	ŭ — cut

Skin

The skin protects underlying structures from injury and provides sensory information to the brain. Beneath the skin's surface is an intricate network of nerve fibers that register sensations of temperature, pain, and pressure. Other important functions of the skin include protecting the body against ultraviolet rays, regulating body temperature, and preventing dehydration. The skin also acts as a reservoir for food and water. It also synthesizes vitamin D when exposed to sunlight. The skin consists of two distinct layers: the epidermis and the dermis. A subcutaneous layer of tissue binds the skin to underlying structures. (See Fig. 5-1.)

Epidermis

The outer layer of the skin, the (1) **epidermis,** is relatively thin over most areas but is thickest on the palms of the hands and the soles of the feet. Although the epidermis is composed of several sublayers called **strata,** the (2) **stratum corneum** and the (3) **basal layer,** which is the deepest layer, are of greatest importance.

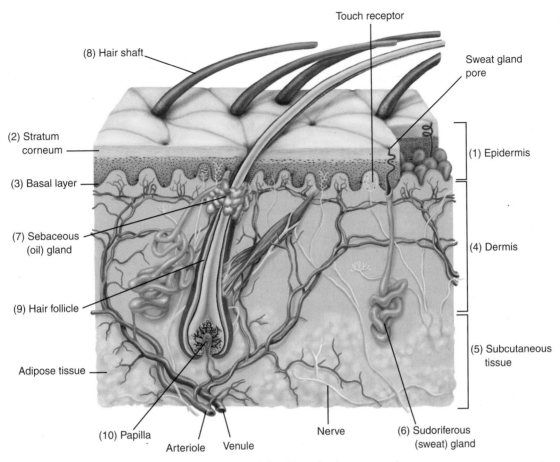

Figure 5-1 Structure of the skin and subcutaneous tissue.

The stratum corneum is composed of dead, flat cells that lack a blood supply and sensory receptors. Its thickness is related to normal wear of the area it covers. The basal layer is the only layer of the epidermis that is composed of living cells where new cells are formed. As these cells move toward the stratum corneum to replace the cells that have been sloughed off, they die and become filled with a hard protein material called **keratin.** The relatively waterproof characteristic of keratin prevents body fluids from evaporating and moisture from entering the body. The entire process by which a cell forms in the basal layer, rises to the surface, becomes keratinized, and sloughs off takes about 1 month.

In the basal layer, special cells called **melanocytes** produce a black pigment called **melanin.** Melanin provides a protective barrier from the damaging effects of the sun's ultraviolet radiation, which can cause skin cancer. Moderate sun exposure increases the rate of melanin production and results in a suntan. However, overexposure results in sunburn caused by melanin's inability to absorb sufficient ultraviolet rays to prevent the burn.

Differences in skin color are attributed to the amount of melanin in each cell. Dark-skinned people produce large amounts of melanin and are less likely to have wrinkles or skin cancer. Production of melanocytes is genetically regulated and, thus, inherited. Local accumulations of melanin are seen in pigmented moles and freckles. An absence of pigment in the skin, eyes, and hair is most likely the result of an inherited inability to produce melanin. An individual who cannot produce melanin, known as an **albino,** has a marked deficiency of pigment in the eyes, hair, and skin.

Dermis

The second layer of the skin, the (4) **dermis,** also called the **corium,** lies directly beneath the epidermis. It is composed of living tissue and contains numerous capillaries, lymphatic vessels, and nerve endings. Hair follicles, **sebaceous** (oil) glands, and **sudoriferous** (sweat) glands are also located in the dermis.

The (5) **subcutaneous layer,** also called the **hypodermis,** binds the dermis to underlying structures. It is composed primarily of loose connective tissue and **adipose** (fat) tissue interlaced with blood vessels. The subcutaneous layer stores fats, insulates and cushions the body, and regulates temperature. The amount of fat in the subcutaneous layer varies with the region of the body and sex, age, and nutritional state.

Accessory Organs of the Skin

The accessory organs of the skin consist of integumentary glands, hair, and nails. The glands play an important role in defending the body against disease and maintaining **homeostasis,** whereas the hair and nails have more limited functional roles.

Glands

Two important glands located in the dermis produce secretions: The (6) **sudoriferous (sweat) glands** produce sweat and the (7) **sebaceous (oil) glands** produce oil. These two glands are **exocrine glands** because they secrete substances through ducts to an outer surface of the body rather than directly into the bloodstream.

The sudoriferous glands secrete perspiration, or sweat, onto the surface of the skin through pores. Pores are most plentiful on the palms, soles, forehead, and **axillae** (armpits). The main functions of the sudoriferous glands are to cool the body by evaporation, excrete waste products, and moisten surface cells.

The sebaceous glands are filled with cells, the centers of which contain fatty droplets. As these cells disintegrate, they yield an oily secretion called **sebum.** The acidic nature of sebum helps destroy harmful organisms on the skin, thus preventing infection. When **ductules** of the sebaceous glands become blocked, acne may result. Congested sebum causes formation of pimples or whiteheads. If the sebum is dark, it forms blackheads. Sex hormones, particularly **androgens,** regulate the production and secretion of sebum. During adolescence, secretions increase; as the person ages, secretions diminish. The loss of sebum, which lubricates the skin, may be one of the reasons for the formation of wrinkles that accompanies old age. Sebaceous glands are present over the entire body except on the soles of the feet and the palms of the hands. They are especially prevalent on the scalp and face; around such openings as the nose, mouth, external ear, and anus; and on the upper back.

Hair

Hair is found on nearly all parts of the body except for the lips, nipples, palms of the hands, soles of the feet, and parts of the external genitalia. The visible part of the hair is the (8) **hair shaft;** the part that is embedded in the dermis is the hair root. The root, together with its coverings, forms the (9) **hair follicle.** At the bottom of the follicle is a loop of capillaries enclosed in a covering called the (10) **papilla.** The cluster of epithelial cells lying over the papilla reproduces and is responsible for the eventual formation of the hair shaft. As long as these cells remain alive, hair will regenerate even if it is cut, plucked, or otherwise removed. Alopecia (baldness) occurs when the hairs of the scalp are not replaced because of death of the papillae (singular, papilla).

Like skin color, hair color is related to the amount of pigment produced by epidermal melanocytes. Melanocytes are found at the base of the hair follicle. Melanin ranges in color from yellow to reddish brown to black. Varying amounts of melanin produce hair ranging in color from blond to brunette to black; the more abundant the melanin, the darker the hair. Heredity and aging affect melanin levels. A decrease or an absence of melanin causes loss of hair color.

Nails

Nails protect the tips of the fingers and toes from bruises and injuries. (See Fig. 5-2.) Each nail is formed in the (1) **nail root** and is composed of keratinized, stratified, squamous epithelial cells producing a very tough covering. As the nail grows, it stays attached and slides forward over the layer of epithelium called the (2) **nailbed.** This epithelial layer is continuous with the epithelium

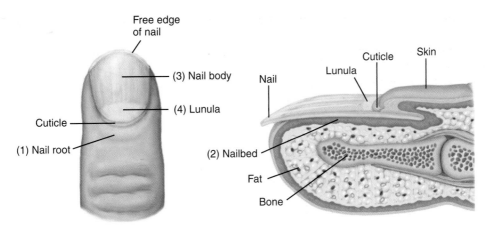

Figure 5-2 Structure of a fingernail.

of the skin. Most of the (3) **nail body** appears pink because of the underlying vascular tissue. The half-moon–shaped area at the base of the nail, the (4) **lunula,** is the region where new growth occurs. The lunula has a whitish appearance because the vascular tissue underneath does not show through.

Anatomy Review: Integumentary System

To review the anatomy of the integumentary system, label the illustration using the listed terms.

dermis

epidermis

hair follicle

hair shaft

papilla

sebaceous (oil) gland

stratum corneum

stratum germinativum

subcutaneous tissue

sudoriferous (sweat) gland

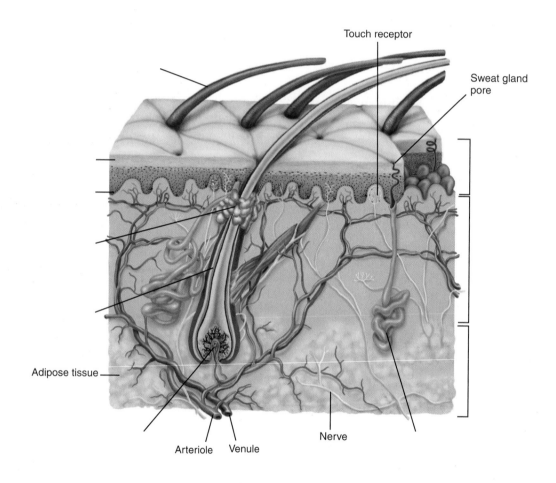

 Check your answers by referring to Figure 5-1 on page 83. Review material that you did not answer correctly.

CONNECTING BODY SYSTEMS—INTEGUMENTARY SYSTEM

The main function of the skin is to protect the entire body, including all of its organs, from the external environment. Specific functional relationships between the skin and other body systems are summarized here.

Blood, Lymphatic, and Immune
- Skin is the first line of defense against the invasion of pathogens into the body.

Cardiovascular
- Cutaneous blood vessels dilate and constrict to help regulate body temperature.

Digestive
- Skin absorbs vitamin D (produced when skin is exposed to sunlight), which is needed for intestinal absorption of calcium.
- Excess calories are stored as subcutaneous fat.

Endocrine
- The subcutaneous layer of the skin stores adipose tissue when insulin secretions cause excess carbohydrate intake to be stored as fat.

Female Reproductive
- Subcutaneous receptors provide pleasurable sensations associated with sexual behavior.
- Skin stretches to accommodate the growing fetus during pregnancy.

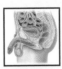
Male Reproductive
- Receptors in the skin respond to sexual stimuli.

Musculoskeletal
- Skin synthesizes the vitamin D needed for absorption of calcium, which is essential for muscle contraction.
- Skin also synthesizes the vitamin D needed for growth, repair, and maintenance of bones.

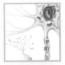
Nervous
- Cutaneous receptors detect stimuli related to touch, pain, pressure, and temperature.

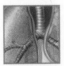
Respiratory
- Skin temperature may influence respiratory rate. As temperature increases, respiratory rate may also increase.
- Hairs of the nasal cavity filter particles from inspired air before it reaches the lower respiratory tract.

Urinary
- Skin provides an alternative route for excreting salts and nitrogenous wastes in the form of perspiration.

Medical Word Elements

This section introduces combining forms, suffixes, and prefixes related to the integumentary system. Word analyses are also provided. From the information provided, complete the meaning of each medical word in the right-hand column. The first one is completed for you.

Element	Meaning	Word Analysis
Combining Forms		
adip/o	fat	**adip**/osis (ăd-ĭ-PŌ-sĭs): *abnormal condition of fat* *-osis:* abnormal condition; increase (used primarily with blood cells) *Adiposis is an abnormal accumulation of fatty tissue in the body.*
lip/o		**lip**/oma (lĭ-PŌ-mă): _____ *-oma:* tumor
steat/o		**steat**/itis (stē-ă-TĪ-tĭs): _____ *-itis:* inflammation
cutane/o	skin	sub/**cutane**/ous (sŭb-kū-TĀ-nē-ŭs): _____ *sub-:* under, below *-ous:* pertaining to
dermat/o		**dermat/o**/plasty (DĔR-mă-tō-plăs-tē): _____ *-plasty:* surgical repair
derm/o		hypo/**derm**/ic (hī-pō-DĔR-mĭk): _____ *hypo-:* under, below, deficient *-ic:* pertaining to *Hypodermic needles are used for subcutaneous injections.*
hidr/o	sweat	**hidr**/aden/itis (hī-drăd-ĕ-NĪ-tĭs): _____ *aden:* gland *-itis:* inflammation *Do not confuse* hidr/o *(sweat) with* hydr/o *(water).*
sudor/o		**sudor**/esis (soo-dō-RĒ-sĭs): _____ *-esis:* condition *Sudoresis is the body's physiological means to regulate body temperature.*
ichthy/o	dry, scaly	**ichthy**/osis (ĭk-thē-Ō-sĭs): _____ *-osis:* abnormal condition; increase (used primarily with blood cells) *Ichthyosis can be any of several dermatological conditions in which the skin is dry and hardened (hyperkeratotic), resembling fish scales. A mild form of ichthyosis, called* winter itch, *is commonly seen on the legs of older patients, especially during the winter months.*
kerat/o	horny tissue; hard; cornea	**kerat**/osis (kĕr-ă-TŌ-sĭs): _____ *-osis:* abnormal condition; increase (used primarily with blood cells) *Keratosis is a thickened area of the epidermis or any horny growth on the skin, such as a callus or wart.*

Medical Word Elements—cont'd

Element	Meaning	Word Analysis
melan/o	black	**melan/oma** (mĕl-ă-NŌ-mă): _____ *-oma:* tumor *Melanoma is a malignant tumor of melanocytes that commonly begins in a darkly pigmented mole and can metastasize widely.*
myc/o	fungus (plural, fungi)	dermat/o/**myc/osis** (dĕr-mă-tō-mī-KŌ-sĭs): _____ *dermat/o:* skin *-osis:* abnormal condition; increase (used primarily with blood cells)
onych/o	nail	**onych/o/malacia** (ŏn-ĭ-kō-mă-LĀ-shē-ă): _____ *-malacia:* softening
ungu/o		**ungu/al** (ŬNG-gwăl): _____ *-al:* pertaining to
pil/o	hair	**pil/o/nid/al** (pī-lō-NĪ-dăl): _____ *nid:* nest *-al:* pertaining to *A pilonidal cyst commonly develops in the skin at the base of the spine. It develops as a growth of hair in a dermoid cyst.*
trich/o		**trich/o/pathy** (trĭk-ŎP-ă-thē): _____ *-pathy:* disease
scler/o	hardening; sclera (white of eye)	**scler/o/derma** (sklĕ-rō-DĔR-mă): _____ *-derma:* skin *Scleroderma is an autoimmune disorder that causes the skin and internal organs to become progressively hardened as a result of deposits of collagen. It may occur as a localized form or as a systemic disease.*
seb/o	sebum, sebaceous	**seb/o/rrhea** (sĕb-ō-RĒ-ă): _____ *-rrhea:* discharge, flow *Seborrhea is an overactivity of the sebaceous glands.*
squam/o	scale	**squam/ous** (SKWĀ-mŭs): _____ *-ous:* pertaining to
xen/o	foreign, strange	**xen/o/graft** (ZĔN-ō-grăft): _____ *-graft:* transplantation *Xenografts are used as a temporary graft to protect the patient against infection and fluid loss.*
xer/o	dry	**xer/o/derma** (zē-rō-DĔR-mă): _____ *-derma:* skin *Xeroderma is a chronic skin condition characterized by dryness and roughness and is a mild form of ichthyosis.*

(continued)

Medical Word Elements—cont'd

Element	Meaning	Word Analysis and Meaning
Suffixes		
-cyte	cell	lip/o/**cyte** (LĬP-ō-sīt): _____ *lip/o:* fat
-derma	skin	py/o/**derma** (pī-ō-DĔR-mă): _____ *py/o:* pus *Pyoderma is an acute, inflammatory, purulent bacterial dermatitis. It may be primary, such as impetigo, or secondary to a previous skin condition.*
-logist	specialist in the study of	dermat/o/**logist** (dĕr-mă-TŎL-ō-jĭst): _____ *dermat/o:* skin
-logy	study of	dermat/o/**logy** (dĕr-mă-TŎL-ō-jē): _____ *dermat/o:* skin
-therapy	treatment	cry/o/**therapy** (krī-ō-THĔR-ă-pē): _____ *cry/o:* cold *Cryotherapy is used to destroy tissue by freezing with liquid nitrogen. Cutaneous warts and actinic keratosis are common skin disorders that respond well to cryotherapy treatment.*
Prefixes		
an-	without, not	**an/**hidr/osis (ăn-hī-DRŌ-sĭs): _____ *hidr:* sweat *-osis:* abnormal condition; increase (used primarily with blood cells)
epi-	above, upon	**epi/**derm/is (ĕp-ĭ-DĔR-mĭs): _____ *derm:* skin *-is:* noun ending *The epidermis is the outermost layer of the skin.*
homo-	same	**homo/**graft (HŌ-mō-grăft): _____ *-graft:* transplantation

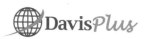

Visit the *Medical Terminology Systems* online resource center at Davis*Plus* for an audio exercise of the terms in this table. Other activities are also available to reinforce content.

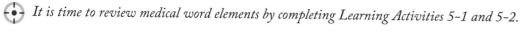

It is time to review medical word elements by completing Learning Activities 5-1 and 5-2.

Disease Focus

The general appearance and condition of the skin are clinically important because they may provide clues to body conditions or dysfunctions. Pale skin may indicate shock; red, flushed, very warm skin may indicate fever and infection. A rash may indicate allergies or local infections. Even chewed fingernails may be a clue to emotional problems. For diagnosis, treatment, and management of skin disorders, the medical services of a specialist may be warranted. **Dermatology** is the medical specialty concerned with diseases that directly affect the skin and systemic diseases that manifest their effects on the skin. The physician who specializes in diagnosis and treatment of skin diseases is known as a **dermatologist.**

Skin Lesions

Lesions are areas of tissue that have been pathologically altered by injury, wound, or infection. Lesions may affect tissue over an area of a definite size **(localized)** or may be widely spread throughout the body **(systemic).** Evaluation of skin lesions, injuries, or changes to tissue helps establish the diagnosis of skin disorders.

Lesions are described as primary or secondary. **Primary skin lesions** are the initial reaction to **pathologically** altered tissue and may be flat or elevated. **Secondary skin lesions** are changes that take place in the primary lesion as a result of infection, scratching, trauma, or various stages of a disease. Lesions are also described by their appearance, color, location, and size as measured in centimeters. Some of the major primary and secondary skin lesions are described and illustrated in Figure 5-3 on page 92.

It is time to review skin lesions by completing Learning Activity 5-3.

PRIMARY LESIONS

FLAT LESIONS
Flat, discolored, circumscribed lesions of any size

Macule
Flat, pigmented, circumscribed area less than 1 cm in diameter.
Examples: freckle, flat mole, or rash that occurs in rubella.

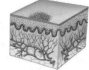

ELEVATED LESIONS

Solid   *Fluid-filled*

Papule
Solid, elevated lesion less than 1 cm in diameter that may be the same color as the skin or pigmented. **Examples:** nevus, wart, pimple, ringworm, psoriasis, eczema.

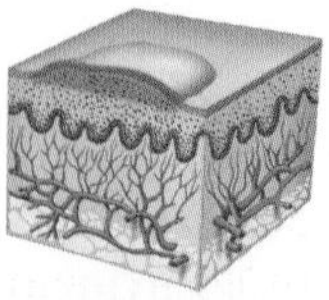

Vesicle
Elevated, circumscribed, fluid-filled lesion less than 0.5 cm in diameter.
Examples: poison ivy, shingles, chickenpox.

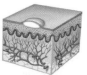

Nodule
Palpable, circumscribed lesion; larger and deeper than a papule (0.6 to 2 cm in diameter); extends into the dermal area. **Examples:** intradermal nevus, benign or malignant tumor.

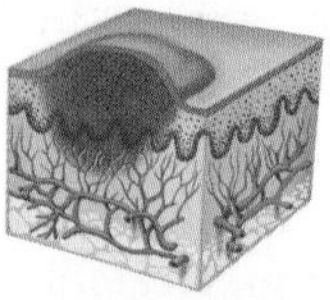

Pustule
Small, raised, circumscribed lesion that contains pus; usually less than 1 cm in diameter. **Examples:** acne, furuncle, pustular psoriasis, scabies.

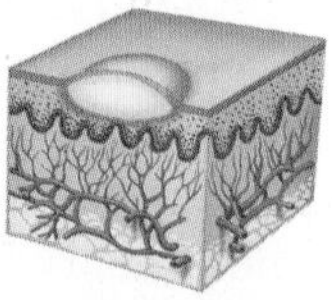

Tumor
Solid, elevated lesion larger than 2 cm in diameter that extends into the dermal and subcutaneous layers.
Examples: lipoma, steatoma, dermatofibroma, hemangioma.

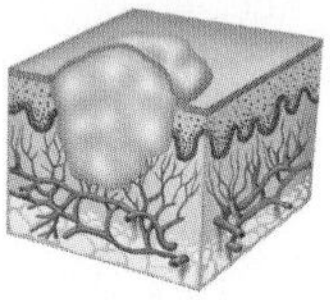

Bulla
A vesicle or blister larger than 1 cm in diameter.
Examples: second-degree burns, severe poison oak, poison ivy.

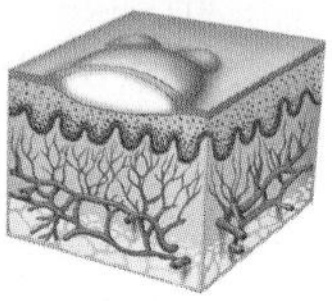

Wheal
Elevated, firm, rounded lesion with localized skin edema (swelling) that varies in size, shape, and color; paler in the center than its surrounding edges; accompanied by itching.
Examples: hives, insect bites, urticaria.

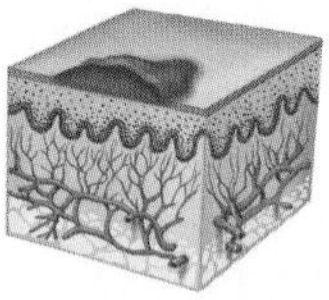

SECONDARY LESIONS

DEPRESSED LESIONS
Depressed lesions caused by loss of skin surface

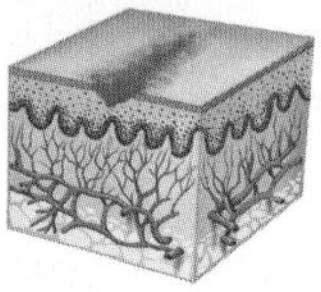

Excoriations
Linear scratch marks or traumatized abrasions of the epidermis.
Examples: scratches, abrasions, chemical or thermal burns.

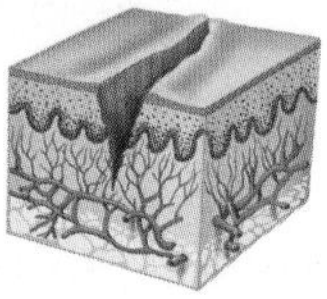

Fissure
Small slit or cracklike sore that extends into the dermal layer; could be caused by continuous inflammation and drying.

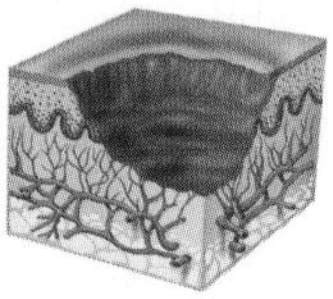

Ulcer
An open sore or lesion that extends to the dermis and usually heals with scarring. **Examples:** pressure sore, basal cell carcinoma.

Figure 5-3 Primary and secondary lesions.

Burns

Burns are tissue injuries caused by contact with thermal, chemical, electrical, or radioactive agents. Although burns generally occur on the skin, they can also affect the respiratory and digestive tract linings. Burns that have a local effect are not as serious as those that have a systemic effect. Systemic effects are life-threatening and may include dehydration, shock, and infection.

Burns are usually classified as first-, second-, or third-degree burns. The extent of injury and degree of severity determine a burn's classification. **First-degree (superficial) burns** are the least serious type of burn because they injure only the top layers of the skin, the epidermis. These burns are most commonly caused by brief contact with dry or moist heat **(thermal burn),** spending too much time in the sun **(sunburn),** or exposure to chemicals **(chemical burn).** Injury is restricted to local effects, such as skin redness **(erythema)** and acute sensitivity to such sensory stimuli as touch, heat, or cold **(hyperesthesia).** Generally, blisters do not form, and the burn heals without scar formation. **Second-degree (partial-thickness)** burns are deep burns that damage the epidermis and part of the dermis. These burns may be caused by contact with flames, hot liquids, or chemicals. Symptoms mimic those of first-degree burns, but fluid-filled blisters **(vesicles or bullae)** form, and the burn may heal with little or no scarring. (See Fig. 5-4.)

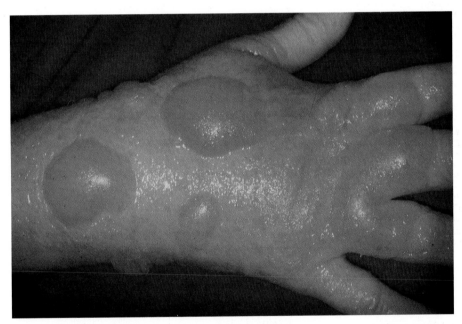

Figure 5-4 Second-degree burn of the hand. From Goldsmith, Lazarus, and Tharp: *Adult and Pediatric Dermatology: A Color Guide to Diagnosis and Treatment.* FA Davis, Philadelphia, 1997, p. 318, with permission.

In **third-degree (full-thickness) burns,** the epidermis and dermis are destroyed, and some of the underlying connective tissue is damaged, leaving the skin waxy and charred with insensitivity to touch. The underlying bones, muscles, and tendons may also be damaged. These burns may be caused by corrosive chemicals, flames, electricity, or extremely hot objects; immersion of the body in extremely hot water; or clothing that catches fire. Because of the extensiveness of tissue destruction, ulcerating wounds develop, and the body attempts to heal itself by forming scar tissue. Skin grafting **(dermatoplasty)** is commonly required to protect the underlying tissue and assist in recovery.

A formula for estimating the percentage of adult body surface area affected by burns is to apply the Rule of Nines. This method assigns values of 9% or 18% of surface area to specific regions. The formula is modified in infants and children because of the proportionally larger head size. (See Fig. 5-5.) To determine treatment, it is important to know the amount of the burned surface area because the patient requires intravenous (IV) fluids for hydration to replace fluids lost from tissue damage.

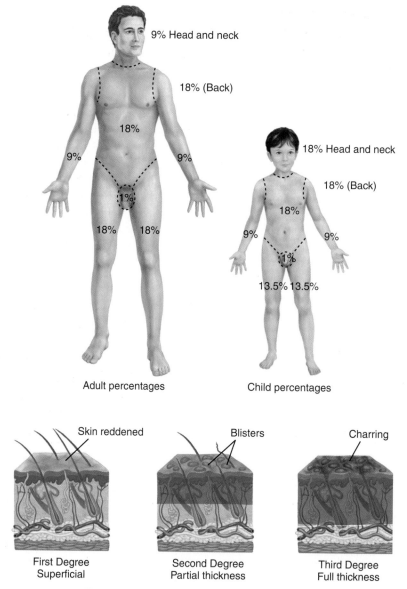

Figure 5-5 Rule of Nines and burn classification.

Oncology

Neoplasms are abnormal growths of new tissue that are classified as benign or malignant. **Benign neoplasms** are noncancerous growths composed of the same type of cells as the tissue in which they are growing. They harm the individual only insofar as they place pressure on or interfere with the functioning of surrounding structures. If the benign neoplasm remains small, it does not commonly require removal. When the tumor enlarges, causes pain, or interferes with other organs or structures, excision is necessary. **Malignant neoplasms,** also called **cancer,** are composed of cells that tend to become invasive and spread to remote regions of the body **(metastasis).** Once the malignant cells from the primary tumor invade surrounding tissues, they tend to enter blood and lymph vessels and travel to remote regions of the body to form secondary tumor sites. If left untreated, cancer tends to be progressive and generally fatal.

Cancer treatment includes surgery, chemotherapy, immunotherapy, and radiation therapy. **Immunotherapy,** also called **biotherapy,** is a newer treatment that stimulates the body's own immune defenses to fight tumor cells. To provide the most effective treatment, the physician may prescribe one of the previously listed treatments or use a combination of them **(combined-modality treatment).**

Grading and Staging Cancer

Pathologists grade and stage tumors to help in diagnosis and treatment planning, provide a possible prognosis, and aid comparison of treatment results when different treatment methods are used.

Tumor Grading

In tumor **grading,** cells from the tumor site are evaluated to determine how closely the biopsied tissue resembles normal tissue. The greater the difference between the normal tissue and the biopsied tissue, the more serious is the grade of cancer. Pathologists commonly describe these changes using four grades of severity based on the microscopic appearance of the cells. (See Table 5-1.) A grade I tumor shows cells that closely resemble the tissue of origin. In other words, most of the cells are well differentiated and able to carry on the function of the tissue. A patient with a grade I tumor has a good prognosis for full recovery. On the other hand, a patient with a grade IV tumor shows cells that are very poorly differentiated and grow rapidly. These cells spread to surrounding tissue, revert back to their primitive state **(anaplasia),** and are incapable of carrying on the normal function of the tissue. A patient with a grade IV tumor has the poorest prognosis.

Table 5-1	**Tumor Grading**
This table defines the four tumor grades and their characteristics.	
Grading	**Tumor Characteristics**
Grade I Tumor cells well differentiated	• Close resemblance to tissue of origin and, thus, retaining some specialized functions
Grade II Tumor cells moderately or poorly differentiated	• Less resemblance to tissue of origin • More variation in size and shape of tumor cells • Increased mitoses
Grade III Tumor cells poorly differentiated	• Increased abnormality in appearance, with only remote resemblance to the tissue of origin • Marked variation in shape and size of tumor cells • Greatly increased mitoses
Grade IV Tumor cells very poorly differentiated	• Abnormal appearance to the extent that recognition of the tumor's tissue origin is difficult • Extreme variation in size and shape of tumor cells

Tumor Staging

The most common system used for staging tumors is the **tumor, node, metastasis (TNM) system.** It is an international system that allows comparison of statistics among cancer centers. The TNM staging system classifies solid tumors by size and degree of spread according to three basic criteria:

- **T**—size and invasiveness of the primary tumor
- **N**—area lymph nodes involved
- **M**—invasiveness (metastasis) of the primary tumor

Numbers are used to indicate size or spread of the tumor. The higher the number, the greater is the extent or spread of the malignancy. For example, *T2* designates a small tumor; *M0* designates no evidence of metastasis. (See Table 5-2.) As with grading, staging provides valuable information to guide treatment plans.

Basal Cell Carcinoma

Basal cell carcinoma, the most common type of skin cancer, is a malignancy of the basal layer of the epidermis, or hair follicles. This type of cancer is commonly caused by overexposure to sunlight. The tumors are locally invasive but rarely metastasize. (See Fig. 5-6.) Basal cell carcinoma

Table 5-2	**TNM System of Staging**	

This table outlines the tumor, node, metastasis (TNM) system of staging, including designations, stages, and degrees of tissue involvement.

Designation	Stage	Tissue Involvement
Tumor		
TX		Primary tumor that cannot be evaluated
T0		No evidence of tumor
Tis	Stage I	Carcinoma in situ, which indicates that the tumor is in a defined location and shows no invasion into surrounding tissues
T1, T2, T3, T4	Stage II	Primary tumor size and extent of local invasion, where T1 is small with minimal invasion, and T4 is large with extensive local invasion into surrounding organs and tissues
Node		
NX		Regional lymph nodes that cannot be evaluated
N0		Regional lymph nodes that show no abnormalities
N1, N2, N3, N4	Stage III	Degree of lymph node involvement and spread to regional lymph nodes, where N1 is less involvement with minimal spreading, and N4 is more involvement with extensive spreading
Metastasis		
MX		Distant metastasis that cannot be evaluated
M0		No evidence of metastasis
M1	Stage IV	Presence of metastasis

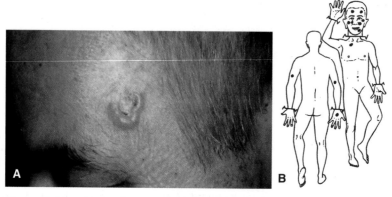

Figure 5-6 Basal cell carcinoma. (A) Basal cell carcinoma with pearly, flesh-colored papule with depressed center and rolled edge. (B) Common sites of basal cell carcinoma. From Goldsmith, Lazarus, and Tharp: *Adult and Pediatric Dermatology: A Color Guide to Diagnosis and Treatment.* F.A. Davis, Philadelphia, 1997, p. 157, with permission.

is most prevalent in blond, fair-skinned men and is the most common malignant tumor affecting white people. Although these tumors grow slowly, they commonly ulcerate as they increase in size and develop crusting that is firm to the touch. Metastases are uncommon with this type of cancer; however, the disease can invade the tissue sufficiently to destroy an ear, nose, or eyelid. Depending on the location, size, and depth of the lesion, treatment may include curettage and electrodesiccation, chemotherapy, surgical excision, irradiation, or chemosurgery.

Squamous Cell Carcinoma

Squamous cell carcinoma arises from skin that undergoes pathological hardening **(keratinizing)** of epidermal cells. It is an invasive tumor with potential for metastasis and occurs most commonly in fair-skinned white men over age 60. (See Fig. 5-7.) Repeated overexposure to the sun's ultraviolet rays greatly increases the risk of squamous cell carcinoma. Other predisposing factors associated with this type of cancer include radiation therapy; chronic skin irritation and inflammation; exposure to cancer-causing agents **(carcinogens),** including tar and oil; hereditary diseases (such as **xeroderma pigmentosum** and **albinism**); and the presence of premalignant lesions (such as **actinic keratosis** or **Bowen disease**).

There are two types of squamous cell carcinoma: those that are confined to the original site **(in situ)** and those that penetrate the surrounding tissue **(invasive).** Depending on the location, size, shape, degree of invasion, and condition of the underlying tissue, treatment is removal by surgical excision, cryotherapy, radiotherapy, or electrodesiccation and curettage. A combination of these treatment methods may be required for a deeply invasive tumor.

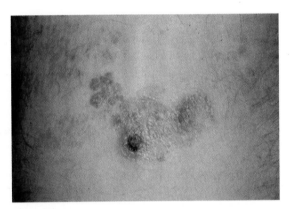

Figure 5-7 Squamous cell carcinoma, in which the surface is fragile and bleeds easily. From Goldsmith, Lazarus, and Tharp: *Adult and Pediatric Dermatology: A Color Guide to Diagnosis and Treatment.* F.A. Davis, Philadelphia, 1997, p. 237, with permission.

Malignant Melanoma

Malignant melanoma, as the name implies, is a malignant growth of melanocytes. (See Fig. 5-8.) This tumor is highly metastatic, with a higher mortality rate than basal or squamous cell carcinomas. It is the most lethal of the skin cancers and can metastasize extensively to the liver, lungs, or brain.

Several factors may influence the development of melanoma, but persons at greatest risk have fair complexions, blue eyes, red or blond hair, and freckles. Excessive exposure to sunlight and severe sunburn during childhood are believed to increase the risk of melanoma in later life. Avoiding the sun and using sunscreen have proved effective in preventing the disease.

Melanomas are diagnosed by **biopsy** and histological examination. Treatment requires surgery to remove the primary cancer, along with adjuvant therapies to reduce the risk of metastasis. The extent of surgery depends on the size and location of the primary tumor and is determined by staging the disease.

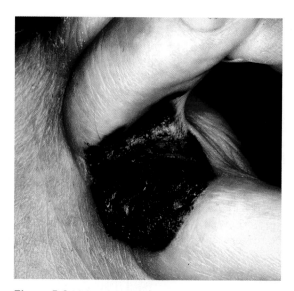

Figure 5-8 Malignant melanoma showing an irregularly pigmented papule with areas of brown, red, white, and blue that can develop anywhere in the body. From Goldsmith, Lazarus, and Tharp: *Adult and Pediatric Dermatology: A Color Guide to Diagnosis and Treatment.* F.A. Davis, Philadelphia, 1997, p. 146, with permission.

 It is time to review burn and oncology terms by completing Learning Activity 5-4.

Diseases and Conditions

This section introduces diseases and conditions of the integumentary system, along with their meanings and pronunciations. Word analyses for selected terms are also provided.

Term	Definition
abscess ĂB-sĕs	Localized collection of pus at the site of an infection (characteristically a staphylococcal infection) *When a localized abscess originates in a hair follicle, it is called a furuncle or boil. A cluster of furuncles in the subcutaneous tissue results in the formation of a carbuncle. (See Fig. 5-9.)*

Figure 5-9 Dome-shaped abscess that has formed a furuncle in the hair follicles of the neck. Large furuncles with connecting channels to the skin surface form a carbuncle.

Diseases and Conditions—cont'd

Term	Definition
acne ĂK-nē	Inflammatory disease of the sebaceous glands and hair follicles of the skin with characteristic lesions that include blackheads (comedos), inflammatory papules, pustules, nodules, and cysts and are usually associated with seborrhea; also called *acne vulgaris* (See Fig. 5-10.) *Acne results from thickening of the follicular opening, increased sebum production, and the presence of bacteria. It is associated with an inflammatory response. The face, neck, and shoulders are common sites for this condition.* **Figure 5-10** Acne vulgaris. From Goldsmith, Lazarus, and Tharp: *Adult and Pediatric Dermatology: A Color Guide to Diagnosis and Treatment.* F.A. Davis, Philadelphia, 1997, p. 227, with permission.
alopecia al-ō-PĒ-shē-ă	Partial or complete loss of hair resulting from normal aging, an endocrine disorder, a drug reaction, anticancer medication, or a skin disease; commonly called *baldness*
Bowen disease BŌ-ĕn	Very early form of skin cancer, which is easily curable and characterized by a red, scaly patch on the skin; also called *squamous cell carcinoma in situ* *Treatment for Bowen disease includes curettage and electrodesiccation.*
cellulitis sĕl-ū-LĪ-tĭs	Diffuse (widespread), acute infection of the skin and subcutaneous tissue *Cellulitis is characterized by a light, glossy appearance of the skin, localized heat, redness, pain, and swelling, occasionally with fever, malaise, and chills.*
chloasma klō-ĂZ-mă	Pigmentary skin discoloration usually occurring in yellowish-brown patches or spots
comedo KŎM-ē-dō	Typical small skin lesion of acne vulgaris caused by accumulation of keratin, bacteria, and dried sebum plugging an excretory duct of the skin *The closed form of comedo, called a whitehead, consists of a papule from which the contents are not easily expressed.*

(continued)

Diseases and Conditions—cont'd

Term	Definition

decubitus ulcer
dĕ-KŪ-bĭ-tŭs ŬL-sĕr

Inflammation, sore, or skin deterioration caused by prolonged pressure from lying in one position that prevents blood flow to the tissues, usually in elderly bedridden persons; also known as *pressure ulcer* (See Fig. 5-11.)

Pressure ulcers are most commonly found in skin overlying a bony projection, such as the hip, ankle, heel, shoulder, and elbow. The wounds are categorized from stage 1 to stage 4. (See Fig. 5-12.)

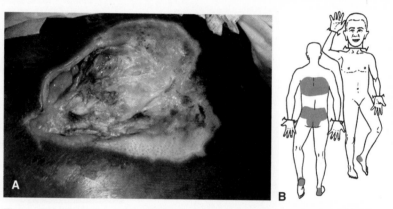

Figure 5-11 Decubitus ulcer. (A) Deep pressure ulcer over a bony prominence in a bedridden patient. (B) Common sites of pressure ulcers. From Goldsmith, Lazarus, and Tharp: *Adult and Pediatric Dermatology: A Color Guide to Diagnosis and Treatment.* F.A. Davis, Philadelphia, 1997, p. 445, with permission.

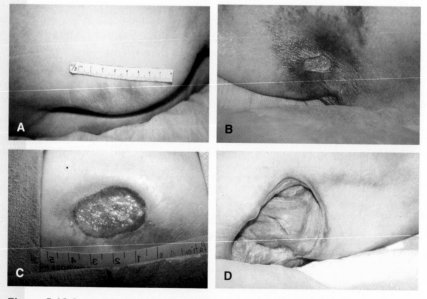

Figure 5-12 Stages of pressure ulcer. (A) Stage 1, with shiny, reddened skin that usually appears over a bony prominence. (B) Stage 2, untreated stage 1 ulcer that becomes more serious when skin is swollen and shows a blister. (C) Stage 3, in which a craterlike ulcer goes deeper into the skin. (D) Stage 4 ulcer that goes into a muscle or bone. From Dillon: *Nursing Health Assessment,* 2nd ed. F.A. Davis, Philadelphia, 2007, p. 239, with permission.

Diseases and Conditions—cont'd

Term	Definition
ecchymosis ĕk-ĭ-MŌ-sĭs	Skin discoloration consisting of a large, irregularly formed hemorrhagic area with colors changing from bluish black to greenish brown or yellow; commonly called a *bruise* (See Fig. 5-13.) **Figure 5-13** Ecchymosis.
eczema ĔK-zĕ-mă	Chronic inflammatory skin condition that is characterized by erythema, papules, vesicles, pustules, scales, crusts, and scabs and accompanied by intense itching (pruritus); also called *atopic dermatitis* *Eczema most commonly occurs during infancy and childhood, with decreasing incidence in adolescence and adulthood. Statistics support a convincing genetic component in that it tends to occur in patients with a family history of allergic conditions.*
erythema ĕr-ĭ-THĒ-mă	Redness of the skin caused by swelling of the capillaries *An example of erythema is a mild sunburn or nervous blushing.*
eschar ĔS-kăr	Dead matter that is sloughed off from the surface of the skin, especially after a burn *Eschar material is commonly crusty or scabbed.*
impetigo ĭm-pĕ-TĪ-gō	Bacterial skin infection characterized by isolated pustules that become crusted and rupture
keratosis kĕr-ă-TŌ-sĭs *kerat:* horny tissue, hard; cornea *-osis:* abnormal condition; increase (used primarily with blood cells)	Thickened area of the epidermis or any horny growth on the skin (such as a callus or wart)
lentigo lĕn-TĪ-gō	Small brown macules, especially on the face and arms, brought on by sun exposure, usually in a middle-aged or older person *Lentigo are benign pigmented lesions of the skin that require no treatment unless cosmetic repair is desired.*
pallor PĂL-or	Unnatural paleness or absence of color in the skin
pediculosis pĕ-dĭk-ū-LŌ-sĭs *pedicul:* lice *-osis:* abnormal condition; increase (used primarily with blood cells)	Infestation with lice, transmitted by personal contact or common use of brushes, combs, or headgear

(continued)

Diseases and Conditions—cont'd

Term	Definition
petechia pē-TĒ-kē-ă	Minute, pinpoint hemorrhage under the skin *A petechia (plural,* petechiae*) is a smaller version of an ecchymosis.*
pruritus proo-RĪ-tŭs	Intense itching
psoriasis sō-RĪ-ă-sĭs	Chronic skin disease characterized by itchy red patches covered by thick, dry, silvery scales and caused by excessive development of the basal layer of the epidermis (See Fig. 5-14.) *New psoriasis lesions tend to appear at sites of trauma. They may be found in any location but commonly occur on the scalp, knees, elbows, umbilicus, and genitalia. Treatment includes topical application of various medications, keratolytics, phototherapy, and ultraviolet light therapy in an attempt to slow hyperkeratosis.*

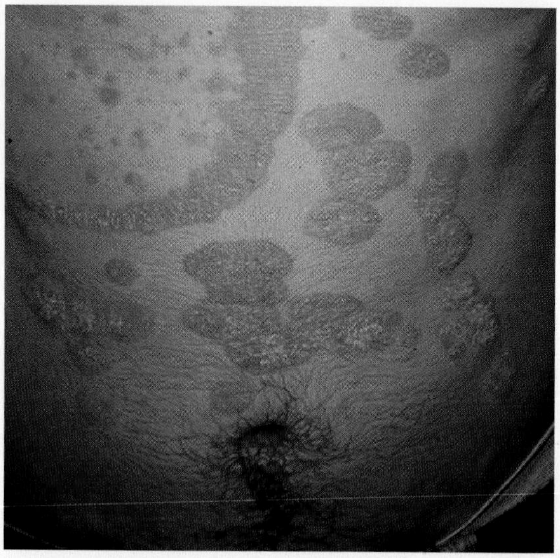

Figure 5-14 Psoriasis. From Goldsmith, Lazarus, and Tharp: *Adult and Pediatric Dermatology: A Color Guide to Diagnosis and Treatment.* F.A. Davis, Philadelphia, 1997, p. 258, with permission.

Term	Definition
purpura PŬR-pŭ-ră	Any of several bleeding disorders characterized by hemorrhage into the tissues, particularly beneath the skin or mucous membranes, producing ecchymoses or petechiae *Hemorrhage into the skin shows red darkening into purple and then brownish yellow and finally disappearing in 2 to 3 weeks. Areas of discoloration do not disappear under pressure.*
scabies SKĀ-bēz	Contagious skin disease transmitted by the itch mite, commonly through sexual contact *Scabies manifests as papules, vesicles, pustules, and burrows and causes intense itching, commonly resulting in secondary infections. The axillae, genitalia, inner aspect of the thighs, and areas between the fingers are most commonly affected.*

Diseases and Conditions—cont'd

Term	Definition
tinea TĬN-ē-ăh	Fungal skin infection whose name commonly indicates the body part affected; also called *ringworm* *Examples of tinea include tinea barbae (beard), tinea corporis (body), tinea pedis (athlete's foot), tinea versicolor (skin), and tinea cruris (jock itch).*
urticaria ŭr-tĭ-KĂR-ē-ă	Allergic reaction of the skin characterized by the eruption of pale red, elevated patches called *wheals* or *hives* (See Fig. 5-15.)

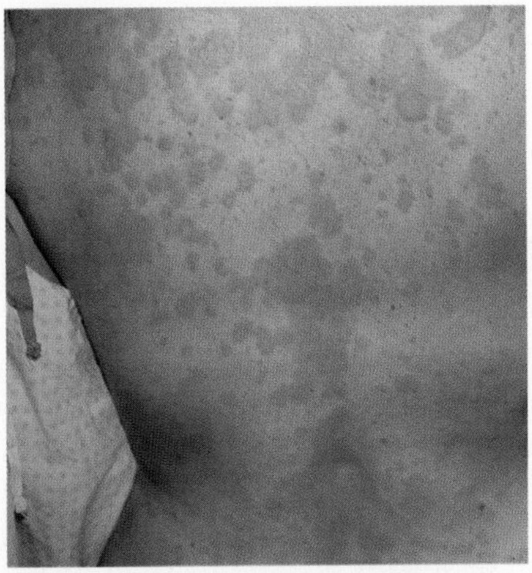

Figure 5-15 Urticaria. From Goldsmith, Lazarus, and Tharp: *Adult and Pediatric Dermatology: A Color Guide to Diagnosis and Treatment.* F.A. Davis, Philadelphia, 1997, p. 209, with permission.

Term	Definition
verruca vĕr-ROO-kă	Epidermal growth caused by a virus; also known as *warts* *Verrucae may be removed by cryosurgery, electrocautery, or acids; however, they may regrow if the virus remains in the skin. Types include plantar warts, juvenile warts, and venereal warts. (See Fig. 5-16.)*

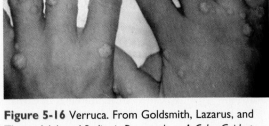

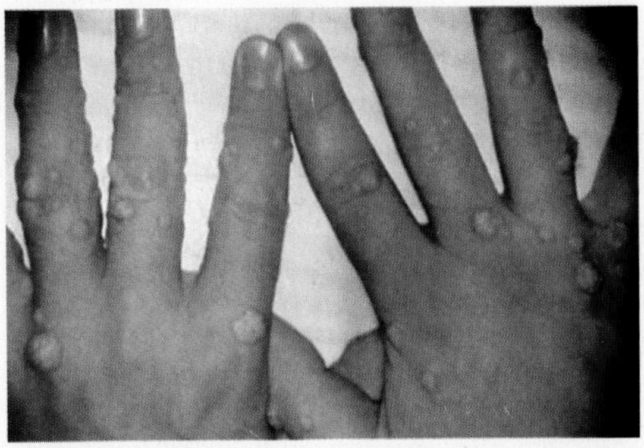

Figure 5-16 Verruca. From Goldsmith, Lazarus, and Tharp: *Adult and Pediatric Dermatology: A Color Guide to Diagnosis and Treatment.* F.A. Davis, Philadelphia, 1997, p. 241, with permission.

(continued)

Diseases and Conditions—cont'd

Term	Definition
vitiligo vĭt-ĭl-Ī-gō	Localized loss of skin pigmentation characterized by milk-white patches (See Fig. 5-17.) 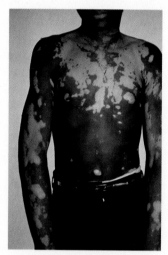 **Figure 5-17** Vitiligo. From Goldsmith, Lazarus, and Tharp: *Adult and Pediatric Dermatology: A Color Guide to Diagnosis and Treatment.* F.A. Davis, Philadelphia, 1997, p. 121, with permission.

 It is time to review pathology, diseases, and conditions by completing Learning Activity 5-5.

Diagnostic, Surgical, and Therapeutic Procedures

This section introduces diagnostic, surgical, and therapeutic procedures used to treat and diagnose skin disorders. Descriptions are provided, along with pronunciations and word analyses for selected terms.

Procedure	Description
Diagnostic	
allergy skin test	Any test in which a suspected allergen or sensitizer is applied to or injected into the skin to determine the patient's sensitivity to it *The most commonly used skin tests are the intradermal, patch, and scratch tests. The intensity of the response is determined by the wheal-and-flare reaction after application of the suspected allergen. Positive and negative controls help verify normal skin reactivity. (See Fig. 5-18.)*
intradermal ĭn-tră-dĕr-măl *intra-:* in, within *derm:* skin *-al:* pertaining to	Skin test that identifies suspected allergens by subcutaneously injecting small amounts of extracts of the suspected allergens and observing the skin for a subsequent reaction *Intradermal skin tests help determine immunity to diphtheria (Schick test) or tuberculosis (Mantoux test).*

Diagnostic, Surgical, and Therapeutic Procedures—cont'd

Procedure	Description
patch	Skin test that identifies allergic contact dermatitis by applying a suspected allergen to a patch, which is then taped on the skin, usually the forearm, and observing the area 24 hours later for an allergic response *After patch removal, a lack of noticeable reaction indicates a negative result; skin reddening or swelling indicates a positive result and means the person is allergic to the suspected allergen.*
scratch	Skin test that identifies suspected allergens by placing a small quantity of the suspected allergen on a lightly scratched area of the skin; also called *puncture test* or *prick test* *Redness or swelling at the scratch sites within 10 minutes indicates an allergy to the substance or a positive test result. If no reaction occurs, the test result is negative.*

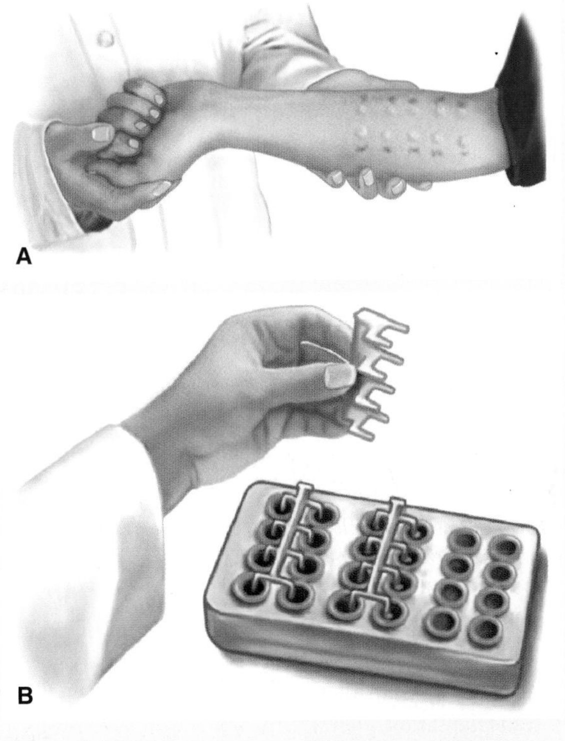

Figure 5-18 Allergy skin tests. (A) Intradermal allergy test reactions. (B) Scratch (prick) skin test kit for allergy testing.

culture & sensitivity (C&S)	Laboratory test to determine the presence of pathogens in patients with suspected wound infections and identify the appropriate drug therapy to which the organism responds (sensitivity)

(continued)

Diagnostic, Surgical, and Therapeutic Procedures—cont'd

Procedure	Description
Surgical	
biopsy (Bx, bx) BĪ-ŏp-sē	Representative tissue sample removed from a body site for microscopic examination *Skin biopsies help establish or confirm a diagnosis, estimate prognosis, or follow the course of a disease. Any lesion suspected of malignancy is removed and sent to the pathology laboratory for evaluation.*
frozen section (FS)	Ultrathin slice of tissue from a frozen specimen for immediate pathological examination *FS is commonly used for rapid diagnosis of malignancy after the patient has been anesthetized to determine treatment options.*
needle	Removal of a small tissue sample for examination using a hollow needle, usually attached to a syringe
punch	Removal of a small core of tissue using a hollow punch
shave	Removal of elevated lesions using a surgical blade
Mohs MŌZ	Procedure that involves progressive removal and examination of layers of cancer-containing skin until only cancer-free tissue remains; also called *micrographic surgery.*
skin graft	Transplantation of healthy tissue to an injured site *Human, animal, or artificial skin can provide a temporary covering or permanent layer of skin over a wound or burn.*
allograft ĂL-ō-grăft *allo-:* other; differing from normal *-graft:* transplantation	Transplantation of healthy tissue from one person to another person; also called *homograft* *In an allograft, the skin donor is usually a cadaver. This type of skin graft is temporary and is used to protect the patient against infection and fluid loss. The allograft is frozen and stored in a skin bank until needed.*
autograft AW-tō-grăft *auto:* self, own *-graft:* transplantation	Transplantation of healthy tissue from one site to another site in the same individual
synthetic sĭn-THĔT-ĭk	Transplantation of artificial skin produced from collagen fibers arranged in a lattice pattern *The recipient's body does not reject synthetic skin (produced artificially), and healing skin grows into it as the graft gradually disintegrates.*
xenograft ZĔN-ō-grăft *xen/o:* foreign *-graft:* transplantation	Transplantation (dermis only) from a foreign donor (usually a pig) and transferred to a human; also called *heterograft* *A xenograft is a temporary graft to protect the patient against infection and fluid loss.*

Diagnostic, Surgical, and Therapeutic Procedures—cont'd

Procedure	Description
Therapeutic	
chemical peel	Chemical removal of the outer layers of skin to treat acne scarring and general keratoses; also called *chemabrasion*
	Chemical peels are also commonly used for cosmetic purposes to remove fine wrinkles on the face.
cryosurgery krī-ō-SĔR-jĕr-ē	Use of subfreezing temperature (commonly liquid nitrogen) to destroy or eliminate abnormal tissue, such as tumors, warts, and unwanted, cancerous, or infected tissue
débridement dĕ-BRĒD-mĕnt	Removal of necrotized tissue from a wound by surgical excision, enzymes, or chemical agents
	Débridement is used to promote healing and prevent infection.
dermabrasion DĔRM-ă-brā-zhŭn	Rubbing (abrasion) using wire brushes or sandpaper to mechanically scrape away (abrade) the epidermis
	Dermabrasion commonly helps remove acne scars, tattoos, and scar tissue.
fulguration fŭl-gū-RĀ-shŭn	Tissue destruction by means of high-frequency electric current; also called *electrodesiccation*
	Fulguration helps remove tumors and lesions in and on the body.
photodynamic therapy (PDT)	Procedure in which cells selectively treated with an agent called a *photosensitizer* are exposed to light to produce a reaction that destroys the cells
	Various forms of photodynamic therapy are used in treatment of cancer, actinic keratosis, and macular degeneration.

Pharmacology

Various medications are available to treat skin disorders. (See Table 5-3.) Because of their superficial nature and location, many skin disorders respond well to topical drug therapy. Such mild, localized skin disorders as contact dermatitis, acne, poison ivy, and diaper rash can be effectively treated with topical agents available as over-the-counter products.

Widespread or particularly severe dermatological disorders may require systemic treatment. For example, poison ivy with large areas of open, weeping lesions may be difficult to treat with topical medication and may require a prescription-strength drug. In such a case, an oral steroid or antihistamine might be prescribed to relieve inflammation and severe itching.

Table 5-3	Drugs Used to Treat Skin Disorders

This table lists classifications of common drugs used to treat skin disorders, their therapeutic actions, and selected generic and trade names.

Classification	Therapeutic Action	Generic and Trade Names
antiacne agents	Reduce acne through multiple mechanisms *Some antiacne medications decrease bacteria in the follicles of the skin to prevent the formation of acne; others disrupt the stickiness of the follicular skin cells and decrease microcomedones (widening of the follicle, which fills with debris and bacteria to form comedones).*	**benzoyl peroxide** BĔN-zō-ĭl pĕr-ŎK-sīd *PanOxyl* **tretinoin** TRĔT-ĭ-noyn *Retin-A*
antifungals ăn-tĭ-FŬN-găls	Alter the cell wall of fungi or disrupt enzyme activity, resulting in cell death *Antifungals help treat ringworm (tinea corporis), athlete's foot (tinea pedis), and fungal infection of the nail (onychomycosis). When topical antifungals are not effective, oral or intravenous antifungal drugs may be necessary.*	**itraconazole** ĭt-ră-KŎN-ă-zōl *Sporanox (oral form only)* **terbinafine** TĔR-bĭn-ă-fēn *Lamisil (available in both oral and topical form)* **fluconazole** flū-KŎ-nă-zōl *Diflucan (available in both intravenous and oral form)*
antihistamines ăn-tĭ-HĬS-tă-mĭns	Inhibit allergic reactions of inflammation, redness, and itching caused by the release of histamine *In a case of severe itching, antihistamines may be given orally. As a group, these drugs are also known as antipruritics (pruritus means "itching").*	**diphenhydramine** dī-fĕn-HĪ-dră-mēn *Benadryl* **hydroxyzine** hī-DRŎKS-ĭzēn *Vistaril, Atarax*
antiparasitics ăn-tĭ-păr-ă-SĬT-ĭks	Kill insect parasites, such as mites and lice *Parasiticides are used to treat scabies (mites) and pediculosis (lice). The drug is applied as a cream or lotion to the body and as a shampoo to treat the scalp.*	**lindane** LĬN-dān *Kwell, Thion* **permethrin** pĕr-MĔTH-rĭn *Nix*
antiseptics ăn-tĭ-SĔP-tĭks	Topically applied agents that inhibit growth of bacteria, thus preventing infections in cuts, scratches, and surgical incisions	**ethyl or isopropyl alcohol** ĔTH-ĭl, ī-sō-PRŌ-pĭl **hydrogen peroxide** HĪ-drō-jĕn pĕ-RŎK-sīd **povidone-iodine** PŌ-vĭ-dōn Ī-ō-dīn *Betadine*

Table 5-3	Drugs Used to Treat Skin Disorders—cont'd		
Classification	**Therapeutic Action**	**Generic and Trade Names**	
corticosteroids kor-tĭ-kō-STĔR-oyds	Decrease inflammation and itching by suppressing the immune system's inflammatory response to tissue damage *Topical corticosteroids are used to treat contact dermatitis, poison ivy, insect bites, psoriasis, seborrhea, and eczema. Oral corticosteroids may be prescribed for systemic treatment of severe or widespread inflammation or itching.*	**hydrocortisone** HĪ-drō-KOR-tĭ-sōn *Cetacort, Cortaid* **triamcinolone** trī-ăm-SĬN-ō-lōn *Azmacort, Kenalog*	
keratolytics kĕr-ă-tō-LĬT-ĭks	Destroy and soften the outer layer of skin so that it is sloughed off or shed *Strong keratolytics remove warts and corns and aid in penetration of antifungal drugs. Milder keratolytics promote shedding of scales and crusts in eczema, psoriasis, seborrheic dermatitis, and other conditions with dry, scaly skin. Weak keratolytics irritate inflamed skin, acting as a tonic to accelerate healing.*	**salicylic acid** săl-ĭ-SĬL-ĭk ĂS-ĭd *Sebasorb, Psoriasin, and so forth* (Multiple brand names based on use) **urea** ū-RĒ-ă *Kerafoam, Keralac*	
protectives prŏ-TĔK-tĭvs	Cover, cool, dry, or soothe inflamed skin *Protectives do not penetrate the skin or soften it. Rather, they allow the natural healing process to occur by forming a long-lasting film that protects the skin from air, water, and clothing.*	**lotions** *Cetaphil moisturizing lotion* **ointments** *Vaseline*	
topical anesthetics ăn-ĕs-THĔT-ĭks	Block sensation of pain by numbing the skin layers and mucous membranes *These topical drugs are administered directly by means of sprays, creams, gargles, suppositories, and other preparations. They provide temporary symptomatic relief of minor burns, sunburns, rashes, and insect bites.*	**lidocaine** LĪ-dō-kān *Xylocaine* **procaine** PRŌ-kān *Novocain*	

Abbreviations

This section introduces integumentary-related abbreviations and their meanings.

Abbreviation	Meaning	Abbreviation	Meaning
Bx, bx	biopsy	**I&D**	incision and drainage
BCC	basal cell carcinoma	**IMP**	impression (synonymous with diagnosis)
C&S	culture and sensitivity	**IV**	intravenous
CA	cancer; chronological age; cardiac arrest	**TNM**	tumor-node-metastasis
FS	frozen section	**ung**	ointment
ID	intradermal	**XP, XDP**	xeroderma pigmentosum

It is time to review procedures, pharmacology, and abbreviations by completing Learning Activities 5-6 and 5-7.

LEARNING ACTIVITIES

The activities that follow provide a review of the integumentary system terms introduced in this chapter. Complete each activity and review your answers to evaluate your understanding of the chapter.

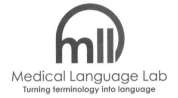

Medical Language Lab
Turning terminology into language

Visit the Medical Language Lab at *medicallanguagelab.com.* Use it to enhance your study and reinforcement of this chapter with the flash-card activity. We recommend that you complete the flash-card activity before starting Learning Activities 5-1 and 5-2.

Learning Activity 5-1

Medical Word Elements

Read the definition in the numbered list. Then select the elements from the table to build medical words. You may use the elements more than once.

Combining Forms		Suffixes		Prefixes
derm/o	myc/o	-al	-osis	an-
dermat/o	py/o	-cyte	-pathy	homo-
hidr/o	scler/o	-derma	-plasty	hypo-
ichthy/o	seb/o	-graft	-rrheap	
kerat/o	trich/o	-ic		
lip/o	xer/o	-logist		
melan/o	-oma			

1. tumor (that is) black _____
2. pertaining to under the skin _____
3. surgical repair of the skin _____
4. cell (composed of) fat _____
5. skin (containing) pus _____
6. specialist in the study of skin disorders _____
7. skin that is dry _____
8. abnormal condition without sweat _____
9. transplantation from the same (species) _____
10. abnormal condition of dry or scaly (skin) _____
11. skin (that has) hardened _____
12. abnormal condition of a fungus _____
13. discharge or flow of sebum _____
14. disease of the hair _____
15. abnormal condition of horny tissue _____

Check your answers in Appendix A. Review any material that you did not answer correctly.

Correct Answers _____ X 6.67 = _____ % Score

Learning Activity 5-2
Building Medical Words

Use *adip/o* or *lip/o* (fat) to build words that mean:

1. tumor consisting of fat _____
2. hernia containing fat _____
3. resembling fat _____
4. fat cell _____

Use *dermat/o* (skin) to build words that mean

5. inflammation of the skin _____
6. abnormal condition of a skin fungus _____

Use *onych/o* (nail) to build words that mean:

7. tumor of the nails _____
8. softening of the nails _____
9. abnormal condition of the nails _____
10. abnormal condition of the nails caused by a fungus _____
11. abnormal condition of a hidden (ingrown) nail _____
12. disease of the nails _____

Use *trich/o* (hair) to build words that mean:

13. disease of the hair _____
14. abnormal condition of hair caused by a fungus _____

Use *-logy* or *-logist* to build words that mean:

15. study of the skin _____
16. specialist in the study of skin (diseases) _____

Build surgical words that mean:

17. excision of fat (adipose tissue) _____
18. removal of a nail _____
19. incision of a nail _____
20. surgical repair (plastic surgery) of the skin _____

✓ *Check your answers in Appendix A. Review material that you did not answer correctly.*

Correct Answers _____ X 5 = _____ % Score

Learning Activity 5-3

Identifying Skin Lesions

Label the skin lesions on the lines provided, using the listed terms.

bulla   *macule*   *pustule*   *vesicle*

excoriations   *nodule*   *tumor*   *wheal*

fissure   *papule*   *ulcer*

PRIMARY LESIONS   **FLAT LESIONS**
Flat, discolored, circumscribed lesions of any size

Flat, pigmented, circumscribed area less than 1 cm in diameter. **Examples:** freckle, flat mole, or rash that occurs in rubella.

ELEVATED LESIONS

Solid   *Fluid-filled*

Solid, elevated lesion less than 1 cm in diameter that may be the same color as the skin or pigmented. **Examples:** nevus, wart, pimple, ringworm, psoriasis, eczema.

Elevated, circumscribed, fluid-filled lesion less than 0.5 cm in diameter. **Examples:** poison ivy, shingles, chickenpox.

Palpable, circumscribed lesion; larger and deeper than a papule (0.6 to 2 cm in diameter); extends into the dermal area. **Examples:** intradermal nevus, benign or malignant tumor.

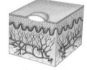

Small, raised, circumscribed lesion that contains pus; usually less than 1 cm in diameter. **Examples:** acne, furuncle, pustular psoriasis, scabies.

Solid, elevated lesion larger than 2 cm in diameter that extends into the dermal and subcutaneous layers. **Examples:** lipoma, steatoma, dermatofibroma, hemangioma.

A vesicle or blister larger than 1 cm in diameter. **Examples:** second-degree burns, severe poison oak, poison ivy.

Elevated, firm, rounded lesion with localized skin edema (swelling) that varies in size, shape, and color; paler in the center than its surrounding edges; accompanied by itching. **Examples:** hives, insect bites, urticaria.

SECONDARY LESIONS   **DEPRESSED LESIONS**
Depressed lesions caused by loss of skin surface

Linear scratch marks or traumatized abrasions of the epidermis. **Examples:** scratches, abrasions, chemical or thermal burns.

Small slit or cracklike sore that extends into the dermal layer; could be caused by continuous inflammation and drying.

An open sore or lesion that extends to the dermis and usually heals with scarring. **Examples:** pressure sore, basal cell carcinoma.

 Check your answers by referring to Figure 5–3 on page 92. Review material that you did not answer correctly.

Learning Activity 5-4

Matching Burn and Oncology Terms

Match each term on the left with its meaning on the right.

_____ erythema	a. develops from keratinizing epidermal cells
_____ T0	b. noncancerous
_____ malignant	c. no evidence of metastasis
_____ first-degree burn	d. extensive damage to underlying connective tissue
_____ grading	e. no evidence of primary tumor
_____ squamous cell carcinoma	f. determines degree of abnormal cancer cells compared with normal cells
_____ benign	g. burn that heals without scar formation
_____ T1	h. cancerous; may be life-threatening
_____ M0	i. redness of skin
_____ third-degree burns	j. primary tumor size, small with minimal invasion

✓ *Check your answers in Appendix A. Review any material that you did not answer correctly.*

Correct Answers _____ X 10 = _____ % Score

Learning Activity 5-5

Diseases and Conditions

Match the terms with the definitions in the numbered list.

abscess	*eschar*	*scabies*
alopecia	*impetigo*	*tinea*
chloasma	*pediculosis*	*urticaria*
ecchymosis	*petechiae*	*verruca*
erythema	*pruritus*	*vitiligo*

1. infestation with lice _____
2. skin depigmentation characterized by milk-white patches _____
3. fungal skin infection, also called *ringworm* _____
4. contagious skin disease transmitted by the itch mite _____
5. bacterial skin infection characterized by pustules that become crusted and rupture _____
6. allergic reaction of the skin, characterized by elevated red patches called hives _____
7. hyperpigmentation of the skin, characterized by yellowish-brown patches or spots _____
8. hemorrhagic spot or bruise on the skin _____
9. minute or small hemorrhagic spots on the skin _____
10. loss or absence of hair _____
11. localized collection of pus at the site of infection (staphylococcal) _____
12. redness of the skin caused by swelling of the capillaries _____
13. damaged tissue following a severe burn _____
14. intense itching _____
15. epidermal growth caused by a virus; also known as *wart* _____

✓ *Check your answers in Appendix A. Review material that you did not answer correctly.*

Correct Answers _____ X 6.67 = _____ % Score

Learning Activity 5-6

Procedures, Pharmacology, and Abbreviations

Match the terms with the definitions in the numbered list.

antifungals   intradermal test   patch test

corticosteroids   keratolytics   ung

dermabrasion   parasiticides   xenograft

fulguration

1. topical agents to treat athlete's foot and onychomycosis _____

2. tissue destruction by means of high-frequency electric current _____

3. agents that decrease inflammation or itching _____

4. use of wire brushes or other abrasive materials to remove scars, tattoos, or fine wrinkles _____

5. agents that kill parasitic skin infestations _____

6. agents that soften the outer layer of skin so that it sloughs off _____

7. procedure in which extracts of suspected allergens are injected subcutaneously _____

8. procedure in which allergens are applied topically, usually on the forearm _____

9. ointment _____

10. transplantation taken from another species (usually a pig) to a human _____

✓ *Check your answers in Appendix A. Review material that you did not answer correctly.*

Correct Answers _____ X 10 = _____ % Score

DOCUMENTING HEALTH-CARE ACTIVITIES

This section provides practical application activities in the form of exercises to help students develop skills in documenting patient care. First, read the medical report. Then complete the activities and exercises that follow.

Documenting Health-Care Activity 5-1

Pathology Report: Skin Lesion

General Hospital

1511 Ninth Avenue ■ ■ Sun City, USA 12345 ■ ■ (555) 802–1887

Pathology Report

Date: April 16, 20xx   Pathology: 43022
Patient: Franks, Robert   Room: 910
Physician: Dante Riox, MD

Specimen: Skin from (a) dorsum left wrist and (b) left forearm, ulnar, near elbow.

Clinical Diagnosis: Bowen disease versus basal cell carcinoma versus dermatitis.

Microscopic Description: (a) There is mild hyperkeratosis and moderate epidermal hyperplasia with full-thickness atypia of squamous keratinocytes. Squamatization of the basal cell layer exists. A lymphocytic inflammatory infiltrate is present in the papillary dermis. Solar elastosis is present. (b) Nests, strands, and columns of atypical neoplastic basaloid keratinocytes grow down from the epidermis into the underlying dermis. Fibroplasia is present. Solar elastosis is noted.

Pathological Diagnosis: (a) Bowen disease of left wrist; (b) nodular and infiltrating basal cell carcinoma of left forearm, near elbow.

Samantha Roberts, MD
Samantha Roberts, MD

sr:bg

D: 4–16-xx
T: 4–16-xx

Terminology

The terms listed in the table that follows are taken from *Pathology Report: Skin Lesion.* Use a medical dictionary such as *Taber's Cyclopedic Medical Dictionary,* the appendices of this book, or other resources to define each term. Then review the pronunciation for each term and practice by reading the medical record aloud.

Term	Definition
atypia ā-TĬP-ē-ă	
atypical ā-TĬP-ĭ-kăl	
basal cell layer BĀ-săl	
Bowen disease BŌ-ĕn	
dermis DĔR-mĭs	
dorsum DOR-sŭm	
epidermal hyperplasia ĕp-ĭ-DĔR-măl hī-pĕr-PLĀ-zē-ă	
fibroplasia fī-brō-PLĀ-sē-ă	
hyperkeratosis hī-pĕr-kĕr-ă- TŌ-sĭs	
infiltrate ĬN-fĭl-trāt	
keratinocytes kĕ-RĂT-ĭ-nō-sīts	
neoplastic nē-ō-PLĂS-tĭk	
papillary PĂP-ĭ-lăr-ē	

(continued)

Term	Definition
pathological păth-ō-LŎJ-ĭk-ăl	
solar elastosis SŌ-lăr ĕ-lăs- TŌ-sĭs	
squamous SKWĀ-m ŭs	

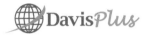 Visit the *Medical Terminology Systems* online resource center at Davis*Plus* to practice pronunciation and reinforce the meanings of the terms in this medical report.

Critical Thinking

Review *Pathology Report: Skin Lesion* to answer the questions.

1. In the specimen section, what does "skin on dorsum left wrist" mean?

_____

_____

_____

_____

2. What was the inflammatory infiltrate?

_____

_____

_____

_____

3. What was the pathologist's diagnosis for the left forearm?

_____

_____

_____

_____

4. Provide a brief description of Bowen disease, the pathologist's diagnosis for the left wrist.

_____

_____

_____

_____

Patient Referral Letter: Onychomycosis

Physician Center

2422 Rodeo Drive ■ ■ **Sun City, USA 12345** ■ ■ **(555)788–2427**

May 3, 20xx

John Roberts, MD
1115 Forest Ave
Sun City, USA 12345

Dear Doctor Roberts:

Thank you for referring Alicia Gonzoles to my office. Mrs. Gonzoles presents to the office for evaluation and treatment of onychomycosis with no previous treatment. Past pertinent medical history does reveal hypertension and breast CA. Pertinent surgical history does reveal mastectomy.

Examination of patient's feet does reveal onychomycosis, 1–5 bilaterally. Vascular and neurological examinations are intact. Previous laboratory work was within normal limits except for an elevated alkaline phosphatase of 100.

Tentative diagnosis: Onychomycosis, 1–5 bilaterally

Treatment consisted of débridement of mycotic nails and bilateral feet and dispensing a prescription for Sporanox Pulse Pack to be taken for 3 months to treat the onychomycotic infection. I have also asked her to repeat her liver enzymes in approximately 4 weeks. Mrs. Gonzoles will make an appointment in 2 months for follow-up, and I will keep you informed of any changes in her progress. If you have any questions, please feel free to contact me.

Sincerely yours,

Juan Perez, MD
Juan Perez, MD

jp:az

Terminology

The terms in the table that follows are taken from *Patient Referral Letter: Onychomycosis*. Use a medical dictionary such as *Taber's Cyclopedic Medical Dictionary*, the appendices of this book, or other resources to define each term. Then review the pronunciation for each term and practice by reading the medical record aloud.

Term	Definition
alkaline phosphatase ĂL-kă-lĭn FŎS-fă-tās	
bilaterally bī-LĂT-ĕr-ăl-ē	
CA	
débridement dĕ-BRĒD-mĕnt	
hypertension hī-pĕr-TĔN-shŭn	
mastectomy măs-TĔK-tŏ-mē	
neurological noor-ō-LŎJ-ĭk-ăl	
onychomycosis ŏn-ĭ-kō-mī-KŌ-sĭs	
Sporanox* SPŎR-ă-nŏks	
vascular VĂS-kū-lăr	

*Refer to Table 5-3 to determine the drug classification and the generic name for Sporanox.

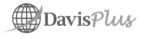

Visit the *Medical Terminology Systems* online resource center at Davis*Plus* to practice pronunciation and reinforce the meanings of the terms in this medical report.

Critical Thinking

Review *Patient Referral Letter: Onychomycosis* to answer the questions.

1. What pertinent disorders were identified in the past medical history?

_____

_____

_____

_____

2. What pertinent surgery was identified in the past surgical history?

_____

_____

_____

_____

3. Did the doctor identify any problems in the vascular system or nervous system?

_____

_____

_____

_____

4. What was the significant finding in the laboratory results?

_____

_____

_____

_____

5. What treatment did the doctor employ for the onychomycosis?

_____

_____

_____

_____

6. What did the doctor recommend regarding the abnormal laboratory finding?

_____

_____

_____

_____

Constructing Chart Notes

To construct chart notes, replace the italicized and boldfaced terms in each of the two case studies with one of the medical terms from the list.

asymptomatic	erythematous	Mohs surgery
biopsy	lymphadenectomy	oncologist
chemotherapy	metastasize	pruritic
dermatologist		

Mr. R. is concerned about a "patch" that developed on the back of his neck. Lately, the patch has become (1) *reddened* and is (2) *itchy*. Now that the patch is crusting and bleeding, his wife advises him to see a (3) *skin specialist.* After various tests are performed, the dermatologist identifies the patch as a basal cell carcinoma. She explains that this type of cancer rarely (4) *spreads to other body sites.* The dermatologist advises that the tumor must be removed using a technique in which (5) *thin layers of cancer-containing skin are progressively removed and microscopically examined until only cancer-free tissue remains.*

1. _____
2. _____
3. _____
4. _____
5. _____

Miss M. noticed that a mole on her neck is increasing in size. Other than the increase in size, Miss M. is experiencing (6) *no other symptoms.* An appointment in the outpatient clinic is scheduled for the (7) *excision of the lesion for microscopic examination.* After evaluation of the biopsy, the pathology report indicates a diagnosis of melanoma. Miss M. is advised to see the (8) *physician who specializes in tumors.* In addition to the melanoma, the surgeon discovers metastasis of adjacent lymph glands (nodes) and (9) *removes the lymph glands (nodes).* After her discharge, Miss M. will begin (10) *treatment using chemicals* to target and destroy any remaining cancer cells.

6. _____
7. _____
8. _____
9. _____
10. _____

✓ *Check your answers in Appendix A. Review any material that you did not answer correctly.*

Correct Answers _____ X 10 = _____ % Score

Digestive System

Chapter Outline

Objectives

Upon completion of this chapter, you will be able to:

- Locate the major organs of the digestive system, and describe their structure and function.
- Describe the functional relationship between the digestive system and other body systems.
- Pronounce, spell, and build words related to the digestive system.
- Describe diseases, conditions, and procedures related to the digestive system.
- Explain pharmacology related to the treatment of digestive disorders.
- Demonstrate your knowledge of this chapter by completing the learning and documenting health-care activities.

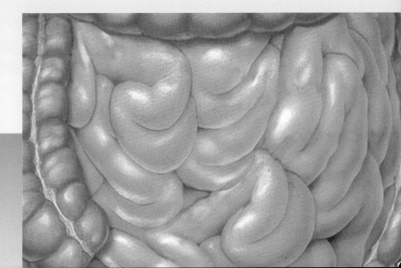

Anatomy and Physiology

The digestive system, also called the *gastrointestinal (GI) system,* consists of a digestive tube called the *GI tract* (or *alimentary canal*) and several accessory organs whose primary function is to break down food, prepare it for absorption, and eliminate waste. The GI tract, extending from the mouth to the anus, varies in size and structure in several distinct regions.

Food passing along the GI tract is mixed with digestive enzymes and broken down into nutrient molecules, which are absorbed in the bloodstream. Undigested waste materials not absorbed by the blood are then eliminated from the body through defecation. Included in the digestive system are the accessory organs of digestion: the liver, gallbladder, and pancreas. The process of digestion breaks down food into nutrients to nourish the body. (See Fig. 6-1.)

Anatomy and Physiology Key Terms

This section introduces important terms, along with their definitions and pronunciations. The key terms are highlighted in color in the Anatomy and Physiology section. Word analyses for selected terms are also provided. Pronounce the term, and place a check mark in the box after you do so.

Term	Definition
bilirubin bĭl-ĭ-ROO-bĭn ☐	Orange-yellow pigment formed during destruction of erythrocytes that is taken up by liver cells and eventually excreted in the feces *Elevated bilirubin in the blood produces yellowing of the skin (jaundice). It also indicates liver damage or disease.*
bolus BŌ-lŭs ☐	Mass of masticated food ready for swallowing
exocrine ĔKS-ō-krĭn ☐ *exo-:* outside, outward *-crine:* secrete	Type of gland that secretes its products through excretory ducts to the surface of an organ or tissue or into a vessel
sphincter SFĬNGK-tĕr ☐	Circular band of muscle fibers that constricts a passage or closes a natural opening of the body *An example of a sphincter is the lower esophageal (cardiac) sphincter, which constricts once food passes into the stomach.*
triglycerides trī-GLĬS-ĕr-īd ☐	Organic compound, a true fat, that is made of one glycerol and three fatty acids *In the blood, triglycerides combine with proteins to form lipoproteins. The liver synthesizes lipoproteins to transport fats to other tissues, where they are a source of energy. Fat in adipose tissue is stored energy.*

Pronunciation Help	Long Sound	ā — rate	ē — rebirth	ī — isle	ō — over	ū — unite
	Short Sound	ă — apple	ĕ — ever	ĭ — it	ŏ — not	ŭ — cut

Mouth

The process of digestion begins in the mouth. (See Fig. 6-2, page 130.) The mouth, also known as the (1) **oral cavity,** is a receptacle for food. It is formed by the cheeks **(bucca),** lips, teeth, tongue, and hard and soft palates. Located around the oral cavity are three pairs of salivary glands that secrete saliva. Saliva contains important digestive enzymes that help begin the chemical breakdown of food. In the mouth, food is broken down mechanically (by the teeth) and chemically (by saliva) and then formed into a **bolus.**

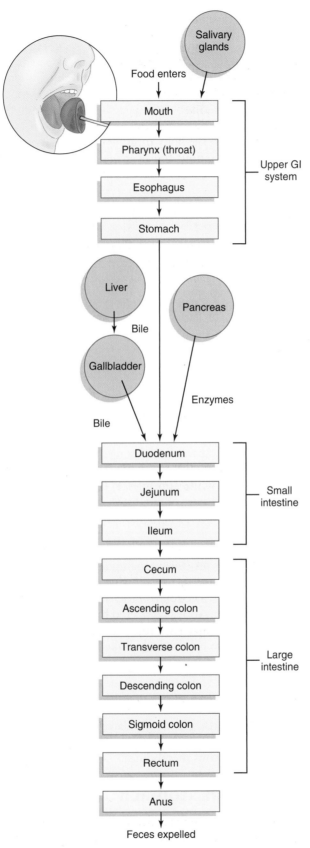

Figure 6-1 Pathway of food through the digestive system.

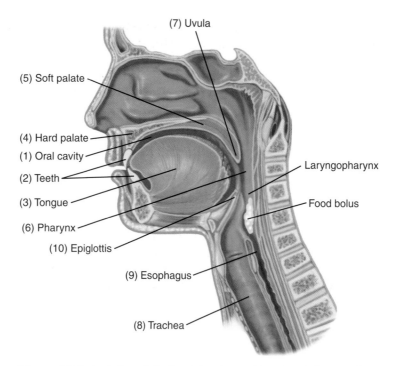

Figure 6-2 Sagittal view of the head showing oral, nasal, and pharyngeal components of the digestive system.

Teeth

The (2) **teeth** play an important role in the initial stages of digestion by mechanically breaking down food **(mastication)** into smaller pieces as they mix it with saliva. Teeth are covered by a hard enamel, giving them a smooth, white appearance. Beneath the enamel is **dentin,** the main structure of the tooth. The innermost part of the tooth is the **pulp,** which contains nerves and blood vessels. The teeth are embedded in pink, fleshy tissue known as **gums (gingiva).**

Tongue

The (3) **tongue** assists in the chewing process by manipulating the bolus of food during chewing and moving it to the back of the mouth for swallowing **(deglutition).** The tongue also aids in speech production and taste. Rough projections on the surface of the tongue called **papillae** contain taste buds. The four basic taste sensations registered by chemical stimulation of the taste buds are sweet, sour, salty, and bitter. All other taste perceptions are combinations of these four basic flavors. In addition, the sense of taste is intricately linked with the sense of smell, making taste perception very complex.

Hard and Soft Palates

The two structures forming the roof of the mouth are the (4) **hard palate** (anterior portion) and the (5) **soft palate** (posterior portion). The soft palate, which forms a partition between the mouth and the nasopharynx, is continuous with the hard palate. The entire oral cavity, like the rest of the GI tract, is lined with mucous membranes.

Pharynx, Esophagus, and Stomach

As the tongue pushes the bolus into the (6) **pharynx** (throat), it is guided by the soft, fleshy, V-shaped structure called the (7) **uvula.** The funnel-shaped pharynx serves as a passageway to the respiratory and GI tracts and provides a resonating chamber for speech sounds. The lowest portion of the pharynx divides into two tubes: one that leads to the lungs, called the (8) **trachea,** and one that leads to the stomach, called the (9) **esophagus.** A small flap of cartilage called the

(10) **epiglottis** folds back to cover the trachea during swallowing, forcing food to enter the esophagus. At all other times, the epiglottis remains upright, allowing air to freely pass through the respiratory structures.

The **stomach,** a saclike structure located in the left upper quadrant (LUQ) of the abdominal cavity, serves as a food reservoir that continues mechanical and chemical digestion. (See Fig. 6-3.) The stomach extends from the (1) **esophagus** to the first part of the small intestine, the (2) **duodenum.** The terminal portion of the esophagus, the (3) **lower esophageal (cardiac) sphincter,** is composed of muscle fibers that constrict once food has passed into the stomach. It prevents the stomach contents from regurgitating back into the esophagus. The (4) **body** of the stomach, the large central portion, together with the (5) **fundus,** the upper portion, are mainly storage areas. Most digestion takes place in the funnel-shaped terminal portion, the (6) **pylorus.** The interior lining of the stomach is composed of mucous membranes and contains numerous macroscopic longitudinal folds called (7) **rugae** that gradually unfold as the stomach fills. Located within the rugae, digestive glands produce hydrochloric acid (HCl) and enzymes. Secretions from these glands coupled with the mechanical churning of the stomach turn the bolus into a semiliquid form called **chyme** that slowly leaves the stomach through the (8) **pyloric sphincter** to enter the duodenum. This **sphincter** regulates the speed and movement of chyme into the small intestine and prohibits backflow. Food is propelled through the entire GI tract by coordinated, rhythmic muscle contractions called **peristalsis.**

Small Intestine

The small intestine is a coiled tube approximately 20 feet long that begins at the pyloric sphincter and ends at the large intestine. (See Fig. 6-4, page 132.) It consists of three parts:

- (1) **duodenum,** the uppermost segment, which is approximately 10 inches long
- (2) **jejunum,** which is approximately 8 feet long
- (3) **ileum,** which is approximately 12 feet long

Digestion is completed in the small intestine with the help of additional enzymes and secretions from the (4) **pancreas** and (5) **liver.** Nutrients in chyme are absorbed through microscopic, finger-like projections called **villi.** Nutrients enter the bloodstream and lymphatic system for distribution

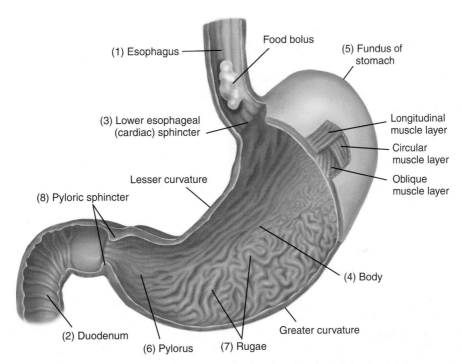

Figure 6-3 Anterior view of the stomach showing muscle layers and rugae of the mucosa.

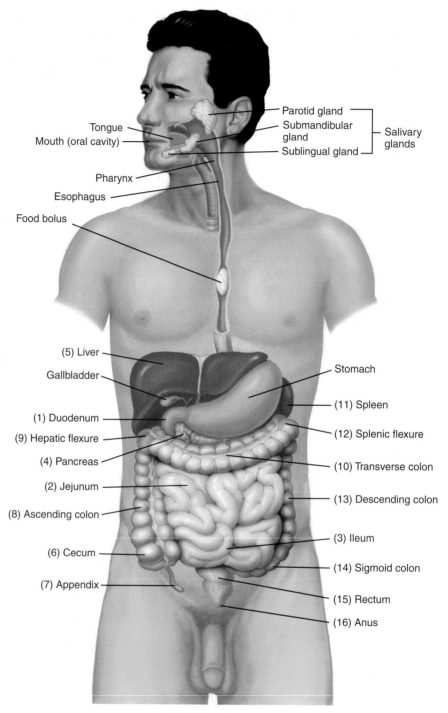

Figure 6-4 Anterior view of the trunk and digestive organs.

to the rest of the body. At the terminal end of the small intestine, a sphincter muscle called the **ileo-cecal valve** allows undigested or unabsorbed material from the small intestine to pass into the large intestine and eventually be excreted from the body.

Large Intestine

The large intestine is approximately 5 feet long. It begins at the end of the ileum and extends to the anus. No digestion takes place in the large intestine. The only secretion is mucus in the colon, which lubricates fecal material so it can pass from the body. The large intestine has three main components: the cecum, colon, and rectum. The first 2 or 3 inches of the large intestine comprise the (6) **cecum,** a small pouch that hangs inferior to the ileocecal valve. Projecting downward from the cecum is the (7) **appendix**, a small, wormlike structure with no apparent function that can become inflamed (**appendicitis**) and infected when blocked. If it becomes infected and inflamed, the appendix can cause considerable pain and must be surgically removed (**appendectomy).** The cecum merges as it becomes the first part of the colon. The main functions of the colon are to absorb water and minerals and eliminate undigested material. The colon is divided into ascending, transverse, descending, and sigmoid portions:

- The (8) **ascending colon** extends from the cecum to the lower border of the liver and turns abruptly to form the (9) **hepatic flexure.**
- The colon continues across the abdomen to the left side as the (10) **transverse colon,** curving beneath the lower end of the (11) **spleen** to form the (12) **splenic flexure.**
- As the transverse colon turns downward, it becomes the (13) **descending colon.**
- The descending colon continues until it forms the (14) **sigmoid colon** and the (15) **rectum.** The rectum, the last part of the GI tract, terminates at the (16) **anus.**

Accessory Organs of Digestion

Although the liver, gallbladder, and pancreas lie outside the GI tract, they play a vital role in the proper digestion and absorption of nutrients. (See Fig. 6-5.)

Liver

The (1) **liver,** the largest glandular organ in the body, weighs approximately 3 to 4 pounds. It is located beneath the diaphragm in the right upper quadrant (RUQ) and the left upper quadrant (LUQ) of the abdominal cavity. The liver performs many vital functions, and death occurs if it ceases to function. Some of its important functions include the following:

- Producing bile, which aids in the digestion of fat
- Removing glucose (sugar) from the blood to synthesize glycogen (starch) and retain it for later use

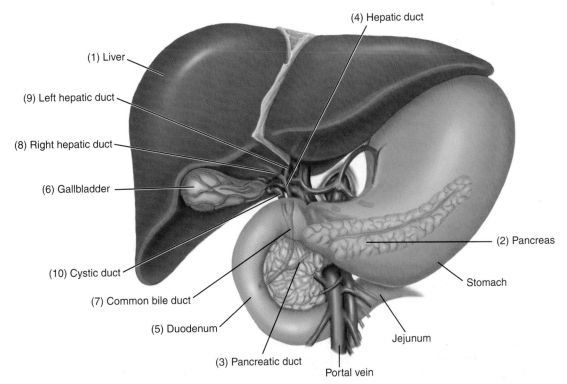

Figure 6-5 Liver, gallbladder, pancreas, and duodenum with associated ducts and blood vessels.

- Storing vitamins, such as B_{12}, A, D, E, and K
- Destroying or transforming toxic products into less harmful compounds
- Maintaining normal glucose levels in the blood
- Destroying old erythrocytes and releasing **bilirubin**
- Synthesizing proteins that circulate in the blood, such as albumin for fluid balance and prothrombin and fibrinogen for coagulation (blood clotting)

Pancreas

The (2) **pancreas** is an elongated, somewhat flattened organ that lies posterior and slightly inferior to the stomach. It performs endocrine and exocrine functions. As an **endocrine** gland, the pancreas secretes insulin directly into the bloodstream to maintain normal blood glucose levels. For a comprehensive discussion of the endocrine function of the pancreas, review Chapter 13. As an **exocrine** gland, the pancreas produces digestive enzymes that pass into the duodenum through the (3) **pancreatic duct.** The pancreatic duct extends along the pancreas and, together with the (4) **hepatic duct** from the liver, enters the (5) **duodenum.** The pancreas produces enzymes, such as trypsin, which digests proteins; amylase, which digests starch; and lipase, which digests **triglycerides**. These pass into the duodenum through the pancreatic duct.

Gallbladder

The (6) **gallbladder,** a saclike structure on the inferior surface of the liver, serves as a storage area for bile, which is produced by the liver. When bile is needed for digestion, the gallbladder releases it into the duodenum through the (7) **common bile duct.** Bile is also drained from the liver through the (8) **right hepatic duct** and the (9) **left hepatic duct.** These two structures eventually form the hepatic duct. The (10) **cystic duct** of the gallbladder merges with the hepatic duct to form the common bile duct, which leads into the duodenum. Bile production is stimulated by hormone secretions, which are produced in the duodenum as soon as food enters the small intestine. Without bile, fat digestion is not possible.

Anatomy Review: Digestive System

To review the anatomy of the digestive system, label the illustration using the listed terms.

anus	*hepatic flexure*	*rectum*
appendix	*ileum*	*sigmoid colon*
ascending colon	*jejunum*	*spleen*
cecum	*liver*	*splenic flexure*
descending colon	*pancreas*	*transverse colon*
duodenum		

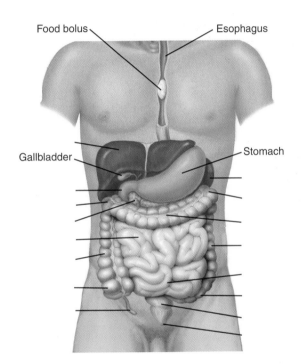

Food bolus   Esophagus

Gallblader   Stomach

Check your answers by referring to Figure 6–4 on page 132. Review material that you did not answer correctly.

Anatomy Review: Accessory Organs of Digestion

To review the anatomy of the accessory organs of digestion, label the illustration using the listed terms.

common bile duct   hepatic duct   pancreas

cystic duct   left hepatic duct   pancreatic duct

duodenum   liver   right hepatic duct

gallbladder

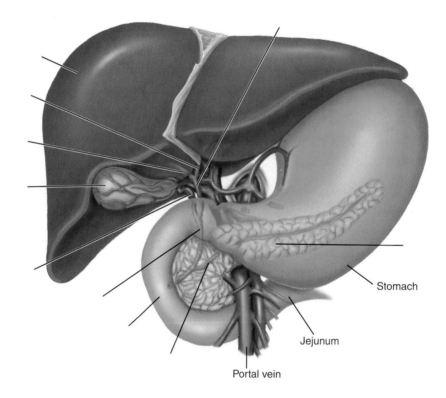

Stomach

Jejunum

Portal vein

 Check your answers by referring to Figure 6-5 on page 133. Review material that you did not answer correctly.

CONNECTING BODY SYSTEMS—DIGESTIVE SYSTEM

The main function of the digestive system is to provide vital nutrients for growth, maintenance, and repair of all organs and body cells. Specific functional relationships between the digestive system and other body systems are discussed here.

Blood, Lymphatic, and Immune

- The liver regulates blood glucose levels.
- The digestive tract secretes acids and enzymes to provide a hostile environment for pathogens.
- The intestinal walls contain lymphoid nodules that help prevent the invasion of pathogens.
- The digestive system absorbs vitamin K, which is necessary for blood clotting.

Cardiovascular

- The digestive system absorbs nutrients needed by the heart.

Endocrine

- The liver eliminates hormones from the blood to end their activity.
- The pancreas contains hormone-producing cells.

Female Reproductive

- The digestive system provides adequate nutrition, including fats, to make conception and normal fetal development possible.
- The digestive system provides nutrients for repair of the endometrium following menstruation.

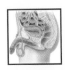

Male Reproductive

- The digestive system provides adequate nutrients in the development of viable sperm.

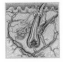

Integumentary

- The digestive system supplies fats that provide insulation in the dermis and subcutaneous tissue.
- The digestive system absorbs nutrients for maintenance, growth, and repair of the skin.

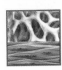

Musculoskeletal

- The digestive system provides the nutrients needed for energy fuel.
- The digestive system absorbs calcium, which is needed for bone salts and muscle contraction.
- The liver removes lactic acid (resulting from muscle activity) from the blood.

Nervous

- The digestive system supplies nutrients necessary for normal neural functioning.
- The digestive system provides nutrients for the synthesis of neurotransmitters and electrolytes for the transmission of a nervous impulse.
- The liver plays a role in maintaining the glucose levels needed for neural function.

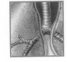

Respiratory

- The digestive system absorbs nutrients needed by cells in the lungs and other tissues in the respiratory tract.
- The pharynx is shared by the digestive and respiratory systems. The lowest portion of the pharynx divides into two tubes: one that leads to the lungs, called the *trachea,* and one that leads to the stomach, called the *esophagus.*

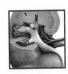

Urinary

- The liver metabolizes hormones, toxins, and drugs into forms that can be excreted in the urine.

Medical Word Elements

This section introduces combining forms, suffixes, and prefixes related to the digestive system. Word analyses are also provided. From the information provided, complete the meaning of the medical words in the right-hand column. The first one is completed for you.

Element	Meaning	Word Analysis and Meaning
Combining Forms		
Mouth		
or/o	mouth	**or**/al (OR-ăl): *pertaining to the mouth* *-al:* pertaining to
stomat/o		**stomat**/itis (stŏ-mă-TĪ-tĭs): _____ *-itis:* inflammation
gloss/o	tongue	**gloss**/ectomy (glŏs-ĔK-tō-mē): _____ *-ectomy:* excision, removal
lingu/o		**lingu**/al (LĬN-gwăl): _____ *-al:* pertaining to
bucc/o	cheek	**bucc**/al (BŬK-ăl): _____ *-al:* pertaining to
cheil/o	lip	**cheil/o**/plasty (KĪ-lō-plăs-tē): _____ *-plasty:* surgical repair
labi/o		**labi**/al (LĀ-bē-ăl): _____ *-al:* pertaining to
dent/o	teeth	**dent**/ist (DĔN-tĭst): _____ *-ist:* specialist
odont/o		orth/**odont**/ist (or-thō-DŎN-tĭst): _____ *orth:* straight *-ist:* specialist *Orthodontists are dentists who specialize in correcting and preventing irregularities of abnormally aligned teeth.*
gingiv/o	gum(s)	**gingiv**/ectomy (jĭn-jĭ-VĔK-tō-mē): _____ *-ectomy:* excision, removal *Gingivectomy is a surgical treatment for periodontal disease.*
sial/o	saliva, salivary gland	**sial/o**/lith (sī-ĂL-ō-lĭth): _____ *-lith:* stone, calculus

Medical Word Elements—cont'd

Element	Meaning	Word Analysis and Meaning
Esophagus, Pharynx, and Stomach		
esophag/o	esophagus	**esophag/o**/scope (ē-SŎF-ă-gō-skōp): _____ *-scope:* instrument for examining
pharyng/o	pharynx (throat)	**pharyng/o**/tonsill/itis (fă-rĭng-gō-tŏn-sĭ-LĪ-tĭs): _____ *tonsill:* tonsils *-itis:* inflammation
gastr/o	stomach	**gastr**/algia (găs-TRĂL-jē-ă): _____ *-algia:* pain *Gastralgia is also called stomachache.*
pylor/o	pylorus	**pylor/o**/spasm (pī-LOR-ō-spăzm): _____ *-spasm:* involuntary contraction, twitching *Pylorospasm occurs in the pyloric sphincter of the stomach.*
Small Intestine		
duoden/o	duodenum (first part of small intestine)	**duoden/o**/scopy (dū-ŏd-ĕ-NŎS-kō-pē): _____ *-scopy:* visual examination
enter/o	intestine (usually small intestine)	**enter/o**/pathy (ĕn-tĕr-ŎP-ă-thē): _____ *-pathy:* disease *Enteropathy typically occurs in the small intestine.*
jejun/o	jejunum (second part of small intestine)	**jejun/o**/rrhaphy (jĕ-joo-NOR-ă-fē): _____ *-rrhaphy:* suture
ile/o	ileum (third part of small intestine)	**ile/o**/stomy (ĭl-ē-ŎS-tō-mē): _____ *-stomy*:* forming an opening (mouth) *An ileostomy creates an opening on the surface of the abdomen to allow feces to be discharged into a bag worn on the abdomen.*
Large Intestine		
append/o	appendix	**append**/ectomy (ăp-ĕn-DĔK-tō-mē): _____ *-ectomy:* excision, removal *An appendectomy removes a diseased appendix that is in danger of rupturing.*
appendic/o		**appendic**/itis (ă-pĕn-dĭ-SĪ-tĭs): _____ *-itis:* inflammation

*When the suffix *-stomy* is used with a combining form that denotes an organ, it refers to a surgical opening to the outside of the body.

(continued)

Medical Word Elements—cont'd

Element	Meaning	Word Analysis and Meaning
col/o	colon	**col/o**/stomy (kō-LŎS-tō-mē): _____ _-stomy:_* forming an opening (mouth) _A colostomy creates a place for fecal matter to exit the body other than through the anus._
colon/o		**colon/o**/scopy (kō-lŏn-ŎS-kō-pē): _____ _-scopy:_ visual examination _Colonoscopy is performed with an elongated flexible endoscope called a colonoscope._
sigmoid/o	sigmoid colon	**sigmoid/o**/tomy (sĭg-moyd-ŎT-ō-mē): _____ _-tomy:_ incision
Terminal End of Large Intestine		
rect/o	rectum	**rect/o**/cele (RĔK-tŏ-sēl): _____ _-cele:_ hernia, swelling _Rectocele is also known as_ proctocele.
proct/o	anus, rectum	**proct/o**/logist (prŏk-TŎL-ō-jĭst): _____ _-logist:_ specialist in the study of _A proctologist is a physician who specializes in treating disorders of the colon, rectum, and anus._
an/o	anus	peri/**an**/al (pĕr-ē-Ā-năl): _____ _peri-:_ around _-al:_ pertaining to
Accessory Organs of Digestion		
hepat/o	liver	**hepat/o**/megaly (hĕp-ă-tō-MĔG-ă-lē): _____ _-megaly:_ enlargement
pancreat/o	pancreas	**pancreat/o**/lysis (păn-krē-ă-TŎL-ĭ-sĭs): _____ _-lysis:_ separation; destruction; loosening _Pancreatolysis may be related to alcohol consumption or result from inflammation, infection, or cancer._
cholangi/o	bile vessel	**cholangi**/ole (kō-LĂN-jē-ōl): _____ _-ole:_ small, minute
chol/e**	bile, gall	**chol/e**/lith (KŌ-lē-lĭth): _____ _-lith:_ calculus, stone _Gallstones are solid masses composed of bile and cholesterol that form in the gallbladder and common bile duct._

*When the suffix -_stomy_ is used with a combining form that denotes an organ, it refers to a surgical opening to the outside of the body.

**The e in _chol/e_ is an exception to the rule of using the connecting vowel _o._

Medical Word Elements—cont'd

Element	Meaning	Word Analysis and Meaning
cholecyst/o	gallbladder	**cholecyst/**ectomy (kō-lē-sĭs-TĔK-tō-mē): _____ *-ectomy:* excision, removal *Cholecystectomy is performed by laparoscopic or open surgery.*
choledoch/o	bile duct	**choledoch/o/**plasty (kō-LĔD-ō-kō-plăs-tē): _____ *-plasty:* surgical repair
Suffixes		
-emesis	vomit	hyper/**emesis** (hī-pĕr-ĔM-ĕ-sĭs): _____ *hyper-:* excessive, above normal
-iasis	abnormal condition (produced by something specified)	chol/e/lith/**iasis** (kō-lē-lĭ-THĪ-ă-sĭs): _____ *chol/e:* bile, gall *lith:* stone, calculus *When gallstones form in the common bile duct, the condition is called* **choledocholithiasis.**
-megaly	enlargement	hepat/o/**megaly** (hĕp-ă-tō-MĔG-ă-lē): _____ *hepat/o:* liver *Hepatomegaly may be caused by hepatitis or infection, fatty infiltration (as in alcoholism), biliary obstruction, or malignancy.*
-orexia	appetite	an/**orexia** (ăn-ō-RĔK-sē-ă): _____ *an-:* without, not *Anorexia can result from various conditions, such as adverse effects of drugs or various physical or psychological causes.*
-pepsia	digestion	dys/**pepsia** (dĭs-PĔP-sē-ă): _____ *dys-:* bad; painful; difficult *Dyspepsia, also called* indigestion, *is an epigastric discomfort felt after eating.*
-phagia	swallowing, eating	aer/o/**phagia** (ĕr-ō-FĀ-jē-ă): _____ *aer/o:* air
-prandial	meal	post/**prandial** (pōst-PRĂN-dē-ăl): _____ *post-:* after, behind
-rrhea	discharge, flow	steat/o/**rrhea** (stē-ă-tō-RĒ-ă): _____ *steat/o:* fat

(continued)

Medical Word Elements—cont'd

Element	Meaning	Word Analysis and Meaning
Prefixes		
dia-	through, across	**dia**/rrhea (dī-ă-RĒ-ă): _____ *-rrhea:* discharge, flow *Diarrhea is a discharge or flow of fluid fecal matter through the bowel.*
peri-	around	**peri**/odont/itis (pĕr-ē-ō-dŏn-TĪ-tĭs): _____ *odont-:* tooth *-itis:* inflammation
sub-	under, below	**sub**/lingu/al (sŭb-LĬN-gwăl): _____ *lingu:* tongue *-al:* pertaining to

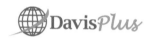

Visit the *Medical Terminology Systems* online resource center at Davis*Plus* for an audio exercise using the terms in this table. Other activities are also available to reinforce content.

 It is time to review medical word elements by completing Learning Activities 6-1, 6-2, and 6-3.

Disease Focus

Although some digestive disorders do not manifest symptoms **(asymptomatic),** many are associated with nausea, vomiting, bleeding, pain, and weight loss. Clinical signs, such as jaundice and edema, may indicate a hepatic disorder. Severe infection, drug toxicity, and changes in fluid and electrolyte balance can cause behavioral abnormalities. Disorders of the GI tract or any of the accessory organs (liver, gallbladder, and pancreas) may result in far-reaching metabolic or systemic problems that can eventually threaten life itself. Assessment of a suspected digestive disorder includes a thorough history and physical examination. A range of diagnostic tests can assist in identifying abnormalities of the GI tract, liver, gallbladder, and pancreas.

For diagnosis, treatment, and management of digestive disorders, the medical services of a specialist may be warranted. **Gastroenterology** is the branch of medicine concerned with digestive diseases. The physician who specializes in the diagnosis and treatment of digestive disorders is known as a **gastroenterologist.** Gastroenterologists do not perform surgeries; however, under the broad classification of surgery, they do perform such procedures as liver biopsy and endoscopic examinations.

Peptic Ulcer Disease (PUD)

An **ulcer** is a circumscribed open sore on the skin or mucous membranes of the body. Peptic ulcers are one of the most common ulcer types that occur in the digestive system. They primarily develop in the stomach and duodenum but may also occur to a lesser extent in the lower esophagus. Ulcers are named by their location in the body: *esophageal ulcer, gastric ulcer,* or *duodenal ulcer.* (See Fig. 6-6.)

A common cause of PUD is the erosion of the protective mucous membrane caused by infection with ***Helicobacter pylori*** bacteria. As the mucous membrane erodes, it exposes the tissue beneath to the strong acids and digestive enzymes of the stomach, and eventually, an ulcer forms. Some individuals have more rapid gastric emptying, which—combined with hypersecretion of acid—creates a large amount of acid moving into the duodenum. As a result, peptic ulcers occur more commonly in the duodenum.

Peptic Ulcers

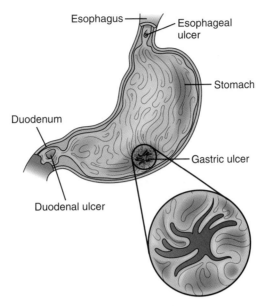

Figure 6-6 Peptic ulcers.

Risk factors that contribute to PUD include smoking, chewing tobacco, stress, caffeine use, and such medications as steroids, aspirin, and nonsteroidal anti-inflammatory drugs (NSAIDs). Peptic ulcer development is influenced by smoking because smoking increases the harmful effects of *H. pylori*, alters protective mechanisms, and decreases gastric blood flow. Treatment includes antibiotics to destroy *H. pylori* and antacids to reduce stomach acids and allow the ulcer to heal. If left untreated, mucosal destruction produces a hole **(perforation)** in the wall lining, with resultant bleeding from the damaged area. At worst, the hole penetrates the entire wall, and the gastric contents leak into the abdominal cavity, possibly leading to inflammation of the peritoneum **(peritonitis).**

Hernia

A **hernia** is a protrusion of any organ, tissue, or structure through the wall of the cavity in which it is naturally contained. (See Fig. 6-7, page 144.) In general, though, the term is applied to protrusions of abdominal organs **(viscera)** through the abdominal wall.

An (1) **inguinal hernia** develops in the groin where the abdominal folds of flesh meet the thighs. In the initial stages, it may be hardly noticeable and appears as a soft lump under the skin, no larger than a marble. In the early stages, an inguinal hernia is usually reducible; that is, it can be pushed gently back into its normal place. With this type of hernia, pain may be minimal. As time passes, the pressure of the abdomen against the weak abdominal wall may increase the size of the opening and the size of the hernia lump. If the blood supply to the hernia is cut off because of pressure, a (2) **strangulated hernia** may develop, leading to necrosis with gangrene. An (3) **umbilical hernia** is a protrusion of part of the intestine at the navel. It occurs more commonly in obese women and among those who have had several pregnancies. Hernias also occur in newborn infants **(congenital)** or during early childhood. If the defect has not corrected itself by age 2, the deformity can be surgically corrected. Treatment consists of surgical repair of the hernia **(hernioplasty)** with suture of the abdominal wall **(herniorrhaphy).**

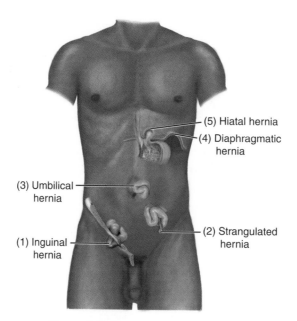

Figure 6-7 Common locations of hernias.

Although hernias most commonly occur in the abdominal region, they may develop in the diaphragm. Two forms of this type include (4) **diaphragmatic hernia,** a congenital disorder, and (5) **hiatal hernia,** in which the lower part of the esophagus and the top of the stomach slide through an opening **(hiatus)** in the diaphragm into the thorax. With a hiatal hernia, stomach acid backs up into the esophagus, causing heartburn, chest pain, and swallowing difficulty. Although many hiatal hernias are asymptomatic, if the disease continues for a prolonged period, it may cause **gastroesophageal reflux disease (GERD).**

Hepatitis

Hepatitis is an inflammatory condition of the liver. The usual causes include exposure to toxic substances, especially alcohol; obstructions in the bile ducts; metabolic diseases; autoimmune diseases; and bacterial or viral infections. A growing public health concern is the increasing incidence of viral hepatitis. Even though its mortality rate is low, the disease is easily transmitted and can cause significant morbidity and prolonged loss of time from school or employment.

Although forms of hepatitis range from hepatitis A through hepatitis E, the three most common forms are hepatitis A **(infectious hepatitis),** hepatitis B **(serum hepatitis),** and hepatitis C. The most common cause of hepatitis A is the ingestion of contaminated food, water, or milk. Hepatitis B and hepatitis C are usually transmitted by routes other than the mouth **(parenteral),** such as from blood transfusions and sexual contact. Because of patient exposure, health-care personnel are at increased risk for contracting hepatitis B, but a vaccine that provides immunity to hepatitis B is available. There is no vaccine available for hepatitis C. Patients with hepatitis C may remain asymptomatic for years, or the disease may produce only mild, flulike symptoms. Treatment for hepatitis includes antiviral drugs; however, there is no cure. As the disease progresses, scarring of the liver may become so serious that liver transplantation is the only recourse.

One of the major symptoms of many liver disorders, including hepatitis and cirrhosis, is a yellowing of the skin, mucous membranes, and sclerae of the eyes **(jaundice** or **icterus).** This condition occurs because the liver is no longer able to remove **bilirubin,** a yellow compound formed during the destruction of erythrocytes. Jaundice may also result when the bile duct is blocked, causing bile to enter the bloodstream.

Diverticulosis

Diverticulosis is a condition in which small, blisterlike pockets **(diverticula)** develop in the inner lining of the large intestine and may balloon through the intestinal wall. These pockets occur most commonly in the sigmoid colon. They usually do not cause any problem unless they become inflamed **(diverticulitis).** (See Fig. 6-8.) Symptoms of diverticulitis include pain, commonly in the left lower quadrant (LLQ) of the abdomen; extreme constipation **(obstipation)** or diarrhea; fever; abdominal swelling; and occasional blood in bowel movements. Treatment for mild cases of diverticulitis includes rest, antibiotics, and changes in diet. Severe cases, however, may require surgical intervention, such as excision of the affected segment of intestine.

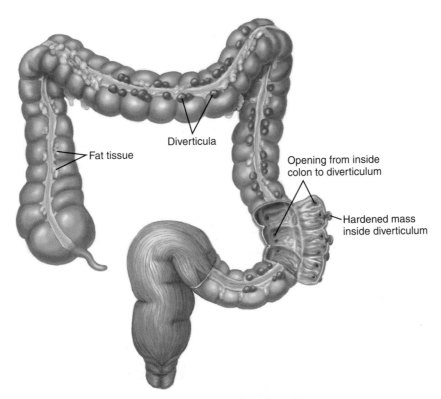

Figure 6-8 Diverticula of the colon.

Oncology

Although stomach cancer is rare in the United States, it is common in many parts of the world where food preservation is problematic. It is an important medical problem because of its high mortality rate. Men are more susceptible to stomach cancer than women. The neoplasm nearly always develops from the epithelial or mucosal lining of the stomach in the form of a cancerous glandular tumor **(gastric adenocarcinoma).** Persistent indigestion is one of the important warning signs of stomach cancer. Other types of GI carcinomas include **esophageal** carcinomas, **hepatocellular** carcinomas, and **pancreatic** carcinomas.

Colorectal cancer is one of the most common types of intestinal cancer in the United States. It originates in the epithelial lining of the colon or rectum and can occur anywhere in the large intestine. Symptoms of carcinoma of the colon depend largely on the location of the malignancy and include changes in bowel habits, passage of blood and mucus in stools, rectal or abdominal pain, anemia, weight loss, obstruction, and perforation. (See Fig. 6-9, page 146.) An obstruction that develops suddenly may be the first symptom of cancer involving the colon

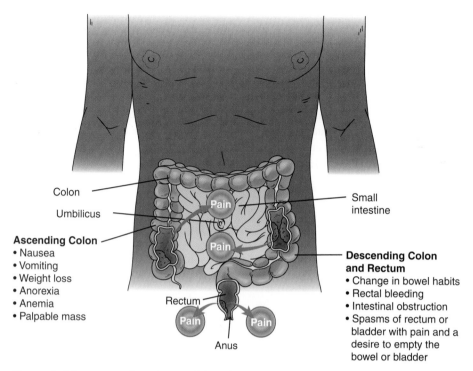

Figure 6-9 Symptoms of carcinoma of the colon, in which pain usually radiates toward the umbilicus or perianal area.

between the cecum and the sigmoid colon. In this region, where bowel contents are liquid, a slowly developing obstruction will not become evident until the lumen is almost closed. Cancer of the sigmoid colon and rectum causes symptoms of partial obstruction with constipation alternating with diarrhea, lower abdominal cramping pain, and distention. The stages of colon cancer are illustrated in Figure 6-10.

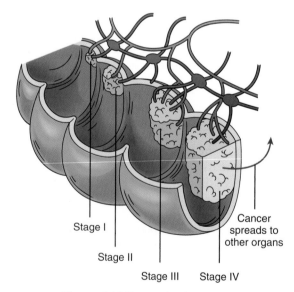

Figure 6-10 Stages of colon cancer.

Diseases and Conditions

This section introduces diseases and conditions of the digestive system, along with their meanings and pronunciations. Word analyses for selected terms are also provided.

Term	Definition
anorexia ăn-ō-RĔK-sē-ă *an-:* without, not *-orexia:* appetite	Lack or loss of appetite, resulting in the inability to eat *Anorexia should not be confused with anorexia nervosa, which is a complex psychogenic eating disorder characterized by an all-consuming desire to remain thin.*
appendicitis ă-pĕn-dĭ-SĪ-tĭs *appendic:* appendix *-itis:* inflammation	Inflammation of the appendix, usually caused by obstruction or infection *Treatment for appendicitis is open or laparoscopic appendectomy. Because of the likelihood of the appendix rupturing and causing a severe, life-threatening infection, the surgeon will remove the appendix as soon as possible. (See Fig. 6-11.)*

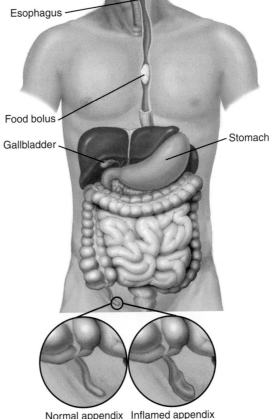

Esophagus

Food bolus

Gallbladder

Stomach

Normal appendix   Inflamed appendix

Figure 6-11 Appendicitis. (A) Normal appendix. (B) Inflamed appendix.

(continued)

Diseases and Conditions—cont'd

Term	Definition
ascites ă-SĪ-tēz	Abnormal accumulation of fluid in the abdominal cavity, usually as a result of chronic liver disease, a neoplasm, or an inflammatory disorder in the abdomen *Ascites is most commonly associated with cirrhosis of the liver, especially when caused by alcoholism. Treatment includes paracentesis to remove the fluid.*
borborygmus bor-bō-RĬG-mŭs	Rumbling or gurgling noises that are audible at a distance and caused by passage of gas through the liquid contents of the intestine
cachexia kă-KĔKS-ē-ă	Physical wasting that includes loss of weight and muscle mass and is commonly associated with acquired immune deficiency syndrome (AIDS) and cancer; also called *wasting syndrome*
cholelithiasis kō-lē-lĭ-THĪ-ă-sĭs *chol/e:* bile, gall *lith:* stone, calculus *-iasis:* abnormal condition (produced by something specified)	Presence or formation of gallstones in the gallbladder *When one or more gallstones are present in the common bile duct, the condition is called* choledocholithiasis. *Gallstones may or may not produce symptoms. (See Fig. 6-12.)*

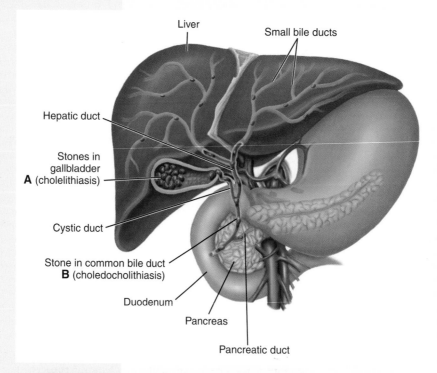

Liver

Small bile ducts

Hepatic duct

Stones in gallbladder
A (cholelithiasis)

Cystic duct

Stone in common bile duct
B (choledocholithiasis)

Duodenum

Pancreas

Pancreatic duct

Figure 6-12 Sites of gallstones. (A) Cholelithiasis. (B) Choledocholithiasis.

cirrhosis sĭr-RŌ-sĭs	Scarring and dysfunction of the liver caused by chronic liver disease *Cirrhosis is most commonly caused by chronic alcoholism. It may also be caused by toxins, infectious agents, metabolic diseases, and circulatory disorders.*

Diseases and Conditions—cont'd

Term	Definition
Crohn disease KRŌN	Form of inflammatory bowel disease (IBD), usually of the ileum but possibly affecting any portion of the intestinal tract; also called *regional enteritis* *Crohn disease is a chronic disease distinguished from closely related bowel disorders by its inflammatory pattern. It may cause fever, cramping, diarrhea, and weight loss.*
dysentery DĬS-ĕn-tĕr-ē	Inflammation of the intestine, especially the colon, that may be caused by ingesting water or food containing chemical irritants, bacteria, protozoa, or parasites and results in bloody diarrhea *Dysentery is common in underdeveloped countries and in times of disaster when sanitary living conditions, clean food, and safe water are not available.*
flatus FLĀ-tŭs	Gas in the GI tract; expelling of air from a body orifice, especially the anus
gastroesophageal reflux disease (GERD) găs-trō-ĕ-sŏf-ă-JĒ-ăl RĒ-flŭks *gastr/o:* stomach *esophag:* esophagus *-eal:* pertaining to	Backflow of gastric contents into the esophagus as a result of a malfunction of the sphincter muscle at the inferior portion of the esophagus *GERD may occur whenever pressure in the stomach is greater than that in the esophagus and may be associated with heartburn, esophagitis, hiatal hernia, or chest pain.*
halitosis hăl-ĭ-TŌ-sĭs	Foul-smelling breath *Halitosis may result from poor oral hygiene; dental or oral infections; ingestion of certain foods, such as garlic or alcohol; use of tobacco; or a systemic disease, such as diabetes or liver disease.*
hematemesis hĕm-ăt-ĔM-ĕ-sĭs *hemat:* blood *-emesis:* vomiting	Vomiting of blood from bleeding in the stomach or esophagus *Hematemesis can be caused by an esophageal ulcer, esophageal varices (dilation of veins), or a gastric ulcer. Treatment requires correction of the underlying cause.*
hemorrhoids HĔM-ō-roydz	Swollen varicose veins in the anorectal region categorized as external or internal *Hemorrhoids are usually caused by abdominal pressure, such as from straining during bowel movement, pregnancy, and standing or sitting for long periods. Consuming a high-fiber diet and drinking plenty of water and juice play a pivotal role in hemorrhoid prevention. Treatment of an advanced condition involves surgical removal of the hemorrhoids (hemorrhoidectomy).*
intestinal obstruction ĭn-TĔS-tĭ-năl	Mechanical or functional blockage of the intestines that occurs when the contents of the intestine cannot move forward through the intestinal tract because of a partial or complete blockage of the bowel *Obstruction of the intestine causes the bowel to become vulnerable to ischemia. The intestinal mucosal barrier can suffer damage, allowing intestinal bacteria to invade the intestinal wall.*

(continued)

Diseases and Conditions—cont'd

Term	Definition
irritable bowel syndrome (IBS)	Symptom complex marked by abdominal pain and altered bowel function (typically constipation, diarrhea, or alternating constipation and diarrhea) for which no organic cause can be determined; also called *spastic colon* *Contributing or aggravating factors of IBS include anxiety and stress.*
malabsorption syndrome măl-ăb-SORP-shŭn SĬN-drŏm	Symptom complex of the small intestine characterized by the impaired passage of nutrients, minerals, or fluids through intestinal villi into the blood or lymph *Malabsorption syndrome may be associated with or caused by a number of diseases, including those affecting the intestinal mucosa. It may also be caused by surgery, such as gastric resection and ileal bypass, or by antibiotic therapy.*
melena MĔL-ĕ-nă	Dark, tarlike feces that contain digested blood from bleeding in the esophagus or stomach *Treatment requires correcting the underlying cause of bleeding.*
obesity ō-BĒ-sĭ-tē	Excessive accumulation of fat that exceeds the body's skeletal and physical standards, usually an increase of 20% or more above ideal body weight *Obesity may be caused by excessive intake of food (exogenous) or metabolic or endocrine abnormalities (endogenous).*
morbid	Obesity in which body mass index (BMI) is greater than 40, and generally 100 lb or more over ideal body weight *Morbid obesity is a disease with serious psychological, social, and medical ramifications and one that threatens necessary body functions such as respiration.*
obstipation ŏb-stĭ-PĀ-shŭn	Severe constipation, which may be caused by an intestinal obstruction
oral leukoplakia OR-ăl loo-kō-PLĀ-kē-ă *leuk/o:* white *-plakia:* plaque	Formation of white spots or patches on the mucous membrane of the tongue, lips, or cheek caused primarily by irritation *Oral leukoplakia is a precancerous condition, usually associated with pipe or cigarette smoking or ill-fitting dentures.*
pancreatitis păn-krē-ă-TĪ-tĭs *pancreat:* pancreas *-itis:* inflammation	Inflammation of the pancreas *Pancreatitis occurs when digestive enzymes attack pancreatic tissue, causing damage to the gland. The most common causes of pancreatitis are alcoholism, gallstone obstruction, drug toxicity, or infection of the pancreas caused by bacteria or viruses.*
pyloric stenosis pī-LOR-ĭk stĕ-NŌ-sĭs *pylor:* pylorus *-ic:* pertaining to *sten:* narrowing, stricture *-osis:* abnormal condition; increase (used primarily with blood cells)	Stricture or narrowing of the pyloric sphincter (circular muscle of the pylorus) at the outlet of the stomach, causing an obstruction that blocks the flow of food into the small intestine
regurgitation rē-gŭr-jĭ-TĀ-shŭn	A backward flow, as in the return of solids or fluids to the mouth from the stomach

Diseases and Conditions—cont'd

Term	Definition
ulcerative colitis kō-LĪ-tĭs	Chronic inflammatory disease of the colon, commonly beginning in the rectum or sigmoid colon and extending upward into the entire colon *Ulcerative colitis is characterized by profuse, watery diarrhea containing varying amounts of blood, mucus, and pus. Severe cases may require surgical creation of an opening (stoma) for bowel evacuation to a bag worn on the abdomen. Ulcerative colitis is associated with an increased risk of colon cancer.*

 It is time to review pathology, diseases, and conditions by completing Learning Activity 6-4.

Diagnostic, Surgical, and Therapeutic Procedures

This section introduces diagnostic, surgical, and therapeutic procedures used to diagnose and treat digestive system disorders. Descriptions are provided, along with pronunciations and word analyses for selected terms.

Procedure	Description
Diagnostic	
Endoscopic	
gastrointestinal endoscopy găs-trō-ĭn-TĔS-tĭn-ăl ĕn-DŎS-kō-pē *endo-:* in, within *-scopy:* visual examination	Visual examination of the gastrointestinal tract using a flexible fiberoptic instrument with a magnifying lens and a light source (endoscope) to identify abnormalities, including bleeding, ulcerations, and tumors *In endoscopy of the esophagus (esophagoscopy), stomach (gastroscopy), and duodenum (duodenoscopy), the endoscope is inserted through the nose or mouth. In endoscopy of the colon (colonoscopy) and sigmoid colon (sigmoidoscopy), the endoscope is inserted through the rectum. (See Fig. 6-13.)*

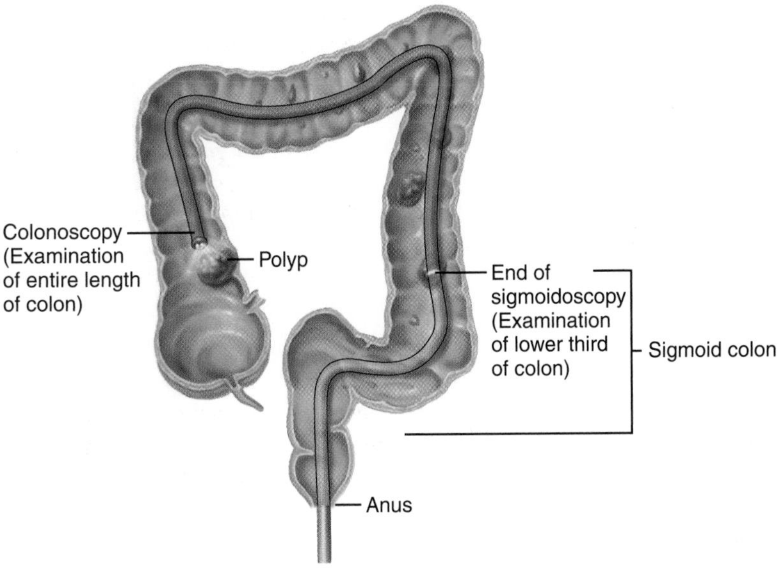

Colonoscopy (Examination of entire length of colon) — Polyp — End of sigmoidoscopy (Examination of lower third of colon) — Sigmoid colon — Anus

Figure 6-13 Colonoscopy and sigmoidoscopy.

(continued)

Diagnostic, Surgical, and Therapeutic Procedures—cont'd

Procedure	Description
Laboratory	
hepatitis panel hĕp-ă-TĪ-tĭs *hepat:* liver *-itis:* inflammation	Panel of blood tests that identifies the specific virus—hepatitis A (HAV), hepatitis B (HBV), or hepatitis C (HCV)—that is causing hepatitis by testing serum using antibodies to each of these antigens
liver function tests (LFTs)	Group of blood tests that evaluate liver injury, liver function, and conditions commonly associated with the biliary tract *LFTs evaluate liver enzymes, bilirubin, and proteins produced by the liver.*
serum bilirubin SĒ-rŭm bĭl-ĭ-ROO-bĭn	Measurement of the level of bilirubin in the blood *Elevated serum bilirubin indicates excessive destruction of erythrocytes, liver disease, or biliary tract obstruction.*
stool culture	Test to identify microorganisms or parasites present in feces that are causing a gastrointestinal infection *Feces are examined microscopically after being placed in a growth medium.*
stool guaiac GWĪ-ăk	Test that applies a substance called *guaiac* to a stool sample to detect the presence of occult (hidden) blood in the feces; also called *Hemoccult* (trade name of a modified guaiac test) *A stool guaiac test helps detect colon cancer and bleeding associated with digestive disorders.*
Imaging	
computed tomography (CT) kŏm-PŪ-tĕd tō-MŎG-ră-fē *tom/o:* to cut *-graphy:* process of recording	Imaging technique achieved by rotating an x-ray emitter around the area to be scanned and measuring the intensity of transmitted rays from different angles *In CT scanning, a computer generates a detailed cross-sectional image that appears as a slice. (See Fig. 4-5D.) In the digestive system, CT scans aid in visualizing the gallbladder, bowel, liver, bile ducts, and pancreas. They also aid in the diagnosis of tumors, cysts, inflammation, abscesses, perforation, bleeding, and obstruction.*
lower gastrointestinal series găs-trō-ĭn-TĔS-tĭn-ăl, BĂ-rē-ŭm ĔN-ĕ-mă	Radiographic images of the rectum and colon following administration of barium into the rectum; also called *lower GI series* or *barium enema* *Barium is retained in the lower GI tract during fluoroscopic and radiographic studies. It helps diagnose obstructions, tumors, and other abnormalities of the colon. (See Fig. 6-14.)*

Diagnostic, Surgical, and Therapeutic Procedures—cont'd

Procedure	Description

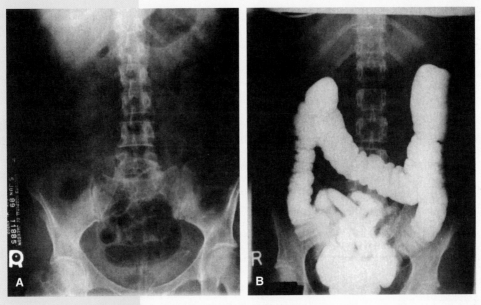

Figure 6-14 Barium enema done poorly (A) and correctly (B).

Procedure	Description
oral cholecystography (OCG) kō-lē-sĭs-TŎG-ră-fē chol/e: bile, gall cyst/o: bladder -graphy: process of recording	Radiographic images taken of the gallbladder after administration of a contrast material containing iodine, usually in the form of a tablet *OCG evaluates gallbladder function and identifies the presence of disease or gallstones.*
magnetic resonance imaging (MRI) RĔZ-ō-năns ĬM-ăj-ĭng	Technique that uses radio waves and a strong magnetic field, rather than an x-ray beam, to produce highly detailed, multiplanar, cross-sectional views of soft tissues
magnetic resonance cholangiopancreatography (MRCP) kō-lăn-jē-ō-păn-krē-ă-TŎG-ră-fē cholangi/o: bile vessel pancreat/o: pancreas -graphy: process of recording	Special MRI technique that produces detailed images of the hepatobiliary and pancreatic systems, including the liver, gallbladder, bile ducts, pancreas, and pancreatic duct *MRCP requires no contrast medium. It can help determine whether gallstones are lodged in any of the ducts surrounding the gallbladder. It may also detect tumors, inflammation, infection, or pancreatitis.*

(continued)

Diagnostic, Surgical, and Therapeutic Procedures—cont'd

Procedure	Description
ultrasonography (US) ŭl-tră-sŏn-ŎG-ră-fē *ultra-:* excess, beyond *son/o:* sound *-graphy:* process of recording	Test in which high-frequency sound waves (ultrasound) are directed at soft tissue and reflected as "echoes" to produce an image on a monitor of an internal body structure; also called *ultrasound, sonography,* and *echo* *US is a noninvasive procedure that does not require a contrast medium. It helps detect diseases and abnormalities in the digestive organs, such as the gallbladder, liver, and pancreas. It also helps locate abdominal masses outside the digestive organs.*
abdominal ăb-DŎM-ĭ-năl *abdomin:* abdomen *-al:* pertaining to	Ultrasound visualization of the abdominal aorta, liver, gallbladder, bile ducts, pancreas, kidneys, ureters, and bladder *An abdominal US helps diagnose and locate cysts, tumors, and malformations; document the progression of various diseases; and guide the insertion of instruments during surgical procedures.*
endoscopic ĕn-dō-SKŎP-ĭk *endo:* in; within *scop:* to view *-ic:* pertaining to	Combination of endoscopy and ultrasound that examines and obtains images of the digestive tract and the surrounding tissues and organs *In endoscopic US, a long, flexible tube (endoscope) inserted via the mouth or rectum emits high-frequency sound waves (ultrasound) that produce images of the organs and structures.*
upper gastrointestinal series (UGIS) gĂS-trō-ĭn-TĔS-tĭn-ăl	Radiographic images of the esophagus, stomach, and small intestine following oral administration of barium; also called *barium swallow* *UGIS is most commonly used with patients who are experiencing difficulty swallowing. It also helps identify ulcers, tumors, or an obstruction in the esophagus, stomach, or small intestine.*
Surgical	
anastomosis ă-năs-tō-MŌ-sĭs	Surgical joining of two ducts, vessels, or bowel segments to allow flow from one to another
ileorectal ĭl-ē-ō-RĔK-tăl *ile/o:* ileum *rect:* rectum *-al:* pertaining to	Surgical connection of the ileum and rectum after total colectomy, as is sometimes performed in the treatment of ulcerative colitis
intestinal ĭn-TĔS-tĭ-năl	Surgical connection of two portions of the intestines
appendectomy ăp-ĕn-DĔK-tō-mē *append:* appendix *-ectomy:* excision, removal	Excision of a diseased appendix using an open or laparoscopic procedure *Appendectomy usually occurs within 24–48 hours of the first symptoms. Delay in treatment may result in rupture of the appendix, causing peritonitis as fecal matter enters the peritoneal cavity. (See Fig. 6–15.)*
open	Excision of a diseased appendix through a 2" to 3" incision in the right lower quadrant of the abdomen
laparoscopic lăp-ă-rō-SKŎP-ĭk	Minimally invasive appendectomy using three small abdominal incisions while monitoring an enlarged image of the surgical site projected on a monitor (See Fig. 6-16.) *Laparoscopic surgery may slightly reduce recovery time. However, the procedure takes longer and has additional risks associated with inflating the abdomen with gas (pneumoperitoneum).*

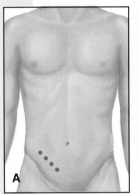 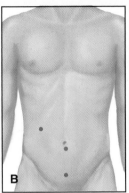

Figure 6-15 Appendectomy incision sites. (A) Open appendectomy. (B) Laparoscopic appendectomy.

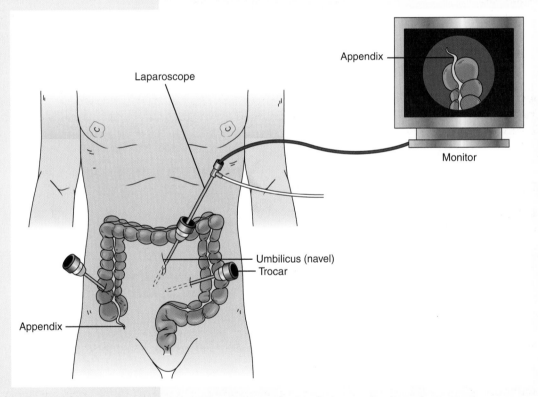

Figure 6-16 Laparoscopic appendectomy with trocars (access devices used to insert laparoscopic instruments).

(continued)

Diagnostic, Surgical, and Therapeutic Procedures—cont'd

Procedure	Description
bariatric surgery băr-ē-Ă-trĭk	Group of procedures that treat morbid obesity, a condition that arises from severe accumulation of excess weight as fatty tissue, and the resultant health problems (See Fig. 6-17.)
vertical banded gastroplasty GĂS-trō-plăs-tē	Bariatric surgery that involves vertical stapling of the upper stomach near the esophagus to reduce it to a small pouch and insertion of a band that restricts food consumption and delays its passage from the pouch, causing a feeling of fullness
Roux-en-Y gastric bypass (RGB) rū-ĕn-WĪ GĂS-trĭk	Bariatric surgery that involves stapling the stomach to decrease its size and then shortening the jejunum and connecting it to the small stomach pouch, causing the base of the duodenum leading from the nonfunctioning portion of the stomach to form a Y configuration, which decreases the pathway of food through the intestine, thus reducing absorption of calories and fats; also called *gastric bypass with gastroenterostomy* *RGB can be performed laparoscopically or as an open procedure (laparotomy), depending on the health of the patient. RGB is currently the most commonly performed weight-loss surgery.*

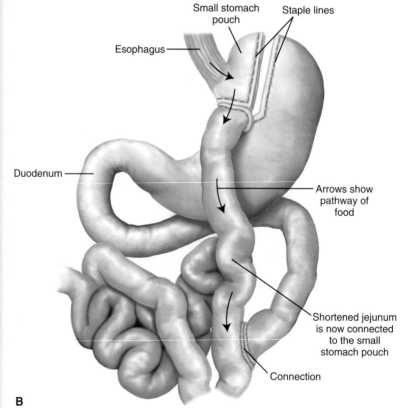

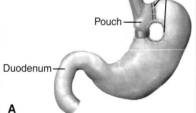

Figure 6-17 Bariatric surgery. (A) Vertical banded gastroplasty. (B) Roux-en-Y gastric bypass.

Diagnostic, Surgical, and Therapeutic Procedures—cont'd

Procedure	Description
colostomy kō-LŎS-tō-mē *col/o:* colon *-stomy:* forming an opening (mouth)	Surgical procedure in which a surgeon forms an opening (stoma) by drawing the healthy end of the colon through an incision in the anterior abdominal wall and suturing it into place *A colostomy diverts fecal flow to a colostomy bag and provides a new path for waste material to leave the body. (See Fig. 6-18.)*

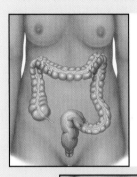 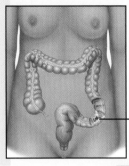 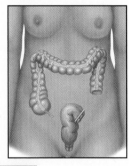

Healthy colon — Intestinal obstruction — Excision of diseased colon

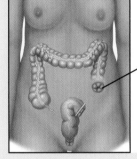 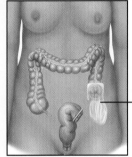

Stoma
Colostomy performed to attach healthy tissue to abdomen — Colostomy bag attached to stoma

Figure 6-18 Colostomy.

Procedure	Description
lithotripsy LĬTH-ō-trĭp-sē *lith/o:* stone, calculus *-tripsy:* crushing	Procedure for crushing a stone and eliminating its fragments surgically or using ultrasonic shock waves
extracorporeal shock-wave lithotripsy (ESWL) ĕks-tră-kor-POR-ē-ăl SHŎK-wāv	Use of shock waves as a noninvasive method to break up stones in the gallbladder or biliary ducts *In ESWL, ultrasound helps locate the stones and monitor their destruction. (See Fig. 11-4.)*
paracentesis păr-ă-sĕn-TĒ-sĭs *para-:* near, beside, beyond *-centesis:* surgical puncture	Procedure to remove fluid from the abdomen using a long, thin needle inserted through the belly; also called *abdominocentesis* *The fluid is sent to a laboratory for analysis to find the cause of the fluid accumulation. Paracentesis may also relieve belly pressure or pain in patients with cancer, cirrhosis, or ascites. (See Fig. 6-19.)*

(continued)

Diagnostic, Surgical, and Therapeutic Procedures—cont'd

Procedure	Description

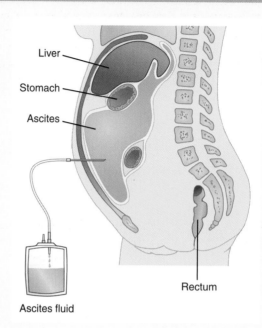

Figure 6-19 Paracentesis.

polypectomy
pŏl-ĭ-PĔK-tō-mē
polyp: small growth
-ectomy: excision, removal

Excision of a polyp

When polyps are discovered during sigmoidoscopy or colonoscopy, they are excised for microscopic tissue examination to detect abnormal or cancerous cells. (See Fig. 6-20.)

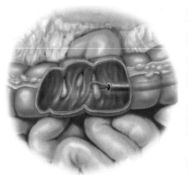

Polyps are removed from
colon for examination

Figure 6-20 Polypectomy.

Therapeutic

nasogastric intubation
nā-zō-GĂS-trĭk ĭn-tū-BĀ-shŭn
nas/o: nose
gastr: stomach
-ic: pertaining to

Insertion of a nasogastric tube through the nose into the stomach to relieve gastric distention by removing gas, food, or gastric secretions; instill medication, food, or fluids; or obtain a specimen for laboratory analysis

Pharmacology

Various pharmaceutical agents are available to counteract abnormal conditions that occur in the GI tract. Antacids counteract or decrease excessive stomach acid, the cause of heartburn, gastric discomfort, and gastric reflux. Antidiarrheals and antiemetics help preserve water and electrolytes, which are essential for body hydration and homeostasis. Medications that increase or decrease peristalsis help regulate the speed at which food passes through the GI tract. These drugs include agents that relieve "cramping" (**antispasmodics**) and those that help in the movement of material through a sluggish bowel (**laxatives**). (See Table 6-1.)

Table 6-1	**Drugs Used to Treat Digestive Disorders**		
This table lists common drug classifications used to treat digestive disorders, their therapeutic actions, and selected generic and trade names.			
Classification	**Therapeutic Action**		**Generic and Trade Names**
antacids ănt-ĂS-ĭds	Counteract or neutralize acidity, usually in the stomach *Antacids treat and prevent heartburn and acid reflux.*		**calcium carbonate** KĂL-sē-ŭm KĂR-bŏn-āt *Rolaids, Tums* **aluminum hydroxide and magnesium hydroxide** ă-LŪ-mĭ-nŭm hī-DRŎKS-īd, măg-NĒ-zē-ŭm hī-DRŎKS-īd *Maalox, Mylanta*
antidiarrheals an-tĭ-dī-ă-RĒ-ăls	Control loose stools and relieve diarrhea by absorbing excess water in the bowel or slowing peristalsis in the intestinal tract		**loperamide** lō-PĔR-ă-mīd *Imodium* **kaolin/pectin** KĀ-ō-lĭn, PĔK-tĭn *Donnagel-MB, Kapectolin*
antiemetics ăn-tĭ-ē-MĔT-ĭks	Control nausea and vomiting by blocking nerve impulses to the vomiting center of the brain *Some antiemetics act by hastening movement of food through the digestive tract.*		**prochlorperazine** prō-klor-PĔR-ă-zēn *Compazine, Compro* **ondansetron** ŏn-DĂN-sĕ-trŏn *Zofran*
antispasmodics ăn-tē-spăz-MŎD-ĭks	Decrease gastrointestinal (GI) spasms by slowing peristalsis and motility throughout the GI tract *Antispasmodics help treat irritable bowel syndrome (IBS), spastic colon, and diverticulitis.*		**glycopyrrolate** glī-kō-PĬR-rō-lāt *Robinul* **dicyclomine** dī-SĪ-klō-mēn *Bentyl*
histamine-2 (H₂) blockers	Inhibit secretion of stomach acid from the gastric cells by blocking the H_2 receptor *H_2 blockers treat acid reflux and gastric or duodenal ulcers.*		**ranitidine** ră-NĬ-tĭ-dēn *Zantac* **famotidine** fă-MŌ-tĭ-dēn *Pepcid*

(continued)

Table 6-1　Drugs Used to Treat Digestive Disorders—cont'd

Classification	Therapeutic Action	Generic and Trade Names
laxatives LĂK-să-tĭvs	Treat constipation by increasing peristaltic activity in the large intestine or increasing water and electrolyte secretion into the bowel to induce defecation	**senna, sennosides** SĔN-ă, SĔN-ō-sīdz *Senokot, Senolax* **psyllium** SĬL-ē-ŭm *Metamucil, Natural Fiber Supplement*
proton pump inhibitors	Suppress basal and stimulated acid production by inhibiting the acid pump in the gastric cells *Proton pump inhibitors treat gastric and duodenal ulcers and acid reflux. These drugs are more potent acid inhibitors than the H$_2$ blockers.*	**omeprazole** ō-MĔP-ră-zōl *Prilosec* **esomeprazole** ĕs-ō-MĔP-ră-zōl *Nexium*

Abbreviations

This section introduces digestive-related abbreviations and their meanings.

Abbreviation	Meaning	Abbreviation	Meaning
AIDS	acquired immune deficiency syndrome	**GI**	gastrointestinal
Ba	barium	**HAV**	hepatitis A virus
BaE, BE	barium enema	**HBV**	hepatitis B virus
BM	bowel movement	**HCV**	hepatitis C virus
BMI	body mass index	**HDV**	hepatitis D virus
CT	computed tomography	**HEV**	hepatitis E virus
EGD	esophagogastroduodenoscopy	**IBS**	irritable bowel syndrome
ESWL	extracorporeal shock-wave lithotripsy	**LFT**	liver function test
EUS	endoscopic ultrasonography (x-ray studies)	**LUQ**	left upper quadrant
GBS	gallbladder series	**MRCP**	magnetic resonance cholangiopancreatography
GER	gastroesophageal reflux	**NG**	nasogastric
GERD	gastroesophageal reflux disease	**NSAID**	nonsteroidal anti-inflammatory drugs

Abbreviation	Meaning	Abbreviation	Meaning
OCG	oral cholecystography	**RGB**	Roux-en-Y gastric bypass
PE	physical examination; pulmonary embolism; pressure-equalizing (tube)	**RUQ**	right upper quadrant
PUD	peptic ulcer disease	**UGIS**	upper gastrointestinal series
R/O	rule out	**US**	ultrasound; ultrasonography

It is time to review procedures, pharmacology, and abbreviations by completing Learning Activity 6-5.

LEARNING ACTIVITIES

The activities that follow provide a review of the digestive system terms introduced in this chapter. Complete each activity and review your answers to evaluate your understanding of the chapter.

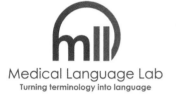

Medical Language Lab
Turning terminology into language

Visit the Medical Language Lab at *medicallanguagelab.com.* Use it to enhance your study and reinforcement of this chapter with the flash-card activity. We recommend that you complete the flash-card activity before starting Learning Activities 6-1 and 6-2.

Learning Activity 6-1

Medical Word Elements

Use the listed elements to build medical words. You may use the elements more than once.

Combining Forms		Suffixes		Prefixes
an/o	jejun/o	-al	-pepsia	an-
colon/o	pharyng/o	-emesis	-phagia	dys-
dent/o	sial/o	-ic	-plasty	hypo-
esophag/o	stomat/o	-itis	-rrhaphy	peri-
gastr/o		-lith	-scope	
gingiv/o		-pathy	-scopy	
hemat/o				

  1. inflammation of the gum(s) _____

  2. visual examination of the colon _____

  3. surgical repair of the stomach _____

  4. pertaining to under or below the stomach _____

  5. bad, painful, or difficult digestion _____

  6. calculus in a salivary gland or duct _____

  7. disease of the mouth _____

  8. pertaining to around the anus _____

  9. suture of the jejunum (second part of the small intestine) _____

10. inflammation of the pharynx _____

11. instrument to examine the esophagus _____

12. without an appetite _____

13. vomiting blood _____

14. pertaining to the teeth _____

15. bad, painful, or difficult swallowing or eating _____

✓ *Check your answers in Appendix A. Review any material that you did not answer correctly.*

Correct Answers _____ X 6.67 = _____ % Score

Building Medical Words

Use *esophag/o* (esophagus) to build words that mean

1. pain in the esophagus _____
2. spasm of the esophagus _____
3. stricture or narrowing of the esophagus _____

Use *gastr/o* (stomach) to build words that mean

4. inflammation of the stomach _____
5. pain in the stomach _____
6. disease of the stomach _____

Use *duoden/o* (duodenum), *jejun/o* (jejunum), or *ile/o* (ileum) to build words that mean

7. excision of all or part of the jejunum _____
8. relating to the duodenum _____
9. inflammation of the ileum _____
10. pertaining to the jejunum and ileum _____

Use *enter/o* (usually small intestine) to build words that mean

11. inflammation of the small intestine _____
12. disease of the small intestine _____
13. inflammation of the small intestine and colon _____

Use *col/o* (colon) to build words that mean

14. inflammation of the colon _____
15. pertaining to the colon and rectum _____
16. prolapse or downward displacement of the colon _____
17. disease of the colon _____

Use *proct/o* (anus, rectum) or *rect/o* (rectum) to build words that mean

18. narrowing or constriction of the rectum _____
19. herniation of the rectum _____
20. paralysis of the anus (anal muscles) _____

Use *chol/e* (bile, gall) to build words that mean

21. inflammation of the gallbladder _____
22. abnormal condition of a gallstone _____

Use *hepat/o* (liver) or *pancreat/o* (pancreas) to build words that mean

23. tumor of the liver _____

24. enlargement of the liver _____

25. inflammation of the pancreas _____

✓ *Check your answers in Appendix A. Review material that you did not answer correctly.*

Correct Answers _____ X 4 = _____ % Score

Building Surgical Words

Build a surgical word that means

1. excision of gums (tissue) _____
2. partial or complete excision of the tongue _____
3. repair of the esophagus _____
4. removal of part or all of the stomach _____
5. forming an opening between the stomach and jejunum _____
6. excision of (part of) the esophagus _____
7. forming an opening between the stomach, small intestine, and colon _____
8. surgical repair of the small intestine _____
9. fixation of the small intestine (to the abdominal wall) _____
10. suture of the bile duct _____
11. forming an opening into the colon _____
12. fixation of a movable liver (to the abdominal wall) _____
13. surgical repair of the anus or rectum _____
14. removal of the gallbladder _____
15. surgical repair of a bile duct _____

✓ *Check your answers in Appendix A. Review material that you did not answer correctly.*

Correct Answers _____ X 6.67 = _____ % Score

Learning Activity 6-4

Diseases and Conditions

Match the terms with the definitions in the numbered list.

anorexia	Crohn disease	hemorrhoids
ascites	dysphagia	leukoplakia
borborygmus	flatus	melena
cachexia	halitosis	obstipation
cirrhosis	hematemesis	steatorrhea

1. vomiting blood _____
2. difficulty swallowing or inability to swallow _____
3. varicose veins in the rectal area _____
4. foul-smelling breath _____
5. loss of appetite _____
6. dark, tarry stools caused by presence of blood in the GI tract _____
7. yellowing of the skin caused by liver disease _____
8. state of ill health, malnutrition, and wasting _____
9. intractable constipation _____
10. gurgling audible noises caused by pass of gas through the liquid contents of the stomach _____
11. abnormal accumulation of fluid in the abdominal cavity _____
12. form of inflammatory bowel disease, usually of the ileum _____
13. passage of fat in large amounts in the feces _____
14. formation of white patches on the mucous membrane of the cheek _____
15. gas in the gastrointestinal tract _____

> ✓ *Check your answers in Appendix A. Review any material that you did not answer correctly.*

Correct Answers _____ X 6.67 = _____ % Score

Learning Activity 6-5
Procedures, Pharmacology, and Abbreviations

Match the terms with the definitions in the numbered list.

anastomosis	*choledochoplasty*	*intubation*	*proctosigmoidoscopy*
antacids	*endoscopy*	*laxatives*	*stat*
antiemetics	*ESWL*	*liver function tests*	*stool culture*
antispasmodics	*gastroscopy*	*lower GI series*	*stool guaiac*
bariatric	*IBS*	*MRCP*	*upper GI series*

1. procedure to visualize biliary and pancreatic ducts by using magnetic resonance imaging _____
2. procedure in which shock waves break up calculi in the biliary ducts _____
3. disorder that affects the colon and causes constipation and diarrhea; also called spastic colon _____
4. agents that alleviate muscle spasms _____
5. surgical reconstruction of a bile duct _____
6. administration of a barium enema while a series of radiographs is taken of the colon _____
7. visual examination of the stomach _____
8. agents that control nausea and vomiting _____
9. insertion of a tube into any hollow organ _____
10. surgical formation of a passage or opening between two hollow viscera or vessels _____
11. detects presence of blood in the feces; also called *Hemoccult* _____
12. visual examination of a cavity or canal using a specialized lighted instrument _____
13. used to treat constipation _____
14. neutralize excess acid in the stomach and help to relieve gastritis and ulcer pain _____
15. test to identify microorganisms present in feces _____
16. measures the levels of certain enzymes, bilirubin, and various proteins _____
17. surgery that treats morbid obesity _____
18. immediately _____
19. endoscopic procedure for visualization of the rectosigmoid colon _____
20. radiographic imaging of the esophagus, duodenum, and stomach after ingestion of barium _____

Check your answers in Appendix A. Review material that you did not answer correctly.

Correct Answers _____ X 5 = _____ % Score

DOCUMENTING HEALTH-CARE ACTIVITIES

This section provides practical application activities in the form of exercises to help students develop skills in documenting patient care. First, read the medical report. Then complete the activities and exercises that follow.

Documenting Health-Care Activity 6-1
Chart Note: GI Evaluation

Jones, Roberta

March 15, 20xx   **Age: 50**

History of Present Illness: Patient's abdominal pain began 2 years ago when she first had intermittent, sharp epigastric pain. Each episode lasted 2–4 hours. Eventually, she was diagnosed as having cholecystitis with cholelithiasis and underwent cholecystectomy. Three to five large calcified stones were found.

Postoperative Course: Her postoperative course was uneventful until 4 months ago when she began having continuous, deep, right-sided pain. This pain followed a crescendo pattern and peaked several weeks ago, at a time when family stress was also at its climax. Since then, the pain has been following a decrescendo pattern. It does not cause any nausea or vomiting, does not trigger any urge to defecate, and is not alleviated by passage of flatus. Her PMH is significant only for tonsillectomy, appendectomy, and the cholecystectomy. Her PE findings indicated that there was no hepatomegaly or splenomegaly. The rectal examination confirmed normal sphincter tone and heme-negative stool.

Impression: Abdominal pain. Rule out hepatomegaly and splenomegaly.

Plan: Schedule a complete barium work-up for possible obstruction.

Joseph Bogata, MD
Joseph Bogata, MD

bcg

Terminology

The terms listed in the table that follows are taken from *Chart Note: GI Evaluation*. Use a medical dictionary such as *Taber's Cyclopedic Medical Dictionary,* the appendices of this book, or other resources to define each term. Then review the pronunciation for each term and practice by reading the medical record aloud.

Term	Definition
appendectomy* ăp-ĕn-DĔK-tō-mē	
cholecystectomy kō-lē-sĭs-TĔK-tō-mē	
cholecystitis kō-lē-sĭs-TĪ-tĭs	
cholelithiasis* kō-lē-lĭ-THĪ-ă-sĭs	
crescendo krĕ-SHĔN-dō	
decrescendo dā-krĕ-SHĔN-dō	
defecate DĔF-ĕ-kāt	
flatus FLĀ-tŭs	
heme-negative stool hēm-NĔG-ă-tĭv	
hepatomegaly hĕp-ă-tō-MĔG-ă-lē	
intermittent ĭn-tĕr-MĬT-ĕnt	
nausea NAW-sē-ă	
PE	
PMH	
postoperative pōst-ŎP-ĕr-ă-tĭv	

(continued)

Term	Definition
R/O	
splenomegaly splē-nō-MĔG-ă-lē	
tonsillectomy tōn-sĭl-ĔK-tō-mē	

*Refer to Figure 6-15 and Figure 6-16 for a visual illustration of this term.

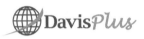

Visit the *Medical Terminology Systems* online resource center at Davis*Plus* to practice pronunciation and reinforce the meanings of the terms in this medical report.

Critical Thinking

Review *Chart Note: GI Evaluation* to answer the questions.

1. Referring to Figure 6-3, describe the location of the gallbladder in relation to the liver.

_____

_____

_____

_____

2. Why did the patient undergo the cholecystectomy?

_____

_____

_____

_____

3. What were the patient's prior surgeries?

_____

_____

_____

_____

4. How does the patient's most recent postoperative episode of discomfort (pain) differ from the initial pain she described?

_____

_____

_____

_____

Documenting Health-Care Activity 6-2

Operative Report: Esophagogastroduodenoscopy with Biopsy

OPERATIVE REPORT

Date: May 14, 20xx   Physician: Dante Riox, MD
Patient: Franks, Roberta   Room: 703

Preoperative Diagnosis: Hematemesis of unknown etiology

Postoperative Diagnosis: Diffuse gastritis and duodenitis

Procedure: Esophagogastroduodenoscopy with biopsy

Specimen: Biopsies from gastric antrum and duodenal bulb

Estimated Blood Loss: Nil

Complications: None

Time Under Sedation: 20 minutes

Procedure and Findings: After obtaining informed consent regarding the procedure, its risks, and its alternatives, the patient was taken to the GI laboratory, where she was placed on the examining table in the left lateral recumbent position. She was given nasal oxygen at 3 liters per minute and monitored with a pulse oximeter throughout the procedure. Through a previously inserted intravenous line, the patient was sedated with a total of 50 mg of Demerol intravenously plus 4 mg of Midazolam intravenously throughout the procedure. The Fujinon computed tomography scan videoendoscope was then readily introduced, and the following organs were evaluated:

Esophagus: The esophageal mucosa appeared normal throughout. No other abnormalities were seen. Specifically, there was prior evidence of esophageal varices.

Stomach: There was diffuse erythema with old blood seen within the stomach. No ulcerations, erosions, or fresh bleeding was seen. A representative biopsy was obtained from the gastric antrum and submitted to the pathology laboratory.

Duodenum: Punctate erythema was noted in the duodenal bulb. There was some friability. No ulcerations, erosions, or active bleeding was seen. A bulbar biopsy was obtained. The second portion of the duodenum appeared normal.

The patient tolerated the procedure well. Patient was transferred to the recovery room in stable condition.

Dante Riox, MD
Dante Riox, MD

dr:bg

D: 5-14-20xx; T: 5-14-20xx

Terminology

The terms listed in the table that follows are taken from *Operative Report: Esophagogastroduodenoscopy with Biopsy.* Use a medical dictionary such as *Taber's Cyclopedic Medical Dictionary,* the appendices of this book, or other resources to define each term. Then review the pronunciation for each term and practice by reading the medical record aloud.

Term	Definition
Demerol DĔM-ĕr-ŏl	
duodenal bulb dū-ō-DĒ-năl bŭlb	
duodenitis dū-ŏd-ĕ-NĪ-tĭs	
erythema ĕr-ĭ-THĒ-mă	
esophageal varices ĕ-sŏf-ă-JĒ-ăl VĂR-ĭ-sēz	
esophagogastro- duodenoscopy ĕ-sŏf-ă-gō-găs-trō- doo-ō-dĕn-ŎS-kō-pē	
etiology ē-tē-ŎL-ō-jē	
friability frī-ă-BĬL-ĭ-tē	
gastric antrum GĂS-trĭk ĂN-trŭm	
gastritis găs-TRĪ-tĭs	
hematemesis hĕm-ăt-ĔM-ĕ-sĭs	
lateral recumbent LĂT-ĕr-ăl rē-KŬM-bĕnt	
Midazolam mĭ-dā-zōl-ăm	
oximeter ŏk-SĬM-ĕ-tĕr	

(continued)

Term	Definition
punctate erythema PŬNK-tāt ĕr-ĭ-THĒ-mă	
tomography tō-MŎG-ră-fē	
videoendoscope vĭd-ē-ō-ĔND-ō-skōp	

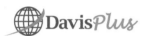

Visit the *Medical Terminology Systems* online resource center at Davis*Plus* to practice pronunciation and reinforce the meanings of the terms in this medical report.

Critical Thinking

Review the medical report *Operative Report: Esophagogastroduodenoscopy with Biopsy* to answer the questions.

1. What caused the hematemesis?

   _____

   _____

   _____

   _____

2. What procedures were carried out to determine the cause of bleeding?

   _____

   _____

   _____

   _____

3. How much blood did the patient lose during the procedure?

   _____

   _____

   _____

   _____

4. Were any ulcerations or erosions found during the exploratory procedure that might account for the bleeding?

   _____

   _____

   _____

   _____

5. What type of sedation was used during the procedure?

   _____

   _____

   _____

   _____

6. What did the doctors find when they examined the stomach and duodenum?

_____

_____

_____

_____

Constructing Chart Notes

To construct chart notes, replace the italicized and boldfaced terms in each of the two case studies with one of the listed medical terms.

anorexia	gastric reflux	jaundice
antacids	hepatomegaly	nausea
dyspepsia	hiatal hernia	sclerae
dysphagia		

During her annual checkup, Mrs. L. complains that she has (1) *difficulty swallowing.* Also, she is awakened at night with a feeling of (2) *difficult or painful digestion.* She further complains of (3) *regurgitation of stomach acid* and has been taking Tums and Rolaids. She feels that the (4) *medications* to neutralize the backflow of acid from her stomach have not been effective. After a thorough examination along with some radiographic procedures, the doctor suspects her symptoms are caused by a (5) *part of her stomach herniating up through the opening of the diaphragm.*

1. _____
2. _____
3. _____
4. _____
5. _____

Mr. K. recently returned from Haiti where he worked with other volunteers from his church. Their purpose was to help homeless families rebuild their communities. Lately, he complains of (6) *no appetite* and feeling feverish. He also complains of (7) *unpleasant queasy sensations of discomfort in the region of his stomach.* Today, he presents to the clinic, and his doctor notes that the (8) *whites of his eyes* are now (9) *yellow in color.* After further examination and a series of blood tests, the doctor suspects that Mr. K. suffers from an (10) *enlarged liver* and should undergo further testing for hepatitis A.

6. _____
7. _____
8. _____
9. _____
10. _____

Check your answers in Appendix A. Review any material that you did not answer correctly.

Correct Answers _____ X 10 = _____ % Score

Respiratory System

Chapter Outline

Objectives

Upon completion of this chapter, you will be able to:

- Locate and describe the structures of the respiratory system.
- Describe the functional relationship between the respiratory system and other body systems.
- Pronounce, spell, and build words related to the respiratory system.
- Describe diseases, conditions, and procedures related to the respiratory system.
- Explain pharmacology related to the treatment of respiratory disorders.
- Demonstrate your knowledge of this chapter by completing the learning and documenting health-care activities.

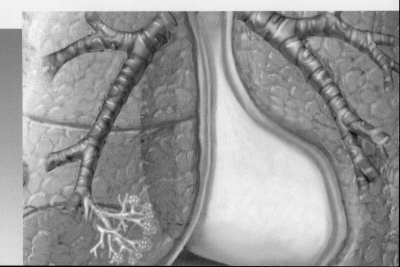

Anatomy and Physiology

The respiratory system is responsible for the exchange of **oxygen (O_2)** and **carbon dioxide (CO_2)**. Oxygen is essential for life. It is carried to all cells of the body in exchange for CO_2, a waste product. The lungs and airways transport oxygen-enriched air from the atmosphere to the lungs and carry waste CO_2 from the lungs to the atmosphere by a process called **breathing (ventilation).** Breathing helps regulate the **pH** (acidity/alkalinity) of the blood, thereby helping maintain a stable internal environment of the body **(homeostasis).**

Anatomy and Physiology Key Terms

This section introduces important respiratory system terms and their definitions. The key terms are highlighted in color in the Anatomy and Physiology section. Word analyses for selected terms are also provided. Pronounce the term, and place a check mark in the box after you do so.

Term	Definition
carbon dioxide (CO_2) KĂR-bŏn dī-ŎK-sīd □	Tasteless, colorless, odorless gas produced by body cells during metabolism *The blood carries CO_2 to the lungs, which then exhale it.*
cartilage KĂR-tĭ-lĭj □	Tough, elastic connective tissue that is more rigid than ligaments but less dense than bone *The tip of the nose and the outer ear are composed of cartilage.*
cilia SĬL-ē-ă □	Minute, hairlike structures that extend from the surface of a cell *Cilia in the trachea move particles upward to the pharynx, a mechanism called the* **cilia escalator.** *Habitual smoking destroys the cilia escalator.*
diffuse dĭ-FŪZ □	To move or spread out a substance at random, rather than by chemical reaction or application of external forces
oxygen (O_2) ŎK-sĭ-jĕn □	Tasteless, odorless, colorless gas essential for human respiration
pH	Symbol that indicates the degree of acidity or alkalinity of a substance *Increasing acidity is expressed as a number less than 7; increasing alkalinity is expressed as a number greater than 7; 7 indicates a neutral substance.*
serous membrane SĒR-ŭs MĔM-brăn □ *ser:* serum *-ous:* pertaining to	Thin layer of tissue that covers internal body cavities and secretes a fluid that keeps the membrane moist; also called *serosa*

Pronunciation Help	Long Sound	ā — rate	ē — rebirth	ī — isle	ō — over	ū — unite
	Short Sound	ă — apple	ĕ — ever	ĭ — it	ŏ — not	ŭ — cut

Upper Respiratory Tract

The breathing process begins with inhalation. (See Fig. 7-1.) Air is drawn into the (1) **nasal cavity,** a chamber lined with **mucous membranes** and tiny hairs called **cilia.** Here, air is filtered, heated, and moistened to prepare it for its journey to the lungs. The nasal cavity is divided into a right and left side by a vertical partition of **cartilage** called the **nasal septum.**

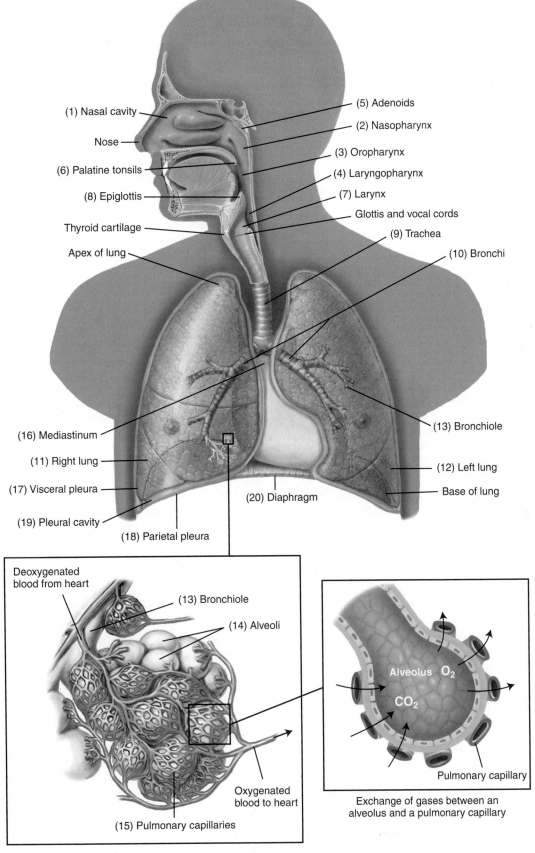

(1) Nasal cavity

Nose

(6) Palatine tonsils

(8) Epiglottis

Thyroid cartilage

Apex of lung

(16) Mediastinum

(11) Right lung

(17) Visceral pleura

(19) Pleural cavity

(18) Parietal pleura

(5) Adenoids

(2) Nasopharynx

(3) Oropharynx

(4) Laryngopharynx

(7) Larynx

Glottis and vocal cords

(9) Trachea

(10) Bronchi

(13) Bronchiole

(12) Left lung

Base of lung

(20) Diaphragm

Deoxygenated blood from heart

(13) Bronchiole

(14) Alveoli

Oxygenated blood to heart

(15) Pulmonary capillaries

Alveolus O_2

CO_2

Pulmonary capillary

Exchange of gases between an alveolus and a pulmonary capillary

Figure 7-1 Anterior view of the upper and lower respiratory tracts.

Olfactory neurons are receptors for the sense of smell. They are covered with a layer of mucus and located deep in the nasal cavity, embedded among the epithelial cells lining the nasal tract. Because they are located higher in the nasal passage than air normally travels during breathing, a person must sniff or inhale deeply to identify weak odors. Air passes from the nasal cavity to the throat **(pharynx),** a muscular tube that serves as a passageway for food and air. The pharynx consists of three sections: the (2) **nasopharynx,** posterior to the nose; the (3) **oropharynx,** posterior to the mouth; and the (4) **laryngopharynx,** superior to the larynx.

Within the nasopharynx is a collection of lymphoid tissue known as (5) **adenoids** (pharyngeal tonsils). The (6) **palatine tonsils,** more commonly known as **tonsils,** are located in the oropharynx. They protect the opening to the respiratory tract from microscopic organisms that may attempt entry by this route. The (7) **larynx** (voice box) contains the structures that make vocal sounds possible. A leaf-shaped structure on top of the larynx, the (8) **epiglottis,** seals off the air passage to the lungs during swallowing. This function ensures that food or liquids do not obstruct the flow of air to the lungs. The larynx is a short passage that joins the pharynx with the (9) **trachea** (windpipe). The trachea is composed of smooth muscle embedded with C-shaped rings of cartilage, which provide rigidity to keep the air passage open.

Lower Respiratory Tract

The trachea divides into two branches called (10) **bronchi** (singular, **bronchus**). One branch leads to the (11) **right lung** and the other to the (12) **left lung.** The inner walls of the trachea and bronchi are composed of **mucous membrane (mucosa)** embedded with cilia. This membrane traps incoming particles, and the cilia move the entrapped material upward into the pharynx, where it is expelled by coughing, sneezing, or swallowing. Like the trachea, bronchi contain C-shaped rings of cartilage.

Each bronchus divides into smaller and smaller branches, eventually forming (13) **bronchioles.** At the end of the bronchioles are tiny air sacs called (14) **alveoli** (singular, **alveolus**). An alveolus resembles a small balloon because it expands and contracts with inflow and outflow of air. The (15) **pulmonary capillaries** lie next to the thin tissue membranes of the alveoli. Carbon dioxide **diffuses** from the blood within the pulmonary capillaries and enters the alveolar spaces, and O_2 from the alveoli diffuses into the blood. After the exchange of gases, freshly oxygenated blood returns to the heart. Oxygen is now ready for delivery to all body tissues.

The lungs are divided into lobes: three lobes in the right lung and two lobes in the left lung. The space between the right and left lungs is called the (16) **mediastinum.** It contains the heart, aorta, esophagus, and bronchi. A **serous membrane,** the pleura, covers the lobes of the lungs and folds over to line the walls of the thoracic cavity. The membrane lying closest to the lung is the (17) **visceral pleura;** the membrane that lines the thoracic cavity is the (18) **parietal pleura.** The space between these two membranes is the (19) **pleural cavity.** It contains a small amount of lubricating fluid, which permits the visceral pleura to glide smoothly over the parietal pleura during breathing.

Ventilation depends on a pressure differential between the atmosphere and chest cavity. A large muscular partition, the (20) **diaphragm,** lies between the chest and abdominal cavities. The diaphragm assists in changing the volume of the thoracic cavity to produce the needed pressure differential for ventilation. When the diaphragm contracts, it partially descends into the abdominal cavity, thus decreasing the pressure within the chest and drawing air into the lungs **(inspiration).** When the diaphragm relaxes, it slowly reenters the thoracic cavity, thus increasing the pressure within the chest. As pressure increases, air leaves the lungs **(expiration).** The intercostal muscles assist the diaphragm in changing the volume of the thoracic cavity by elevating and lowering the rib cage. (See Fig. 7-2.)

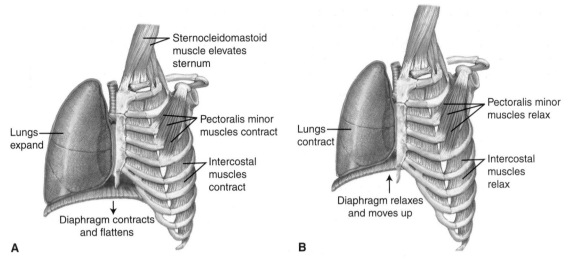

Figure 7-2 Breathing muscles. (A) Inspiration. (B) Expiration.

Pulmonary Respiration

Pulmonary respiration is the process by which O_2 is taken from air and carried to body cells for their use, and CO_2 and water, the waste products generated by these cells, are carried to the lungs and returned to the environment. Respiration includes four separate processes:

- **pulmonary ventilation (breathing),** a largely involuntary action that moves air into (inspiration) and out of (expiration) the lungs in response to changes in blood O_2 and CO_2 levels and nervous stimulation of the diaphragm and intercostal muscles
- **external respiration,** the exchange of O_2 and CO_2 between the alveoli and the blood in the pulmonary capillaries
- **transport of respiratory gases,** the movement of O_2 to body cells and CO_2 to the lungs by means of the cardiovascular system
- **internal respiration,** the exchange of O_2 and CO_2 between body cells and the blood in systemic capillaries.

Anatomy Review: Respiratory System

To review the anatomy of the respiratory system, label the illustration using the listed terms.

adenoids   *epiglottis*   *nasal cavity*   *pleural cavity*

alveoli   *laryngopharynx*   *nasopharynx*   *pulmonary capillaries*

bronchi   *larynx*   *oropharynx*   *right lung*

bronchiole   *left lung*   *palatine tonsils*   *trachea*

diaphragm   *mediastinum*   *parietal pleura*   *visceral pleura*

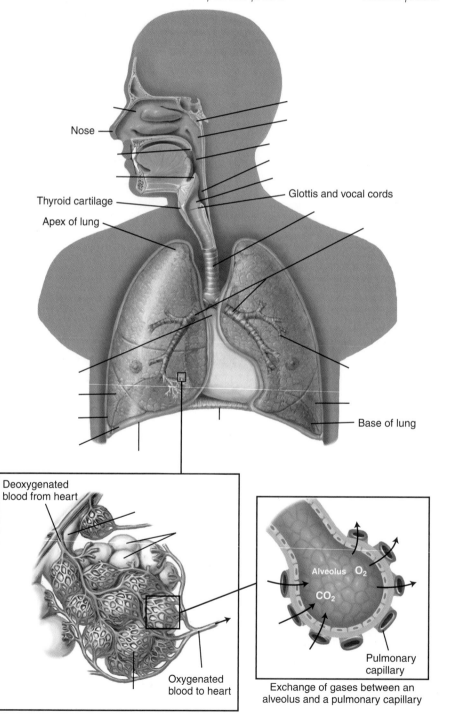

Nose

Thyroid cartilage

Apex of lung

Glottis and vocal cords

Base of lung

Deoxygenated blood from heart

Oxygenated blood to heart

Alveolus O₂

CO₂

Pulmonary capillary

Exchange of gases between an alveolus and a pulmonary capillary

Check your answers by referring to Figure 7-1 on page 181. Review material that you did not answer correctly.

CONNECTING BODY SYSTEMS—RESPIRATORY SYSTEM

The main function of the respiratory system is to provide oxygen to the entire body and expel carbon dioxide from the body. Specific functional relationships between the respiratory system and other body systems are summarized here.

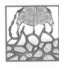

Blood, Lymphatic, and Immune

- The tonsils, adenoids, and other immune structures in the respiratory tract protect against pathogens that attempt entry through respiratory passageways.

Cardiovascular

- The respiratory system provides O_2 and removes CO_2 from cardiac tissue.

Digestive

- The respiratory system provides O_2 needed for digestive functions.
- The respiratory system removes CO_2 produced by the organs of digestion.
- The respiratory and digestive systems share the pharynx, an anatomic structure of digestion.

Endocrine

- The respiratory system helps maintain a stable pH required for proper functioning of the endocrine glands.

Female Reproductive

- Respiratory rate increases in response to sexual activity.
- Fetal respiration occurs during pregnancy.

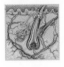

Integumentary

- The respiratory system furnishes O_2 and disposes of CO_2 to maintain healthy skin.

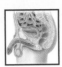

Male Reproductive

- Respiratory rate increases in response to sexual activity.
- The respiratory system helps maintain pH for gonadal hormone function.
- Oxygen is supplied to reproductive structures to maintain viable sperm.

Musculoskeletal

- The respiratory system provides O_2 for muscle contraction.
- The respiratory system eliminates CO_2 produced by muscles.
- The respiratory system provides O_2 for bone development.

Nervous

- The respiratory system provides O_2 for brain, spinal cord, and sensory organ functions.
- The respiratory system helps maintain a stable pH for neural function.

Urinary

- The respiratory system supplies O_2 and removes CO_2 to maintain proper functioning of urinary structures.
- The respiratory system assists the urinary structures in regulating pH by removing CO_2.

Medical Word Elements

This section introduces combining forms, suffixes, and prefixes related to the respiratory system. Word analyses are also provided. From the information provided, complete the meaning of the medical words in the right-hand column. The first one is completed for you.

Element	Meaning	Word Analysis
Combining Forms		
Upper Respiratory Tract		
nas/o	nose	**nas**/al (NĀ-zl): *pertaining to the nose* -*al:* pertaining to
rhin/o		**rhin/o**/plasty (RĪ-nō-plăs-tē): _____ -*plasty:* surgical repair *Rhinoplasty is performed to correct birth defects or for cosmetic purposes.*
sept/o	septum	**sept/o**/plasty (SĔP-tō-plăs-tē): _____ -*plasty:* surgical repair *Septoplasty is commonly performed to correct a deviated septum.*
sinus/o	sinus, cavity	**sinus/o**/tomy (sī-nŭs-ŎT-ō-mē): _____ -*tomy:* incision *Sinusotomy is performed to improve breathing or for drainage in unresponsive sinusitis.*
pharyng/o	pharynx (throat)	**pharyng/o**/scope (făr-ĬN-gō-skōp): _____ -*scope:* instrument for examining
adenoid/o	adenoids	**adenoid**/ectomy (ăd-ĕ-noyd-ĔK-tō-mē): _____ -*ectomy:* excision, removal
tonsill/o	tonsils	peri/**tonsill**/ar (pĕr-ĭ-TŎN-sĭ-lăr): _____ *peri-:* around -*ar:* pertaining to
epiglott/o	epiglottis	**epiglott**/itis (ĕp-ĭ-glŏt-Ī-tĭs): _____ -*itis:* inflammation *Because the epiglottis seals the opening to the lungs, inflammation can lead to severe airway obstruction and death. Epiglottitis is treated as a medical emergency.*
laryng/o	larynx (voice box)	**laryng/o**/plegia (lă-rĭn-gō-PLĒ-jē-ă): _____ -*plegia:* paralysis
trache/o	trachea (windpipe)	**trache/o**/plasty (TRĀ-kē-ō-plăs-tē): _____ -*plasty:* surgical repair *Tracheoplasty is performed to correct a narrow or stenotic trachea.*

Medical Word Elements—cont'd

Element	Meaning	Word Analysis
Lower Respiratory Tract		
bronchi/o	bronchus (plural, bronchi)	**bronchi**/ectasis (brŏng-kē-ĔK-tă-sĭs): _____ *-ectasis:* dilation, expansion *Bronchiectasis is associated with various lung conditions and is commonly accompanied by chronic infection.*
bronch/o		**bronch/o**/scope (BRŎNG-kō-skōp): _____ *-scope:* instrument for examining *A bronchoscope is a flexible tube that is passed through the nose or mouth to enable inspection of the lungs and collection of tissue biopsies and secretions for analysis.*
bronchiol/o	bronchiole	**bronchiol**/itis (brŏng-kē-ō-LĪ-tĭs): _____ *-itis:* inflammation
alveol/o	alveolus; air sac	**alveol**/ar (ăl-VĒ-ō-lăr): _____ *-ar:* pertaining to
pleur/o	pleura	**pleur/o**/scopy (ploo-RŎS-kō-pē): _____ *-scopy:* visual examination *Pleuroscopy involves insertion of a specialized endoscope through a small incision in the chest to allow an inspection of the pleural space, obtain lung tissue for analysis, inject medications, and perform other diagnostic or therapeutic procedures.*
pneum/o	air; lung	**pneum/o**/lith (NŪ-mō-lĭth): _____ *-lith:* stone, calculus
pneumon/o		**pneumon**/ia (nū-MŌ-nē-ă): _____ *-ia:* condition
pulmon/o	lung	**pulmon/o**/logist (pŭl-mŏ-NŎL-ŏ-jĭst): _____ *-logist:* specialist in the study of
Other		
anthrac/o	coal, coal dust	**anthrac**/osis (ăn-thră-KŌ-sĭs): _____ *-osis:* abnormal condition; increase (used primarily with blood cells) *Anthracosis (black lung disease) is a chronic occupational disease found in coal miners and those associated with the coal industry.*
atel/o	incomplete; imperfect	**atel**/ectasis (ăt-ĕ-LĔK-tă-sĭs): _____ *-ectasis:* dilation, expansion *Atelectasis (airless or collapsed lung) is usually caused by a blocked airway, trauma to the chest cavity, or infection.*

(continued)

Medical Word Elements—cont'd

Element	Meaning	Word Analysis
coni/o	dust	pneum/o/**coni**/osis (nū-mō-kō-nē-Ō-sĭs): _____ *pneum/o:* air; lung *-osis:* abnormal condition; increase (used primarily with blood cells) *Pneumoconiosis is caused by mineral dusts of occupational or environmental origin and includes silicosis, asbestosis, and anthracosis.*
cyan/o	blue	**cyan**/osis (sī-ă-NŌ-sĭs): _____ *-osis:* abnormal condition; increase (used primarily with blood cells) *Cyanosis results from poor circulation or inadequate oxygenation of the blood.*
lob/o	lobe	**lob**/ectomy (lō-BĔK-tō-mē): _____ *-ectomy:* excision *Lobectomies are performed when a malignancy is confined to a single lobe of any lobed organ, such as the lungs, liver, and thyroid gland.*
orth/o	straight	**orth**/o/pnea (or-THŎP-nē-ă): _____ *-pnea:* breathing *Discomfort in breathing that is relieved by sitting or standing in an erect position.*
ox/o	oxygen (O_2)	hyp/**ox**/emia (hī-pŏks-Ē-mē-ă): _____ *hyp-:* under, below, deficient *-emia:* blood condition *Hypoxemia is an abnormal decrease of oxygen in arterial blood.*
pector/o	chest	**pector**/algia (pĕk-tō-RĂL-jē-ă): _____ *-algia:* pain *Pectoralgia is also called* thoracalgia *or* thoracodynia.
steth/o		**steth**/o/scope (STĔTH-ō-skōp): _____ *-scope:* instrument for examining *A stethoscope enables evaluation of sounds in the chest and the abdomen, an assessment technique known as auscultation.*
thorac/o		**thorac**/o/pathy (thō-răk-ŎP-ă-thē): _____ *-pathy:* disease
phren/o	diaphragm; mind	**phren**/o/spasm (FRĔN-ō-spăzm): _____ *-spasm:* involuntary contraction, twitching
spir/o	breathe	**spir**/o/meter (spī-RŎM-ĕt-ĕr): _____ *-meter:* instrument for measuring *A spirometer evaluates the movement of air into and out of the lungs (ventilation).*

Medical Word Elements—cont'd

Element	Meaning	Word Analysis
Suffixes		
-capnia	carbon dioxide (CO$_2$)	hyper/**capnia** (hī-pĕr-KĂP-nē-ă): _____ *hyper-*: excessive, above normal
-osmia	smell	an/**osmia** (ăn-ŎZ-mē-ă): _____ *an-*: without, not *Anosmia is a loss, usually partial, of the sense of smell. It can be temporary or permanent, depending on the cause.*
-phonia	voice	dys/**phonia** (dĭs-FŌ-nē-ă): _____ *dys-*: bad; painful; difficult *Dysphonia usually signifies dysfunction in the muscles needed to produce sound.*
-pnea	breathing	a/**pnea** (ĂP-nē-ă): _____ *a-*: without, not
-ptysis	spitting	hem/o/**ptysis** (hē-MŎP-tĭ-sĭs): _____ *hem/o*: blood *Hemoptysis is usually a sign of a serious condition of the lungs.*
-thorax	chest	hem/o/**thorax** (hē-mō-THŌ-răks): _____ *hem/o*: blood *Hemothorax is a type of pleural effusion containing blood and commonly associated with severe trauma to the chest.*
Prefixes		
brady-	slow	**brady**/pnea (brăd-ĭp-NĒ-ă): _____ *-pnea*: breathing
dys-	bad; painful; difficult	**dys**/pnea (DĬSP-nē-ă): _____ *-pnea*: breathing
eu-	good, normal	**eu**/pnea (ŪP-nē-ă): _____ *-pnea*: breathing
tachy-	rapid	**tachy**/pnea (tăk-ĭp-NĒ-ă): _____ *-pnea*: breathing

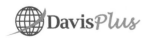

Visit the *Medical Terminology Systems* online resource center at Davis*Plus* for an audio exercise of the terms in this table. Other activities are also available to reinforce content.

⊕ *It is time to review medical word elements by completing Learning Activities 7-1 and 7-2.*

Disease Focus

Common signs and symptoms of many respiratory disorders include cough (dry or productive), chest pain **(thoracodynia)**, altered breathing patterns, shortness of breath (SOB), cyanosis, fever, and exercise intolerance. Many disorders of the respiratory system, including bronchitis and emphysema, begin as an acute problem but become chronic over time. Chronic respiratory diseases are difficult to treat. Their damaging effects are often irreversible.

For diagnosis, treatment, and management of respiratory disorders, the medical services of a specialist may be warranted. **Pulmonology** is the medical specialty concerned with disorders of the respiratory system. The physician who treats these disorders is called a **pulmonologist.**

Chronic Obstructive Pulmonary Disease

Chronic obstructive pulmonary disease (COPD) includes respiratory disorders that produce a chronic partial obstruction of the air passages. Because of its chronic nature, the disease leads to limited airflow into and out of the lungs, with increased difficulty in breathing **(dyspnea).** COPD is insidious and is commonly first diagnosed after the patient has already lost some lung capacity. It is possible to have early stages of COPD without knowing it. (See Table 7-1.) The three major disorders of COPD are asthma, chronic bronchitis, and emphysema. (See Fig. 7-3.)

Asthma

Asthma produces spasms in the bronchial passages **(bronchospasms)** that may be sudden and violent **(paroxysmal)**, causing dyspnea. Asthma is caused by exposure to allergens or irritants. Other causes include stress, cold, and exercise. During recovery, coughing episodes produce large amounts of mucus **(productive cough)**. Over time, the epithelium of the bronchial passages thickens, breathing becomes more difficult, and flare-ups **(exacerbations)** occur more frequently. Treatment includes agents that loosen and break down mucus **(mucolytics)** and medications that expand the bronchi **(bronchodilators)** by relaxing their smooth muscles. Most cases of asthma can be treated effectively. However, when treatment does not reverse bronchospasm, a life-threatening condition called **status asthmaticus** can occur, requiring hospitalization.

Table 7-1	Stages of COPD	
This table lists the levels of severity of COPD and describes their characteristics.		
Severity Level	**Description**	
At risk, mild	• Minor difficulty with airflow	
	• Possible presence of chronic cough with sputum production	
	• Patient possibly unaware of disease	
Moderate	• Apparent limitation in airflow	
	• Possible shortness of breath	
	• Patient possibly seeking medical intervention at this level	
Severe	• Inadequate airflow	
	• Increase in shortness of breath with activity	
	• Patient experiencing diminished quality of life	
Very severe	• Severe airflow limitations	
	• Significant impairment in quality of life	
	• Possible life-threatening exacerbations	
	• Possible development of complications, such as respiratory or heart failure	

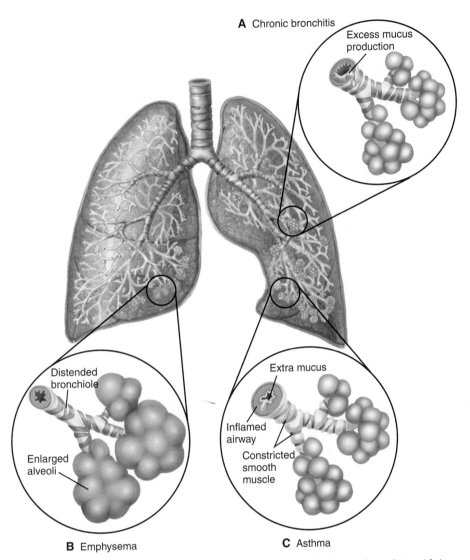

A Chronic bronchitis

Excess mucus production

Distended bronchiole

Enlarged alveoli

B Emphysema

Extra mucus

Inflamed airway

Constricted smooth muscle

C Asthma

Figure 7-3 Chronic obstructive pulmonary disease (COPD). (A) Chronic bronchitis with inflamed airways and excessive mucus. (B) Emphysema with distended bronchioles and alveoli. (C) Asthma with narrowed bronchial tubes and swollen mucous membranes.

Chronic Bronchitis

Chronic bronchitis is an inflammation of the bronchi caused mainly by smoking and air pollution. However, other agents, such as viruses and bacteria, may also cause the disorder. Bronchitis is characterized by swelling of the mucosa and a heavy, productive cough accompanied by chest pain. Patients commonly seek medical help when they suffer exercise intolerance, wheezing, and SOB. Bronchodilators and medications that aid in the removal of mucus **(expectorants)** help widen air passages. Steroids are prescribed if the disease progresses or becomes chronic.

Emphysema

Emphysema is characterized by decreased elasticity of the alveoli. The alveoli expand **(dilate)** but are unable to contract to their original size, making it difficult to exhale. The air that remains trapped in the chest results in a characteristic "barrel-chested" appearance. Emphysema commonly occurs with another respiratory disorder, such as asthma, tuberculosis, or chronic bronchitis, and in long-term heavy smokers. Most emphysema sufferers find it easier to breathe when sitting upright or standing erect **(orthopnea)**. As the disease progresses, relief—even in the orthopneic position—is not possible. Treatment for emphysema is similar to that for chronic bronchitis.

Pneumonia

Pneumonia is an inflammatory condition affecting the lungs, primarily the microscopic air sacs **(alveoli).** As inflammatory fluids collect in the alveoli, lung tissue loses its spongy texture and becomes swollen and engorged **(consolidation),** and oxygen exchange becomes difficult. Causes of pneumonia include bacterial and viral infections, but fungi, chemicals, and even inhaled substances such as food, vomitus, or liquids **(aspiration pneumonias)** can also cause pneumonia.

Lobar pneumonia is generally of bacterial origin and affects a large portion or an entire lobe of a lung. Typically this disease occurs in young, healthy adults and thus is considered a *primary pneumonia.* Antibiotic therapy is effective in the treatment of this disease.

Bronchopneumonia is caused by a wider variety of organisms and is centered in the bronchi and surrounding alveoli. It tends to occur in infants, the elderly, and those suffering from other illnesses, including cancer, heart failure, and immune disorders. Because of this association, it is considered a *secondary pneumonia.*

Pneumocystis pneumonia (PCP) is a type of pneumonia closely associated with AIDS. Recent evidence suggests that it is caused by an organism that resides in or on most people **(normal flora)** but causes no harm as long as the individual remains healthy. When the immune system begins to fail, this organism becomes infectious **(opportunistic).**

Thoracodynia, dyspnea, hemoptysis, and coughing up sputum containing white blood cells **(mucopurulent sputum)** are common signs and symptoms of pneumonia.

Auscultation, percussion, chest x-ray, and blood tests help diagnose pneumonia. For elderly patients, especially those who are hospitalized with other health issues, a pleural fluid culture and computed tomography (CT) scan aid in determining a diagnosis.

Acute Respiratory Distress Syndrome

Acute respiratory distress syndrome (ARDS) is a condition in which the lungs no longer function effectively, threatening the life of the patient. It usually occurs as a result of very serious lung conditions, such as trauma, severe pneumonia, and other major infections that affect the entire body **(systemic infections)** or blood **(sepsis).** In ARDS, the alveoli fill with fluid **(edema)** caused by inflammation and then collapse, making oxygen exchange impossible. Mechanical ventilation is commonly required to save the life of the patient.

Neonatal respiratory distress syndrome (NRDS) is a form of respiratory distress syndrome seen in preterm infants or infants born to diabetic mothers. It is caused by insufficient **surfactant,** a phospholipid substance that helps keep alveoli open. With insufficient surfactant, the alveoli collapse, and breathing becomes labored. Clinical signs may include blueness **(cyanosis)** of the extremities. Flaring of the nostrils **(nares),** rapid breathing **(tachypnea),** and a characteristic grunt audible during exhalation are signs of this disorder. Radiography shows a membrane that has a ground-glass appearance **(hyaline membrane),** bilateral decrease in lung volume, and fluid in the alveoli **(alveolar consolidation).** Although severe cases of hyaline membrane disease (HMD) result in death, some forms of therapy are effective.

Oncology

Lung cancer, also called **bronchogenic carcinoma,** is a malignancy that arises from the epithelium of the bronchial tree. As masses form, they block air passages and alveoli. Within a short time, they spread **(metastasize)** to other areas of the body, usually lymph nodes, liver, bones, brain, and kidneys. Cigarette smoking causes most lung cancers. High levels of pollution, radiation, and asbestos exposure may also increase risk.

Very few lung cancers are found in the early stages when the cure rate is high. Treatment depends on the type, stage, and general health of the patient and includes surgery, radiation, chemotherapy, or a combination of these methods. The prognosis for patients with lung cancer is generally poor.

Diseases and Conditions

This section introduces diseases and conditions of the respiratory system, along with their definitions and pronunciations. Word analyses for selected terms are also provided.

Term	Definition
abnormal breath sounds	Abnormal sounds or noises heard over the lungs and airways, commonly leading to a diagnosis of a respiratory or cardiac condition; also called *adventitious breath sounds*
crackle KRĂK-ĕl	Intermittent sounds caused by exudates, spasms, hyperplasia, or when air enters moisture-filled alveoli; also called *rale*
rhonchus RŎNG-kŭs	Continuous sound heard during inspiration and expiration caused by secretions in the larger airways and commonly resembling snoring
stridor STRĪ-dor	High-pitched, harsh sound caused by a spasm or swelling of the larynx or an obstruction in the upper airway *The presence of stridor may be life-threatening and requires immediate intervention.*
wheeze HWĒZ	Whistling or sighing that results from narrowing of the lumen of the respiratory passageway *Wheezing is a sign of asthma, croup, hay fever, obstructive emphysema, and other obstructive respiratory conditions.*
acidosis ăs-ĭ-DŌ-sĭs *acid:* acid *-osis:* abnormal condition; increase (used primarily with blood cells)	Excessive acidity of body fluids *Respiratory acidosis is commonly associated with pulmonary insufficiency and the subsequent retention of carbon dioxide.*
anosmia ăn-ŎZ-mē-ă *an-:* without, not *-osmia:* smell	Absence of the sense of smell *Anosmia usually occurs as a temporary condition resulting from an upper respiratory infection (URI) or a condition that causes intranasal swelling.*
apnea ĂP-nē-ă *a-:* without, not *-pnea:* breathing	Disorder in which breathing stops repeatedly during sleep, resulting in blood deoxygenation, causing the patient to awaken, gasping for air; also called *sleep apnea* *Apneic episodes may be as seldom as once per hour or as often as once every 5 minutes.*
central (CSA)	A form of sleep apnea that occurs when the brain fails to stimulate breathing muscles, causing brief pauses in breathing *Cheyne-Stokes, a type of periodic respiration related to CSA, is commonly associated with heart failure.*
obstructive (OSA)	Most common form of sleep apnea caused by an upper airway blockage that prevents an adequate flow of air to the lungs *Causes of OSA include enlarged tonsils or adenoids or decreased muscle tone of the soft palate that causes it to collapse over the airway, blocking air passages and resulting in loud snoring. Continuous positive airway pressure (CPAP) is ventilatory support used to keep airways open. (See Fig. 7-4, page 194.)*
mixed	Type of sleep apnea that occurs when central sleep apnea and obstructive sleep apnea occur simultaneously

(continued)

Diseases and Conditions—cont'd

Term	Definition

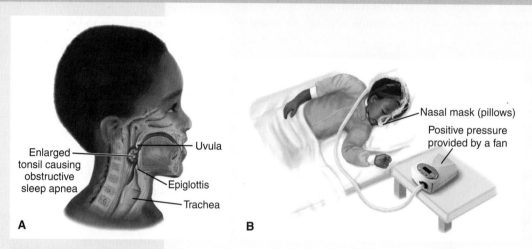

Figure 7-4 Apnea. (A) Airway obstruction caused by enlarged tonsils, which eventually leads to obstructive sleep apnea. (B) Continuous positive airway pressure (CPAP) machine used to treat sleep apnea.

Term	Definition
atelectasis ăt-ĕ-LĔK-tă-sĭs *atel:* incomplete; imperfect *-ectasis:* dilation, expansion	Collapsed or airless state of the lung, which may be acute or chronic and affects all or part of a lung *Atelectasis is a potential complication of some surgical procedures, especially those of the chest, because of shallow breathing to avoid pain from the surgical incision.*
coryza kŏ-RĪ-ză	Acute inflammation of the membranes of the nose; also called *rhinitis* *Causes of coryza include bacteria, viruses, irritants, and allergens.*
croup CROOP	Common childhood condition involving inflammation of the larynx, trachea, and bronchial passages and sometimes involving the lungs *Signs and symptoms of croup include a resonant, barking cough with suffocative, difficult breathing; laryngeal spasms; and, sometimes, the narrowing of the top of the air passages.*
cystic fibrosis (CF) SĬS-tĭk fĭ-BRŌ-sĭs *cyst:* bladder *-ic:* pertaining to *fibr:* fiber, fibrous tissue *-osis:* abnormal condition; increase (used primarily with blood cells)	Life-threatening genetic disease causing mucus to become unusually thick and sticky, plugging tubes and ducts, especially in the lungs and pancreas *There is no cure for cystic fibrosis. Treatment consists of supportive measures that help the patient lead a normal life to the extent possible and that prevent pulmonary infection.*
deviated nasal septum DĒ-vē-āt-ĕd NĀ-zl SĔP-tŭm *nas:* nose *-al:* pertaining to	Displacement of the cartilage dividing the nostrils that causes reduced airflow and sometimes causes nosebleed

Diseases and Conditions—cont'd

Term	Definition
epiglottitis ĕp-ĭ-glŏt-Ī-tĭs *epiglott:* epiglottis *-itis:* inflammation	Severe, life-threatening infection of the epiglottis and supraglottic structures that occurs most commonly in children between ages 2 and 12 years *Signs and symptoms of epiglottitis include fever, dysphagia, inspiratory stridor, and severe respiratory distress. Intubation or tracheostomy may be required to open the obstructed airway.*
epistaxis ĕp-ĭ-STĂK-sĭs	Nasal hemorrhage; also called *nosebleed*
hypoxemia hī-pŏks-Ē-mē-ă *hyp-:* under, below, deficient *ox:* oxygen *-emia:* blood condition	Oxygen deficiency in arterial blood, which is usually a sign of respiratory impairment and commonly causes hypoxia
hypoxia hī-PŎKS-ē-ă *hyp-:* under, below, deficient *-oxia:* oxygen	Oxygen deficiency in the body or a region of the body that commonly causes cyanosis
influenza ĭn-floo-ĔN-ză	Acute, contagious viral disorder of the respiratory tract, characterized by weakness, fever, chills, and muscle pain, especially in the back, arms, and legs; also called *flu* *Flu viruses are constantly changing, with new strains appearing regularly. Guidelines recommend vaccination each flu season because flu can cause serious complications, including pneumonia, bronchitis, sinusitis, and asthma flare-up.*
pertussis pĕr-TŬS-ĭs	Acute, infectious disease characterized by a cough that has a characteristic "whoop" sound; also called *whooping cough* *Immunization of infants as part of the diphtheria-pertussis-tetanus (DPT) vaccination is effective in preventing pertussis.*
pleural effusion PLOO-răl ĕ-FŪ-zhŭn *pleur:* pleura *-al:* pertaining to	Abnormal accumulation of fluid in the pleural cavity that impairs breathing by limiting the expansion of the lungs *Pleural effusions are described as exudates when the effusion is high in protein and immune cells or as transudates when the fluid resembles serum and does not contain inflammatory cells.*
empyema ĕm-pī-Ē-mă	Exudative effusion characterized by collection of pus in the pleural cavity, commonly as a result of bacterial pneumonia that spreads from the lungs; also called *pyothorax*
pneumothorax nū-mō-THŌ-răks *pneum/o:* air; lung *-thorax:* chest	Presence of air in the pleural cavity, commonly caused by a blunt or penetrating chest injury or as the result of a thoracic surgery *Pneumothorax commonly causes a partial or complete collapse of a lung (atelectasis). (See Fig. 7-5, page 196.)*

(continued)

Diseases and Conditions—cont'd

Term	Definition

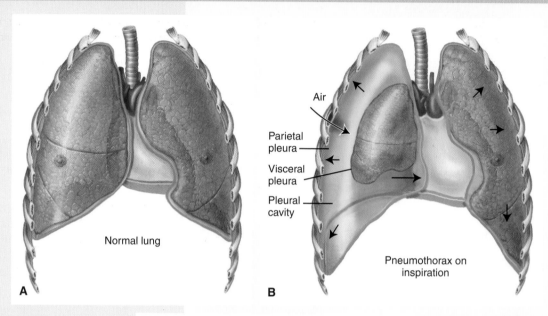

Normal lung

Air
Parietal pleura
Visceral pleura
Pleural cavity
Pneumothorax on inspiration

A   B

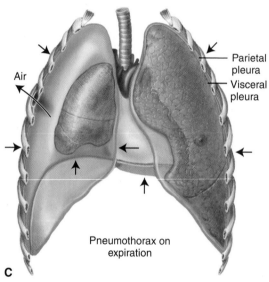

Parietal pleura
Visceral pleura
Air
Pneumothorax on expiration

C

Figure 7-5 Pneumothorax. (A) Normal. (B) Open pneumothorax during inspiration. (C) Open pneumothorax during expiration.

pleurisy PLOO-rĭs-ē *pleur:* pleura *-isy:* state of; condition	Inflammation of the pleural membrane characterized by a stabbing pain that is intensified by coughing or deep breathing; also called *pleuritis*
pulmonary edema PŬL-mō-nĕ-rē ĕ-DĒ-mă *pulmon:* lung *-ary:* pertaining to	Accumulation of extravascular fluid in lung tissues and alveoli, most commonly caused by heart failure *Excessive fluid in the lungs induces coughing and dyspnea.*

Diseases and Conditions—cont'd

Term	Definition

pulmonary embolism
PŬL-mō-nĕ-rē ĔM-bō-lĭzm
pulmon: lung
-*ary:* pertaining to
embol: plug
-*ism:* condition

Blockage in an artery of the lungs caused by a mass of undissolved matter (such as a blood clot, tissue, air bubbles, and bacteria) that has traveled to the lungs from another part of the body.

Pulmonary embolism is commonly caused by a deep vein thrombosis (DVT) that travels from the leg to the lungs. (See Fig. 7-6.)

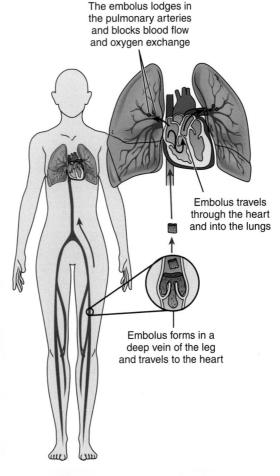

The embolus lodges in the pulmonary arteries and blocks blood flow and oxygen exchange

Embolus travels through the heart and into the lungs

Embolus forms in a deep vein of the leg and travels to the heart

Figure 7-6 Pulmonary embolism.

sudden infant death syndrome (SIDS)

Completely unexpected and unexplained death of an apparently normal, healthy infant, usually less than age 12 months; also called *crib death*

The rate of SIDS has decreased more than 30% since parents have been instructed to place babies on their backs for sleeping, rather than on their stomachs.

tuberculosis (TB)
tū-bĕr-kū-LŌ-sĭs
tubercul: little swelling
-*osis:* abnormal condition; increase (used primarily with blood cells)

Potentially fatal contagious disease spread through respiratory droplets, affecting any organ of the body but primarily the lungs and causing chest pain, hemoptysis, weight loss, fatigue, and night sweats

Many strains of TB are resistant to treatment. Therefore, patients with TB require administration of multiple antibiotics taken for several months to eradicate the organism.

 It is time to review diseases and conditions by completing Learning Activity 7-3.

Diagnostic, Surgical, and Therapeutic Procedures

This section introduces diagnostic, surgical, and therapeutic procedures used to diagnose and treat respiratory disorders. Descriptions are provided, along with pronunciations and word analyses for selected terms.

Procedure	Description
Diagnostic	
Clinical	
Mantoux test măn-TŪ	Tuberculosis screening test in which an injection of tuberculin purified protein derivative (PPD) is placed just beneath the surface of the skin to identify a previous exposure to tuberculosis *A positive test result is indicated by a lump that is hardened, red, and swollen at the injection site after 2 days. A positive test is followed up with a chest x-ray to confirm whether or not the patient has active tuberculosis.*
oximetry ŏk-SĬM-ĕ-trē *ox/i:* oxygen *-metry:* act of measuring	Noninvasive method of monitoring the percentage of hemoglobin (Hb) saturated with oxygen; also called *pulse oximetry* *In oximetry, a probe attached to the patient's finger or earlobe links to a computer that displays the percentage of hemoglobin saturated with oxygen.*
polysomnography pŏl-ē-sŏm-NŎG-ră-fē *poly-:* many, much *somn/o:* sleep *-graphy:* process of recording	Test of sleep cycles and stages using electroencephalograms (EEGs), which are continuous recordings of brain waves, as well as electrical activity of muscles, eye movement, respiratory rate, blood pressure, blood oxygen saturation, heart rhythm and, sometimes, direct observation of the person during sleep using a video camera (See Fig. 7-7.)

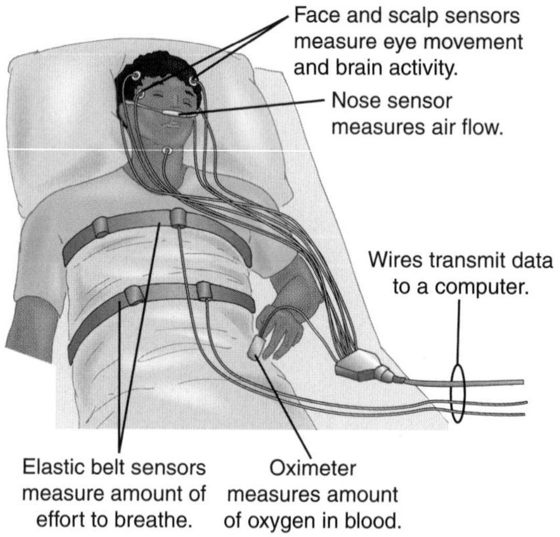

Face and scalp sensors measure eye movement and brain activity.

Nose sensor measures air flow.

Wires transmit data to a computer.

Elastic belt sensors measure amount of effort to breathe.

Oximeter measures amount of oxygen in blood.

Figure 7-7 Polysomnography.

Diagnostic, Surgical, and Therapeutic Procedures—cont'd

Procedure	Description
pulmonary function tests (PFTs) PŬL-mō-nĕ-rē *pulmon:* lung *-ary:* pertaining to	Series of tests to aid in the diagnosis of lung diseases and evaluate effectiveness of treatments *PFTs help evaluate patients with shortness of breath and assess lung function before surgery.*
spirometry spī-RŎM-ĕ-trē *spir/o:* breathe *-metry:* act of measuring	PFT that measures how much and how quickly air moves in and out of the lungs (See Fig. 7-8.) *A spirometer produces a graphic record of spirometry results for placement in the patient's chart.* 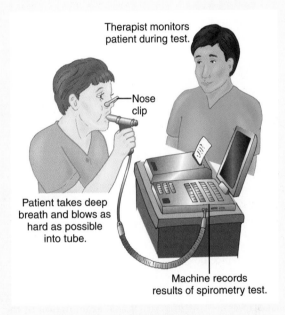 Therapist monitors patient during test. Nose clip Patient takes deep breath and blows as hard as possible into tube. Machine records results of spirometry test. **Figure 7-8** Spirometry.

Endoscopy

bronchoscopy brŏng-KŎS-kō-pē *bronch/o:* bronchus *-scopy:* visual examination	Visual examination of the bronchi using an endoscope (flexible fiberoptic or rigid) inserted through the mouth and trachea for direct viewing of structures or for projection on a monitor (See Fig. 7-9.) *Attachments on the bronchoscope can help suction mucus, remove foreign bodies, collect sputum, or perform biopsy.*

(continued)

Diagnostic, Surgical, and Therapeutic Procedures—cont'd

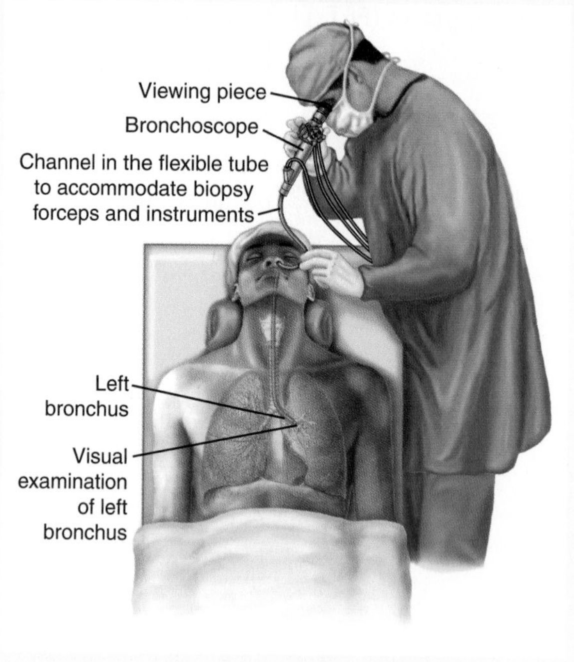

Procedure	Description

Viewing piece
Bronchoscope
Channel in the flexible tube
to accommodate biopsy
forceps and instruments

Left
bronchus

Visual
examination
of left
bronchus

Figure 7-9 Bronchoscopy of the left bronchus.

laryngoscopy
lăr-ĭn-GŎS-kō-pē
laryng/o: larynx (voice box)
-scopy: visual examination

Visual examination of the larynx to detect tumors, foreign bodies, nerve or structural injury, or other abnormalities

mediastinoscopy
mē-dē-ăs-tĭ-NŎS-kō-pē
mediastin/o: mediastinum
-scopy: visual examination

Visual examination of the mediastinal structures, including the heart, trachea, esophagus, bronchus, thymus, and lymph nodes

The mediastinoscope is inserted through a small incision made above the sternum. The attached camera projects images on a monitor. The surgeon may make additional incisions to remove nodes or perform other diagnostic or therapeutic procedures.

Laboratory

arterial blood gas (ABG)
ăr-TĒ-rē-ăl
arteri/o: artery
-al: pertaining to

Test that measures dissolved oxygen and carbon dioxide in arterial blood

ABG analysis evaluates acid–base state and how well oxygen is being carried to body tissues.

sputum culture
SPŪ-tŭm

Microbial test used to identify disease-causing organisms of the lower respiratory tract, especially those that cause pneumonias

sweat test

Measurement of the amount of salt (sodium chloride) in sweat

A sweat test is used almost exclusively in children to confirm cystic fibrosis and is commonly considered the gold standard in diagnosis.

throat culture

Test used to identify pathogens, especially group A streptococci

Untreated streptococcal infections may lead to serious secondary complications, including kidney and heart disease.

Diagnostic, Surgical, and Therapeutic Procedures—cont'd

Procedure	Description

Imaging

Procedure	Description
chest x-ray (CXR)	Radiographic test that aids in identifying lung conditions such as pneumonia, lung cancer, COPD, and pneumothorax *When CXR results are inconclusive, other imaging tests are performed.*

computed tomography pulmonary angiography (CTPA)
kŏm-PŪ-tĕd tō-MŎG-ră-fē
PŬL-mō-nĕr-ē ăn-jē-ŎG-ră-fē
  tom/o: to cut
  -graphy: process of recording
  pulmon: lung
  -ary: pertaining to
  angi/o: vessel (usually blood or lymph)
  -graphy: process of recording
	Minimally invasive imaging that combines computed tomography scanning and angiography to produce images of the pulmonary arteries
	CTPA is highly sensitive and specific for the presence of pulmonary emboli.

ventilation-perfusion (V-Q) scan	Nuclear test scan that evaluates airflow (ventilation) and blood flow (perfusion) in the lungs for evidence of a blood clot in the lungs; also called *V-Q lung scan*

Surgical

Procedure	Description

pleurectomy
ploor-ĔK-tō-mē
  pleur: pleura
  -ectomy: excision, removal
	Excision of part of the pleura, usually the parietal pleura
	Pleurectomy helps reduce pain caused by a tumor mass or prevent the recurrence of pleural effusion but is generally ineffective in the treatment of malignancy of the pleura.

(continued)

Diagnostic, Surgical, and Therapeutic Procedures—cont'd

Procedure	Description
pneumonectomy nū-mŏn-ĔK-tō-mē *pneumon:* air; lung *-ectomy:* excision, removal	Excision of a lung or a portion of the lung, commonly for treatment of cancer (See Fig. 7-10.) 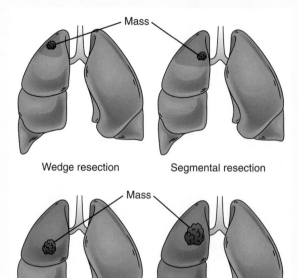 **Figure 7-10** Types of pneumonectomy.
septoplasty sĕp-tō-PLĂS-tē *sept/o:* septum *-plasty:* surgical repair	Surgical repair of a deviated nasal septum that is usually performed when the septum is encroaching on the breathing passages or nasal structures *Common complications of a deviated septum include interference with breathing and a predisposition to sinus infections.*
thoracentesis thō-ră-sĕn-TĒ-sĭs	Surgical puncture and drainage of the pleural cavity; also called *pleurocentesis* or *thoracocentesis* *Thoracentesis as a diagnostic procedure helps determine the nature and cause of an effusion; as a therapeutic procedure, it relieves the discomfort caused by the effusion. (See Fig. 7-11.)*

Diagnostic, Surgical, and Therapeutic Procedures—cont'd

Procedure	Description

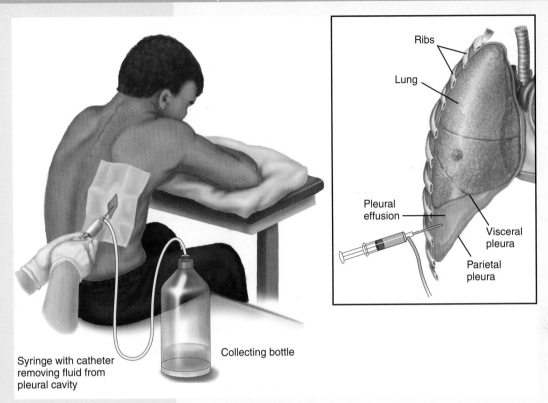

Figure 7-11 Thoracentesis.

tracheostomy
trā-kē-ŎS-tō-mē
trache/o: trachea
-stomy: forming an opening (mouth)

Surgical procedure in which an opening is made in the neck and into the trachea into which a breathing tube may be inserted (See Fig. 7-12.)

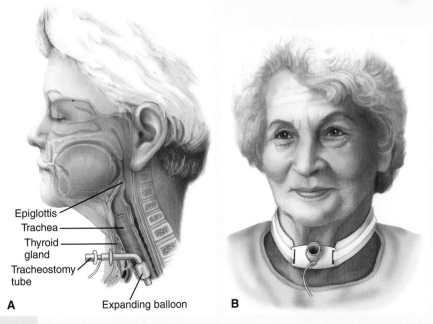

Figure 7-12 Tracheostomy. (A) Lateral view with tracheostomy tube in place. (B) Frontal view.

(continued)

Diagnostic, Surgical, and Therapeutic Procedures—cont'd

Procedure	Description
Therapeutic	

aerosol therapy
ĂR-ō-sŏl THĔR-ă-pē

Lung treatment using various techniques to deliver medication in mist form directly to the lungs or air passageways

Techniques include nebulizer mist treatments (NMTs), metered-dose inhalers (MDIs), and dry powder inhalers (DPIs). Nebulizers change liquid medications into droplets to be inhaled through a mouthpiece. (See Fig. 7-13.) MDIs deliver a specific amount when activated. Children and the elderly can use a spacer to synchronize inhalation with medication release. (See Fig. 7-14.) DPIs are activated by a quick inhalation by the user.

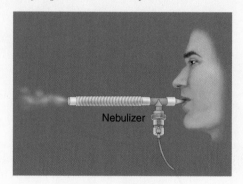

Figure 7-13 Nebulizer.

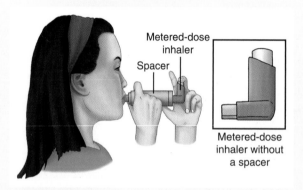

Figure 7-14 Metered-dose inhaler.

antral lavage
ĂN-trăl lă-VĂZH

Washing or irrigating of the paranasal sinuses to remove mucopurulent material in an immunosuppressed patient or one with known sinusitis that has failed to respond to medical management

endotracheal intubation
ĕn-dŏ-TRĀ-kē-ăl
ĭn-tū-BĀ-shŭn
 endo-: in, within
 trache: trachea
 -al: pertaining to

Procedure in which a plastic tube is inserted into the trachea to maintain an open airway

Endotracheal intubation is commonly performed before surgery when the patient is first placed under sedation or in emergency situations to facilitate ventilation if necessary. (See Fig. 7-15.)

Diagnostic, Surgical, and Therapeutic Procedures—cont'd

Procedure	Description

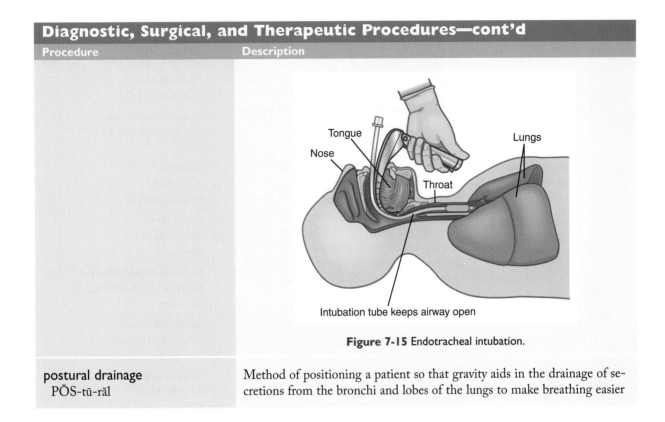

Figure 7-15 Endotracheal intubation.

Procedure	Description
postural drainage PŎS-tū-răl	Method of positioning a patient so that gravity aids in the drainage of se-cretions from the bronchi and lobes of the lungs to make breathing easier

Pharmacology

Several classes of drugs are prescribed to treat pulmonary disorders. These include antibiotics, which are used to treat respiratory infections, and bronchodilators, which are especially effective in treating COPD and exercise-induced asthma. (See Table 7-2.) Steroidal and nonsteroidal anti-inflammatory drugs are important in the control and management of many pulmonary disorders.

Table 7-2 Drugs Used to Treat Respiratory Disorders

This table lists common drug classifications used to treat respiratory disorders, their therapeutic actions, and selected generic and trade names.

Classification	Therapeutic Action	Generic and Trade Names
antibiotics ăn-tĭ-bī-ĂW-tĭks	Destroy or inhibit the growth of bacteria by disrupting their membranes or one or more of their metabolic processes	**azithromycin** ā-ZĬTH-rō-mī-sĭn *Zithromax* **amoxicillin clavulanate** ă-MŎX-ĭ-cĭl-ĭn clă-vū-LĂN-āt *Augmentin*
antihistamines ăn-tĭ-HĬS-tă-mēnz	Block histamines from binding with histamine receptor sites in tissues *Histamines cause sneezing, runny nose, itchiness, and rashes. Antihistamines are commonly combined with decongestants, antitussives, or analgesics for cold and flu symptom relief.*	**fexofenadine** fĕk-sō-FĔN-ă-dēn *Allegra* **loratadine** lor-ĂH-tă-dēn *Claritin*

(continued)

Table 7-2	Drugs Used to Treat Respiratory Disorders—cont'd	
Classification	**Therapeutic Action**	**Generic and Trade Names**
antitussives ăn-tĭ-TŬS-ĭvz	Relieve or suppress coughing by blocking the cough reflex in the medulla of the brain *Antitussives alleviate nonproductive dry coughs and should not be used with productive coughs.*	**hydrocodone*** hī-drō-KŌ-dōn **dextromethorphan** dĕk-strō-mĕth-OR-făn *Delsym*
bronchodilators brŏng-kō-DĪ-lă-torz	Stimulate bronchial muscles to relax, thereby expanding air passages, resulting in increased airflow *Bronchodilators help treat chronic symptoms and prevent acute attacks in respiratory diseases, such as asthma and COPD, and may be delivered by an inhaler, orally, or intravenously. Because bronchodilators are commonly used in conjunction with corticosteroids, combination products are available.*	**albuterol** ăl-BŪ-tĕr-ŏl *Proventil, Ventolin* **salmeterol** săl-MĔT-ĕr-ŏl *Serevent* **budesonide/formoterol** bū-DĔS-ō-nīd for-MŌ-tĕr-ŏl *Symbicort*
corticosteroids kor-tĭ-kō-STĔR-oyds	Act on the immune system by blocking production of substances that trigger allergic and inflammatory actions *Corticosteroids are available as nasal sprays, in metered-dose inhalers (inhaled steroids), and in oral forms (pills or syrups) to treat chronic lung conditions, such as asthma and COPD.*	**beclomethasone** bĕ-klō-MĔTH-ă-sōn *Qvar (metered-dose inhaler)* **mometasone** mō-MĔT-ă-sōn *Nasonex (nasal spray)*
decongestants dē-kŏn-JĔST-ănts	Constrict blood vessels of nasal passages and limit blood flow, which causes swollen tissues to shrink so that air can pass more freely through the passageways *Decongestants are commonly prescribed for allergies and colds and are usually combined with antihistamines in cold remedies. They can be administered orally or topically as nasal sprays and nasal drops.*	**oxymetazoline** ŏks-ē-mĕt-ĂZ-ō-lēn *Afrin (available for nasal instillation only)* **pseudoephedrine** soo-dō-ĕ-FĔD-rĭn *Sudafed (oral product)*
expectorants ĕk-SPĔK-tō-rănts	Liquefy respiratory secretions so that they are more easily dislodged during coughing episodes *Expectorants are prescribed for productive coughs.*	**guaifenesin** gwī-FĔN-ĕ-sĭn *Robitussin, Mucinex*

*Available only in generic form

Abbreviations

This section introduces respiratory-related abbreviations and their meanings.

Abbreviation	Meaning	Abbreviation	Meaning
ABG	arterial blood gas(es)	HMD	hyaline membrane disease
AIDS	acquired immunodeficiency syndrome	MDI	metered-dose inhaler
ARDS	acute respiratory distress syndrome	NMT	nebulized mist treatment
CF	cystic fibrosis	O_2	oxygen
CO_2	carbon dioxide	OSA	obstructive sleep apnea
COPD	chronic obstructive pulmonary disease	Pco_2	partial pressure of carbon dioxide
CPAP	continuous positive airway pressure	PCP	*Pneumocystis* pneumonia; primary care physician
CT	computed tomography	PFT	pulmonary function test
CTPA	computed tomography pulmonary angiography	pH	degree of acidity or alkalinity
CXR	chest x-ray, chest radiograph	Po_2	partial pressure of oxygen
DPI	dry powder inhaler	PPD	purified protein derivative
DPT	diphtheria, pertussis, tetanus	SIDS	sudden infant death syndrome
DVT	deep vein thrombosis	SOB	shortness of breath
EEG	electroencephalogram	TB	tuberculosis
Hb, Hgb	hemoglobin	URI	upper respiratory infection

It is time to review procedures, pharmacology, and abbreviations by completing Learning Activity 7-4.

LEARNING ACTIVITIES

The activities that follow provide a review of the respiratory system terms introduced in this chapter. Complete each activity and review your answers to evaluate your understanding of the chapter.

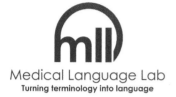

Medical Language Lab
Turning terminology into language

Visit the Medical Language Lab at *medicallanguagelab.com*. Use it to enhance your study and reinforcement of this chapter with the flash-card activity. We recommend that you complete the flash-card activity before starting Learning Activities 7-1 and 7-2.

Learning Activity 7-1
Medical Word Elements

Use the listed elements to build medical words. You may use these elements more than once.

Combining Forms		Suffixes		Prefixes
bronch/o	pneumon/o	-capnia	-phonia	brady-
bronchi/o	rhin/o	-centesis	-plasty	dys-
cyan/o	sept/o	-ectasis	-plegia	eu-
laryng/o	sinus/o	-ectomy	-pnea	hyper-
ox/o	tonsill/o	-ia	-scope	hyp-
pleur/o		-osis	-tomy	

1. surgical puncture of the pleura _____
2. instrument for examining the bronchus _____
3. excision of the tonsils _____
4. slow breathing _____
5. difficult voice _____
6. abnormal condition of blue(ness) _____
7. condition of decrease of oxygen _____
8. paralysis of the voice box _____
9. surgical repair of the septum _____
10. incision of the sinus _____
11. excessive carbon dioxide _____
12. good, normal breathing _____
13. expansion of a bronchi _____
14. surgical repair of the nose _____
15. condition of the lungs _____

✓ *Check your answers in Appendix A. Review any material that you did not answer correctly.*

Correct Answers _____ X 6.67 = _____ % Score

Learning Activity 7-2
Building Medical Words

Use *rhin/o* (nose) to build words that mean:

1. discharge from the nose _____
2. inflammation of (mucous membranes of the) nose _____

Use *laryng/o* (larynx [voice box]) to build words that mean:

3. visual examination of the larynx _____
4. inflammation of the larynx _____
5. stricture or narrowing of the larynx _____

Use *bronch/o* or *bronchi/o* (bronchus) to build words that mean:

6. dilation or expansion of the bronchus _____
7. disease of the bronchus _____
8. spasm of the bronchus _____

Use *pneumon/o* or *pneum/o* (air; lung) to build words that mean:

9. air in the chest (pleural space) _____
10. inflammation of the lungs _____

Use *pulmon/o* (lung) to build words that mean:

11. specialist in lung (diseases) _____
12. pertaining to the lung _____

Use *-pnea* (breathing) to build words that mean:

13. difficult breathing _____
14. slow breathing _____
15. rapid breathing _____
16. absence of breathing _____

Build surgical words that mean:

17. surgical repair of the nose _____
18. surgical puncture of the chest _____
19. removal of a lung _____
20. forming an opening (mouth) in the trachea _____

Check your answers in Appendix A. Review material that you did not answer correctly.

Correct Answers _____ X 5 = _____ % Score

Learning Activity 7-3

Diseases and Conditions

Match the terms with the definitions in the numbered list.

anosmia	deviated septum	hemoptysis	pleurisy
atelectasis	emphysema	hypoxemia	pulmonary edema
consolidation	empyema	hypoxia	rhonchus
coryza	epistaxis	influenza	transudate
cystic fibrosis	exudate	pertussis	tuberculosis

1. collapsed or airless lung _____

2. pus in the pleural cavity _____

3. abnormal breath sound commonly resembling snoring _____

4. deficiency of oxygen (in the tissues) _____

5. inflammatory fluid high in protein with blood and immune cells _____

6. absence or decrease in the sense of smell _____

7. deficiency of oxygen in atrial blood _____

8. genetic disease causing mucus to become unusually thick and sticky _____

9. acute, contagious viral disorder of the respiratory tract _____

10. disease characterized by a decrease in alveolar elasticity _____

11. spitting of blood _____

12. nosebleed; nasal hemorrhage _____

13. excessive fluid in the lungs that induces cough and dyspnea _____

14. noninflammatory fluid that resembles serum but with less protein _____

15. displacement of the cartilage dividing the nostrils _____

16. acute inflammation of the membranes of the nose; also called *rhinitis* _____

17. potentially fatal disease spread through respiratory droplets _____

18. inflammation of the pleural membrane _____

19. loss of sponginess of lungs due to engorgement _____

20. whooping cough _____

Check your answers in Appendix A. Review material that you did not answer correctly.

Correct Answers _____ X 5 = _____ % Score

Learning Activity 7-4
Procedures, Pharmacology, and Abbreviations

Match the terms with the definitions in the numbered list.

ABGs	CXR	oximetry	septoplasty
aerosol therapy	decongestant	pneumonectomy	sputum culture
antihistamine	expectorant	polysomnography	sweat test
antitussive	laryngoscopy	pulmonary function tests	thoracentesis
antral lavage	Mantoux test	rhinoplasty	throat culture

1. microbial test used to identify disease-causing organisms of the lower respiratory tract _____

2. test of sleep cycles and stages _____

3. imaging procedure to evaluate the lungs _____

4. washing or irrigating sinuses _____

5. relieves sneezing, runny nose, itchiness, and rashes _____

6. relieves or suppresses coughing _____

7. used primarily in children to confirm cystic fibrosis _____

8. noninvasive test used to monitor the percentage of hemoglobin saturated with oxygen _____

9. surgical puncture and drainage of the pleural cavity _____

10. inhalation of medication directly into the respiratory system via a nebulizer _____

11. decreases mucous membrane swelling by constricting blood vessels _____

12. intradermal test to determine tuberculin sensitivity _____

13. laboratory tests to assess gases and pH of arterial blood _____

14. reduces the viscosity of sputum to facilitate productive coughing _____

15. used to identify pathogens, especially group A streptococci _____

16. multiple tests used to determine the ability of lungs and capillary membranes to exchange oxygen _____

17. visual examination of the voice box to detect tumors and other abnormalities _____

18. procedure to correct a deviated nasal septum _____

19. excision of the entire lung _____

20. reconstructive surgery of the nose, commonly for cosmetic purposes _____

✓ *Check your answers in Appendix A. Review any material that you did not answer correctly.*

Correct Answers _____ X 5 = _____ % Score

DOCUMENTING HEALTH-CARE ACTIVITIES

This section provides practical application activities in the form of exercises to help develop skills in documenting patient care. First, read the medical report. Then complete the activities and exercises that follow.

Documenting Health-Care Activity 7-1
SOAP Note: Respiratory Evaluation

Emergency Department Record

Date: February 1, 20xx   Time Registered: 1345 hours
Patient: Flowers, Richard   Physician: Samara Batichara, MD
Chief Complaint: SOB

S: This 49-year-old married, Caucasion male presents with chief complaint of shortness of breath over the past few days. Patient was a heavy smoker and states that he quit smoking for a short time but now smokes 3–4 cigarettes a day. He has a history of difficult breathing, hypertension, COPD, and peripheral vascular disease. The patient underwent triple bypass surgery in 19xx.

O: T: 98.9 F. BP: 180/90. Pulse: 80 and regular. R: 20 and shallow. PE indicates scattered bilateral wheezes and rhonchi heard anteriorly and posteriorly. Compared with a portable chest film taken 22 months earlier, the current study most likely indicates interstitial vascular congestion. Some superimposed inflammatory change cannot be excluded. There may also be some pleural reactive change.

A: 1. Acute exacerbation of chronic obstructive pulmonary disease.
2. Heart failure.
3. Hypertension.
4. Peripheral vascular disease.

P: Admit to hospital. Continue the following medication: Vytorin 10/20 mg daily; Toprol-XL 50 mg daily; Azmacort 2 puffs three times a day; Proventil 2 puffs every six hours.

Samara Batichara, MD
Samara Batichara, MD

SB:icc

D: 2/1/20xx; T: 2/1/20xx

Terminology

The terms listed in the table that follows are taken from *SOAP Note: Respiratory Evaluation.* Use a medical dictionary such as *Taber's Cyclopedic Medical Dictionary,* the appendices of this book, or other resources to define each term. Then review the pronunciation for each term and practice by reading the medical record aloud.

Term	Definition
anteriorly ăn-TĒR-ē-or-lē	
bilateral bī-LĂT-ĕr-ăl	
COPD	
exacerbation ĕks-ăs-ĕr-BĀ-shŭn	
heart failure	
Hx	
hypertension hī-pĕr-TĔN-shŭn	
interstitial ĭn-tĕr-STĬSH-ăl	
PE	
peripheral vascular disease pĕr-ĬF-ĕr-ăl VĂS-kū-lăr	
pleural PLOO-răl	
posteriorly pŏs-TĒR-ē-or-lē	
rhonchi RŎNG-kī	
SOB	
wheezes HWĒZ-ĕz	

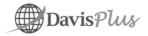

Visit the *Medical Terminology Systems* online resource center at Davis*Plus* to practice pronunciation and reinforce the meanings of the terms in this medical report.

Critical Thinking

Review *SOAP Note: Respiratory Evaluation* to answer the questions.

1. What symptom caused the patient to seek medical help?

_____

_____

_____

_____

2. What was the patient's previous history?

_____

_____

_____

_____

3. What were the abnormal findings of the physical examination?

_____

_____

_____

_____

4. What changes were noted from the previous film?

_____

_____

_____

_____

5. What are the present assessments?

_____

_____

_____

_____

6. What new diagnosis was made that did not appear in the previous medical history?

_____

_____

_____

_____

SOAP Note: Chronic Interstitial Lung Disease

O'Malley, Robert   09/01/20xx

S: Patient is an 84-year-old male with chief complaint of dyspnea with activity and pedal edema. He carries the dx cardiomyopathy, renal insufficiency, COPD, and pulmonary fibrosis. He also has peripheral neuropathy, which has improved with Elavil therapy.

O: BP: 140/70. Pulse: 76. Neck is supple without thyromegaly or adenopathy. Mild kyphosis without scoliosis is present. Chest reveals basilar crackles without wheezing or rhonchi. Cardiac examination shows trace edema without clubbing or murmur. Abdomen is soft and nontender. ABGs on room air demonstrate a Po_2 of 55, Pco_2 of 45, and pH of 7.42.

A: Chronic interstitial lung disease, likely a combination of pulmonary fibrosis and heart failure. We do believe he would benefit from further diuresis, which was implemented by Dr. Lu. Should there continue to be concerns about his volume status or lack of response to Lasix therapy, then he might benefit from right heart catheterization.

P: Supplemental oxygen will be (continued). We plan no change in his pulmonary medication at this time and will see him in return visit in 4 months. He has been told to contact us should he worsen in the interim.

Samara Batichara, MD
Samara Batichara, MD

SB:icc

Terminology

The terms listed in the table that follows are taken from *SOAP Note: Chronic Interstitial Lung Disease.* Use a medical dictionary such as *Taber's Cyclopedic Medical Dictionary,* the appendices of this book, or other resources to define each term. Then review the pronunciations for each term and practice by reading the medical record aloud.

Term	Definition
adenopathy ăd-ĕ-NŎP-ă-thē	
basilar crackles BĂS-ĭ-lăr KRĂK-ĕlz	
cardiomyopathy kăr-dē-ō-mī-ŎP-ă-thē	
diuresis dī-ū-RĒ-sĭs	
fibrosis fī-BRŌ-sĭs	
interstitial ĭn-tĕr-STĬSH-ăl	
kyphosis kī-FŌ-sĭs	
Lasix LĀ-sĭks	
neuropathy nū-RŎP-ă-thē	
pedal edema PĔD-ăl ĕ-DĒ-mă	
pulmonary fibrosis PŬL-mō-nĕ-rē fī-BRŌ-sĭs	
renal insufficiency RĒ-năl ĭn-sŭ-FĬSH-ĕn-sē	
silicosis sĭl-ĭ-KŌ-sĭs	

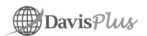 **DavisPlus**

Visit the *Medical Terminology Systems* online resource center at Davis*Plus* to practice pronunciation and reinforce the meanings of the terms in this medical report.

Critical Thinking

Review *SOAP Note: Chronic Interstitial Lung Disease* to answer the following questions.

1. When did the patient notice dyspnea?

_____

_____

_____

_____

2. Other than the respiratory system, what other body systems are identified in the history of present illness?

_____

_____

_____

_____

3. What were the findings regarding the neck?

_____

_____

_____

_____

4. What was the finding regarding the chest?

_____

_____

_____

_____

5. What appears to be the likely cause of the chronic interstitial lung disease?

_____

_____

_____

_____

6. What did the cardiac examination reveal?

_____

_____

_____

_____

Documenting Health-Care Activity 7-3

Constructing Chart Notes

To construct chart notes, replace the italicized and boldfaced terms in each of the two case studies with one of the listed medical terms.

antitussive	dyspnea	septoplasty
cephalodynia	myalgia	sinusitis
coryza	pharyngitis	T&A
deviated nasal septum		

Billy P., a 2-year-old boy, was referred to the ENT Clinic by his pediatrician. His mother states that when he is sleeping, Billy experiences (1) *difficult breathing*, starts gasping for air, and then wakes up crying. This is especially true when he has a (2) *head cold*. The examination of his nasal passages shows a (3) *septum displaced to one side*, causing impaired airflow through the nostrils. His tonsils and adenoids are also enlarged, making breathing even more difficult. The physician schedules a (4) *surgical repair of the septum* and (5) *removal of the tonsils and adenoids*.

1. _____
2. _____
3. _____
4. _____
5. _____

Betty L. presents to the Student Health Services on campus. She complains of (6) *muscle pain* and (7) *headache*. Betty states that she was up the entire night with a dry, hacking cough. Upon examination, the physician confirms that Betty has the flu and stated that her headache was probably a result of (8) *inflamed sinuses*. He further notes an (9) *inflammation of the throat* without evidence of strep infection. Betty is advised to drink clear fluids and take Tylenol, as needed, to reduce fever and general discomfort. The physician also prescribes Hycodan, a (10) *medication to control coughing*.

6. _____
7. _____
8. _____
9. _____
10. _____

✔ *Check your answers in Appendix A. Review any material that you did not answer correctly.*

Correct Answers _____ X 10 = _____ % Score

Cardiovascular System

Chapter Outline

Objectives

Upon completion of this chapter, you will be able to:

- Locate and describe the structures of the cardiovascular system.
- Describe the functional relationship between the cardiovascular system and other body systems.
- Pronounce, spell, and build words related to the cardiovascular system.
- Describe diseases, conditions, and procedures related to the cardiovascular system.
- Explain pharmacology related to the treatment of cardiovascular disorders.
- Demonstrate your knowledge of this chapter by completing the learning and documenting health-care activities.

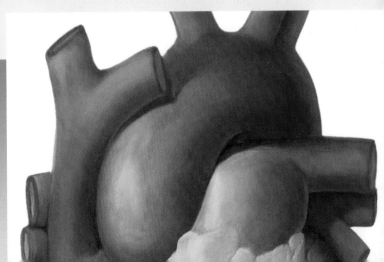

Anatomy and Physiology

The cardiovascular (CV) system is composed of the heart and blood vessels. The heart is a hollow, muscular organ lying in the mediastinum, the center of the thoracic cavity between the lungs. The pumping action of the heart propels blood that contains oxygen (O_2), nutrients, and other vital products from the heart to body cells through a vast network of blood vessels called **arteries.** Arteries branch into smaller vessels until they become microscopic vessels called **capillaries.** At the capillary level, an exchange of products occurs between body cells and blood. Capillaries merge to form larger blood vessels called **venules,** which then combine to form **veins,** the vessels that return blood to the heart to begin the cycle again. Millions of body cells rely on the CV system for their survival. When it fails, life at the cellular level is not possible and, ultimately, death occurs.

Anatomy and Physiology Key Terms

This section introduces important terms, along with their definitions and pronunciations. The key terms are highlighted in color in the Anatomy and Physiology section. Word analyses for selected terms are also provided. Pronounce the term, and place a check mark in the box after you do so.

Term	Definition
leaflets	Flat, leaf-shaped structures that comprise the valves of the heart and prevent the backflow of blood
lumen LŪ-mĕn ☐	Tubular space or channel within an organ or structure of the body; space within an artery, vein, intestine, or tube
regurgitation rē-gŭr-jĭ-TĀ-shŭn ☐	Backflow or ejecting of contents through an opening
sphincters SFĬNGK-tĕr ☐	Circular muscles found in a tubular structure or hollow organ that constrict or dilate to regulate passage of substances through its opening
vasoconstriction văs-ō-kŏn-STRĬK-shŭn ☐	Narrowing of the lumen of a blood vessel that limits blood flow, usually as a result of diseases, medications, or physiological processes
vasodilation văs-ō-dī-LĀ-shŭn ☐	Widening of the lumen of a blood vessel caused by the relaxing of the muscles of the vascular walls
viscosity vĭs-KŎS-ĭ-tē ☐	Thickness or a measure of how resistant a liquid is to flowing *A solution that has a high viscosity is relatively thick and flows slowly.*

Pronunciation Help	Long Sound	ā — rate	ē — rebirth	ī — isle	ō — over	ū — unite
	Short Sound	ă — apple	ĕ — ever	ĭ — it	ŏ — not	ŭ — cut

Vascular System

Three major types of vessels—(1) **artery,** (2) **capillary,** and (3) **vein**—carry blood throughout the body. (See Fig. 8-1.) Each type of vessel differs in structure, depending on its function.

Arteries

Arteries carry blood from the heart to all cells of the body. Because the pumping action of the heart propels blood through the arteries, the walls of the arteries must be strong and flexible enough to withstand the surge of blood that results from each contraction.

The walls of large arteries have three layers to provide toughness and elasticity. The (4) **tunica externa** is the outer coat, composed of connective tissue that provides strength and flexibility. The

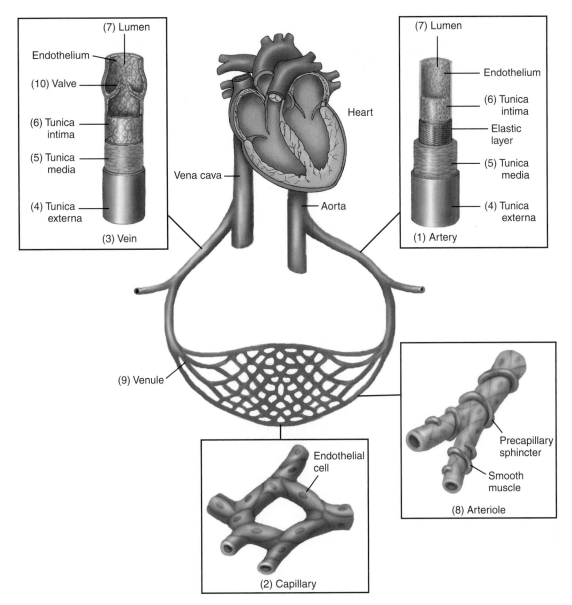

Figure 8-1 Vascular structures.

(5) **tunica media** is the middle layer, composed of smooth muscle. Depending on the needs of the body, this muscle can alter the size of the (7) **lumen** of the vessel. When it contracts, the tunica media causes **vasoconstriction**, resulting in decreased blood flow. When it relaxes, it causes **vasodilation**, resulting in increased blood flow. The (6) **tunica intima** is the thin, inner lining of the lumen of the vessel, composed of endothelial cells that provide a smooth surface on the inside of the vessel.

The surge of blood felt in the arteries when blood is pumped from the heart is referred to as a **pulse.** Because of the pressure against arterial walls associated with the pumping action of the heart, a cut or severed artery may lead to profuse bleeding.

Arterial blood (except for that found in the pulmonary artery) contains a high concentration of **oxygen** (O_2) and appears bright red in color. Oxygenated blood travels to smaller arteries called (8) **arterioles** and, finally, to the smallest vessels, the capillaries.

Capillaries

Capillaries are microscopic vessels that join the arterial system with the venous system. Although they might seem like the most insignificant of the three vessel types because of their microscopic size, they are actually the most important because of their function. Because capillary walls are composed of only a single layer of endothelial cells, they are very thin. This thinness enables the exchange of water, respiratory gases, macromolecules, metabolites, and wastes between the blood and the cells adjacent to the capillary bed. The vast number of capillaries branching from arterioles causes blood to flow very slowly, providing sufficient time for exchange of essential substances.

Blood flow through the capillary networks is slow and intermittent, rather than steady, and is regulated by the precapillary **sphincters**. When tissues require more blood, these sphincters open; when less blood is required, they close. Once the exchange of products is complete, blood enters the venous system for its return to the heart.

Veins

Veins return blood to the heart. They are formed from smaller vessels called (9) **venules** that develop from the union of capillaries. Because the extensive network of capillaries absorbs the propelling pressure exerted by the heart, veins use other methods to return blood to the heart, including the following:

• skeletal muscle contraction
• gravity
• respiratory activity
• valves

The (10) **valves** are small structures within veins that prevent the backflow of blood. Valves are found mainly in the extremities and are especially important for returning blood from the legs to the heart because blood must travel a long distance against the force of gravity to reach the heart from the legs. Large veins, especially in the abdomen, contain smooth muscle that provides peristalsis and helps propel blood toward the heart.

Blood carried in veins (except for the blood in the pulmonary veins) contains a low concentration of O_2 and a correspondingly high concentration of carbon dioxide (CO_2). This blood takes on a characteristic purple color and is said to be deoxygenated. It continuously circulates from the heart to the lungs so that CO_2 can be exchanged for O_2.

Heart

The **heart** is a muscular pump that propels blood to the entire body through a closed vascular network. It allows a dual circulatory system: pulmonary circulation provided by the right side of the heart and systemic circulation provided by the left side of the heart. Pulmonary circulation delivers blood to the lungs, where CO_2 is exchanged for O_2. Systemic circulation delivers blood to body tissues, where O_2 is exchanged for CO_2, a waste product that will be expelled by the lungs. Both systemic and pulmonary circulatory activities occur simultaneously. (See Fig. 8-2.)

The heart is enclosed in a sac called the **pericardium** and is composed of three distinct layers:

• **endocardium,** a serous membrane that lines the four chambers of the heart and its valves and is continuous with the endothelium of the arteries and veins
• **myocardium,** the muscular layer of the heart
• **epicardium,** the outermost layer of the heart.

The heart is divided into four chambers. (See Fig. 8-3, page 226.) The two upper chambers, the (1) **right atrium (RA)** and (2) **left atrium (LA),** collect blood. The two lower chambers, the (3) **right ventricle (RV)** and (4) **left ventricle (LV),** pump blood from the heart. The right ventricle pumps blood to the lungs **(pulmonary circulation)** for oxygenation, and the left ventricle pumps oxygenated blood to the entire body **(systemic circulation).**

Deoxygenated blood from the body returns to the right atrium by way of two large veins: the (5) **superior vena cava,** which collects and carries blood from the upper body, and the (6) **inferior vena cava,** which collects and carries blood from the lower body. From the right atrium, blood passes through the (7) **tricuspid valve,** consisting of three **leaflets,** to the right ventricle. When the heart contracts, blood leaves the right ventricle by way of the (8) **left pulmonary artery** and (9) **right pulmonary artery** and travels to the lungs. During contraction of the ventricle, the tricuspid

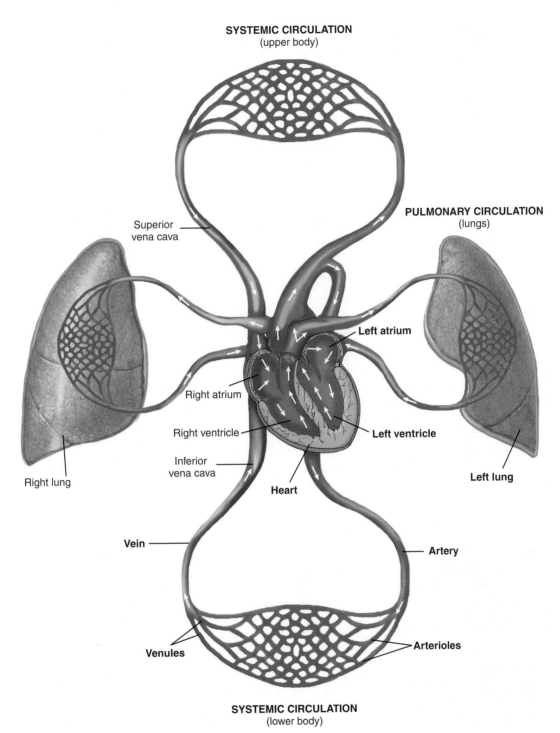

SYSTEMIC CIRCULATION
(upper body)

PULMONARY CIRCULATION
(lungs)

Superior
vena cava

Left atrium

Right atrium

Right ventricle

Left ventricle

Inferior
vena cava

Right lung

Left lung

Heart

Vein

Artery

Venules

Arterioles

SYSTEMIC CIRCULATION
(lower body)

Figure 8-2 Systemic and pulmonary circulation.

valve closes to prevent a backflow of blood to the right atrium. The (10) **pulmonic valve** (or **pulmonary semilunar valve**) prevents **regurgitation** of blood into the right ventricle from the pulmonary artery. In the lungs, the pulmonary artery branches into millions of capillaries, each lying close to an alveolus. Here, carbon dioxide in the blood is exchanged for oxygen that has been drawn into the lungs during inhalation.

Pulmonary capillaries unite to form four pulmonary veins—two (11) **right pulmonary veins** and two (12) **left pulmonary veins.** These vessels carry oxygenated blood back to the heart. They

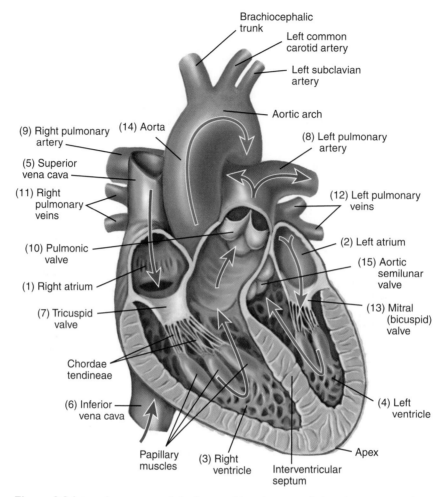

Brachiocephalic
trunk

Left common
carotid artery

Left subclavian
artery

Aortic arch

(9) Right pulmonary
artery

(14) Aorta

(8) Left pulmonary
artery

(5) Superior
vena cava

(11) Right
pulmonary
veins

(12) Left pulmonary
veins

(10) Pulmonic
valve

(2) Left atrium

(15) Aortic
semilunar
valve

(1) Right atrium

(7) Tricuspid
valve

(13) Mitral
(bicuspid)
valve

Chordae
tendineae

(6) Inferior
vena cava

(4) Left
ventricle

Apex

Papillary
muscles

(3) Right
ventricle

Interventricular
septum

Figure 8-3 Internal structures of the heart, with red arrows designating oxygen-rich blood flow and blue arrows designating oxygen-poor blood flow.

deposit blood in the left atrium. From there, blood passes to the left ventricle through the (13) **mitral (bicuspid) valve,** a structure consisting of two leaflets. Upon contraction of the ventricles, the oxygenated blood leaves the heart through the largest artery of the body, the (14) **aorta.** The aorta contains the (15) **aortic semilunar valve (aortic valve)** that permits blood to flow in only one direction—from the left ventricle to the aorta. The aorta branches into many smaller arteries that carry blood to all parts of the body.

It is important to understand that the myocardium cannot use the blood that passes through the chambers of the heart as a source of oxygen and nutrients. Instead, an arterial system composed of the coronary arteries branches from the aorta and provides the myocardium with its own blood supply. (See Fig. 8-4.) The artery vascularizing the right side of the heart is the (1) **right coronary artery.** The artery vascularizing the left side of the heart is the (2) **left coronary artery.** The left coronary artery divides into two branches, the (3) **left anterior descending artery** and the (4) **circumflex artery.** If blood flow in the coronary arteries is diminished, damage to the heart muscle may result. When severe damage occurs, part of the heart muscle may die.

Conduction System of the Heart

Within the heart, specialized cardiac tissue known as **conduction tissue** has the sole function of initiating and spreading contraction impulses. (See Fig. 8-5.) This tissue consists of the following four masses of highly specialized cells that possess characteristics of both nervous and cardiac tissue:

- sinoatrial (SA) node
- atrioventricular (AV) node

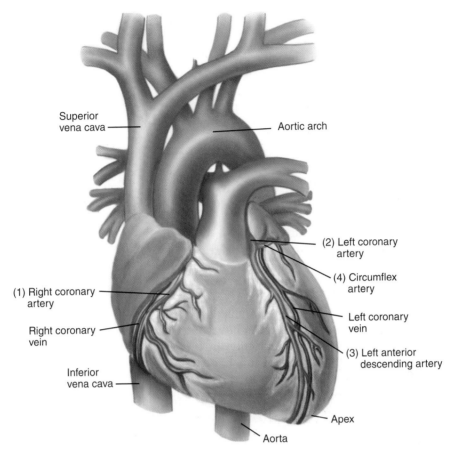

Figure 8-4 Anterior view of the heart showing coronary arteries.

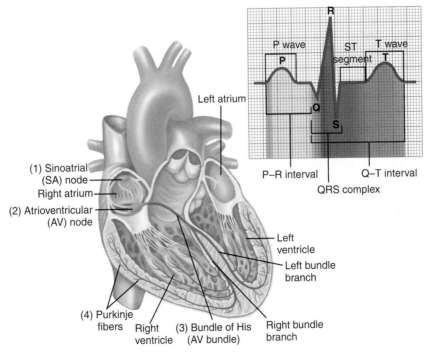

Figure 8-5 Conduction system.

• bundle of His (AV bundle)
• Purkinje fibers

The (1) **sinoatrial (SA) node** is located in the upper portion of the right atrium and possesses its own intrinsic rhythm. Without being stimulated by external nerves, it has the ability to initiate and propagate each heartbeat, thereby setting the basic pace for the cardiac rate. For this reason, the SA node is commonly known as the **pacemaker** of the heart. The cardiac rate may be altered by impulses from the **autonomic nervous system.** Such an arrangement allows outside influences to accelerate or decelerate heart rate. For example, the heart beats more quickly during physical exertion and more slowly during rest. Each electrical impulse discharged by the SA node is transmitted to the (2) **atrioventricular (AV) node,** causing the atria to contract. The AV node is located at the base of the right atrium. From this point, a tract of conduction fibers called the (3) **bundle of His (or AV bundle),** composed of a right and left branch, relays the impulse to the (4) **Purkinje fibers.** These fibers extend up the ventricle walls. The Purkinje fibers transmit the impulse to the right and left ventricles, causing them to contract. Blood is now forced from the heart through the pulmonary artery and aorta. Thus, the sequence of the four structures responsible for conduction of a contraction impulse is as follows:

SA node → AV node → bundle of His → Purkinje fibers

Impulse transmission through the conduction system generates weak electrical impulses on the surface of the body. These impulses can be recorded on graph paper by an instrument called an **electrocardiograph.** The needle deflection of the electrocardiograph produces waves or peaks designated by the letters P, Q, R, S, and T, each of which is associated with a specific electrical event, as follows:

• The **P wave** is the depolarization (contraction) of the atria.
• The **QRS complex** is the depolarization (contraction) of the ventricles.
• The **T wave**, which appears a short time later, is the repolarization (recovery) of the ventricles.

Blood Pressure

Blood pressure (BP) is the force exerted by blood against the arterial walls during two phases of a heartbeat: the contraction phase **(systole)** when the blood is forced out of the heart and the relaxation phase **(diastole)** when the ventricles are filling with blood. Systole produces the maximum force; diastole, the weakest. A **sphygmomanometer** measures blood pressure, which you record as two figures separated by a diagonal line. When recording a blood pressure reading, list systolic pressure first, followed by diastolic pressure. For instance, a blood pressure of *120/80 mm Hg* means a systolic pressure of 120 with a diastolic pressure of 80.

Several factors influence blood pressure:

• resistance of blood flow in blood vessels
• pumping action of the heart
• **viscosity** of blood
• elasticity of arteries
• quantity of blood in the vascular system

Anatomy Review: Cardiovascular System

To review the anatomy of the heart, label the illustration using the listed terms.

aorta

aortic semilunar valve

inferior vena cava

left atrium

left pulmonary artery

left pulmonary veins

left ventricle

mitral (bicuspid) valve

pulmonic valve

right atrium

right pulmonary artery

right pulmonary veins

right ventricle

superior vena cava

tricuspid valve

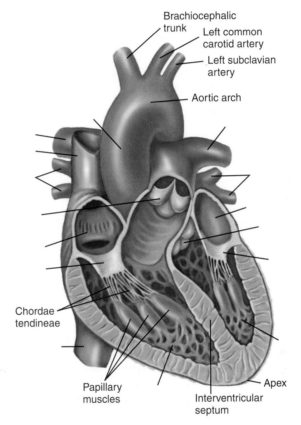

Brachiocephalic trunk

Left common carotid artery

Left subclavian artery

Aortic arch

Chordae tendineae

Papillary muscles

Interventricular septum

Apex

 Check your answers by referring to Figure 8–3 on page 226. Review material that you did not answer correctly.

CONNECTING BODY SYSTEMS—CARDIOVASCULAR SYSTEM

The main function of the cardiovascular (CV) system is to provide a network of vessels through which blood is pumped by the heart to all body cells. Specific functional relationships between the CV system and other body systems are discussed here.

Blood, Lymphatic, and Immune
- The CV system transports the products of the immune system.

Digestive
- The CV system delivers hormones that affect the glandular activity of the digestive tract.
- The vessels of the CV system in the walls of the small intestine absorb nutrients.

Endocrine
- The CV system delivers oxygen and nutrients to the endocrine glands.
- The CV system transports hormones from glands to target organs.

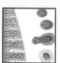

Female Reproductive
- The CV system transports hormones that regulate the menstrual cycle.
- The CV system influences the normal function of sex organs, especially erectile tissue.
- During pregnancy, the vessels of the CV system in the placenta exchange nutrients and waste products.

Integumentary
- The blood vessels of the CV system in the skin regulate body temperature.
- The CV system transports clotting factors to the skin to control bleeding.

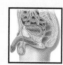

Male Reproductive
- The CV system transports reproductive hormones.
- The CV system influences the normal function of sex organs, especially erectile tissue.

Musculoskeletal
- The CV system removes heat and waste products generated by muscle contraction.
- The CV system delivers oxygen for energy to sustain muscle contraction.
- The CV system delivers calcium and nutrients and removes metabolic wastes from skeletal structures.
- The CV system delivers hormones that regulate skeletal growth.

Nervous
- The CV system carries electrolytes for transmission of electrical impulses.

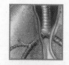

Respiratory
- The CV system transports oxygen and carbon dioxide between lungs and tissues.

Urinary
- The CV system delivers oxygen and nutrients.
- Blood pressure maintains kidney function.

Medical Word Elements

This section introduces combining forms, suffixes, and prefixes related to the cardiovascular system. Word analyses are also provided. From the information provided, complete the meaning of the medical words in the right-hand column. The first one is completed for you.

Element	Meaning	Word Analysis
Combining Forms		
aneurysm/o	aneurysm (widened blood vessel)	**aneurysm/o**/rrhaphy (ăn-ū-rĭz-MOR-ă-fē): *suture of an aneurysm* *-rrhaphy:* suture
angi/o	vessel (usually blood or lymph)	**angi/o**/plasty (ĂN-jē-ō-plăs-tē): _____ *-plasty:* surgical repair *Angioplasty is a procedure that reopens narrowed blood vessels and restores blood flow using a balloon-tipped catheter.*
vascul/o		**vascul**/itis (văs-kū-LĪ-tĭs): _____ *-itis:* inflammation
aort/o	aorta	**aort/o**/stenosis (ā-or-tō-stĕ-NŌ-sĭs): _____ *-stenosis:* narrowing, stricture
arteri/o	artery	**arteri/o**/rrhexis (ăr-tē-rē-ō-RĔK-sĭs): _____ *-rrhexis:* rupture
arteriol/o	arteriole	**arteriol**/itis (ăr-tēr-ē-ō-LĪ-tĭs): _____ *-itis:* inflammation
atri/o	atrium	**atri/o**/megaly (ā-trē-ō-MĔG-ă-lē): _____ *-megaly:* enlargement
ather/o	fatty plaque	**ather**/oma (ăth-ĕr-Ō-mă): _____ *-oma:* tumor *Atheromas are formed when fatty plaque builds up on the inner lining of arterial walls.*
cardi/o	heart	**cardi/o**/megaly (kăr-dē-ō-MĔG-ă-lē): _____ *-megaly:* enlargement
coron/o		**coron**/ary (KOR-ō-nă-rē): _____ *-ary:* pertaining to *Coronary artery disease (CAD) is the most common type of heart disease and the leading cause of death in the United States in men and women.*
electr/o	electricity	**electr/o**/cardi/o/gram (ē-lĕk-trō-KĂR-dē-ō-grăm): _____ *cardi/o:* heart *-gram:* record, recording *An electrocardiogram helps detect many heart problems including heart attacks, arrhythmias, and heart failure.*

(continued)

Medical Word Elements—cont'd

Element	Meaning	Word Analysis
embol/o	embolus (plug)	**embol**/ectomy (ĕm-bō-LĔK-tō-mē): _____ *-ectomy:* excision, removal *An embolectomy is performed in emergency situations to open blood vessels and reestablish blood flow.*
hemangi/o	blood vessel	**hemangi**/oma (hē-măn-jē-Ō-mă): _____ *-oma:* tumor *Hemangiomas, also called strawberry marks and found mostly in neonates, are benign tumors of cells that line blood vessels and usually disappear over time.*
my/o	muscle	**my/o**/cardi/al (mī-ō-KĂR-dē-ăl): _____ *cardi:* heart *-al:* pertaining to
phleb/o	vein	**phleb**/ectasis (flĕ-BĔK-tă-sĭs): _____ *-ectasis:* dilation, expansion
ven/o		**ven/o**/stasis (vē-nō-STĀ-sĭs): _____ *-stasis:* standing still *Venostasis, also called phlebostasis, is an abnormally slow blood flow in the veins and is a major risk factor for clot formation.*
scler/o	hardening; sclera (white of eye)	**arteri/o**/scler/osis (ăr-tē-rē-ō-sklĕ-RŌ-sĭs): _____ *arteri/o:* artery *-osis:* abnormal condition; increase (used primarily with blood cells) *The most common cause of arteriosclerosis is the presence of an atheroma in the vessel. Other causes include smoking, diabetes, high blood pressure, obesity, and familial tendency.*
sept/o	septum	**sept/o**/stomy (sĕp-TŎS-tō-mē): _____ *-stomy:* forming an opening (mouth) *Septostomy is a temporary procedure performed to increase systemic oxygenation in infants with congenital heart defects until corrective surgery can be performed.*
sphygm/o	pulse	**sphygm**/oid (SFĬG-moyd): _____ *-oid:* resembling
sten/o	narrowing, stricture	**sten/o**/tic (stĕ-NŎT-ĭk): _____ *-tic:* pertaining to
thromb/o	blood clot	**thromb/o**/lysis (thrŏm-BŎL-ĭ-sĭs): _____ *-lysis:* separation; destruction; loosening *In thrombolysis, enzymes that destroy blood clots are infused into the occluded vessel.*

Medical Word Elements—cont'd

Element	Meaning	Word Analysis
valv/o	valve	**valv/o**/tomy (văl-VŎT-ō-mē): _____ *-tomy:* incision *Valvotomy commonly involves use of a balloon catheter passed through a blood vessel in the groin to gain access to a stenosed valve of the heart.*
valvul/o	'	**valvul/o**/plasty (VĂL-vū-lō-plăs-tē): _____ *-plasty:* surgical repair
ventricul/o	ventricle (of the heart or brain)	**ventricul**/ar (v ĕn-TRĬK-ū-lăr): _____ *-ar:* pertaining to

Suffixes

Element	Meaning	Word Analysis
-cardia	heart condition	tachy/**cardia** (tăk-ē-KĂR-dē-ă): _____ *tachy-:* rapid
-stenosis	narrowing, stricture	aort/o/**stenosis** (ā-or-tō-st ĕ-NŌ-s ĭs): _____ *aort/o:* aorta

Prefixes

Element	Meaning	Word Analysis
brady-	slow	**brady**/cardia (brăd-ē-KĂR-dē-ă): _____ *-cardia:* heart condition
endo-	in, within	**endo**/vascul/ar (ĕn-dō-VĂS-kū-lăr): _____ *vascul:* vessel (usually blood or lymph) *-ar:* pertaining to *Endovascular procedures are those that occur within the lumen of a vessel.*
extra-	outside	**extra**/vascul/ar (ĕks-tră-VĂS-kū-lăr): _____ *vascul:* vessel (usually blood or lymph) *-ar:* pertaining to
peri-	around	**peri**/cardi/al (pĕr-ĭ-KĂR-dē-ăl): _____ *cardi:* heart *-al:* pertaining to *Pericardial refers to the membrane that surrounds the heart, the pericardium.*
trans-	across	**trans**/sept/al (trăns-SĔP-tăl): _____ *sept:* septum *-al:* pertaining to

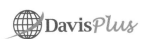

Visit the *Medical Terminology Systems* online resource center at Davis*Plus* for an audio exercise of the terms in this table. Other activities are also available to reinforce content.

It is time to review medical word elements by completing Learning Activities 8-1 and 8-2.

Disease Focus

Many cardiac disorders, especially coronary artery disease, and valvular disorders are associated with a genetic predisposition. Although some of the most serious cardiovascular diseases have few signs and symptoms, when they occur they may include chest pain, breathing difficulties, cardiac irregularities, and loss of consciousness.

For diagnosis, treatment, and management of cardiovascular disorders, the medical services of a **cardiologist** may be warranted. **Cardiology** is the medical specialty concerned with disorders of the cardiovascular system.

Arteriosclerosis

Arteriosclerosis is a progressive degenerative disease of arterial walls that causes them to become thickened and brittle, restricting the flow of blood to tissues and organs. Its most common cause is the buildup of a plaquelike substance composed of cholesterol, lipids, and cellular debris (**atheroma**) on the interior arterial wall. Over time, the atheroma hardens (**atherosclerosis**) and increases in size, causing the lumen of the artery to narrow. (See Fig. 8-6.) In some instances, blood hemorrhages into the plaque and forms a clot (**thrombus**) that may break loose, travel through the vascular system, and lodge in a more distal area of the artery. Arterial emboli that completely block circulation cause localized tissue death (**infarction**) in the surrounding area. A partial blocking of circulation causes localized tissue anemia (**ischemia**).

Arteries usually affected by arteriosclerosis include the coronary, carotid, cerebral, and femoral arteries and the aorta. Depending on the artery involved, signs and symptoms vary. Arteriosclerosis in the coronary arteries causes chest pain and tightness (**angina**), commonly with excessive sweating (**diaphoresis**). Arteriosclerosis in the carotid and cerebral arteries causes weakness or paralysis on one side of the body (**hemiplegia**), blurred vision, and confusion. Arteriosclerosis in the femoral arteries causes muscle pain (**myalgia**) in calves, thighs, and feet.

Major risk factors for developing arteriosclerosis include an elevated level of fatty substances in the blood (**hyperlipidemia**), age, family history, smoking, hypertension, and diabetes. Treatment for arteriosclerosis varies depending on the location and symptoms. Drugs that slow down or reverse fat buildup (**statins**) in arteries, those that control blood pressure (**antihypertensives**), and those that reduce thrombus formation (**anticoagulants**) are helpful. Surgical treatments include repairing the affected vessels (**angioplasty**) and surgical removal of fatty deposits from the inside of the artery (**endarterectomy**). Physicians commonly use endarterectomy to treat carotid artery disease, peripheral artery disease, and diseases of the renal artery and aortic arch. (See Fig. 8-7.)

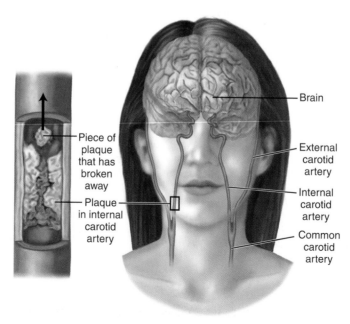

Figure 8-6 Atherosclerosis of the internal carotid artery.

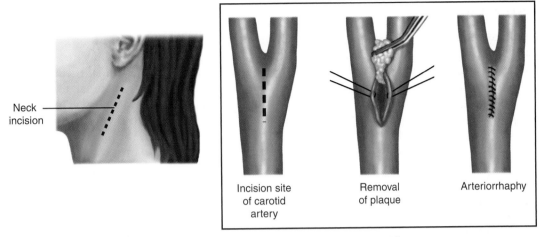

Neck incision

Incision site of carotid artery

Removal of plaque

Arteriorrhaphy

Figure 8-7 Endarterectomy of the common carotid artery.

Coronary Artery Disease (CAD)

For the heart to function effectively, the myocardium must receive an adequate and uninterrupted supply of blood from the coronary arteries. Any disease that interferes with the ability of the coronary arteries to supply blood to the myocardium is called **coronary artery disease (CAD)**. The major cause of CAD is arteriosclerosis. Other causes include hypertension, diabetes, hyperlipidemia, and radiation therapy to the chest associated with certain types of cancers. An inadequate blood supply to the myocardium **(ischemia)** may lead to death **(necrosis)** of the heart muscle **(myocardial infarction [MI]).** (See Fig. 8-8.)

As the heart muscle undergoes necrotic changes, it releases several highly specific substances, including enzymes, proteins, and hormones. Rapid elevation in the levels of these substances at predictable times following MI helps differentiate MI from pericarditis, abdominal aortic aneurysm (AAA), and acute pulmonary embolism.

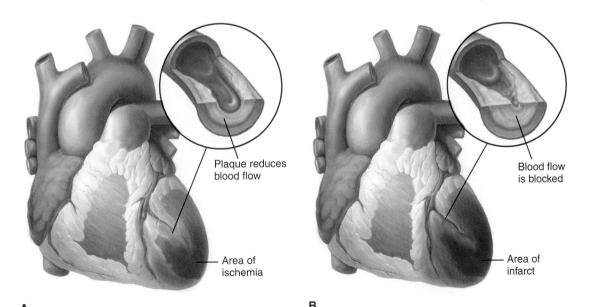

Plaque reduces blood flow

Area of ischemia

Blood flow is blocked

Area of infarct

A

B

Figure 8-8 Coronary artery occlusions. (A) Partial occlusion showing area of ischemia. (B) Complete occlusion showing myocardial infarction.

Endocarditis

Endocarditis is an inflammation of the inner lining of the heart and its valves. It is usually caused by bacteria **(infective endocarditis)** that have entered the bloodstream from infections in remote regions of the body (gut, skin, mouth) and have lodged on damaged endocardial tissue or abnormal valves. Once established in the heart, bacteria and other cellular material form clumps **(vegetations)** on the valves, especially the mitral valve, causing it to narrow **(mitral valve stenosis)** and impeding blood flow to the ventricle or not to close properly **(mitral valve insufficiency)**, commonly causing a backflow of blood into the atrium **(regurgitation)**. (See Fig. 8-9.) Although medications may prove helpful, if heart failure develops as a result of damaged heart valves, surgery to correct the damaged valves **(valvuloplasty)** may be the only treatment option. Whenever possible, the original valve is repaired. When the damage is extensive, a mechanical device or one made of human or animal tissue **(bioprosthetic)** may be used.

Congenital valvular defects, scarlet fever, rheumatic fever, mitral valve prolapse, and prosthetic valves are predisposing factors for developing endocarditis. Patients susceptible to endocarditis are given antibiotic treatment to protect against infection before invasive procedures **(prophylactic treatment)**.

Varicose Veins

Varicose veins are enlarged, engorged, twisted, superficial veins. They develop when the valves of the veins do not function properly **(incompetent)** and fail to prevent the backflow of blood. Varicose veins may develop in almost any part of the body, including the esophagus **(varices)** and rectum **(hemorrhoids)**, but occur most commonly in the greater and lesser saphenous veins of the lower legs. (See Fig. 8-10.) Varicose veins of the legs are not typically painful but may be unsightly in appearance. Treatment of mild cases of varicose veins includes use of elastic stockings and rest periods, during which the legs are elevated.

However, if pain, open lesions, or inflammation of the vein **(phlebitis)** develops, treatment may be required. Destroying the tissue within the vein **(endovenous ablation)** is an effective and minimally

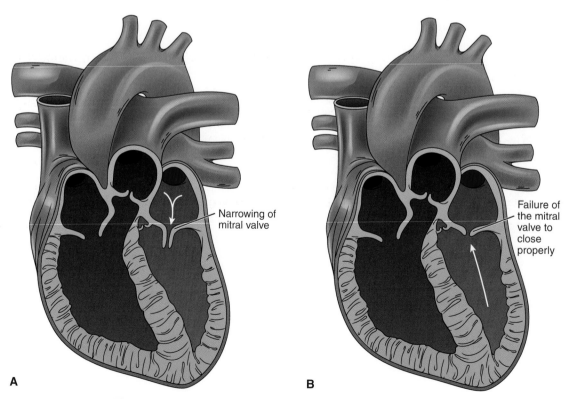

A   B

Figure 8-9 Valvular defects. (A) Mitral stenosis. (B) Mitral insufficiency.

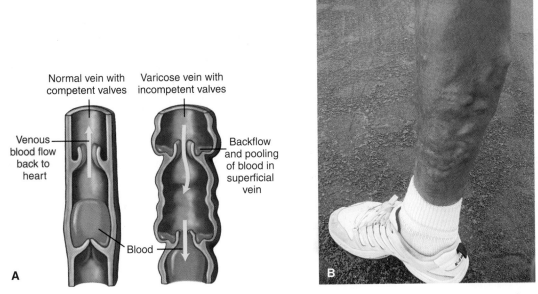

Figure 8-10 Healthy and unhealthy veins and valves. (A) Valve function in competent and incompetent valves. (B) Varicose veins.

invasive technique in treating varicose veins. Common endovenous options include treatments that employ lasers, heat **(radiofrequency ablation),** extreme cold **(cryoablation),** or chemicals **(sclerotherapy).** These treatments destroy the vein wall and coagulate blood inside the vessel, causing it to collapse and seal. Later, the vessels dissolve within the body, becoming less visible or disappearing altogether. Endovascular methods of treatment are replacing the more invasive, complicated ligation and stripping, which is more painful and requires a longer convalescent time.

Oncology

Although rare, the most common primary tumor of the heart is composed of mucous connective tissue **(myxoma);** however, these tumors tend to be benign. Although some myxomas originate in the endocardium of the heart chambers, most arise in the left atrium. Occasionally, they impede mitral valve function and cause a decrease in exercise tolerance, dyspnea, fluid in the lungs **(pulmonary edema),** and systemic problems, including joint pain **(arthralgia),** malaise, and anemia. These tumors are usually identified and located by two-dimensional echocardiography. When present, they should be excised surgically.

Most cancers of the heart are the result of a malignancy originating in another area of the body **(primary tumor)** that spreads **(metastasizes)** to the heart. The most common primary tumor site is a darkly pigmented mole or tumor **(malignant melanoma)** of the skin, bone marrow, or lymphatic tissue. Treatment of the metastatic tumor of the heart involves treating the primary tumor.

Diseases and Conditions

This section introduces diseases and conditions of the cardiovascular system, along with their meanings and pronunciations. Word analyses for selected terms are also provided.

Term	Definition

aneurysm
ĂN-ū-rĭzm

Localized abnormal dilation of a vessel, usually an artery (See Fig. 8-11.)

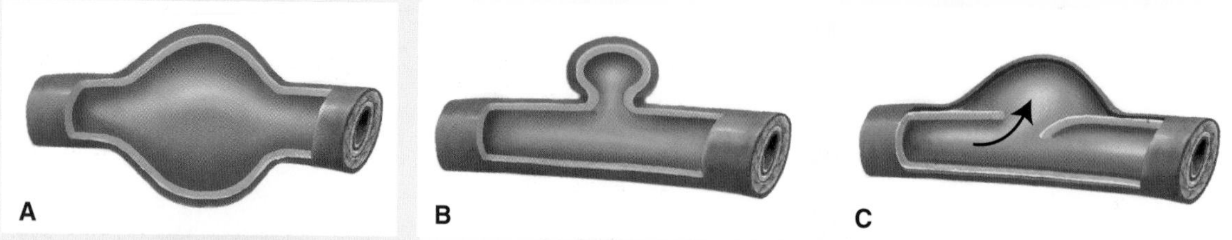

A   B   C

Figure 8-11 Types of aneurysm. (A) Fusiform, with dilation of the entire circumference of the artery. (B) Saccular, with dilation of one side of the artery. (C) Dissecting, in which a tear in the inner layer causes a cavity to form between the layers of the artery that fills with blood and expands with each heartbeat.

angina
ĂN-jĭ-nă
angin: choking pain
-a: noun ending

Chest pain caused by obstructions or spasms of the coronary arteries that decrease blood flow to the myocardium; also called *angina pectoris*

Anginal pain typically radiates down the left arm or into the shoulder, neck, jaw, or back. (See Fig. 8-12.)

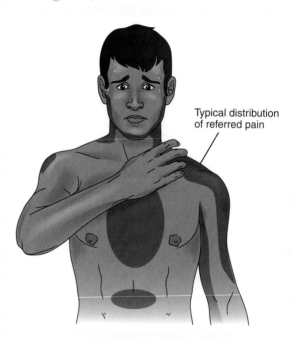

Typical distribution of referred pain

Figure 8-12 Common locations of anginal pain, which may vary in combination and intensity.

Diseases and Conditions—cont'd

Term	Definition
arrhythmia ă-RĬTH-mē-ă	Irregularity in the rate or rhythm of the heart; also called *dysrhythmia*

bradycardia
  brăd-ē-KĂR-dē-ă
   brady-: slow
   -cardia: heart condition
	Abnormally slow heart rate, usually fewer than 60 beats per minute in a resting adult

fibrillation fĭ-brĭl-Ā-shŭn	Abnormally rapid, uncoordinated quivering of the myocardium that can affect the atria or the ventricles
heart block	Interference with the normal transmission of electrical impulses from the SA node to the Purkinje fibers

tachycardia
  tăk-ē-KĂR-dē-ă
   tachy-: rapid
   -cardia: heart condition
	Abnormally fast but regular rhythm, with the heart possibly beating up to 200 beats/minute
	Patients with tachycardia may experience palpitations.

bruit BRWĒ	Soft, blowing sound heard on auscultation and associated valvular action, the movement of blood as it passes an obstruction, or both; also called *murmur*
cardiomyopathy kăr-dē-ō-mī-ŎP-ă-thē *cardi/o:* heart *my/o:* muscle *-pathy:* disease	Disease or weakening of heart muscle that diminishes cardiac function *Causes of cardiomyopathy include viral or bacterial infections, metabolic disorders, and general systemic disease.*
coarctation kō-ărk-TĀ-shŭn	Narrowing of a vessel, especially the aorta
embolism ĔM-bō-lĭzm *embol:* embolus (plug) *-ism:* condition	Intravascular mass that dislodges from one part of the body and causes a blockage in another area, commonly leading to life-threatening situations *The deadliest form of embolism is a pulmonary embolism that blocks blood flow to the lungs, causing chest pain, hypoxemia, tachycardia, and even sudden death. When treated, mortality rate drops considerably.*
heart failure (HF)	Disorder that occurs when the heart is unable to effectively pump the quantity of blood required by the body *Common causes of HF include coronary artery disease, hypertension, diabetes, and obesity. When, blood returning to the heart backs up, causing congestion in the lungs, liver, abdomen and lower extremities, the disease is called congestive heart failure (CHF).*
hyperlipidemia hī-pĕr-lĭp-ĭ-DĒ-mē-ă *hyper-:* excessive, above normal *lipid:* fat *-emia:* blood condition	Excessive amounts of lipids (cholesterol, phospholipids, and triglycerides) in the blood *Hyperlipidemia is associated with an increased risk of atherosclerosis.*

(continued)

Diseases and Conditions—cont'd

Term	Definition
hypertension (HTN) hī-pĕr-TĔN-shŭn *hyper-:* excessive, above normal *-tension:* to stretch	Elevated blood pressure persistently higher than 140/90 mm Hg (See Table 8-1.)
hypotension hī-pō-TĔN-shŭn *hypo-:* under, below, deficient *-tension:* to stretch	Low blood pressure persistently lower than 90/60 mm Hg
mitral valve prolapse (MVP) MĪ-trăl, PRŌ-lăps	Structural defect in which the mitral (bicuspid) valve leaflets prolapse into the left atrium during ventricular contraction (systole), resulting in incomplete closure and backflow of blood *Common signs and symptoms of MVP include a characteristic murmur heard on auscultation and palpitations of the heart.*
palpitation păl-pĭ-TĀ-shŭn	Sensation of an irregular heartbeat, commonly described as pounding, racing, skipping a beat, or flutter
peripheral artery disease (PAD) pĕr-ĬF-ĕr-ăl ĂR-tĕr-ē	Common circulatory disorder characterized by a reduced flow of blood to the extremities, especially the legs, resulting in muscle cramping and pain, and commonly the result of atherosclerosis *If PAD is caused by plaque, it may signal disease in the arteries of vital organs, including the heart (heart attack) and brain (stroke).*
phlebitis flĕ-BĪ-tĭs *phleb:* vein *-itis:* inflammation	Inflammation of a deep or superficial vein of the arms or legs (more commonly the legs) *Thrombophlebitis, a more serious condition, is vein inflammation caused by the development of thrombi within the veins.*
rheumatic heart disease (RHD) roo-MĂT-ĭk	Serious pathological condition resulting from rheumatic fever, commonly causing permanent scarring of the heart valves, especially the mitral valve *Chronic rheumatic heart disease remains the leading cause of mitral valve stenosis and valve replacement in adults.*
syncope SĬN-kō-pē	Partial or complete loss of consciousness usually caused by a decreased supply of blood to the brain; also called *fainting*
thrombosis thrŏm-BŌ-sĭs *thromb:* blood clot *-osis:* abnormal condition; increase (used primarily with blood cells)	Abnormal condition in which a blood clot develops in a vessel and obstructs it at the site of its formation
deep vein thrombosis (DVT) thrŏm-BŌ-sĭs *thromb:* blood clot *-osis:* abnormal condition; increase (used primarily with blood cells)	Blood clot that forms in the deep veins of the body, especially those in the legs or thighs; also called *deep venous thrombosis* (See Fig. 8-13.) *In DVT, blood clots may break away from the vein wall and travel in the body, especially to the lungs.*

Diseases and Conditions—cont'd

Term	Definition

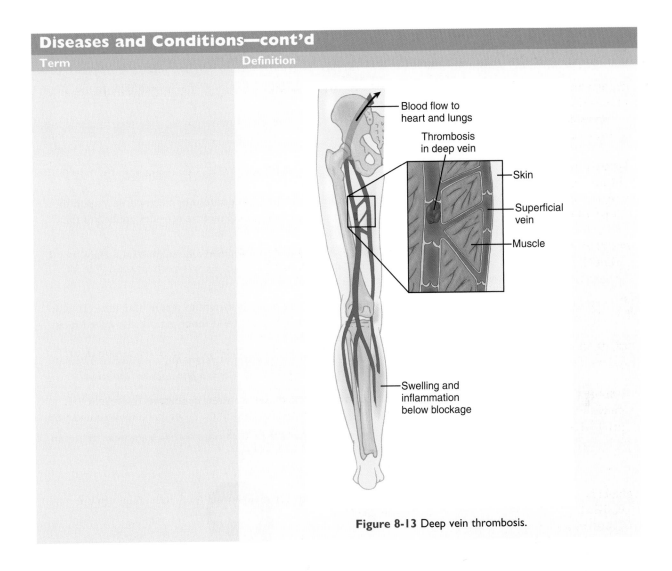

Figure 8-13 Deep vein thrombosis.

Table 8-1	Hypertensive Blood Pressure Levels		

This table lists blood pressure levels with their corresponding systolic and diastolic readings.

Level	Systolic	Diastolic
Normal	Less than 120 mm Hg	Less than 80 mm Hg
Prehypertension (HTN)*	120–139 mm Hg	80–89 mm Hg
Stage 1 HTN	140–159 mm Hg	90–99 mm Hg
Stage 2 HTN	160 mm Hg or higher	100 mm Hg or higher

*A blood pressure of 130/80 mm Hg or higher is considered hypertension in persons with diabetes and chronic kidney disease.

 It is time to review pathology, diseases, and conditions by completing Learning Activity 8–3.

Diagnostic, Surgical, and Therapeutic Procedures

This section introduces diagnostic, surgical, and therapeutic procedures used to diagnose and treat cardiovascular disorders. Descriptions are provided, along with pronunciations and word analyses for selected terms.

Procedure	Description
Diagnostic Procedures	
Clinical	
electrocardiography (ECG, EKG) ē-lĕk-trō-kăr-dē-ŎG-ră-fē *electr/o:* electricity *cardi/o:* heart *-graphy:* process of recording	Procedure that graphically records the spread of electrical excitation to different parts of the heart using small metal electrodes applied to the chest, arms, and legs *ECG helps diagnose abnormal heart rhythms and myocardial damage.*
Holter monitor test HŌL-tĕr	Procedure that uses a small, portable system to record and store the electrical activity of the heart over a 24- to 48-hour period; also called *event monitor test* (See Fig. 8-14.) *Holter monitoring is particularly useful in diagnosing a cardiac arrhythmia that would be missed during an ECG of only a few minutes' duration.*
stress test	ECG taken under controlled exercise stress conditions (bicycle or treadmill) *A stress test may show abnormal ECG tracings that do not appear during an ECG taken when the patient is resting.*

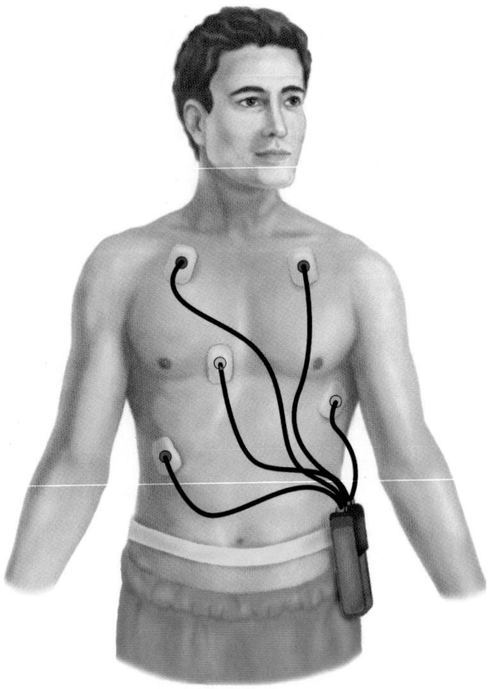

Figure 8-14 Holter monitor.

Diagnostic, Surgical, and Therapeutic Procedures—cont'd

Procedure	Description
Laboratory	
cardiac biomarkers KĂR-dē-ăk BĪ-ō-măr-kĕrz *cardi:* heart *-ac:* pertaining to	Blood test that measures the presence and amount of several substances released by the heart when it is damaged or under stress; also called *cardiac enzyme test* *When the presence of cardiac biomarkers is first detected in a blood specimen, it helps diagnose and differentiate various cardiac conditions.*
lipid panel LĬP-ĭd	Series of blood tests (total cholesterol, high-density lipoprotein, low-density lipoprotein, and triglycerides) used to assess risk factors of ischemic heart disease
Imaging	
angiography ăn-jē-ŎG-ră-fē *angi/o:* vessel (usually blood or lymph) *-graphy:* process of recording	Procedure that records a radiographic image of the inside of a blood vessel (angiogram) after injection of a contrast medium *Angiography of an artery is called arteriography. Angiography of a vein is called venography.*
aortography ā-or-TŎG-ră-fē *aort/o:* aorta *-graphy:* process of recording	Angiography of the aorta and its branches after injection of a contrast medium *Aortography helps diagnose aortic insufficiency.*
coronary angiography KOR-ō-nă-rē *coron:* heart *-ary:* pertaining to	Specialized type of angiography that helps diagnose stenosis or obstruction of the arteries that supply blood to the heart muscle
Doppler US DŎP-lĕr	Ultrasonography used to assess the direction and speed of blood flow through blood vessels by reflecting sound waves off red blood cells; also called *ultrasonography using sound pitch* *Various Doppler techniques help diagnose blood clots, valvular disorders, arterial occlusions, and aneurysms.*
carotid artery US kă-RŎT-ĭd ĂR-tĕr-ē	Ultrasound procedure that determines blood flow problems caused by blood clots, plaque, or tears on the walls of the carotid arteries (See Fig. 8-15, page 244.)

(continued)

Diagnostic, Surgical, and Therapeutic Procedures—cont'd

Procedure	Description

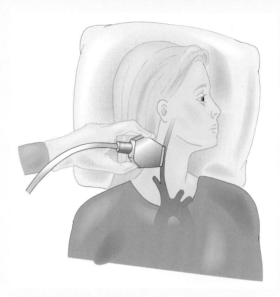

Figure 8-15 Doppler ultrasound of the carotid artery in which a handheld transducer sends and receives sound waves that are processed by a computer to provide information regarding blood flow through the vessel.

echocardiography (ECHO)
ĕk-ō-kăr-dē-ŎG-ră-fē

echo-: repeated sound
cardi/o: heart
-graphy: process of recording

Ultrasound test that produces moving images of blood passing through the heart, valves, and chambers, and assesses cardiac output

ECHO involves placement of a transducer on the chest to direct ultrahigh-frequency sound waves toward cardiac structures. Reflected echoes are displayed on a monitor.

myocardial perfusion imaging (MPI)
mī-ō-KĂR-dē-ăl pĕr-FŪ-zhŭn

my/o: muscle
cardi: heart
-al: pertaining to

Noninvasive imaging test using a radioactive tracer in conjunction with a stress test to show how well blood flows through (perfuses) the heart muscle at rest and during exercise; also called *nuclear stress test*

Typically, MPI involves intravenous administration of such radioactive substances as Cardiolite and thallium during the test. A gamma camera identifies areas of reduced blood flow that show up as "cold spots," an indication of myocardial damage.

single-photon emission computed tomography (SPECT)
tō-MŎG-ră-fē

tom/o: to cut
-graphy: process of recording

Myocardial perfusion test that involves injection of a radioactive tracer into the blood while a gamma camera moves in a circle around the patient to create individual images as "slices" of the heart (tomography)

SPECT shows how well blood is flowing to the heart and how efficiently the heart is pumping with the patient at rest or during exercise.

cardiac magnetic resonance imaging (MRI)
KĂR-dē-ăk

cardi: heart
-ac: pertaining to

Specialized MRI procedure that provides images of the heart chambers, valves, major vessels, and pericardium

Cardiac MRI helps evaluate the effects of coronary heart disease, plan treatment strategies, and monitor the progression of disorders over time.

Diagnostic, Surgical, and Therapeutic Procedures—cont'd

Procedure	Description
magnetic resonance angiography (MRA) măg-NĔT-ĭk RĔZ-ĕn-ăns ăn-jē-ŎG-ră-fē *angi/o:* vessel (usually blood or lymph *-graphy:* process of recording	Type of MRI that provides highly detailed images of blood vessels *Unlike angiography, MRA detects blood flow, the condition of blood vessel walls, and blockages without using a contrast medium.*
multiple-gated acquisition (MUGA) scan	Nuclear procedure that uses radioactive tracers to detect how effectively the heart walls move as they contract and then calculates the ejection fraction rate (amount of blood the ventricle can pump out in one contraction) *The ejection fraction rate is the most accurate predictor of overall heart function. The gamma camera is coordinated (gated) with the patient's ECG.*

Other

Procedure	Description
cardiac catheterization (CC) KĂR-dē-ăk kăth-ĕ-tĕr-ĭ-ZĀ-shŭn *cardi:* heart *-ac:* pertaining to	Passage of a catheter into the heart through a vein or artery to provide a comprehensive evaluation of the heart *CC gathers information about the heart, including blood supply through the coronary arteries and blood flow and pressure through the heart's chambers, and enables blood sample collection and x-rays of the heart. (See Fig. 8-16.)*
electrophysiology study (EPS) ē-lĕk-trō-fĭz-ē-ŎL-ō-jē	Special catheterization test that involves insertion of electrode catheters into the heart to study and map the conduction system and safely reproduce the abnormal heart rhythm affecting the patient's heart *The information derived from EPS helps determine the best medication, treatment, or device to control or correct the abnormal rhythm.*

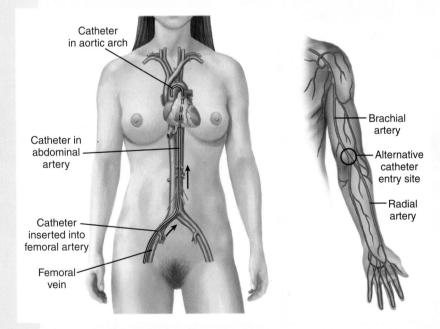

Catheter in aortic arch

Catheter in abdominal artery

Catheter inserted into femoral artery

Femoral vein

Brachial artery

Alternative catheter entry site

Radial artery

Figure 8-16 Cardiac catheterization.

(continued)

Diagnostic, Surgical, and Therapeutic Procedures—cont'd

Procedure	Description
Surgical	

angioplasty

ĂN-jē-ō-plăs-tē

angi/o: vessel (usually blood or lymph)

-plasty: surgical repair

Endovascular procedure that reopens narrowed blood vessels to restore forward blood flow

Angioplasty is most commonly performed on coronary, carotid, renal, or peripheral arteries occluded by atherosclerosis.

percutaneous transluminal coronary angioplasty (PTCA)

pĕr-kū-TĀ-nē-ŭs

trăns-LŪ-mĭ-năl

KOR-ō-nă-rē

ĂN-jē-ō-plăs-tē

per-: through

cutane: skin

-ous: pertaining to

Angioplasty of the coronary arteries that involves insertion of a balloon catheter through the right femoral artery to the site of the stenosis to enlarge the lumen of the artery and restore blood flow

After the balloon opens the lumen, the practitioner deflates and removes it. This procedure is commonly performed in conjunction with stent placement, a device that remains in the artery after the procedure is complete. (See Fig. 8-17.)

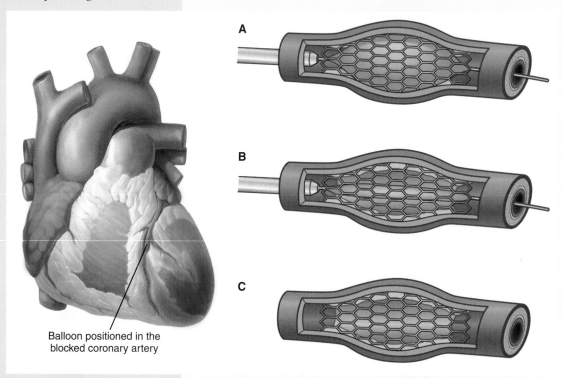

Balloon positioned in the blocked coronary artery

A

B

C

Figure 8-17 Percutaneous transluminal coronary angioplasty (PTCA) with stent placement. (A) Balloon is inflated when positioned at the site of stenosis. (B) Deflation and removal of the balloon after enlargement of the artery. (C) Stent remaining in the artery to hold it open after the procedure is complete.

Diagnostic, Surgical, and Therapeutic Procedures—cont'd

Procedure	Description
cardiac ablation KĂR-dē-ăk ăb-LĀ-shŭn *cardi:* heart *-ac:* pertaining to	Procedure in which a catheter is inserted through a vein in the groin and threaded to the heart to correct structural problems in the heart that cause an arrhythmia *Cardiac ablation employs radiofrequency (heat) laser, or cryoenergy (very cold) to cause scarring of abnormal areas, thus correcting arrhythmias of the heart.*
coronary artery bypass graft (CABG) KOR-ō-nă-rē ĂR-tĕr-ē *coron:* heart *-ary:* pertaining to	Placement of a vessel graft from another part of the body to bypass the blocked area of a coronary artery and restore blood supply to the heart muscle (See Fig. 8-18.) *The two most common vessels for coronary grafts are the internal mammary arteries and the saphenous veins of the leg.* 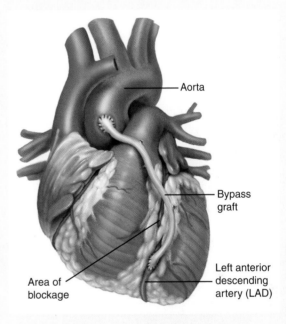 **Figure 8-18** Coronary artery bypass graft.

(continued)

Diagnostic, Surgical, and Therapeutic Procedures—cont'd

Procedure	Description
implantable cardioverter-defibrillator (ICD) KĂR-dē-ō-vĕr-tĕr dē-FĬB-rĭ-lā-tor	Small, battery-powered device inserted within the chest of a patient who is at high risk for developing an arrhythmia, such as ventricular tachycardia, ventricular fibrillation, or cardiac arrest; also called *automatic implantable cardioverter-defibrillator (AICD)* *The ICD monitors and restores the heart to a normal rhythm by delivering an electrical shock to the heart. (See Fig. 8-19.)* **Figure 8-19** Implantable cardioverter defibrillator.
open heart surgery	Surgical procedure in which the sternum is cut in half vertically to open the chest and expose the heart, its valves, or the arteries *During the operation, a heart-lung machine takes over circulation and oxygen exchange to allow surgery on the resting (nonbeating) heart. Types of open heart surgery include CABG, valve replacement, and heart transplant.*
pacemaker insertion PĀS-māk-ĕr	Implantation of a battery-powered device inside the chest to control the heart rate and rhythm *The pacemaker uses a wire positioned in the heart to coordinate the heartbeat with an electrical pulse.*
Therapeutic	
defibrillation dē-fĭb-rĭ-LĀ-shŭn	Lifesaving emergency treatment to restart the heart in cardiorespiratory arrest by delivering high-voltage electrical current through the heart *An automated external defibrillator (AED) analyzes heart rhythm and delivers an electrical shock to stimulate a heart in cardiac arrest. These devices are designed for use by laypersons and are located in ambulances and at airports, sports stadiums, health fitness centers, and other areas where large numbers of people congregate.*

Diagnostic, Surgical, and Therapeutic Procedures—cont'd

Procedure	Description

cardioversion
  KĂR-dē-ō-vĕr-zhŭn
  cardi/o: heart
  –version: turning

Defibrillation technique using low-energy shocks to reset the heart's rhythm back to its normal pattern

Cardioversion helps treat arrhythmias that antiarrhythmic drugs cannot treat. This procedure is not typically performed in an emergency situation but as a scheduled outpatient procedure. (See Fig. 8-20.)

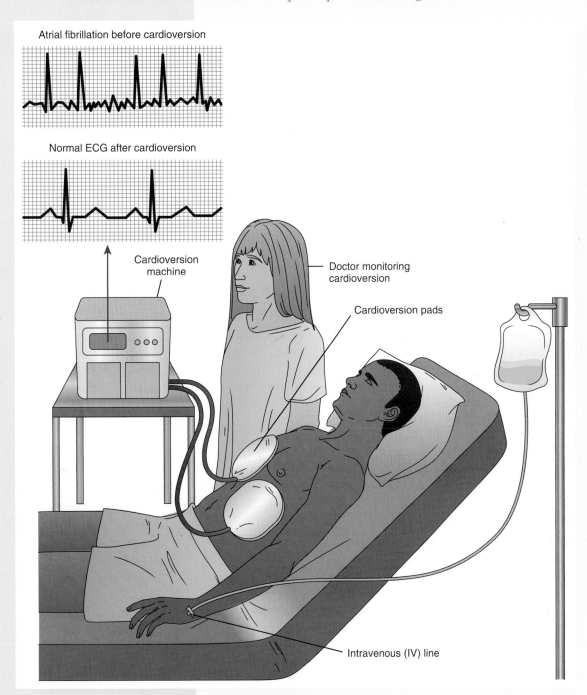

Atrial fibrillation before cardioversion

Normal ECG after cardioversion

Cardioversion machine

Doctor monitoring cardioversion

Cardioversion pads

Intravenous (IV) line

Figure 8-20 Cardioversion.

Pharmacology

A healthy, functional cardiovascular system ensures adequate blood circulation and efficient delivery of oxygen and nutrients to all parts of the body. When any part of the cardiovascular system malfunctions or becomes diseased, drug therapy plays an integral role in establishing and maintaining perfusion and homeostasis.

Medications treat a variety of cardiovascular conditions, including angina pectoris, myocardial infarction, heart failure (HF), arrhythmias, hypertension, hyperlipidemia, and vascular disorders. (See Table 8-2.) Many cardiovascular drugs treat multiple problems simultaneously.

Table 8-2 Drugs Used to Treat Cardiovascular Disorders

This table lists common drug classifications used to treat cardiovascular disorders, their therapeutic actions, and selected generic and trade names.

Classification	Therapeutic Action	Generic and Trade Names
angiotensin-converting enzyme (ACE) inhibitors ăn-jē-ō-TĔN-sĭn ĔN-zīm ĭn-HĬB-ĭ-tōrs	Lower blood pressure by inhibiting the conversion of angiotensin I (an inactive enzyme) to angiotensin II (a potent vasoconstrictor) *ACE inhibitors treat hypertension alone or with other agents and aid in the management of heart failure.*	benazepril bĕn-Ā-ză-prĭl *Lotensin* lisinopril lī-SĬN-ō-prĭl *Prinivil, Zestril*
angiotensin II receptor blockers (ARBs)	Lower blood pressure by blocking the angiotensin II enzyme from causing vasoconstriction	losartan lō-SĂR-tăn *Cozaar* valsartan văl-SĂR-tăn *Diovan*
antiarrhythmics ăn-tē-ă-RĬTH-mĭks	Prevent, alleviate, or correct cardiac arrhythmias (dysrhythmias) by stabilizing the electrical conduction of the heart *Antiarrhythmics help treat atrial and ventricular arrhythmias.*	amiodarone ă-mē-Ō-dă-rōn *Cordarone* digoxin dī-JŎX-ĭn *Lanoxin*
anticoagulants ăn-t ĭ-kō-ĂG-ū-lăntz	Inhibit the body's natural coagulation response to prevent the formation of clots in blood vessels *Clots can embolize, or travel, to vital organs and cause heart attacks or strokes.*	warfarin WĂR-fa-rĭn *Coumadin* dabigatran dă-BĬG-ă-trăn *Pradaxa*
beta blockers BĀ-tă	Block the effect of adrenaline, which slows nerve pulses through the heart, causing a decrease in heart rate *Beta blockers are prescribed for hypertension, angina, and arrhythmias (dysrhythmias).*	atenolol ă-TĔN-ō-lŏl *Tenormin* metoprolol mĕ-TŌ-prō-lŏl *Lopressor, Toprol-XL*

Table 8-2 Drugs Used to Treat Cardiovascular Disorders—cont'd

Classification	Therapeutic Action	Generic and Trade Names
calcium channel blockers KĂL-sē-ŭm	Block movement of calcium (required for blood vessel contraction) into myocardial cells and arterial walls, causing heart rate and blood pressure to decrease *Calcium channel blockers help treat angina pectoris, hypertension, arrhythmias, and heart failure.*	amlodipine ăm-LŌ-dĭ-pēn *Norvasc* diltiazem dĭl-TĪ-ă-zĕm *Cardizem CD* nifedipine nī-FĔD-ĭ-pēn *Adalat CC, Procardia*
diuretics dī-ū-RĔT-ĭks	Act on kidneys to increase excretion of water and sodium *Diuretics reduce fluid buildup in the body, including fluid in the lungs, a common symptom of heart failure. Diuretics also help treat hypertension.*	furosemide fū-RŌ-sĕ-mīd *Lasix* hydrochlorothiazide hī-drō-klō-rō-THĪ-a-zīd *Hydrodiuril*
nitrates NĪ-trāts	Dilate blood vessels of the heart, causing an increase in the amount of oxygen delivered to the myocardium, and widen blood vessels of the body, allowing more blood flow to the heart *Nitrate administration can be sublingual as a spray or tablet, oral as a tablet, transdermal as a patch, topical as an ointment, or intravenous in an emergency setting.*	nitroglycerin nī-trō-GLĬS-ĕr-ĭn *Nitrolingual, Nitrogard, Nitrostat* isosorbide mononitrate ī-sō-SŌR-bīd mŏn-ō-NĪ-trāt *Imdur*
statins STĂ-tĭnz	Lower cholesterol in the blood and reduce its production in the liver by blocking the enzyme that produces it *A combination of Vytorin, a statin drug, with a cholesterol absorption inhibitor not only lowers cholesterol in the blood and reduces its production in the liver but also decreases absorption of dietary cholesterol from the intestine.*	atorvastatin ăh-tor-vă-STĂ-tĭn *Lipitor* simvastatin SĬM-vă-stă-tĭn *Zocor* simvastatin and ezetimibe SĬM-vă-stă-tĭn, ĕ-ZĔ-tĭ-mīb *Vytorin*

Abbreviations

This section introduces cardiovascular-related abbreviations and their meanings.

Abbreviation	Meaning	Abbreviation	Meaning
AAA	abdominal aortic aneurysm	EPS	electrophysiology studies
ACE	angiotensin-converting enzyme (inhibitor)	HTN	hypertension
AED	automated external defibrillator	ICD	implantable cardioverter-defibrillator
AICD	automatic implantable cardioverter-defibrillator	LA	left atrium
ARB	angiotensin receptor blocker	LV	left ventricle
AV	atrioventricular; arteriovenous	MI	myocardial infarction
BP, B/P	blood pressure	MPI	myocardial perfusion imaging
CA	cancer; cardiac arrest; chronological age	MRA	magnetic resonance angiogram, magnetic resonance angiography
CABG	coronary artery bypass graft	MRI	magnetic resonance imaging
CAD	coronary artery disease	MUGA scan	multiple-gated acquisition scan
CC	cardiac catheterization	MVP	mitral valve prolapse
CHF	congestive heart failure	O_2	oxygen
CK	creatine kinase (cardiac enzyme); conductive keratoplasty	PAD	peripheral artery disease
CO_2	carbon dioxide	PTCA	percutaneous transluminal coronary angioplasty
CV	cardiovascular	RA	right atrium
DVT	deep vein thrombosis, deep venous thrombosis	RHD	rheumatic heart disease
ECG, EKG	electrocardiogram, electrocardiography	RV	residual volume; right ventricle
ECHO	echocardiogram, echocardiography; echoencephalogram, echoencephalography	SA, S-A	sinoatrial

Abbreviation	Meaning	Abbreviation	Meaning
HF	heart failure	SPECT	single photon emission computed tomography
Hg	mercury	US	ultrasound

It is time to review procedures, pharmacology, and abbreviations by completing Learning Activity 8-4.

LEARNING ACTIVITIES

The activities that follow provide a review of the cardiovascular system terms introduced in this chapter. Complete each activity and review your answers to evaluate your understanding of the chapter.

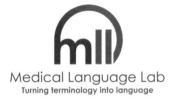

Medical Language Lab
Turning terminology into language

Visit the Medical Language Lab at *medicallanguagelab.com*. Use it to enhance your study and reinforcement of this chapter with the flash-card activity. We recommend that you complete the flash-card activity before starting Learning Activities 8-1 and 8-2.

Learning Activity 8-1
Medical Word Elements

Use the listed elements to build medical words. You may use the elements more than once.

Combining Forms		Suffixes		Prefixes
aneurysm/o	scler/o	-ar	-lysis	a-
aort/o	sept/o	-al	-megaly	trans-
arteri/o	thromb/o	-algia	-oma	peri-
ather/o	valvul/o	-ectasis	-osis	
cardi/o	ventricul/o	-ectomy	-plasty	
phleb/o		-gram	-rrhexis	
rrhythm/o		-ia	-therapy	

1. enlargement of the heart _____
2. tumor composed of fatty plaque _____
3. rupture of an artery _____
4. pertaining to a ventricle _____
5. pertaining to across (or through) the septum _____
6. dilation or expansion of a vein _____
7. record of the aorta _____
8. surgical repair of a valve _____
9. abnormal condition of hardening _____
10. treatment that hardens (a varicose vein) _____
11. destruction of a blood clot _____
12. condition (of the heart) without a rhythm _____
13. pertaining to around an artery _____
14. pain in the heart _____
15. excision of an aneurysm _____

✓ *Check your answers in Appendix A. Review any material that you did not answer correctly.*

Correct Answers _____ X 6.67 = _____ % Score

Learning Activity 8-2

Building Medical Words

Use *ather/o* (fatty plaque) to build words that mean:

1. tumor of fatty plaque _____
2. abnormal condition of fatty plaque hardening _____

Use *phleb/o* (vein) to build words that mean:

3. inflammation of a vein (wall) _____
4. abnormal condition of a blood clot in a vein _____

Use *ven/o* (vein) to build words that mean:

5. pertaining to a vein _____
6. spasm of a vein _____

Use *cardi/o* (heart) to build words that mean:

7. specialist in the study of the heart _____
8. rupture of the heart _____
9. poisonous to the heart _____
10. enlargement of the heart _____

Use *angi/o* (vessel) to build words that mean:

11. softening of a vessel (wall) _____
12. tumor of a vessel _____

Use *thromb/o* (blood clot) to build words that mean:

13. beginning or formation of a blood clot _____
14. abnormal condition of a blood clot _____

Use *aort/o* (heart) to build words that mean:

15. abnormal condition of narrowing or stricture of the aorta _____
16. process of recording the aorta _____

Build surgical words that mean:

17. puncture of the heart _____
18. suture of an artery _____
19. removal of an embolus _____
20. separation, destruction, or loosening of a blood clot _____

✓ *Check your answers in Appendix A. Review material that you did not answer correctly.*

Correct Answers _____ X 5 = _____ % Score

Learning Activity 8-3

Diseases and Conditions

Match the terms with the definitions in the numbered list.

aneurysm	bradycardia	embolism	insufficiency	stenosis
angina	bruit	hyperlipidemia	ischemia	tachycardia
arrhythmia	coarctation	hypertension	palpitation	thrombosis
arteriosclerosis	diaphoresis	infarction	regurgitation	varices

1. area of tissue that undergoes necrosis _____

2. pain, usually in the chest, that is associated with lack of oxygen to the myocardium _____

3. failure of a valve to close completely _____

4. abnormally rapid heart rate _____

5. varicose veins of the esophagus _____

6. soft, blowing sound heard on auscultation; murmur _____

7. abnormally slow heart rate _____

8. sensation of an irregular heartbeat _____

9. abnormal condition in which a blood clot develops in a blood vessel _____

10. localized abnormal dilation of a vessel _____

11. condition in which a mass (usually a blood clot) blocks a blood vessel _____

12. inability of the heart to maintain a normal rhythm _____

13. backflow of blood due to valve failure _____

14. profuse sweating _____

15. hardening of the wall of an artery _____

16. persistent elevated blood pressure _____

17. excessive amounts of lipids in the blood _____

18. narrowing of a vessel, especially the aorta _____

19. deficiency of blood in tissues _____

20. narrowing of a valve _____

Check your answers in Appendix A. Review any material that you did not answer correctly.

Correct Answers _____ X 5 = _____ % Score

Learning Activity 8-4

Procedures, Pharmacology, and Abbreviations

Match the terms with the definitions in the numbered list.

anticoagulants	defibrillation	echocardiography	nitrates	statins
CABG	diuretics	endarterectomy	open heart	stent placement
cardiac biomarkers	Doppler	Holter monitor test	PTCA	stress test
cardioversion	ECG	ICD	sclerotherapy	valvotomy

1. 24-hour ECG tracing taken with a small, portable recording system _____

2. ultrasound test used to visualize internal cardiac structures _____

3. incision to increase the opening of a valve _____

4. agents used to treat angina _____

5. drugs that have lipid-lowering properties _____

6. agents that increase urine output _____

7. evaluates substances released into the blood by the heart when it is under stress; also called *cardiac enzyme studies* _____

8. ultrasound procedure that assesses blood flow direction and speed through blood vessels _____

9. ECG taken under controlled exercise conditions _____

10. lifesaving emergency treatment to restart the heart _____

11. defibrillation technique that resets the normal heart rhythm _____

12. graphically records the electrical activity of the heart _____

13. device inserted in the chest that corrects potential fatal arrhythmias _____

14. insertion of a device that holds open tubular structures _____

15. prevent the formation of clots in blood vessels _____

16. treatment of a varicose vein using a chemical irritant _____

17. surgery that creates a bypass around a blocked segment of a coronary artery _____

18. removal of occluding material from the interior of an artery _____

19. abbreviation for a type of coronary angioplasty _____

20. surgery requiring a heart-lung machine to maintain circulation _____

Check your answers in Appendix A. Review any material that you did not answer correctly.

Correct Answers _____ X 5 = _____ % Score

DOCUMENTING HEALTH-CARE ACTIVITIES

This section provides practical application activities in the form of exercises to help students develop skills in documenting patient care. First, read the medical report. Then complete the activities and exercises that follow.

Documenting Health-Care Activity 8-1

Chart Note: Acute Myocardial Infarction

Gately, Mary   March 15, 20xx

PRESENT ILLNESS: Patient is a 68-year-old woman hospitalized for acute anterior myocardial infarction. She has a history of sudden onset of chest pain. Approximately 2 hours before hospitalization, she had severe substernal pain with radiation to the back. ECG showed evidence of abnormalities. She was given streptokinase and treated with heparin at 800 units per hour. She will be evaluated with a partial thromboplastin time and cardiac enzymes in the morning.

PAST HISTORY: Patient was seen in 20xx, with a history of an inferior MI in 19xx, but she was stable and underwent a treadmill test. Test results showed no ischemia and she had no chest pain. Her records confirmed an MI with enzyme elevation and evidence of a previous inferior MI.

IMPRESSION: Acute lateral anterior myocardial infarction and a previous healed inferior myocardial infarction.

PLAN: At this time the patient is stable, is in the CCU, and will be given appropriate follow-up and supportive care.

Juan Perez, MD
Juan Perez, MD

D: 03–15–20xx
T: 03–15–20xx

bg

Terminology

The terms listed in the table that follows are taken from *Chart Note: Acute Myocardial Infarction.* Use a medical dictionary such as *Taber's Cyclopedic Medical Dictionary,* the appendices of this book, or other resources to define each term. Then review the pronunciation for each term and practice by reading the medical record aloud.

Term	Definition
acute	
cardiac enzymes KĂR-dē-ăk ĔN-zīmz	
ECG	
heparin HĔP-ă-rĭn	
infarction ĭn-FĂRK-shŭn	
ischemia ĭs-KĒ-mē-ă	
lateral LĂT-ĕr-ăl	
MI	
myocardial mī-ō-KĂR-dē-ăl	
partial thromboplastin time thrŏm-bō-PLĂS-tĭn	
streptokinase strĕp-tō-KĪ-nās	
substernal sŭb-STĔR-năl	

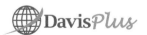 Davis*Plus*

Visit the *Medical Terminology Systems* online resource center at DavisPlus to practice pronunciation and reinforce the meanings of the terms in this medical report.

Critical Thinking

Review *Chart Note: Acute Myocardial Infarction* to answer the questions.

1. How long had the patient experienced chest pain before she was seen in the hospital?

_____

_____

_____

_____

2. Did the patient have a previous history of chest pain?

_____

_____

_____

_____

3. Initially, what medications were administered to stabilize the patient?

_____

_____

_____

_____

4. What two laboratory tests will be used to evaluate the patient?

_____

_____

_____

_____

5. During the current admission, what part of the heart was damaged?

_____

_____

_____

_____

6. Was the location of damage to the heart for this admission the same as that for the initial MI?

_____

_____

_____

_____

Operative Report: Right Temporal Artery Biopsy

General Hospital

1511 Ninth Avenue ■ ■ **Sun City, USA 12345** ■ ■ **(555) 802–1887**

OPERATIVE REPORT

Date: May 14, 20xx   Physician: Dante Riox, MD
Patient: Gonzolez, Roberto   Room: 703

PREOPERATIVE DIAGNOSIS: Rule out right temporal arteritis.

POSTOPERATIVE DIAGNOSIS: Rule out right temporal arteritis.

PROCEDURE: Right temporal artery biopsy

SPECIMEN: 1.5-cm segment of right temporal artery

ESTIMATED BLOOD LOSS: Nil

COMPLICATIONS: None

TIME UNDER SEDATION: 25 minutes

PROCEDURE AND FINDINGS: Informed consent was obtained. Patient was taken to the surgical suite and placed in the supine position. IV sedation was administered. Patient was turned to his left side, and the preauricular area was prepped for surgery using Betadine. Having been draped in sterile fashion, 1% Xylocaine was infiltrated along the palpable temporal artery and a vertical incision was made. Dissection was carried down through the subcutaneous tissue and superficial fascia, which was incised. The temporal artery was located and dissected proximally and distally. Then the artery was ligated with 6-0 Vicryl proximally and distally and a large segment of approximately 1.5 cm was removed. The specimen was sent to the pathology laboratory, and then the superficial fascia was closed with interrupted stitches of 6-0 Vicryl, and the skin was closed with interrupted stitches of 6-0 Prolene. A sterile dressing was applied. Patient tolerated the procedure well and was transferred to the postanesthesia care unit in stable condition.

Dante Riox, MD
Dante Riox, MD

dr:bg

D: 5–14–20xx; T: 5–14–20xx

Terminology

The terms listed in the table that follows are taken from *Operative Report: Right Temporal Artery Biopsy.* Use a medical dictionary such as *Taber's Cyclopedic Medical Dictionary,* the appendices of this book, or other resources to define each term. Then review the pronunciation for each term and practice by reading the medical record aloud.

Term	Definition
arteritis ăr-tĕ-RĪ-tĭs	
Betadine BĀ-tă-dĭn	
dissected dī-SĔKT-ĕd	
distally DĬS-tă-lē	
incised ĭn-SĪZD	
ligated LĪ-gā-tĕd	
palpable PĂL-pă-b'l	
preauricular prē-aw-RĬK-ū-lăr	
proximally PRŎK-sĭ-mă-lē	
superficial fascia soo-pĕr-FĬSH-ăl FĂSH-ē-ă	
supine sū-PĪN	
temporal TĔM-por-ăl	
Xylocaine ZĪ-lō-kān	

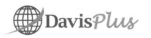

Visit the *Medical Terminology Systems* online resource center at Davis*Plus* to practice pronunciation and reinforce the meanings of the terms in this medical report.

Critical Thinking

Review *Operative Report: Right Temporal Artery Biopsy* to answer the questions.

1. Why was the right temporal artery biopsied?

_____

_____

_____

_____

2. In what position was the patient placed?

_____

_____

_____

_____

3. What was the incision area?

_____

_____

_____

_____

4. How was the temporal artery located for administration of Xylocaine?

_____

_____

_____

_____

5. How was the dissection carried out?

_____

_____

_____

_____

6. What was the size of the specimen?

_____

_____

_____

_____

Documenting Health-Care Activity 8-3

Constructing Chart Notes

To construct chart notes, replace the italicized and boldfaced terms in each of the two case studies with one of the listed medical terms.

angina pectoris	*edema*	*myocardial infarction*
angioplasty	*hypertension*	*palpitations*
catheter	*ischemia*	*stent*
diaphoresis		

Mr. J. presented to the emergency room with complaints of (1) ***chest pains,*** (2) ***profuse sweating,*** and (3) ***an awareness of his heart skipping beats.*** He takes medication for (4) ***persistent high blood pressure.*** He also takes diuretics to promote urine excretion and to control fluid retention that is causing (5) ***puffiness*** in his ankles and legs.

1. _____
2. _____
3. _____
4. _____
5. _____

Mrs. R. has a family history of coronary artery disease. Her 60-year-old uncle died of a (6) ***heart attack*** 2 years ago. Last year, her father was diagnosed with an occlusion of the coronary artery. He was also diagnosed with (7) ***decreased blood flow*** of the coronary vessels. He was admitted to the hospital for a (8) ***surgical repair of the vessel.*** During this surgery, the surgeon threaded a (9) ***tube*** with a deflated balloon into the blocked vessel and used it to press the fatty plaque against the arterial walls. The surgeon then inserted an (10) ***expandable mesh tube*** to keep the artery open after surgery.

6. _____
7. _____
8. _____
9. _____
10. _____

✓ *Check your answers in Appendix A. Review any material that you did not answer correctly.*

Correct Answers _____ X 10 = _____ % Score

CHAPTER

Blood, Lymphatic, and Immune Systems

9

Chapter Outline

Objectives

Upon completion of this chapter, you will be able to:

- Identify and describe the components of blood.
- Locate and identify the structures associated with the lymphatic system.
- Explain the various types of immune processes.
- List the cells associated with the acquired immune response and describe their function.
- Describe the functional relationships among the blood, lymphatic, and immune systems and other body systems.
- Pronounce, spell, and build words related to the blood, lymphatic, and immune systems.
- Describe diseases, conditions, and procedures related to the blood, lymphatic, and immune systems.
- Explain pharmacology related to the treatment of blood, lymphatic, and immune disorders.
- Demonstrate your knowledge of this chapter by completing the learning and documenting health-care activities.

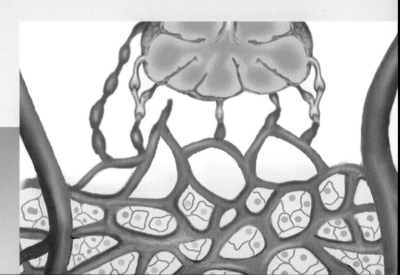

Anatomy and Physiology

The **blood, lymphatic, and immune systems** have separate but interrelated functions in maintaining a healthy environment within the body **(homeostasis).**

Blood is responsible for transporting oxygen (O_2) and carbon dioxide (CO_2) and provides cells that defend against disease. It also protects the body from loss of blood by the action of clotting.

The lymphatic system is responsible for cellular communication by delivering nutrients, hormones, and other needed products to body cells while removing their waste products as it drains tissue fluid back to the vascular system. It also provides the cells of the immune system needed to defend the body against disease.

The immune system defends the body against disease. In its most simple form, it uses barriers that exclude unwanted substances from entering the body. In its most complex form, it uses cells of the lymphatic system to undertake the complex processes that identify and destroy pathogens and protect the body against future encounters by these same pathogens.

Anatomy and Physiology Key Terms

This section introduces important blood, lymphatic, and immune system terms and their definitions. The key terms are highlighted in color in the Anatomy and Physiology section. Word analyses for selected terms are also provided. Pronounce the term, and place a check mark in the box after you do so.

Term	Definition
antibody ĂN-tĭ-bŏd-ē ☐	Protective protein produced by B lymphocytes in response to the presence of a specific foreign substance called an *antigen* *Antibodies combine with antigens to destroy or neutralize them.*
antigen ĂN-tĭ-jĕn ☐	Substance, recognized as harmful to the host, that stimulates formation of antibodies in an immunocompetent individual
bile pigment BĪL ☐	Substance derived from the breakdown of hemoglobin and excreted by the liver *Interference with the excretion of bile may lead to jaundice.*
cytokine SĪ-tō-kīn ☐	Chemical substance produced by certain cells that initiates, inhibits, increases, or decreases activity in other cells *Cytokines are important chemical communicators in the immune response, regulating many activities associated with immunity and inflammation.*
dendritic cell dĕn-DRĬT-ĭk ☐ *dendr:* tree *-itic:* pertaining to	Specialized type of monocyte that displays antigens on its cell surface and presents them to components of the immune system
immunocompetent ĭm-ū-nō-KŎM-pĕ-tĕnt ☐	Possessing the ability to develop an immune response
natural killer (NK) cells	Specialized lymphocytes that destroy virally infected cells and tumor cells by releasing chemicals that disrupt their cell membranes, causing their intercellular fluid to leak out *NK cells are components of the innate immune system and do not require prior sensitization to engage in cell destruction.*

Blood

Blood is connective tissue composed of a liquid medium called **plasma** in which solid components are suspended. The solid components of blood include the following:

- red blood cells **(erythrocytes)**
- white blood cells **(leukocytes)**
- platelets **(thrombocytes)** (See Fig. 9-1.)

The body produces millions of blood cells every second to replace those that are destroyed or worn out. In adults, blood cells form in the bone marrow of the skull, ribs, sternum, vertebrae, pelvis, and ends of the long bones of the arms and legs. The stem cells in the bone marrow give rise to embryonic **(blastic)** forms of all blood cell types. In the embryonic stages, monocytes and lymphocytes migrate to the lymphatic system for maturation and specialization. All other embryonic cells remain in the bone marrow to complete their development. Once blood cells mature, they enter the circulatory system. The development of blood cells into their mature forms is called **hematopoiesis** or **hemopoiesis.** (See Fig. 9-2, page 270.)

Red Blood Cells

Red blood cells (RBCs), or **erythrocytes,** transport oxygen (O_2) and carbon dioxide (CO_2). They are the most numerous of the circulating blood cells. During RBC development **(erythropoiesis),** they decrease in size and, just before reaching maturity, extrude their nuclei. They also develop a specialized iron-containing compound called **hemoglobin (Hb, Hgb)** that gives them their red color. Hemoglobin carries oxygen to body tissues and exchanges it for carbon dioxide. When mature, RBCs are shaped like biconcave disks of approximately the same size and hemoglobin concentration.

RBCs live about 120 days and then rupture, releasing hemoglobin and cell fragments. Hemoglobin breaks down into an iron compound called **hemosiderin** and several **bile pigments.** Most hemosiderin returns to the bone marrow for reuse in a different form to manufacture new blood cells. The liver eventually excretes bile pigments.

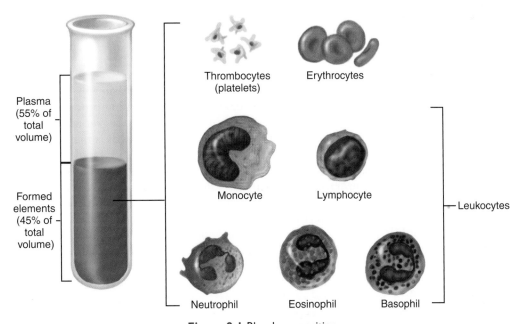

Figure 9-1 Blood composition.

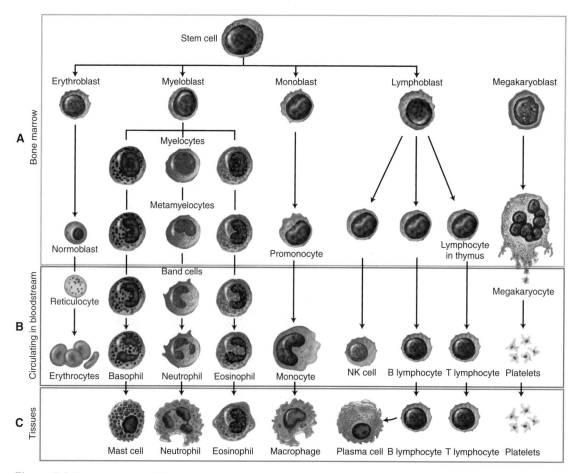

Figure 9-2 Hematopoiesis. (A) Bone marrow: site where all blood cells develop from undifferentiated stem cells. (B) Bloodstream; site of mature circulating blood cells. (C) Tissues: site where blood defense and protection activities occur.

White Blood Cells

White blood cells (WBCs), or **leukocytes,** protect the body against invasion by pathogens and foreign substances, remove debris from injured tissue, and aid in the healing process. Leukocytes are crucial to the body's defense against disease because of their ability to ingest and destroy bacteria and other foreign particles **(phagocytosis).** (See Fig. 9-3.) Unlike RBCs that remain in the bloodstream, WBCs migrate through endothelial walls of capillaries and venules **(diapedesis)** and enter tissue spaces. (See Fig. 9-4.)

The two major types of leukocytes are classified according to the presence of granules in their cytoplasm **(granuloctyes)** or absence of granules in their cytoplasm **(agranulocytes)** when observed microscopically. The granulocytic leukocytes are further classified as **neutrophils, eosinophils,** and **basophils** according to the staining reaction of their cytoplasmic granules during the preparation of blood smears for microscopic examination. The nuclei of mature granulocytes are so deeply lobed, especially in neutrophils, that these cells appear to have multiple nuclei, providing an alternative naming classification as **polymorphonuclear leukocytes (PMNLs, polys).** This nuclear characteristic is not typical of agranulocytes; consequently, agranulocytes are more commonly called **mononuclear lymphocytes (MNLs).** Because each type of leukocyte performs a different function, it is important for diagnostic purposes to identify their type and know whether their number falls within a normal range. Table 9-1 summarizes important information regarding the five major types of leukocytes.

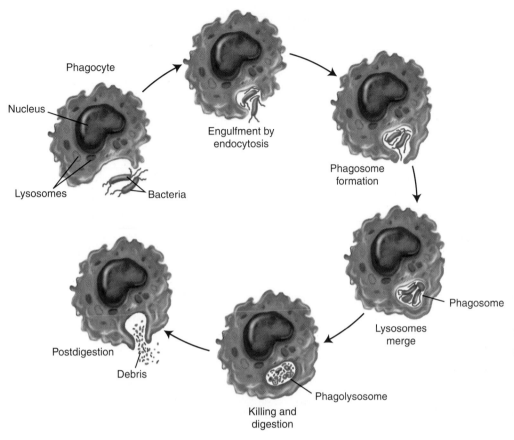

Figure 9-3 Phagocytosis.

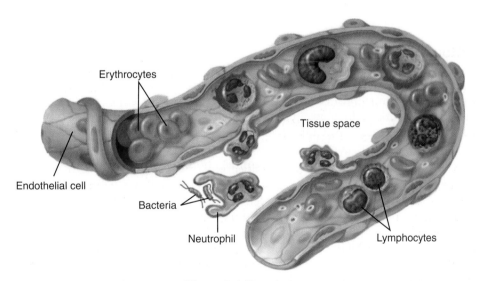

Figure 9-4 Diapedesis.

Table 9-1	**White Blood Cells**		

This table lists the five types of leukocytes, their identifying morphology, and their function.

Cell Type	Nucleus	Cytoplasm	Function
Granulocytes			
Neutrophil	Polymorphonuclear	Lilac granules	• First cell to arrive at a site of injury • Provides nonspecific protection by phagocytosis • Dies as a result of phagocytosis
Eosinophil	Polymorphonuclear	Red granules	• Combats multicellular parasites (worm infestations) • Controls mechanisms associated with allergies
Basophil	Polymorphonuclear	Purple granules	• Initiates inflammation
Agranulocytes			
Lymphocytes	Mononuclear	Agranular	• Provides acquired (specific) immunity
Monocytes	Mononuclear	Agranular	• Performs mildly phagocytic function • Becomes a macrophage when it enters tissues and functions in immunity

Platelets

Platelets (thrombocytes) are the smallest formed elements found in blood. They are not true cells but merely cell fragments. Platelets initiate blood clotting when they encounter vessel walls that have been injured or traumatized. Initially, platelets become sticky and aggregate at the injury site to form a barrier to control blood loss. Clotting factors in platelets and injured tissue release **thromboplastin,** a substance that initiates clot formation. In the final step of coagulation, **fibrinogen** (a soluble blood protein) becomes insoluble and forms fibrin strands that act as a net, entrapping blood cells. This jellylike mass of blood cells and fibrin **(thrombus, blood clot)** impedes the flow of blood **(hemostasis)** into the surrounding tissues.

Plasma

Plasma is the liquid portion of blood in which blood cells are suspended. Without blood cells, plasma appears as a thin, almost colorless fluid. It is composed of about 92% water and contains such products as albumins, globulins, fibrinogen **(plasma proteins),** clotting factors, gases, nutrients, salts, and hormones. A small amount of plasma continuously leaks from capillaries and delivers these products to surrounding cells and exchanges them for waste material produced by body cells. This exchange makes cellular communication possible throughout the body. **Blood serum** is a product of blood plasma formed when fibrinogen and clotting factors are removed from blood plasma.

Blood Types

Human blood is divided into four types, A, B, AB, and O, based on the presence or absence of specific **antigens** on the surface of RBCs. In each of these four blood types, the erythrocyte carries the antigen that gives the name of the blood type. The plasma contains the opposite **antibodies.** Thus, type A blood contains A antigen on the surface of the RBC, and the plasma contains B **antibody.** (See Fig. 9-5.)

Blood types are medically important in transfusions, transplants, and maternal-fetal incompatibilities. In addition to antigens of the four blood types, there are numerous other antigens that may be present on RBCs, but most of these are not of medical concern.

Blood Group	A	B	AB	O
% Population	41	10	4	45
Red blood cell type	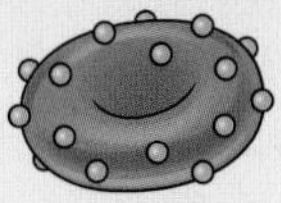 A	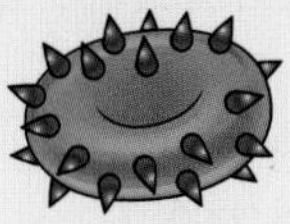 B	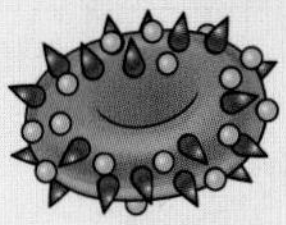 AB	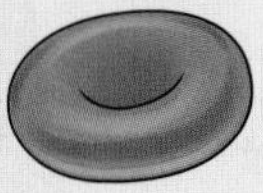 O
Antibodies in Plasma	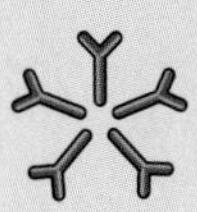 Anti-B	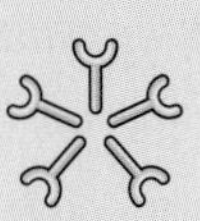 Anti-A	None	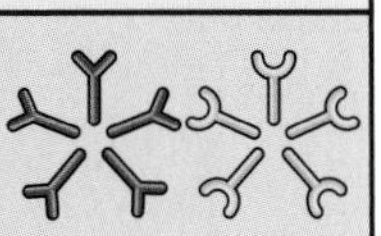 Anti-A and Anti-B
Antigens on the surface of the Red Blood Cell	A antigen	B antigen	A and B antigens	None

Figure 9-5 ABO blood types.

Lymphatic System

The lymphatic system consists of a fluid called **lymph** that contains lymphocytes and monocytes, a network of transporting vessels called **lymph vessels,** and a multiplicity of other structures, including nodes, the spleen, the thymus, and the tonsils. Functions of the lymphatic system include the following:

• maintaining fluid balance of the body by draining interstitial fluid from tissue spaces and returning it to the blood
• transporting lipids away from the digestive organs for use by body tissues
• filtering and removing unwanted or infectious products in lymph nodes

Lymph vessels begin as closed-ended capillaries in tissue spaces and terminate at the right lymphatic duct and the thoracic duct in the chest cavity. (See Fig. 9-6, page 274.) As whole blood circulates, a small amount of plasma seeps from (1) **blood capillaries** and enters surrounding tissue. This fluid, now called **interstitial** or **tissue fluid,** resembles plasma but contains slightly less protein. Interstitial fluid carries needed products to tissue cells while removing their wastes. As interstitial fluid moves through tissues, it collects cellular debris, bacteria, and particulate matter. Upon completing these functions, interstitial fluid returns to the surrounding venules to become plasma or enters closed-ended microscopic vessels called (2) **lymph capillaries** to become lymph. Lymph passes into larger and larger vessels on its return trip to the bloodstream. Before it reaches its final destination, it first enters (3) **lymph nodes** through afferent vessels. In the node, macrophages phagocytize bacteria and other harmful material, and T cells and B cells exert their protective influence. When a local infection exists, the number of bacteria entering a node is so great and the destruction by T cells and B cells so powerful that the node commonly enlarges and becomes tender. Once filtered, lymph exits the node by way of efferent vessels to continue its return to the circulatory system.

Lymph vessels from the right chest and arm join the (4) **right lymphatic duct.** This duct drains into the (5) **right subclavian vein,** a major vessel in the cardiovascular system. Lymph from all other areas of the body enters the (6) **thoracic duct** and drains into the (7) **left subclavian vein.**

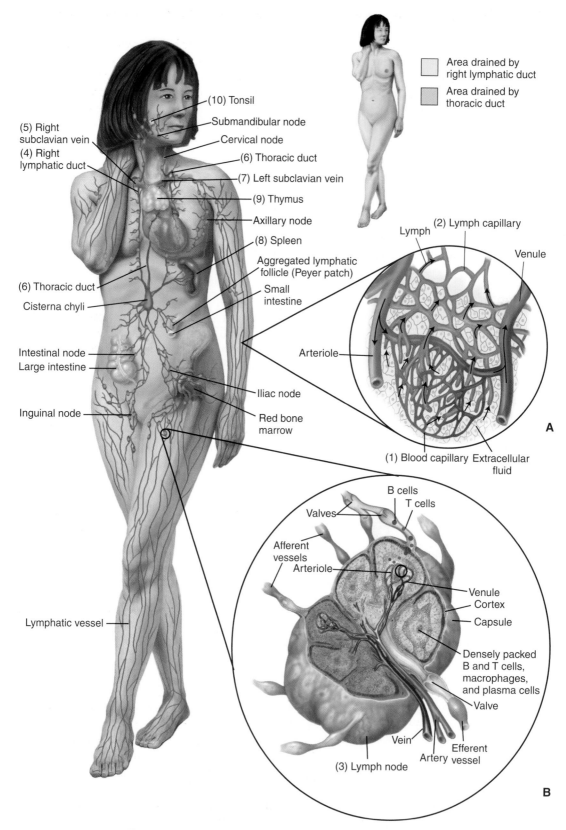

Area drained by right lymphatic duct

Area drained by thoracic duct

(10) Tonsil
Submandibular node
(5) Right subclavian vein
Cervical node
(4) Right lymphatic duct
(6) Thoracic duct
(7) Left subclavian vein
(9) Thymus
Axillary node
(8) Spleen
Aggregated lymphatic follicle (Peyer patch)
(6) Thoracic duct
Small intestine
Cisterna chyli
Intestinal node
Large intestine
Inguinal node
Iliac node
Red bone marrow
Lymphatic vessel

Lymph   (2) Lymph capillary
Venule
Arteriole
(1) Blood capillary Extracellular fluid

A

B cells
T cells
Valves
Afferent vessels
Arteriole
Venule
Cortex
Capsule
Densely packed B and T cells, macrophages, and plasma cells
Valve
Vein
Efferent vessel
Artery
(3) Lymph node

B

Figure 9-6 Lymphatic system. (A) Lymph capillary. (B) Lymph node.

Lymph is redeposited into the circulating blood and becomes plasma. This cycle continually repeats itself.

The (8) **spleen** resembles a lymph node because it acts as a filter by removing cellular debris, bacteria, parasites, and other infectious agents. However, the spleen also destroys old RBCs and serves as a repository for healthy blood cells. The (9) **thymus** is located in the upper part of the chest **(mediastinum).** It partially controls the immune system by transforming certain lymphocytes into T cells to function in the immune system. The (10) **tonsils** are masses of lymphatic tissue located in the pharynx. They act as filters to protect the upper respiratory structures from invasion by pathogens.

Immune System

There are two major immune defenses that protect the body against disease-causing organisms **(pathogens).** The first type of immune defense, called **innate immunity,** includes barriers designed to keep the pathogen from gaining entry into the body. The second type of immune defense, called **acquired immunity,** identifies and specifically destroys pathogens once they have gained entry.

Innate Immunity

Although exposed to a vast number of harmful substances, most people suffer relatively few diseases throughout their lifetime. Numerous body defenses called **immunity** work together to protect against disease. One type of immunity begins functioning at birth or immediately afterward. Because it is present at the very beginning of life, it is called the **innate immune system.** It provides protective barriers to the entry of pathogens into the body and stops their spread should they successfully overcome the barriers. This system does not differentiate the various types of pathogens and is always ready to defend the body, no matter the type or nature of the pathogen. As such, the innate immune system is also considered **nonspecific.** The innate immune system provides two types of barriers:

- **first-line barriers** that keep pathogens from entering the body, including the skin and mucous membranes, tears, saliva, and gastric secretions
- **second-line barriers** that stop the spread of pathogens once they have gained entry, including phagocytic cells, **natural killer cells,** and inflammation

Acquired Immunity

Acquired or **adaptive immunity** develops only after birth in an **immunocompetent** individual and is a lifelong monitoring system. During each encounter with an antigen, the acquired immune system produces unique cells and processes that destroy that particular antigen. The method of destroying the antigen is "custom made" for each specific antigenic encounter. As such, the acquired immune system is considered **specific.** The white blood cells chiefly responsible for the acquired immune response are monocytes and lymphocytes

Monocytes

After a brief stay in the vascular system, monocytes enter tissue spaces and become highly phagocytic **macrophages.** In this form, the macrophage ingests pathogens and other harmful substances. The macrophage processes them in such a way that their unique antigenic properties are preserved and then displayed on the surface of the macrophage. This alerts the immune system to the presence of a pathogen. As such, the macrophage is now considered an **antigen-presenting cell (APC). Dendritic cells,** specialized macrophages, also have the ability to act as APCs. APCs, armed with the antigenic property of the pathogen displayed on their surface, await an encounter by an immune cell capable of responding to the unique antigen. At this encounter, the acquired immune system begins the operations required for the systematic destruction of the antigen.

Lymphocytes

Two types of lymphocytes, B cells **(B lymphocytes)** and T cells **(T lymphocytes),** are the active cells of the acquired immune response. When B cells respond as the principal defense, the form of immunity that develops is **humoral** or **antibody immunity.** When T cells respond as the main defense system, the form of immunity is **cellular immunity.** Although each of these defenses is identified singly, there is a great deal of interaction between them. **Cytokines,** hormonelike chemicals, act as messengers between the two defense systems. They regulate the intensity and duration of their responses and provide cell-to-cell communication among their various cells. Table 9-2 provides information on the cells associated with the acquired immune system.

| Table 9-2 | **Lymphocytes and Immune Response** |

This table provides the functions of B cells and T cells, the major cells of the immune system.

Lymphocyte	Function
B cells	• Function in humoral immunity
	• Originate and mature in bone marrow
	• Protect against extracellular antigens
	• Respond to stimulation by a compatible T cell and begin producing plasma cells
plasma cells	• Create highly specific antibodies that bind to their corresponding antigens forming unique molecules called **antigen–antibody complexes** that lead to the destruction of the antigen by the immune system
memory B cells	• Retreat to lymphatic system and remain prepared to repeat the same procedure upon a subsequent encounter with the same antigen
T cells	• Function in cellular immunity
	• Originate in bone marrow and mature in lymphatic system
	• Protect against intracellular pathogens and cancer cells
cytotoxic T (CD8) cells	• Determine and attack the specific weakness of the cell and destroys it
helper T (CD4) cells	• Provide essential assistance to maintain B-cell activity
	• Produce cytokines that activate, direct and regulate most of the other components of the immune system
	• Require a threshold number to avoid a shutdown of the entire immune system
suppressor T cells	• Monitor and terminate humoral and cellular response when infection resolves
memory T cells	• Migrate to lymphatic system and remain prepared for a second encounter should the same antigen reappear

The memory component is unique to the acquired immune response. Memory B and memory T cells are able to "recall" how they previously disposed of a particular antigen and are able to repeat the process without going through a "learning curve." The repeat performance is immediate, powerful, and sustained. Disposing of the antigen during the second and all subsequent exposures is extremely rapid and much more effective than it was during the first exposure. This long-lasting immunity is referred to as **active immunity.**

Anatomy Review: Lymphatic System

To review the anatomy of the lymphatic system, label the illustration that follows using the listed terms.

blood capillary

left subclavian vein

lymph capillary

lymph node

right lymphatic duct

right subclavian vein

spleen

thoracic duct

thymus

tonsil

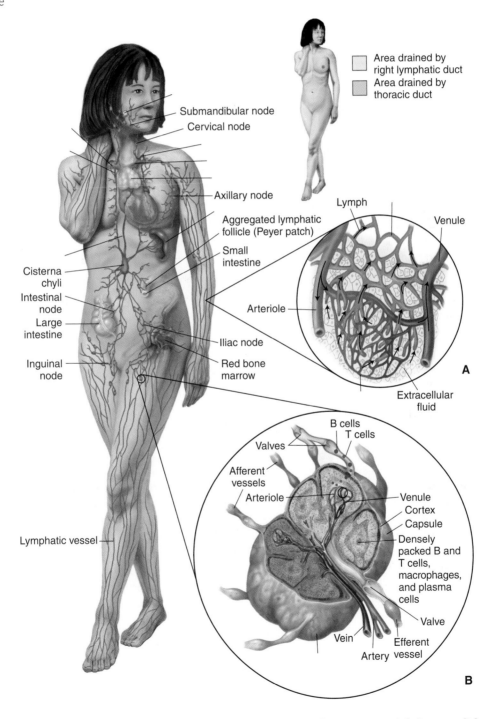

 Check your answers by referring to Figure 9-6 on page 274. Review material that you did not answer correctly.

CONNECTING BODY SYSTEMS—BLOOD, LYMPHATIC, AND IMMUNE SYSTEMS

The main functions of the blood, lymphatic, and immune systems are to provide a way to transport and exchange products throughout the body and protect and repair cells that are damaged by disease or trauma. Specific functional relationships between the blood, lymphatic, and immune systems and other body systems are summarized here.

Cardiovascular
- Blood delivers oxygen needed for contraction of the heart.
- The lymphatic system returns interstitial fluid to the vascular system to maintain blood volume.
- The immune system protects against infections.

Digestive
- Blood transports products of digestion to nourish body cells.
- The immune system provides surveillance mechanisms to detect and destroy cancer cells in the digestive tract.
- An innate component of the immune system, the acidic environment of the stomach helps control pathogens in the digestive tract.

Endocrine
- The blood and lymphatic systems transport hormones to target organs.
- The immune system protects against infection in endocrine glands.

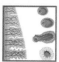

Female Reproductive
- The blood, lymphatic, and immune systems transport nourishing and defensive products across the placental barrier for the developing fetus.
- The immune system provides specific defense against pathogens that enter the body through the reproductive tract.
- The immune system supplies antibodies for breast milk that protect the baby until its immune system is established.

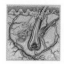

Integumentary
- Blood provides leukocytes, especially neutrophils, to the integumentary system when breaches or injury occurs in the skin.
- The lymphatic system supplies antibodies to the dermis for defense against pathogens.
- Blood in the skin, the largest organ of the body, helps maintain temperature homeostasis.

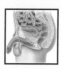

Male Reproductive
- The immune system provides surveillance against cancer cells.
- Blood delivers hormones and other essential products for male fertility.
- Lymph maintains fluid balance in the male organs of reproduction.

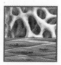

Musculoskeletal
- Blood removes lactic acid that accumulates in muscles during strenuous exercise.
- Blood transports calcium to bones for strength and healing.
- The lymphatic system maintains interstitial fluid balance in muscle tissue.
- The immune system aids in the repair of muscle tissue following trauma.

Nervous
- The immune system responds to nervous stimuli to identify injury or infection sites and initiate tissue defense and repair.
- Plasma and lymph provide the media in which nervous stimuli cross from one neuron to another.
- The lymphatic system removes excess interstitial fluid from tissues surrounding nerves.

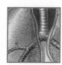

Respiratory
- Red blood cells transport respiratory gases to and from the lungs.
- The tonsils harbor immune cells to combat pathogens that enter through the nose and mouth.

Urinary
- Blood transports waste products, especially urea, to the kidneys for removal via the production of urine.
- Blood in peritubular capillaries reabsorbs essential products that have been filtered by the nephron.

Medical Word Elements

This section introduces combining forms, suffixes, and prefixes related to the blood, lymphatic, and immune systems. Word analyses are also provided. From the information provided, complete the meaning of the medical words in the right-hand column. The first one is completed for you.

Element	Meaning	Word Analysis
Combining Forms		
aden/o	gland	**aden/o**/pathy (ăd-ĕ-NŎP-ă-thē): *disease of a gland* *-pathy:* disease
agglutin/o	clumping, gluing	**agglutin**/ation (ă-gloo-tĭ-NĀ-shŭn): _____ *-ation:* process (of)
blast/o	embryonic cell	erythr/o/**blast**/osis (ĕ-rĭth-rō-blăs-TŌ-sĭs): _____ *erythr/o:* red *-osis:* abnormal condition; increase (used primarily with blood cells) *Erythroblasts are normally found only in bone marrow and develop into mature erythrocytes during hematopoiesis.*
chrom/o	color	hypo/**chrom**/ic (hī-pō-KRŌM-ĭk): _____ *hypo-:* under, below, deficient *-ic:* pertaining to *Hypochromic cells are erythrocytes that appear lighter in color than normal because of a deficiency of hemoglobin, a compound that gives erythrocytes their red color.*
erythr/o	red	**erythr/o**/cyte (ĕ-RĬTH-rō-sīt): _____ *-cyte:* cell *An erythrocyte is an RBC.*
granul/o	granule	**granul/o**/cyte (GRĂN-ū-lō-sīt): _____ *-cyte:* cell
hem/o	blood	**hem/o**/phobia (hē-mō-FŌ-bē-ă): _____ *-phobia:* fear *People who suffer from hemophobia commonly faint at the sight of blood.*
hemat/o		**hemat**/oma (hē-mă-TŌ-mă): _____ *-oma:* tumor *A hematoma is a mass of extravasated, usually clotted, blood caused by a break or leak in a blood vessel. It may be found in any organ, tissue, or space within the body.*
immun/o	immune, immunity, safe	**immun/o**/logy (ĭm-ū-NŎL-ō-jē): _____ *-logy:* study of *Immunology includes the study of autoimmune diseases, hypersensitivities, and immune deficiencies.*
leuk/o	white	**leuk**/emia (loo-KĒ-mē-ă): _____ *-emia:* blood condition *Leukemia causes a profoundly elevated white blood cell (WBC) count and a very low RBC count.*

(continued)

Medical Word Elements—cont'd

Element	Meaning	Word Analysis
lymph/o	lymph	**lymph**/oid (LĬM-foyd): _____ *-oid:* resembling
lymphaden/o	lymph gland (node)	**lymphaden/o**/pathy (lĭm-făd-ĕ-NŎP-ă-thē): _____ *-pathy:* disease *Lymphadenopathy is characterized by changes in the size, consistency, or number of lymph nodes.*
lymphangi/o	lymph vessel	**lymphangi**/oma (lĭm-făn-jē-Ō-mă): _____ *-oma:* tumor
morph/o	form, shape, structure	**morph/o**/logy (mor-FŎL-ō-jē): _____ *-logy:* study of

myel/o	bone marrow; spinal cord	**myel/o**/gen/ic (mī-ĕ-lō-JĔN-ĭk): _____
		  gen: forming, producing, origin
		  -ic: pertaining to
		
		Acute myelogenic leukemia is the most common form of leukemia; also called acute myelogenous *leukemia.*

nucle/o	nucleus	mono/**nucle**/ar (mŏn-ō-NŪ-klē-ăr): _____
		  mono-: one
		  -ar: pertaining to
		
		Mononuclear WBCs, the monocytes and lymphocytes, are also called agranulocytes.

phag/o	swallowing, eating	**phag/o**/cyte (FĂG-ō-sīt): _____ *-cyte:* cell *The neutrophil is an important phagocytic leukocyte of the innate immune system*
poikil/o	varied, irregular	**poikil/o**/cyte (POY-kĭl-ō-sīt): _____ *-cyte:* cell *A poikilocyte is an irregularly shaped RBC, such as a sickle cell.*
ser/o	serum	**ser/o**/logy (sē-RŎL-ō-jē): _____ *-logy:* study of *Serology includes the study of antigens and antibodies in serum and sources other than serum, including plasma, saliva, and urine.*
sider/o	iron	**sider/o**/penia (sĭd-ĕr-ō-PĒ-nē-ă): _____ *-penia:* decrease, deficiency *Common causes of sideropenia include inadequate iron uptake and hemorrhage.*
splen/o	spleen	**splen/o**/megaly (splē-nō-MĔG-ă-lē): _____ *-megaly:* enlargement *Serious forms of infectious mononucleosis commonly cause enlargement of the spleen and liver.*

Medical Word Elements—cont'd

Element	Meaning	Word Analysis
thromb/o	blood clot	**thromb**/osis (thrŏm-BŌ-sĭs): _____ *-osis:* abnormal condition; increase (used primarily with blood cells)
thym/o	thymus gland	**thym/o**/pathy (thī-MŎP-ă-thē): _____ *-pathy:* disease

Suffixes

Element	Meaning	Word Analysis
-blast	embryonic cell	hem/o/cyt/o/**blast** (hē-mō-SĪ-tō-blăst): _____ *hem/o:* blood *cyt/o:* cell *A hemocytoblast is a bone marrow cell capable of giving rise to all types of blood cells.*
-globin	protein	hem/o/**globin** (HĒ-mō-glō-bĭn): _____ *hem/o:* blood *Hemoglobin is an iron-containing protein found in RBCs that transports oxygen and gives blood its red color.*
-penia	decrease, deficiency	*monocyt/o/**penia** (mŏn-ō-sī-tō-PĒ-nē-ă):* _____ *monocyt/o:* monocyte *Some of the causes of monocytopenia include acute infections, leukemia, and reactions to certain drugs.*
-phil	attraction for	neutr/o/**phil** (NŪ-trō-fĭl): _____ *neutr/o:* neutral, neither *Neutrophils are the most numerous type of leukocyte. They provide phagocytic protection for the body.*
-phylaxis	protection	ana/**phylaxis** (ăn-ă-fĭ-LĂK-sĭs): _____ *ana-:* against; up; back *Anaphylaxis is an exaggerated, life-threatening hypersensitivity reaction to a previously encountered antigen. It is treated as a medical emergency.*
-poiesis	formation, production	hem/o/**poiesis** (hē-mō-poy-Ē-sĭs): _____ *hem/o:* blood
-stasis	standing still	hem/o/**stasis** (hē-mō-STĀ-sĭs): _____ *hem/o:* blood *Hemostasis is the control or arrest of bleeding, commonly using chemical agents.*

Prefixes

Element	Meaning	Word Analysis
aniso-	unequal, dissimilar	**aniso**/cyt/osis (ăn-ī-sō-sĭ-TŌ-sĭs): _____ *cyt:* cell *-osis:* abnormal condition; increase (used primarily with blood cells) *Normally, RBCs do not vary in size. When abnormally large RBCs (macrocytes) or abnormally small RBCs (microcytes) are present, the condition is called anisocytosis.*

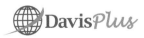 **DavisPlus**   Visit the *Medical Terminology Systems* online resource center at Davis*Plus* for an audio exercise of the terms in this table. Other activities are also available to reinforce content.

It is time to review medical word elements by completing Learning Activities 9–1 and 9–2.

Disease Focus

Anemias, leukemias, and coagulation disorders typically share common signs and symptoms that include paleness, weakness, shortness of breath, and heart palpitations. Lymphatic disorders are commonly associated with edema and lymphadenopathy. Immune disorders include abnormally heightened immune responses **(hypersensitivities),** depressed responses **(immunodeficiencies, or immune deficiencies)**, and responses where the immune system fails to recognize its own tissue **(autoimmunity).**

For diagnosis, treatment, and management of diseases that affect blood and blood-forming organs, the medical services of a specialist may be warranted. **Hematology** is the branch of medicine that studies blood cells, blood-clotting mechanisms, bone marrow, and lymph nodes. The physician who specializes in this branch of medicine is called a **hematologist. Allergy and immunology** is the branch of medicine involving disorders of the immune system, including asthma and anaphylaxis, adverse reactions to drugs, autoimmune diseases, organ transplantations, and malignancies of the immune system. Physicians who specialize in this combined branch of medicine are called **allergists** and **immunologists.**

Anemias

Anemia (erythropenia, erythrocytopenia) is a deficiency in the number of erythrocytes or in the amount of hemoglobin within the red blood cells **(hypochromia).** It is not a disease but a symptom of other illnesses.

An important hereditary anemia that primarily affects individuals of African ancestry is sickle cell anemia. This anemia results from a defective hemoglobin molecule **(hemoglobinopathy)** that causes RBCs to assume bizarre shapes, commonly resembling a crescent, or sickle, when oxygen levels are low. Sickle cells are fragile and easily break apart **(hemolyze).** They have difficulty passing through the small capillaries. (See Fig. 9-7.) Tissue distal to the blockage undergoes ischemia, resulting in severe pain called a **sickle cell crisis** that can last from several hours to several days. Sickle cell anemia affects only those who have inherited the trait from both parents. If the trait is inherited from only one parent, the offspring will be a carrier but will not have the disorder. Treatment is designed to control or limit the number of crises. Folic acid is commonly recommended, and some medications are proving to be helpful in controlling the disease. Table 9-3 provides information on common anemias.

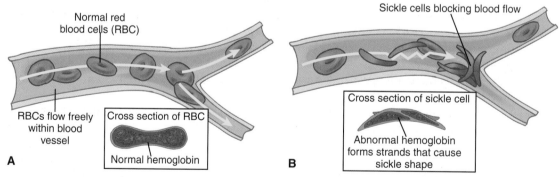

Figure 9-7 Sickle cell anemia. (A) Normal red blood cells (RBCs) passing easily through capillaries. (B) Sickle cells becoming trapped and obstructing normal blood flow.

Table 9-3 Common Anemias

This table lists various types of anemia, along with descriptions and causes.

Type of Anemia	Description	Causes
Aplastic (hypoplastic)	Serious form of anemia associated with bone marrow failure, resulting in erythropenia, leukopenia, and thrombocytopenia	Commonly caused by some autoimmune disorders, chemotherapy, radiation therapy, and exposure to certain cytotoxic agents
Folic-acid deficiency anemia	Inability to produce sufficient red blood cells (RBCs) because of the lack of folic acid, a B vitamin essential for erythropoiesis	Caused by insufficient folic acid intake resulting from poor diet, impaired absorption, prolonged drug therapy, or increased requirements (pregnancy or rapid growth as seen in children)
Hemolytic	Destruction of RBCs, commonly resulting in jaundice	Associated with some inherited immune and blood (sickle cell anemia) disorders, medications, and incompatible transfusions
Iron-deficiency anemia	Lack of sufficient iron in RBCs	Caused by a greater demand for stored iron than can be supplied, usually as a result of inadequate dietary iron intake or malabsorption of iron
Pernicious anemia (PA)	Chronic, progressive anemia found mostly in people older than age 50 resulting from a lack of sufficient vitamin B_{12} needed for blood cell development	Commonly the result of insufficient intrinsic factor in the stomach essential for absorption of vitamin B_{12}
Sickle cell anemia	Inherited anemia that causes RBCs to become crescent- or sickle-shaped when oxygen levels are low	Caused by a defect in the gene responsible for hemoglobin synthesis

Allergy

An **allergy** is an acquired abnormal immune response. It requires an initial exposure (**sensitization**) to an allergen (**antigen**). Subsequent exposures to the allergen produce increasing allergic reactions that cause a broad range of inflammatory changes, including hives (**urticaria**), eczema, allergic rhinitis, asthma, and, in the extreme, **anaphylaxis**, a life-threatening condition.

Allergy-sensitivity tests in which a suspension of the allergen is introduced into the skin identify offending allergens. If the patient has an allergy to the suspected allergen, the area becomes red, swollen, and hardened (**indurated**).

Allergy shots (**immunotherapy, biotherapy**) can help with an allergy response to pollens, pet dander, molds, dust mites, and venom (bee stings) but not to foods. Immunotherapy involves repeated injections of the allergen, beginning with a highly diluted solution and increasing the concentration over a period of weeks or months. When administered as an injection, the body treats the allergen like a vaccine and begins to produces antibodies against the allergen. The newly formed antibodies desensitize the patient and reduce the reaction of the patient to the offending allergen. Allergy shots have been very successful in reducing or even eliminating the symptoms associated with the allergy.

Autoimmune Disease

When the immune system fails to accurately differentiate foreign antigens from the body's own antigens found on cells and tissues **(autoantigens)** and begins its destructive behavior to the detriment of the individual, the disorder is considered an **autoimmune disease.** In this abnormal response, the immune system produces **autoantibodies** directed at one or more of the individual's cells or tissues until they are destroyed. Types of autoimmune disorders range from those that affect only a single organ to those that affect many organs and systems **(multisystemic).** Autoimmune diseases include rheumatoid arthritis **(RA),** systemic lupus erythematosus **(SLE),** multiple sclerosis, myasthenia gravis, vasculitis, and various thyroid disorders. Most autoimmune diseases have periods of flare-ups **(exacerbations)** and latencies **(remissions).**

Treatment goals include reducing symptoms and controlling the autoimmune process while maintaining the body's ability to fight disease. Autoimmune diseases are usually chronic, requiring lifelong care and monitoring, even when the person may look or feel well. Currently, few autoimmune diseases can be cured; however, with treatment, those afflicted can live relatively normal lives.

Oncology

The major types of blood cancers include multiple myelomas that affect a single type of bone marrow cell, lymphomas that arise in the lymphatic system, and leukemias that affect blood and bone marrow.

Leukemia

Leukemia is an oncological disorder of blood and blood-forming organs and is characterized by an overgrowth (proliferation) of blood cells. It is the most common cancer in children, adolescents, and young adults. With this condition, the body replaces healthy blood and bone marrow cells with immature, nonfunctional cells, leading to anemias, infections, and bleeding disorders. The various types of leukemia are generally identified by the type of leukocyte population affected as either granulocytic (myelogenous) or lymphocytic. They are further classified as chronic or acute.

In the acute form, the disease has a sudden onset and blood cells are highly embryonic (blastic) with few mature forms. Severe anemia, infections, and bleeding disorders appear early in the disease. This form of leukemia is life-threatening.

In the chronic form, signs and symptoms are slow to develop because there are usually enough mature cells to carry on the functions of the various cell types. As the chronic form progresses, signs and symptoms develop.

Although the causes of leukemia are unknown, research has implicated viruses, environmental conditions, high-dose radiation, and genetic factors. Bone marrow aspiration and bone marrow biopsy help diagnose leukemia. Treatment includes chemotherapy, radiation, bone marrow transplant, or a combination of these modalities. Recent advances in treatment, such as monoclonal antibody therapy, cancer vaccines, and donor lymphocyte infusions, are becoming more prevalent in treatment. Leukemias are fatal if left untreated.

Diseases and Conditions

This section introduces diseases and conditions of the blood, lymphatic, and immune systems, along with their meanings and pronunciations. Word analyses for selected terms are also provided.

Term	Definition
acquired immunodeficiency syndrome (AIDS) ĭm-ūn dĕ-FĬSH-ĕn-sē SĬN-drōm	Infectious disease caused the human immunodeficiency virus (HIV) that destroys the CD4 (helper T) cells of the immune system to such an extent that the patient falls victim to infections that usually do not affect healthy individuals (opportunistic infections) *Early stages of HIV infection (HIV disease) may remain asymptomatic for many years, especially when the patient receives medical care. Untreated, the disease ultimately develops into full-blown AIDS, a potentially fatal disease.*
coagulation disorders kō-ăg-ū-LĀ-shŭn	Any disruption or impairment in the ability to form blood clots or control bleeding *Causes include deficiency in coagulating factors, certain plasma proteins, or platelet production.*
disseminated intravascular coagulation (DIC) ĭn-tră-VĂS-kū-lăr kō-ăg-ū-LĀ-shŭn *intra-:* in, within *vascul:* vessel, (usually blood or lymph) *-ar:* pertaining to	Abnormal blood clotting in small vessels throughout the body that cuts off the supply of oxygen to distal tissues, resulting in damage to body organs *Increased clotting uses up platelets and proteins, leading to profuse bleeding, even with the slightest trauma. (See Fig. 9-8.)*

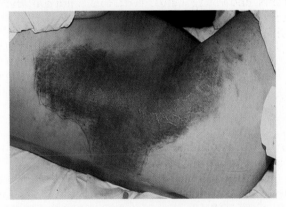

Figure 9-8 Extensive hemorrhage into the skin in disseminated intravascular coagulation (DIC), with an area outlined in pen to assess whether the hemorrhage is spreading. From Harmening: *Clinical Hematology and Fundamentals of Hemostasis*, 3rd ed. F.A. Davis, Philadelphia, 1997, p. 520, with permission.

(continued)

Diseases and Conditions—cont'd

Term	Definition

hemophilia
hē-mō-FĬL-ē-ă
hem/o: blood
philia: attraction for

Congenital hereditary disorder characterized by a deficiency in clotting factor VIII (hemophilia A) or clotting factor IX (hemophilia B), resulting in prolonged bleeding; also called *bleeder's disease*

Mild symptoms include nosebleed and hematomas. Severe symptoms include bleeding into the joints (hemarthrosis) and sudden shock; death is possible. Treatment is intravenous administration of the lacking blood factor.

thrombocytopenia
thrŏm-bō-sī-tō-PĒ-nē-ă
thromb/o: blood clot
cyt/o: cell
-penia: decrease, deficiency

Abnormal decrease in platelets caused by low production of platelets or their increased destruction in the blood vessels, spleen, or liver

A common sign of thrombocytopenia is the development of pinpoint hemorrhages (petechiae) that appear primarily on the lower leg. (See Fig. 9-9.)

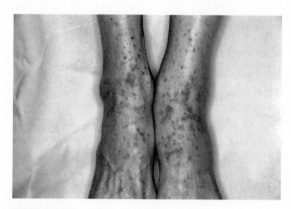

Figure 9-9 Petechiae on the skin from thrombocytopenia. From Goldsmith and Tharp: *Adult and Pediatric Dermatology: A Color Guide to Diagnosis and Treatment.* F.A. Davis, Philadelphia, 1997, p. 61, with permission.

graft rejection
GRĂFT

Process in which a recipient's immune system identifies the transplanted graft as "foreign" and attacks or destroys it

Rejection can be lessened by a close tissue match between donor and recipient or administration of medications that depress the immune system.

graft-versus-host disease (GVHD)
GRĂFT

Complication that occurs following a stem cell or bone marrow transplant in which the transplant produces antibodies against the recipient's organs, commonly severely enough to cause death

hemoglobinopathy
hē-mō-glō-bĭ-NŎP-ă-thē
hem/o: blood
globin/o: protein
-pathy: disease

Any disorder caused by abnormalities in the hemoglobin molecule
One of the most common hemoglobinopathies is sickle cell anemia.

Diseases and Conditions—cont'd

Term	Definition
infectious mononucleosis ĭn-FĔK-shŭs mŏn-ō-nū-klē-Ō-sĭs *mono-:* one *nucle:* nucleus *-osis:* abnormal condition; increase (used primarily with blood cells)	Acute infectious disease caused by the Epstein-Barr virus (EBV) that primarily affects young adults and children and causes fatigue, malaise, sore throat, and lymphadenopathy of the neck or armpits; also called *mono* and *kissing disease* *Rest and adequate fluid intake are important to recovery. Infectious mononucleosis usually resolves spontaneously and without complications. Recovery usually ensures lasting immunity.*
Kaposi sarcoma (KS) KĂP-ō-sē săr-KŌ-mă *sarc:* flesh, connective tissue *-oma:* tumor	Cancer caused by the human herpes virus 8 (HHV-8) that mainly affects the skin and mucous membranes but may also cause extensive visceral organ involvement; also called *malignant neoplasm of soft tissue* *Although several forms of KS are clinically identified, AIDS-related KS is the most common and most aggressive form.*
lymphedema lĭmf-ĕ-DĒ-mă *lymph:* lymph *-edema:* swelling	Swelling, primarily in a single arm or leg, resulting from an accumulation of lymph within tissues caused by obstruction or disease in the lymph vessels *The most common causes of lymphedema are surgery, radiation therapy, and infection of the lymph vessels.*
lymphoma lĭm-FŌ-mă *lymph:* lymph *-oma:* tumor	Any malignancy involving lymphocytes (B cells, T cells, or both) that commonly affects lymph nodes and other lymphatic tissue
Hodgkin (HL) HŎJ-kĭn	Malignancy of B cells that occurs in lymph nodes of the neck or chest and may spread to nearby lymph nodes and the spleen and sometimes to the bone marrow; also called *classical Hodgkin lymphoma, Hodgkin disease* *HL is characterized by the presence of Reed-Sternberg cells. Symptoms include a painless swelling of cervical nodes, fever, chills, and itchy skin. Treatment includes radiation therapy, chemotherapy, or bone marrow transplant.*
non-Hodgkin (NHL)	Any malignancy of B cells, T cells, or NK cells that does not involve Reed-Sternberg cells *More than 60 subtypes of NHL have been identified. Prognosis depends on the type, stage, grade of the disease, and age and general health of the patient.*
multiple myeloma mī-ĕ-LŌ-mă *myel:* bone marrow; spinal cord *-oma:* tumor	Malignancy of the bone marrow that affects plasma cells, leading to proliferation of abnormal antibodies, destruction of healthy bone marrow cells, and weakening of bone tissue *Serious consequences of the disease include low blood counts, bone and kidney disorders, and infections.*
sepsis SĔP-sĭs	Presence of bacteria or their toxins in the blood; also called *septicemia* or *blood poisoning* *Usual causes of sepsis are peritonitis, urinary tract infections, meningitis, cellulitis, and bacterial pneumonias.*

(continued)

Diseases and Conditions—cont'd

Term	Definition
systemic lupus erythematosus (SLE) sĭs-TĔM-ĭk LŪ-pŭs ĕr-ĭ-thē-mă-TŌ-sŭs	Widespread autoimmune disease that affects the skin, brain, kidneys, and joints and causes chronic inflammation; also called *discoid lupus* if symptoms are limited to the skin *A typical "butterfly rash" appears over the nose and cheeks in about 50% of people afflicted with SLE and tends to get worse in direct sunlight. (See Fig. 9–10.)*

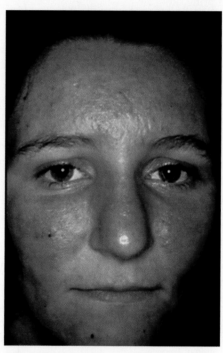

Figure 9-10 Red papules and plaques of systemic lupus erythematosus (SLE) in a butterfly pattern on the face. From Goldsmith and Tharp: *Adult and Pediatric Dermatology: A Color Guide to Diagnosis and Treatment.* F.A. Davis, Philadelphia, 1997, p. 230, with permission.

Term	Definition
thrombocythemia thrŏm-bō-sī-THĒ-mē-ă	Overproduction of platelets, leading to thrombosis or bleeding disorders as a result of platelet malformations

 It is time to review pathology, diseases, and conditions by completing Learning Activity 9-3.

Diagnostic, Surgical, and Therapeutic Procedures

This section introduces diagnostic, surgical, and therapeutic procedures used to treat and diagnose blood, lymphatic, and immune system disorders. Descriptions are provided, along with pronunciations and word analyses for selected terms.

Procedure	Description
Diagnostic	
Laboratory	
antinuclear antibody (ANA) ăn-tĭ-NŪ-klē-ăr ĂN-tĭ-bŏd-ē *anti-:* against *nucle:* nucleus *-ar:* pertaining to	Test that identifies the antibodies that attack the nucleus of the individual's own body cells (autoantibodies) *The presence of ANAs indicates the potential for autoimmunity and directs the physician to explore possible autoimmune diseases.*
blood culture	Test to determine the presence of pathogens in the bloodstream
complete blood count (CBC)	Series of tests that includes hemoglobin, hematocrit, red and white blood cell counts, platelet count, and differential (diff) count; also called *hemogram* *CBC is a broad screening test for anemias, coagulation disorders, and infections.*
monospot	Nonspecific rapid serological test for the presence of the heterophile antibody, which develops several days after infection by Epstein-Barr virus, the organism that causes infectious mononucleosis
partial thromboplastin time (PTT) thrŏm-bō-PLĂS-tĭn	Screening test for deficiencies in clotting factors by measuring the length of time it takes blood to clot; also called *activated partial thromboplastin time (APTT)* *PTT is a valuable tool in preoperative screening for bleeding tendencies.*
prothrombin time (PT) prō-THRŎM-bĭn	Test used to detect and diagnose bleeding disorders or excessive clotting disorders; also called *pro time* *PT is commonly used to monitor blood thinning medications, diagnose liver problems, and assess the blood's ability to clot before undertaking surgical procedures.*
Imaging	
bone marrow magnetic resonance imaging (MRI)	Highly sensitive imaging procedure that detects lesions and changes in bone tissue and bone marrow, especially in diagnosing multiple myeloma
lymphangiography lĭm-făn-jē-ŎG-ră-fē *lymph:* lymph *angi/o:* vessel *-graphy:* process of recording	Visualization of lymph channels and lymph nodes using a contrast medium to determine blockages or other pathologies of the lymphatic system *Because lymph nodes filter and trap cancer cells, this test is commonly used to determine lymph flow in areas that contain malignancy.*

(continued)

Diagnostic, Surgical, and Therapeutic Procedures—cont'd

Procedure	Description
lymphoscintigraphy lĭm-fō-sĭn-TĬG-ră-fē	Introduction of a radioactive tracer into the lymph channels to determine lymph flow, identify obstructions, and locate the sentinel node *Lymphoscintigraphy is also used to biopsy the sentinel node, assess the stage of cancer, and determine a plan of treatment.*
Surgical	
bone marrow aspiration BŌN MĂR-ō ăs-pĭ-RĀ-shŭn	Removal of bone marrow (usually from the pelvis) for microscopic examination using a thin aspirating needle (See Fig. 9-11.) *Bone marrow aspiration aids in identifying blood disorders (leukemias or anemias), infections, and fevers of unknown origin.*

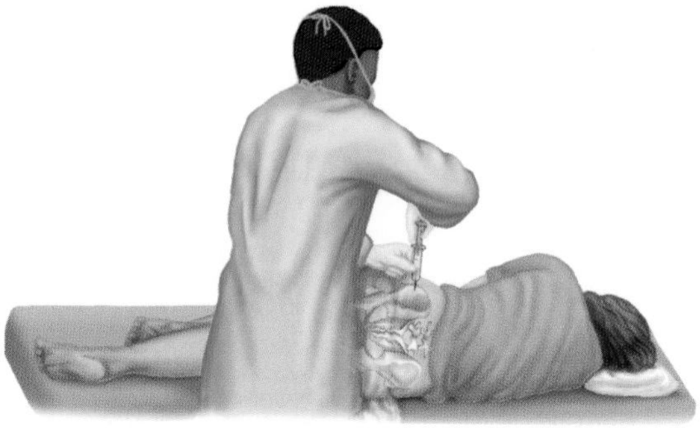

Figure 9-11 Bone marrow aspiration.

bone marrow transplant (BMT) BŌN MĂR-ō TRĂNS-plănt	Infusion of healthy bone marrow stem cells after destroying the diseased bone marrow by chemotherapy, radiation therapy, or both and commonly used to treat leukemia, aplastic anemia, and certain cancers; also called *stem cell transplant* *In an autologous transplant, the donor and recipient are the same individual. In a homologous transplant, the donor and recipient are different individuals.*

lymphadenectomy
lĭm-făd-ĕ-NĔK-tō-mē
  lymph: lymph
  aden: gland
  -ectomy: excision
	Removal of lymph nodes, especially in surgical procedures undertaken to remove malignant tissue, in an effort to control the spread of cancer
	
	A limited or modified lymphadenectomy removes only some of the lymph nodes in the area around a tumor; a total, or radical, lymphadenectomy removes all of the lymph nodes in the area.

Diagnostic, Surgical, and Therapeutic Procedures—cont'd

Procedure	Description
sentinel node excision SĔNT-ĭ-nĕl NŌD	Removal of the first node (sentinel node) that receives drainage from cancer-containing areas and the one most likely to contain malignant cells *If the sentinel node does not contain malignant cells, there may be no need to remove regional lymph nodes during cancer surgery. (See Fig. 9-12.)*

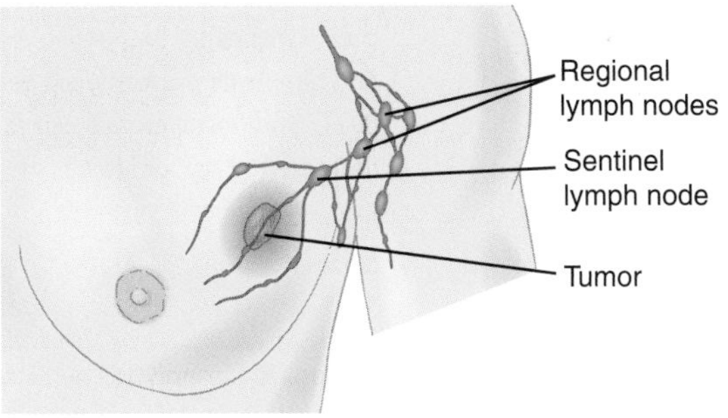

Figure 9-12 Sentinel node.

Therapeutic

Procedure	Description
immunotherapy ĭm-ū-nō-THĔR-ă-pē *immun/o:* immune, immunity, safe *-therapy:* treatment	Any form of treatment that alters, enhances, stimulates, or restores the body's own natural immune mechanisms to treat diseases; also called *biological therapy*
immunoglobulin (IG) therapy ĭm-ū-nō-GLŎB-ū-lĭn THĔR-ă-pē	Treatment using antibody mixtures, administered via intravenous, subcutaneous, or intramuscular routes *IG therapy is commonly used to treat immunodeficiencies and autoimmune diseases.*
plasmapheresis plăz-mă-fĕr-Ē-sĭs	Dialysis procedure that removes and discards the patient's plasma containing the autoantibodies responsible for tissue destruction in autoimmunity and returns the blood cells to the patient suspended in the plasma of a donor *Autoimmune diseases treated using plasmapheresis include myasthenia gravis, Guillain-Barre syndrome, multiple sclerosis, and muscular dystrophy.*
transfusion trăns-FŪ-zhŭn	Infusion of blood or blood products from one person (donor) to another (recipient) *Transfusion is usually performed as a lifesaving maneuver when there is serious blood loss or for the treatment of severe anemias.*

Pharmacology

Various pharmaceutical agents are available to treat blood, lymphatic, and immune system disorders. These drugs act directly on individual components of each system. For example, anticoagulants help prevent clot formation but are ineffective in destroying formed clots. Instead, thrombolytics help dissolve clots that obstruct coronary, cerebral, or pulmonary arteries. Conversely, hemostatics help prevent or control hemorrhage. In addition, chemotherapy and radiation are common treatments for diseases of the blood and immune system. For example, antineoplastics prevent cellular replication to halt the spread of cancer in the body; antiretrovirals prevent viral replication within cells and have been effective in slowing the progression of HIV and AIDS. (See Table 9-4.)

Table 9-4 Drugs Used to Treat Blood, Lymphatic, and Immune Disorders

This table lists common drug classifications used to treat blood, lymphatic, and immune disorders, along with their therapeutic actions and selected generic and trade names.

Classification	Therapeutic Action	Generic and Trade Names
anticoagulants an-tĭ-kō-ĂG-ū-lănts	Prevent blood clot formation by inactivating one or more clotting factors or inhibiting their synthesis *Anticoagulants prevent deep vein thrombosis (DVT) and postoperative clot formation and decrease the risk of stroke.*	**heparin** HĔP-ă-rĭn *heparin sodium* **warfarin** WĂR-făr-ĭn *Coumadin* **dabigatran** dă-BĬG-ă-trăn *Pradaxa*
antifibrinolytics ăn-tĭ-fī-brĭ-nō-LĬT-ĭks	Neutralize fibrinolytic chemicals in the mucous membranes of the mouth, nose, and urinary tract to prevent the breakdown of blood clots *Antifibrinolytics are used to treat serious bleeding following certain surgeries and dental procedures, especially in patients with hemophilia.*	**aminocaproic acid** a-mē-nō-kă-PRŌ-ĭk ĂS-ĭd *Amicar*
antimicrobials ăn-tĭ-mī-KRŌ-bē-ălz	Destroy bacteria, fungi, and protozoa, depending on the particular drug, generally by interfering with the functions of the cell membrane or the reproductive cycle *HIV patients are commonly treated prophylactically with antimicrobials to prevent the development of Pneumocystis pneumonia (PCP).*	**trimethoprim, sulfamethoxazole** trĭ-MĔTH-ō-prĭm, sŭl-fă-mĕth-ŎK-să-zōl *Bactrim, Septra* **metronidazole** mĕ-trō-NĬ-dă-zōl *Flagyl*
antiretrovirals ăn-tĭ-rĕ-trō-VĪ-rălz	Prevent replication of viruses within host cells *Antiretrovirals are used in the treatment of HIV infection and AIDS. Resistance to these agents is common, so they are generally given in combination to avoid this problem.*	**nelfinavir** nĕl-FĬN-ă-vēr *Viracept* **lamivudine/zidovudine** lă-MĬV-ū-dēn, zī-DŌ-vū-dēn *Combivir*
immunosuppressants ĭm-ū-nō-sū-PRĔSS-ănts	Decrease inflammation by suppressing the body's natural immune response *Immunosuppressants are used to treat autoimmune disorders that cause inflammation, such as rheumatoid arthritis; they are also used in transplant patients to prevent graft rejection.*	**prednisone** PRĔD-n ĭ-zōn **cyclosporine** SĪ-klō-spor-ēn *Neoral* **mycophenolate mofetil** mī-cō-FĔN-ō-lāt MŎF-ĕ-tĭl *CellCept*
thrombolytics thrŏm-bō-LĬT-ĭks	Dissolve blood clots by destroying their fibrin strands *Thrombolytics are used to break apart, or lyse, thrombi, especially those that obstruct coronary, pulmonary, and cerebral arteries.*	**alteplase** ĂL-tĕ-plās *Activase, t-PA* **streptokinase** strĕp-tō-KĪ-nās *Streptase*

Abbreviations

This section introduces blood, lymphatic, and immune system abbreviations and their meanings.

Abbreviation	Meaning	Abbreviation	Meaning
AB, Ab, ab	antibody, abortion	Ig	immunoglobulin
A, B, AB, O	blood types in ABO blood group	IVIG	intravenous immunoglobulin
AIDS	acquired immunodeficiency syndrome	KS	Kaposi sarcoma
ANA	antinuclear antibody	MNL	mononuclear leukocytes
APC	antigen-presenting cell	MRI	magnetic resonance imaging
APTT	activated partial thromboplastin time	NHL	non-Hodgkin lymphoma
BMT	bone marrow transplant	NK cell	natural killer cell
CBC	complete blood count	O_2	oxygen
CO_2	carbon dioxide	PA	pernicious anemia
DIC	disseminated intravascular coagulation	PCP	*Pneumocystis* pneumonia; primary care physician
diff	differential count (white blood cells)	PMN	polymorphonuclear
DVT	deep vein thrombosis	PMNL, poly	polymorphonuclear leukocyte
EBV	Epstein-Barr virus	PT	prothrombin time, physical therapy
GVHD	graft-versus-host disease	PTT	partial thromboplastin time
Hb, Hgb	hemoglobin	RA	right atrium; rheumatoid arthritis
HHV-8	human herpes virus 8	RBC, rbc	red blood cell
HIV	human immunodeficiency virus	SLE	systemic lupus erythematosus
HL	Hodgkin lymphoma	WBC, wbc	white blood cell

It is time to review procedures, pharmacology, and abbreviations by completing Learning Activity 9–4.

LEARNING ACTIVITIES

The activities that follow provide a review of the blood, lymphatic, and immune system terms introduced in this chapter. Complete each activity and review your answers to evaluate your understanding of the chapter.

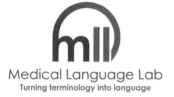

Medical Language Lab
Turning terminology into language

Visit the Medical Language Lab at *medicallanguagelab.com.* Use it to enhance your study and reinforcement of this chapter with the flash-card activity. We recommend that you complete the flash-card activity before starting Learning Activities 9-1 and 9-2.

Learning Activity 9-1
Medical Word Elements

Use the listed elements to build medical words. You may use elements more than once.

Combining Forms		Suffixes		Prefixes
aden/o	lymphangi/o	-ar	-oid	a-
chrom/o	morph/o	-blast	-oma	hypo-
cyt/o	nucle/o	-ectomy	-osis	micro-
erythr/o	sider/o	-ic	-pathy	
granul/o	splen/o	-logy	-penia	
hem/o	thromb/o	-lysis	-poiesis	
lymphaden/o	thym/o	-megaly		

1. tumor of a lymph vessel _____
2. decrease in iron _____
3. enlargement of the spleen _____
4. abnormal condition of a blood clot _____
5. study of shapes (of cells) _____
6. excision of the thymus _____
7. pertaining to deficient color (of red blood cells) _____
8. pertaining to small (red blood) cells _____
9. disease of a lymph gland _____
10. embryonic red (blood cell) _____
11. destruction of blood _____
12. pertaining to a nucleus _____
13. resembling a gland _____
14. pertaining to without granules _____
15. formation (production) of blood _____

Check your answers in Appendix A. Review any material that you did not answer correctly.

Correct Answers _____ X 6.67 = _____ % Score

Learning Activity 9-2
Building Medical Words

Use -*osis* (abnormal condition; increase [used primarily with blood cells]) to build words that mean:

1. abnormal increase in erythrocytes _____
2. abnormal increase in leukocytes _____
3. abnormal increase in lymphocytes _____
4. abnormal increase in reticulocytes _____

Use -*penia* (deficiency, decrease) to build words that mean:

5. decrease in leukocytes _____
6. decrease in erythrocytes _____
7. decrease in thrombocytes _____
8. decrease in lymphocytes _____

Use –*poiesis* (formation, production) to build words that mean:

9. production of blood: _____
10. production of white blood cells _____
11. production of thrombocytes _____

Use *immun/o* (immune, immunity, safe) to build words that mean:

12. specialist in the study of immunity _____
13. study of immunity _____

Use *splen/o* (spleen) to build words that mean

14. herniation of the spleen _____
15. destruction of the spleen _____

Build surgical words that mean

16. excision of the spleen _____
17. removal of the thymus _____
18. removal of a lymph node _____
19. incision of the spleen _____
20. fixation of (a displaced) spleen _____

✓ *Check your answers in Appendix A. Review any material that you did not answer correctly.*

Correct Answers _____ X 5 = _____ % Score

Learning Activity 9-3

Diseases and Conditions

Match the terms with the definitions in the numbered list.

anaphylaxis	hemolytic	lymphedema	sepsis
aplastic	hemophilia	mononucleosis	sensitization
erythropenia	Hodgkin disease	multiple myeloma	sickle cell
graft rejection	Kaposi sarcoma	myelogenous	thrombocythemia
hemoglobinopathy	lymphadenopathy	opportunistic	thrombocytopenia

1. any disorder caused by abnormalities in the hemoglobin molecule _____

2. swelling of tissue in limb(s) usually due to obstruction or disease of a lymph vessel _____

3. disease of a lymph node _____

4. anemia associated with bone marrow failure _____

5. life-threatening allergic response _____

6. denotes an infection that affects only those who are immunocompromised _____

7. malignant disease of the lymph nodes characterized by Reed-Sternberg cells _____

8. initial exposure to an allergen _____

9. deficiency in RBCs or hemoglobin _____

10. malignancy of plasma cells in the bone marrow _____

11. infectious disorder caused by the Epstein-Barr virus _____

12. presence of bacteria or their toxins in blood _____

13. leukemia that affects granulocytes _____

14. malignancy associated with HIV _____

15. hereditary anemia found mostly in the those of African descent _____

16. decrease of platelets in the circulatory system _____

17. anemia caused by destruction of erythrocytes _____

18. excessive number of platelets in circulation _____

19. hereditary bleeding disorder caused by deficiency in clotting factors _____

20. destruction of a transplanted organ or tissue by the recipient's immune system _____

✓ *Check your answers in Appendix A. Review any material that you did not answer correctly.*

Correct Answers _____ X 5 = _____ % Score

Learning Activity 9-4

Procedures, Pharmacology, and Abbreviations

Match the terms with the definitions in the numbered list.

ANA	homologous	plasmapheresis
anticoagulants	lymphadenectomy	RBC
antimicrobials	lymphangiography	thrombolytics
autologous	lymphoscintigraphy	transfusion
biological	monospot	WBC

1. immunotherapy that uses stimulators to enhance the immune system _____
2. procedure that uses a contrast dye to determine blockages of the lymph vessels _____
3. serological test for infectious mononucleosis _____
4. used to prevent blood clot formation _____
5. leukocyte _____
6. transplant from a compatible donor _____
7. test that identifies antibodies that attack an individual's own cells _____
8. procedure that uses a radioactive tracer to identify the location of the sentinel node _____
9. dialysis procedure used to treat autoimmune diseases _____
10. excision of lymph nodes _____
11. transplant using the recipient's own stem cells _____
12. destroy bacteria, fungi, and protozoa _____
13. erythrocyte _____
14. used to dissolve blood clots _____
15. lifesaving procedure to replenish blood loss or for treatment of severe anemia _____

Check your answers in Appendix A. Review any material that you did not answer correctly.

Correct Answers _____ X 6.67 = _____ % Score

DOCUMENTING HEALTH-CARE ACTIVITIES

This section provides practical application activities in the form of exercises to help students develop skills in documenting patient care. First, read the medical report. Then complete the activities and exercises that follow.

Documenting Health-Care Activity 9-1

Discharge Summary: Sickle Cell Crisis

General Hospital

1511 Ninth Avenue ■ ■ Sun City, USA 12345 ■ ■ (555) 802–1887

DISCHARGE SUMMARY

ADMISSION DATE: June 21, 20xx   **DISCHARGE DATE:** June 23, 20xx

ADMITTING AND DISCHARGE DIAGNOSES:
1. Sickle cell crisis
2. Abdominal pain

PROCEDURES: Two units of packed red blood cells and CT scan of the abdomen.

REASON FOR ADMISSION: This is a 46-year-old African American man who reports a history of sickle cell anemia, which results in abdominal cramping when he is in crisis. His hemoglobin was 6 upon admission. He says his baseline runs 7–8. The patient states that he has not had a splenectomy. He describes the pain as midabdominal and cramplike. He denied any chills, fevers, or sweats.

HOSPITAL COURSE BY PROBLEM:
Problem 1. Sickle cell crisis. Patient was admitted to a medical-surgical bed, and placed on oxygen and IV fluids. He received morphine for analgesia as well as Vicodin. At discharge, his abdominal pain had resolved; however, he reported weakness. He was kept for an additional day for observation.

Problem 2. CT scan was performed on the belly and showed evidence of ileus in the small bowel with somewhat dilated small-bowel loops and also an abnormal enhancement pattern in the kidney. The patient has had no nausea or vomiting. He is moving his bowels without any difficulty. He is ambulating. He even goes outside to smoke cigarettes, which he has been advised not to do. Certainly, we should obtain some information on his renal function and have his regular doctor assess this problem.

DISCHARGE INSTRUCTIONS: Patient advised to stop smoking and to see his regular doctor for follow-up on renal function.

Michael R. Saadi, MD
Michael R. Saadi, MD

MRS:dp

D: 6–23–20xx; T: 6–23–20xx

Patient: Evans, Joshua   Physician: Michael R. Saadi, MD
Room #: 609 P   Patient ID#: 532657

Terminology

The terms listed in the table that follows are taken from *Discharge Summary: Sickle Cell Crisis.* Use a medical dictionary such as *Taber's Cyclopedic Medical Dictionary,* the appendices of this book, or other resources to define each term. Then review the pronunciation for each term and practice by reading the medical record aloud.

Term	Definition
ambulating ĂM-bū-lāt-ĭng	
analgesia ăn-ăl-JĒ-zē-ă	
anemia ă-NĒ-mē-ă	
crisis KRĪ-sĭs	
CT	
hemoglobin HĒ-mō-glō-bĭn	
ileus ĬL-ē-ŭs	
infarction ĭn-FĂRK-shŭn	
morphine MOR-fēn	
sickle cell SĬK-ăl SĚL	
splenectomy splē-NĚK-tō-mē	
Vicodin VĪ-kō-dĭn	

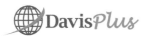 Davis*Plus*

Visit the *Medical Terminology Systems* online resource center at Davis*Plus* to practice pronunciation and reinforce the meanings of the terms in this medical report.

Critical Thinking

Review *Discharge Summary: Sickle Cell Crisis* to answer the questions.

1. What blood product was administered to the patient?

_____

_____

_____

_____

2. Why was this blood product given to the patient?

_____

_____

_____

_____

3. Why was a CT scan performed on the patient?

_____

_____

_____

_____

4. What were the three findings of the CT scan?

_____

_____

_____

_____

5. Why should the patient see his regular doctor?

_____

_____

_____

_____

Discharge Summary: PCP and HIV

General Hospital

1511 Ninth Avenue ■ ■ Sun City, USA 12345 ■ ■ (544) 802–1887

DISCHARGE SUMMARY

ADMISSION DATE: March 5, 20xx   **DISCHARGE DATE:** March 6, 20xx

ADMITTING AND DISCHARGE DIAGNOSES:
1. *Pneumocystis* pneumonia.
2. Human immunodeficiency virus infection.
3. Wasting

SOCIAL HISTORY: Patient's husband is deceased from AIDS 1 year ago with progressive multifocal leukoencephalopathy and Kaposi sarcoma. She denies any history of intravenous drug use or transfusion and identifies three lifetime sexual partners.

PAST MEDICAL HISTORY: Patient's past medical history is significant for HIV and several episodes of diarrhea, sinusitis, thrush, and vaginal candidiasis. She gave a history of a 10-pound weight loss. The chest x-ray showed diffuse lower lobe infiltrates, and she was diagnosed with presumptive *Pneumocystis* pneumonia and placed on Bactrim. She was admitted for a bronchoscopy with alveolar lavage to confirm the diagnosis.

PROCEDURE: The antiretroviral treatment was reinitiated, and she was counseled as to the need to strictly adhere to her therapeutic regimen.

DISCHARGE INSTRUCTIONS: Complete medication regimen. Patient discharged to the care of Dr. Amid Shaheen.

Michael R. Saadi, MD
Michael R. Saadi, MD

MRS:dp

D: 3–06–20xx; T: 3–06–20xx

Patient: Smart, Joann   Physician: Michael R. Saadi, MD
Room #: 540   Patient ID#: 532850

Terminology

The terms listed in the table that follows are taken from *Discharge Summary: PCP and HIV*. Use a medical dictionary such as *Taber's Cyclopedic Medical Dictionary*, the appendices of this book, or other resources to define each term. Then review the pronunciation for each term and practice by reading the medical record aloud.

Term	Definition
alveolar lavage ăl-VĒ-ō-lăr lă-VĂZH	
Bactrim BĂK-trĭm	
bronchoscopy brŏng-KŎS-kō-pē	
diffuse dĭ-FŪS	
human immun- odeficiency virus ĭm-ū-nō-dē- FĬSH-ĕn-sē	
infiltrate ĬN-fĭl-trāt	
Kaposi sarcoma KĂP-ō-sē săr-KŌ-mă	
leukoencephalop- athy loo-kō-ĕn-sĕf-ă- LŎP-ă-thē	
multifocal mŭl-tĭ-FŌ-kăl	
Pneumocystis pneumonia nū-mō-SĬS-tĭs nū-MŌ-nē-ă	
thrush THRŬSH	
vaginal candidiasis VĂJ-ĭn-ăl kăn-dĭ-DĪ-ă-sĭs	

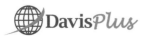

Critical Thinking

Review the medical report *Discharge Summary: PCP and HIV* to answer the questions.

1. How do you think the patient acquired the HIV infection?

_____

_____

_____

_____

2. What were the two diagnoses of the husband?

_____

_____

_____

_____

3. What four disorders in the medical history are significant for HIV?

_____

_____

_____

_____

4. What was the x-ray finding?

_____

_____

_____

5. What two procedures are going to be performed to confirm the diagnosis of *Pneumocystis* pneumonia?

_____

_____

_____

_____

Documenting Health-Care Activity 9-3

Constructing Chart Notes

To construct chart notes, replace the italicized and boldfaced terms in each of the two case studies with one of the listed medical terms.

arthralgia	hematomas	leukocytosis
erythropenia	hemophilia	lymphadenopathy
hemarthrosis	hemostasis	splenomegaly
hematologist		

Mr. X., a 53-year-old male, presents with complaints of feeling "poorly" and not sleeping well for the past 3 months. Upon examination, the physician notes that Mr. X's gums are red and swollen. Also, there is evidence of (1) *disease in the lymph glands* under the patient's left arm and on the back of his neck. Upon palpation, the physician also notes an (2) *enlarged spleen*. The patient's CBC shows an (3) *abnormal increase of leukocytes* and a moderate (4) *decrease of erythrocytes*. The patient is referred to Dr. Jordan, a (5) *specialist in blood diseases*.

1. _____
2. _____
3. _____
4. _____
5. _____

Mr. J. states that his father and uncle have (6) *"bleeder's disease."* The patient also states that he often develops (7) *large bruises* under his skin even with a minimal "bump or scrape." Today he presents with swelling and (8) *pain in his joints,* especially the knees. His present complaints are likely the result of (9) *abnormal bleeding into the joint* cavity. The physician prescribes an infusion of Mr. J.'s deficient clotting factor to (10) *control the bleeding*.

6. _____
7. _____
8. _____
9. _____
10. _____

✅ *Check your answers in Appendix A. Review any material that you did not answer correctly.*

Correct Answers _____ X 10 = _____ % Score

Musculoskeletal System

Chapter Outline

Objectives

Upon completion of this chapter, you will be able to:

- Locate and describe the structures of the musculoskeletal system.
- Describe the functional relationship between the musculoskeletal system and other body systems.
- Pronounce, spell, and build words related to the musculoskeletal system.
- Describe diseases, conditions, and procedures related to the musculoskeletal system.
- Explain pharmacology related to the treatment of musculoskeletal disorders.
- Demonstrate your knowledge of this chapter by completing the learning and documenting health-care activities.

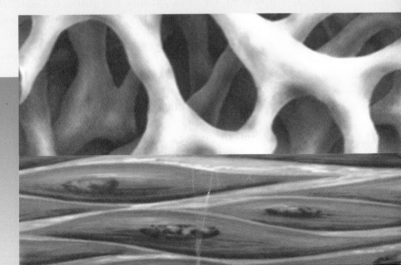

Anatomy and Physiology

The musculoskeletal system includes muscles, bones, joints, and related structures, such as the tendons and connective tissue that function in the support and movement of body parts and organs. (See Fig. 10-1.)

Anatomy and Physiology Key Terms

This section introduces important terms, along with their definitions and pronunciations. The key terms are highlighted in color in the Anatomy and Physiology section. Word analyses for selected terms are also provided. Pronounce the term, and place a check mark in the box after you do so.

Term	Definition
articulation ăr-tĭk-ū-LĀ-shŭn ☐	Place of union between two or more bones; also called *joint*
hematopoiesis hĕm-ă-tō-poy-Ē-sĭs ☐ *hemat/o:* blood *-poiesis:* formation, production	Production and development of blood cells, normally in the bone marrow
ligaments LĬG-ă-mĕnts ☐	Connective tissue that surrounds the joint capsule to bind bones to other bones
tendons TĔN-dŭns ☐	Connective tissue that binds muscle to bone on either side of a joint *Contraction of the muscle attached to the bone by tendon forces the bones in the joint to move.*

Pronunciation Help	Long Sound	ā — rate	ē — rebirth	ī — isle	ō — over	ū — unite
	Short Sound	ă — apple	ĕ — ever	ĭ — it	ŏ — not	ŭ — cut

Muscles

Muscle tissue is composed of contractile cells, or **fibers,** that provide movement of an organ or body part. Muscles contribute to posture, produce body heat, and act as a protective covering for internal organs. Muscles make up the bulk of the body. They have the ability to contract, relax, and return to their original size and shape. Whether muscles are attached to bones or found in internal organs and blood vessels, their primary responsibility is movement. (See Table 10-1, pages 308 and 309.) Apparent motions provided by muscles include walking and talking. Less apparent motions include the passage and elimination of food through the digestive system, propulsion of blood through the arteries, and contraction of the bladder to eliminate urine.

There are three types of muscle tissue in the body:

- **Skeletal muscles** are attached to bones and provide the means for movement. Skeletal muscles are **voluntary muscles** that contract and relax in response to conscious thought. Because of their striped appearance on microscopic examination, they are also called **striated muscles.** Some examples of voluntary muscles are muscles that move the eyeballs, tongue, and bones.
- **Smooth muscles** are mainly responsible for assisting internal processes, such as digestion, circulation, and urination. Thus, they are called **visceral muscles.** Because their movement

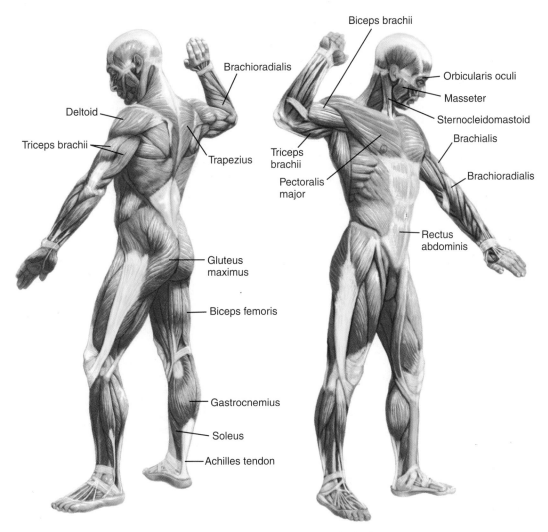

Figure 10-1 Selected muscles of the body.

is not under conscious control but functions under the control of the autonomic (involuntary) nervous system, they are also known as **involuntary muscles.** Some examples of involuntary muscles are those in the digestive tract that propel food through the alimentary canal and those in the urinary system that control urination.

- **Cardiac muscle** is found only in the heart wall, where it forms the myocardium. It is striated like skeletal muscle, but it also produces rhythmic involuntary contractions like smooth muscle.

Table 10-1	Body Movements Produced by Muscle Action

This table lists body movements and the resulting muscle action. With the exception of rotation, these movements are in pairs of opposing functions.

Motion	Action
Adduction	Moves closer to the midline
Abduction	Moves away from the midline

Adduction   Abduction

| **Flexion** | Decreases the angle of a joint |
| **Extension** | Increases the angle of a joint |

Flexion   Extension

Table 10-1	**Body Movements Produced by Muscle Action—cont'd**
Motion	**Action**
Rotation	Moves a bone around its own axis

Rotation

Pronation	Turns the palm downward
Supination	Turns the palm upward

Pronation   Supination

Inversion	Moves the sole of the foot inward
Eversion	Moves the sole of the foot outward

Inversion   Eversion

Dorsiflexion	Elevates the foot
Plantar flexion	Lowers the foot (points the toes)

Dorsiflexion   Plantar flexion

Anatomy Review: Muscular System

To review the anatomy of the muscular system, label the illustration using the listed terms.

Achilles tendon	*gastrocnemius*	*rectus abdominis*
biceps brachii	*gluteus maximus*	*soleus*
biceps femoris	*masseter*	*sternocleidomastoid*
brachioradialis	*orbicularis oculi*	*trapezius*
deltoid	*pectoralis major*	

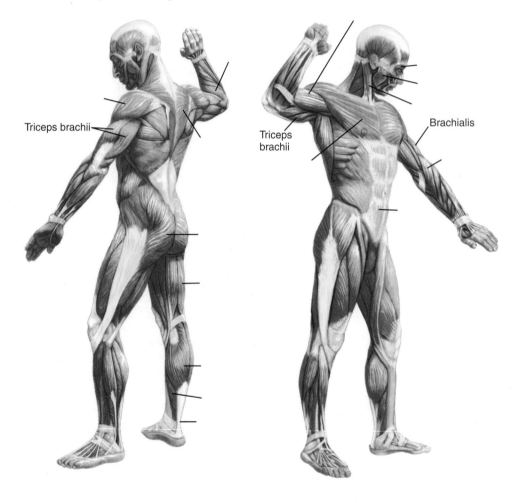

Triceps brachii

Triceps brachii

Brachialis

Check your answers by referring to Figure 10–1 on page 307. Review material that you did not answer correctly.

Bones

Bones provide the framework of the body, protect internal organs, allow for movement, store calcium and other minerals, and produce blood cells within bone marrow **(hematopoiesis)**. The bones of the skull protect the brain; the rib cage protects the heart and lungs; the pelvic bones protect the developing fetus and reproductive organs. Movement is possible because bones provide points of attachment for muscles, **tendons**, and **ligaments**. As muscles contract, tendons and ligaments pull on bones and cause skeletal movement. Bones serve as a storehouse for minerals, particularly phosphorus and calcium.

Bone Types

There are four principal types of bone:

- **Short bones** are somewhat cube-shaped and are nearly equal in length and width. Examples of short bones include the bones of the wrist (carpals) and ankles (tarsals).
- **Irregular bones** include the bones that cannot be classified as short or long because of their complex shapes. Examples of irregular bones include vertebrae and the bones of the middle ear.
- **Flat bones** are exactly what their name suggests. They provide broad surfaces for muscular attachment or protection for internal organs. Examples of flat bones include bones of the skull, shoulder blades, and sternum.
- **Long bones** are found in the extremities of the body, such as the legs, arms, and fingers. The long bones have regular, well-defined shapes. (See Fig. 10-2, page 312.) Each long bone has three main parts:
- The (1) **diaphysis** is the shaft, or long, main portion of a bone. It consists of **compact bone** that forms a cylinder and surrounds a central canal called the (2) **medullary cavity.** The medullary cavity is filled with "yellow bone marrow," so named because it is composed mainly of blood vessels and fatty tissue.
- The (3) **distal epiphysis** and (4) **proximal epiphysis** (plural, **epiphyses**) are the two ends of the bones. Both ends have a somewhat bulbous shape to provide space for muscle and ligament attachments near the joints. Each epiphysis consists of three layers of tissue:
  - (5) **articular cartilage,** which is a thin outer layer of cartilage where bones meet to form joints, and the (6) **epiphyseal line (growth plate),** an area of cartilage constantly being replaced by new bone tissue as the bone grows and that is responsible for lengthening bones during childhood and adolescence and calcifies and disappears when the bone has achieved its full growth
  - thick, dense layer of hard (7) **compact bone**
  - inner layer of porous tissue called (8) **spongy** or **cancellous bone** that is less dense than compact bone and is filled with *red bone marrow,* so named because it is composed mainly of blood cells in various stages of development.
- The (9) **periosteum,** a dense, white, fibrous membrane, covers the remaining surface of the bone. It contains numerous blood and lymph vessels and nerves. In growing bones, the inner layer contains the bone-forming cells known as **osteoblasts.** The periosteum provides a means for bone repair and general bone nutrition. The periosteum also serves as a point of attachment for muscles, ligaments, and tendons.

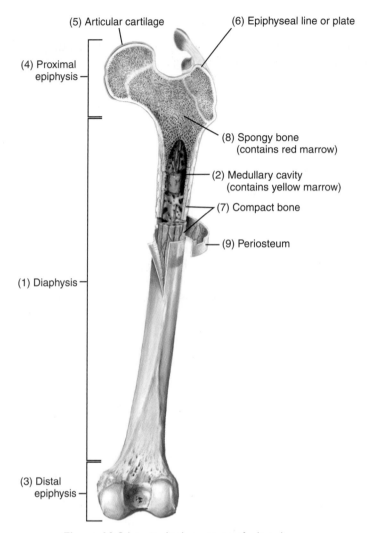

Figure 10-2 Longitudinal structure of a long bone.

Surface Features of Bones

Surfaces of bones are rarely smooth but consist of projections, articulating surfaces, depressions, and openings. These surfaces provide sites for muscle and ligament attachment. They also provide pathways and openings for blood vessels and nerves. Various types of projections are evident in bones, some of which serve as points of **articulation**. Table 10-2 lists common bone markings and their descriptions.

Table 10-2	**Surface Features of Bones**

This table lists the most common types of bone projections, articulating surfaces, depressions, and openings, along with the bones involved, descriptions, and examples for each. Becoming familiar with these terms will help you identify the parts of individual bones described in medical reports related to orthopedics.

Surface Type	Bone Marking	Description	Example
Projections			
• Nonarticulating surfaces	• Trochanter	• Very large, irregularly shaped process found only on the femur	• Greater trochanter of the femur
• Sites of muscle and ligament attachment	• Tubercle	• Small, rounded process	• Tubercle of the femur
	• Tuberosity	• Large, rounded process	• Tuberosity of the humerus
Articulating Surfaces			
• Projections that form joints	• Condyle	• Rounded, articulating knob	• Condyle of the humerus
	• Head	• Prominent, rounded, articulating end of a bone	• Head of the femur
Depressions and Openings			
• Sites for blood vessel, nerve, and duct passage	• Foramen	• Rounded opening through a bone to accommodate blood vessels and nerves	• Foramen of the skull through which cranial nerves pass
	• Fissure	• Narrow, slitlike opening	• Fissure of the sphenoid bone
	• Meatus	• Opening or passage into a bone	• External auditory meatus of the temporal bone
	• Sinus	• Cavity or hollow space in a bone	• Cavity of the frontal sinus containing a duct that carries secretions to the upper part of the nasal cavity

Divisions of the Skeletal System

The skeletal system of a human adult consists of 206 individual bones. For anatomical purposes, the human skeleton is divided into the axial skeleton and appendicular skeleton. (See Fig. 10-3.)

Axial Skeleton

The axial skeleton is divided into three major regions: skull, rib cage, and vertebral column. It contributes to the formation of body cavities and provides protection for internal organs, such as the brain, spinal cord, and organs enclosed in the thorax. Figure 10-3 depicts the axial bones in a light tan color.

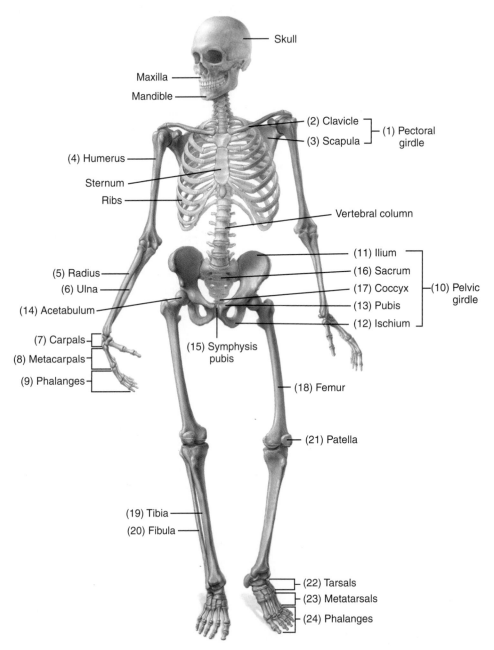

Figure 10-3 Anterior view of the axial (tan) and appendicular (blue) skeleton.

Skull

The bony structure of the skull consists of cranial bones and facial bones. (See Fig. 10-4.) With the exception of one facial bone, all other bones of the skull are joined together by sutures. Sutures are the lines of junction between two bones, especially of the skull, and are usually immovable.

Cranial Bones

Eight bones, collectively known as the **cranium (skull),** enclose and protect the brain and the organs of hearing and equilibrium. Cranial bones are connected to muscles to provide head movements, chewing motions, and facial expressions.

At birth, the skull is incompletely developed, with fibrous membranes connecting the cranial bones. These membranous areas are called **fontanels** or, more commonly, *soft spots.* They permit some movement between the bones that enables an infant's skull to pass more easily through the

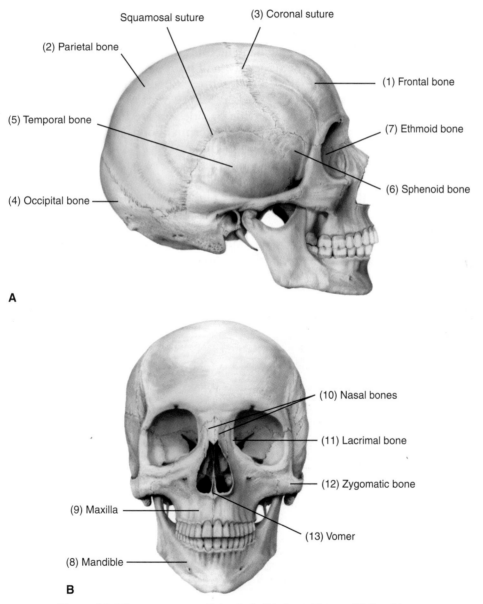

Figure 10-4 Bony structures of the skull. (A) Cranial bones. (B) Facial bones.

birth canal. Eventually, the fontanels close as the cranial bones grow together. The (1) **frontal bone** forms the anterior portion of the skull **(forehead)** and the roof of the bony cavities that contain the eyeballs. One (2) **parietal bone** is situated on each side of the skull just behind the frontal bone. Together they form the upper sides and roof of the cranium. Each parietal bone meets the frontal bone along the (3) **coronal suture.** A single (4) **occipital bone** forms the back and base of the skull. It contains an opening in its base through which the spinal cord passes. Two (5) **temporal bone(s),** one on each side of the skull, form part of the lower cranium. Each temporal bone has a complicated shape that contains various cavities and recesses associated with the internal ear, the essential part of the organ of hearing and balance. The temporal bone projects downward to form the **mastoid process,** which provides a point of attachment for several neck muscles. The (6) **sphenoid bone,** located at the middle part of the base of the skull, forms a central wedge that joins with all other cranial bones, holding them together. The (7) **ethmoid bone** is the anterior cranial bone located between the nasal cavity and parts of the orbits of the eyes.

Facial Bones

All facial bones, with the exception of the (8) **mandible** (lower jaw bone), are joined together by sutures and are immovable. Movement of the mandible is necessary for speaking and chewing **(mastication).** The (9) **maxillae** (singular, **maxilla**), paired upper jawbones, are fused in the midline by a suture. They form the upper jaw and **hard palate** (roof of the mouth). If the maxillary bones do not fuse properly before birth, a congenital defect called **cleft palate** results. The maxillae and mandible contain sockets for the roots of the teeth. Two thin, nearly rectangular bones, the (10) **nasal bones,** lie side by side and are fused medially, forming the shape and the bridge of the nose. Two paired (11) **lacrimal bones** are located at the corner of each eye. These thin, small bones unite to form the groove for the lacrimal sac and canals through which the tear ducts pass into the nasal cavity. The paired (12) **zygomatic bones** (cheekbones) are located on the side of the face below the eyes and form the higher portion of the cheeks below and to the sides of the eyes. The (13) **vomer** is a single, thin bone that forms the lower part of the nasal septum.

Other important structures, the **paranasal sinuses,** are cavities located within the cranial and facial bones. As their names imply, the frontal, ethmoidal, sphenoidal, and maxillary sinuses are named after the bones in which they are located. (See Fig. 10-5.)

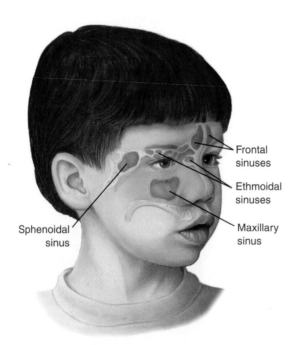

Figure 10-5 Paranasal sinuses.

Thorax

The term *thorax* refers to the entire chest. The internal organs of the thorax include the heart and lungs, which are enclosed in and protected by the **thoracic cage (rib cage).** The thoracic cage consists of 12 pairs of ribs, all attached to the spine. (See Fig. 10-6.) The first seven pairs, the (1) **true ribs,** are attached directly to the (2) **sternum** by a strip of (3) **costal cartilage.** The costal cartilage of the next five pairs of ribs is not fastened directly to the sternum, so these ribs are known as (4) **false ribs.** The last two pairs of false ribs are not joined, even indirectly, to the sternum but attach posteriorly to the thoracic vertebrae. These last two pairs of false ribs are known as (5) **floating ribs.**

Vertebral Column

The vertebral column of the adult is composed of 26 bones called **vertebrae** (singular, **vertebra**). The vertebral column supports the body and provides a protective bony canal for the spinal cord. A healthy, normal spine has four curves that help make it resilient and maintain balance. The cervical and lumbar regions curve forward, whereas the thoracic and sacral regions curve backward. (See Fig. 10-7, page 318.)

The vertebral column consists of five regions of bones, each deriving its name from its location within the spinal column. The seven (1) **cervical vertebrae** form the skeletal framework of the neck. The first cervical vertebra, the (2) **atlas,** supports the skull. The second cervical vertebra, the (3) **axis,** makes possible the rotation of the skull on the neck. Under the cervical vertebra are 12 (4) **thoracic vertebrae,** which support the chest and serve as a point of articulation for the ribs. The next five vertebrae, the (5) **lumbar vertebrae,** are situated in the lower back area and carry most of the weight of the torso. Below this area are five sacral vertebrae, which are fused into a single bone in the adult and are referred to as the (6) **sacrum.** The tail of the vertebral column consists of four or five fragmented fused vertebrae referred to as the (7) **coccyx.**

Vertebrae are separated by flat, round structures, the (8) **intervertebral disks,** which are composed of a fibrocartilaginous substance with a gelatinous mass in the center **(nucleus pulposus).**

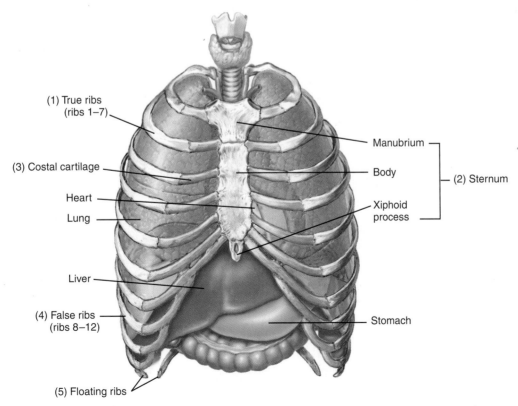

Figure 10-6 Thorax.

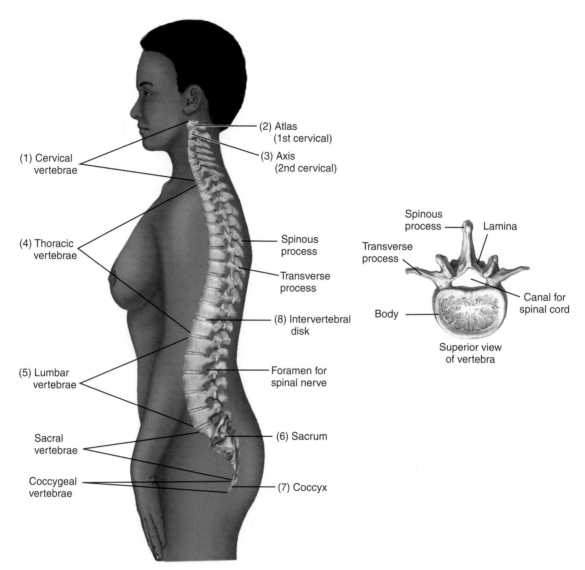

Figure 10-7 Lateral view of the vertebral column.

Appendicular Skeleton

The appendicular skeleton consists of bones of the upper and lower limbs and their girdles, which attach the limbs to the axial skeleton. The appendicular skeleton is distinguished with a blue color in Figure 10-3. The axial skeleton protects internal organs and provides central support for the body; the appendicular skeleton enables body movement. The ability to walk, run, or catch a ball is possible because of the movable joints of the limbs that make up the appendicular skeleton.

Pectoral Girdle

The (1) **pectoral (shoulder) girdle** consists of two bones, the anterior (2) **clavicle** (collarbone) and the posterior (3) **scapula** (triangular shoulder blade). The primary function of the pectoral girdle is to attach the bones of the upper limbs to the axial skeleton and provide attachments for muscles that aid upper limb movements. The paired pectoral structures and their associated muscles form the shoulders of the body.

Upper Limbs

The skeletal framework of each upper limb includes the arm, forearm, and hand. Anatomically speaking, the arm is only that part of the upper limb between the shoulder and elbow. Each **appendage** consists of the (4) **humerus** (upper arm bone) as well as the (5) **radius** and (6) **ulna,** the two bones that constitute the forearm and articulate at the elbow with the humerus. The bones of each hand include eight (7) **carpals** (wrist), five radiating (8) **metacarpals** (palm), and ten radiating (9) **phalanges** (fingers).

Pelvic Girdle

The (10) **pelvic girdle** (hip bone) is a basin-shaped structure that attaches the lower limbs to the axial skeleton. Along with its associated ligaments, it supports the trunk of the body and provides protection for lower organs of digestion and urinary and reproductive structures.

Male and female **pelves** (singular, **pelvis**) differ considerably in size and shape but share the same basic structures. Generally, the bones of males are larger and heavier and possess larger surface markings than those of females of comparable age and physical stature. Some of the differences are attributable to the function of the female pelvis during childbearing. The female pelvis is shallower than the male pelvis but wider in all directions. The female pelvis not only supports the enlarged uterus as the fetus matures but also provides a large opening to allow the infant to pass through during birth. Regardless of these differences, the female and male pelves are divided into the (11) **ilium,** (12) **ischium,** and (13) **pubis.** These three bones fuse together in the adult to form a single hip bone called the **innominate bone.** The ilium travels inferiorly to form part of the (14) **acetabulum,** the deep socket of the hip joint, and joins the pubis. The bladder is located behind the (15) **symphysis pubis;** the rectum is in the curve of the (16) **sacrum** and (17) **coccyx.** In the female, the uterus, fallopian tubes, ovaries, and vagina are located between the bladder and the rectum.

Lower Limbs

The lower limbs support the complete weight of the erect body and are subjected to exceptional stresses, especially in running or jumping. To accommodate for these forces, the lower limb bones are stronger and thicker than comparable bones of the upper limbs.

There are three parts of each lower limb: the thigh, the leg, and the foot. The thigh consists of a single bone called the (18) **femur.** It is the largest, longest, and strongest bone in the body. The leg is formed by two parallel bones: the (19) **tibia** and the (20) **fibula.** A small triangular bone, the (21) **patella** (kneecap), is located anterior to the knee joint. The seven (22) **tarsals** (ankle bones) resemble metacarpals (wrist bones) in structure. Lastly, the bones of each foot include the (23) **metatarsals,** which consists of five small long bones numbered 1 to 5 beginning with the great toe on the medial side of the foot, and the much smaller (24) **phalanges** (toes).

Joints or Articulations

To allow for body movements, bones must have points where they meet **(articulate).** These articulating points form joints that have various degrees of mobility. The **joint capsule** contains a lubrication fluid **(synovial fluid)** that nourishes and protects the joint. The need for greater or lesser flexibility determines the type of joint in any specific location. There are three types of joints. All three types are necessary for smooth, coordinated body movements. Freely movable joints **(diarthroses)** are encased in a sleevelike extension of the periosteum, such as the hinge joints of the elbow (between the humerus and ulna). Slightly movable joints **(amphiarthroses)** are articulations between two bones connected by ligaments or elastic cartilage, such as those between the vertebrae. Immovable joints **(synarthroses)** are joints that have no mobility, such as those that constitute the sutures of the skull.

Anatomy Review: Long Bone

To review the anatomy of a typical long bone, label the illustration of the femur using the listed terms.

articular cartilage   *distal epiphysis*   *proximal epiphysis*

compact bone   *medullary cavity*   *spongy bone*

diaphysis   *periosteum*

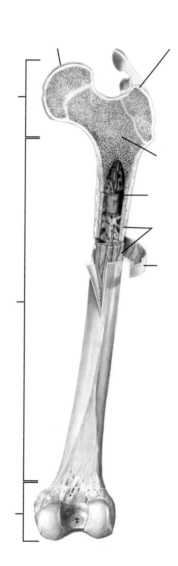

 Check your answers by referring to Figure 10-2 on page 312. Review material that you did not answer correctly.

Anatomy Review: Skeletal System

To review the skeletal structures, label the illustration using the listed terms.

acetabulum	humerus	pelvic girdle	sternum
carpals	ilium	phalanges	symphysis pubis
clavicle	ischium	pubis	tarsals
coccyx	metatarsals	radius	tibia
femur	metacarpals	sacrum	ulna
fibula	pectoral girdle	scapula	

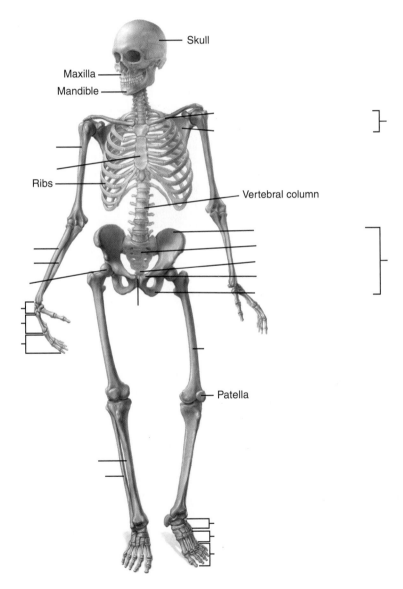

Skull

Maxilla —

Mandible —

Ribs —

Vertebral column

Patella

 Check your answers by referring to Figure 10–3 on page 314. Review material that you did not answer correctly.

CONNECTING BODY SYSTEMS—MUSCULOSKELETAL SYSTEM

The main function of the musculoskeletal system is to provide support, protection, and movement of body parts. Specific functional relationships between the musculoskeletal system and other body systems are summarized here.

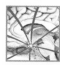

Blood, Lymphatic, and Immune
- Muscle action pumps lymph through lymphatic vessels.
- Bone marrow provides a place for cells of the immune system to develop.

Cardiovascular
- Bone helps regulate blood calcium levels, which are important to heart function.

Digestive
- Muscles play an important role in swallowing and propelling food through the digestive tract.
- Muscles of the stomach mechanically break down food to prepare it for chemical digestion.

Endocrine
- Exercising skeletal muscles stimulates release of hormones to increase blood flow.

Female Reproductive
- Muscles are important in sexual activity and during delivery of the fetus.
- Bones provide a source of calcium during pregnancy and lactation if dietary intake is lacking or insufficient.
- The pelvis helps support the enlarged uterus during pregnancy.

Integumentary
- Involuntary muscle contractions (shivering) help regulate body temperature.

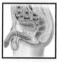

Male Reproductive
- Muscles play an important role in sexual activity.

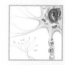

Nervous
- Bones protect the brain and spinal cord.

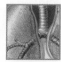

Respiratory
- Muscles elevate ribs and contract the diaphragm to assist in the breathing process.

Urinary
- Bones work in conjunction with the kidneys to help regulate blood calcium levels.
- Skeletal muscles help control urine elimination.

Medical Word Elements

This section introduces combining forms, suffixes, and prefixes related to the musculoskeletal system. Word analyses are also provided. From the information provided, complete the meaning of the medical words in the right-hand column. The first one is completed for you.

Element	Meaning	Word Analysis and Meaning
Combining Forms		
Muscular System		
leiomy/o	smooth (visceral) muscle	**leiomy**/oma (lī-ō-mī-Ō-mǎ): *tumor of smooth muscle* *-oma:* tumor
muscul/o	muscle	**muscul**/ar (MŬS-kū-lǎr): _____ *-ar:* pertaining to
my/o		**my**/oma (mī-Ō-mǎ): _____ *-oma:* tumor
rhabd/o	rod-shaped (striated)	**rhabd**/oid (RĂB-doyd): _____ *-oid:* resembling
rhabdomy/o	rod-shaped (striated) muscle	**rhabdomy**/oma (rǎb-dō-mī-Ō-mǎ): _____ *-oma:* tumor
Skeletal System		
Bones of the Upper Body		
brachi/o	arm	**brachi**/algia (brā-kē-ĂL-jē-ǎ): _____ *-algia:* pain
carp/o	carpus (wrist bone)	**carp/o**/ptosis (kǎr-pŏp-TŌ-sĭs): _____ *-ptosis:* prolapse, downward displacement *Carpoptosis is commonly called* wrist drop.
cephal/o	head	**cephal**/ad (SĔF-ǎ-lǎd): _____ *-ad:* toward
cervic/o	neck; cervix uteri (neck of the uterus)	**cervic/o**/dynia (sĕr-vĭ-kō-DĬN-ē-ǎ): _____ *-dynia:* pain *Cervicodynia is also called* cervical neuralgia.
clavicul/o	clavicle (collar bone)	**clavicul**/ar (klǎ-VĬK-ū-lǎr): _____ *-ar:* pertaining to

(continued)

Medical Word Elements—cont'd

Element	Meaning	Word Analysis and Meaning
cost/o	ribs	**cost**/ectomy (kŏs-TĔK-tō-mē): _____ -*ectomy:* excision, removal
crani/o	cranium (skull)	**crani/o**/tomy (krā-nē-ŎT-ō-mē): _____ -*tomy:* incision
dactyl/o	fingers; toes	**dactyl**/itis (dăk-tĭl-Ī-tĭs): _____ -*itis:* inflammation
humer/o	humerus (upper arm bone)	**humer/o**/scapul/ar (hū-mĕr-ō-SKĂP-ū-lăr): _____ *scapul:* scapula (shoulder blade) -*ar:* pertaining to
metacarp/o	metacarpus (hand bones)	**metacarp**/ectomy (mĕt-ă-kăr-PĔK-tō-mē): _____ -*ectomy:* excision, removal
phalang/o	phalanges (bones of the fingers and toes)	**phalang**/ectomy (făl-ăn-JĔK-tō-mē): _____ -*ectomy:* excision, removal
radi/o	radiation, x-ray; radius (lower arm bone on the thumb side)	**radi**/al (RĀ-dē-ăl): _____ -*al:* pertaining to
spondyl/o	vertebrae (backbone)	**spondyl**/itis (spŏn-dĭl-Ī-tĭs): _____ -*itis:* inflammation *The combining form* spondyl/o *describes diseases and conditions.*
vertebr/o		inter/**vertebr**/al (ĭn-tĕr-VĔRT-ĕ-brĕl): _____ *inter-:* between -*al:* pertaining to *The combining form* vertebr/o *indicates anatomical terms.*
stern/o	sternum (breastbone)	**stern**/ad (STĔR-năd): _____ -*ad:* toward
thorac/o	chest	**thorac/o**/dynia (thō-răk-ō-DĬN-ē-ă): _____ -*dynia:* pain
Bones of the Lower Body		
calcane/o	calcaneum (heel bone)	**calcane/o**/dynia (kăl-kā-nē-ō-DĬN-ē-ă): _____ -*dynia:* pain
femor/o	femur (thigh bone)	**femor**/al (FĔM-or-ăl): _____ -*al:* pertaining to

Medical Word Elements—cont'd

Element	Meaning	Word Analysis and Meaning
fibul/o	fibula (smaller bone of the lower leg)	**fibul/o**/calcane/al (fĭb-ū-lō-kăl-KĀ-nē-ăl): _____ *calcane:* calcaneum (heel bone) *-al:* pertaining to
ili/o	ilium (lateral, flaring portion of the hip bone)	**ili/o**/pelv/ic (ĭl-ē-ō-PĔL-vĭk): _____ *pelv:* pelvis *-ic:* pertaining to
ischi/o	ischium (lower portion of the hip bone)	**ischi/o**/dynia (ĭs-kē-ō-DĬN-ē-ă): _____ *-dynia:* pain
lumb/o	loins (lower back)	**lumb/o**/dynia (lŭm-bō-DĬN-ē-ă): _____ *-dynia:* pain
metatars/o	metatarsus (foot bones)	**metatars**/algia (mĕt-ă-tăr-SĂL-jē-ă): _____ *-algia:* pain *Metatarsalgia radiates from the head of the metatarsus and worsens with weight-bearing activity or palpation.*
patell/o	patella (kneecap)	**patell**/ectomy (păt-ĕ-LĔK-tō-mē): _____ *-ectomy:* excision, removal
pelv/i	pelvis	**pelv/i**/metry* (pĕl-VĬM-ĕt-rē): _____ *-metry:* act of measuring *Pelvimetry is routinely performed in obstetrical management.*
pelv/o		**pelv**/ic (PĔL-vĭc): _____ *-ic:* pertaining to *A woman's pelvis is usually less massive but wider and more circular than a man's pelvis.*
pod/o	foot	**pod**/iatry (pō-DĪ-ă-trē): _____ *-iatry:* medicine, treatment
pub/o	pubis (anterior part of the pelvic bone)	**pub/o**/coccyg/eal (pū-bō-k ŏk-SĬJ-ē-ăl): _____ *coccyg:* coccyx (tailbone) *-eal:* pertaining to
tibi/o	tibia (larger bone of the lower leg)	**tibi/o**/femor/al (tĭb-ē-ō-FĔM-or-ăl): _____ *femor:* femur *-al:* pertaining to

*The *i* in *pelv/i/metry* is an exception to the rule of using the connecting vowel o.

(continued)

Medical Word Elements—cont'd

Element	Meaning	Word Analysis and Meaning
Other		
ankyl/o	stiffness; bent, crooked	**ankyl**/osis (ăng-kĭ-LŌ-sĭs): _____ -_osis:_ abnormal condition; increase (used primarily with blood cells) _Ankylosis results in immobility and stiffness of a joint. It may be the result of trauma, surgery, or disease and most commonly occurs in rheumatoid arthritis._
arthr/o	joint	**arthr**/itis (ăr-THRĪ-tĭs): _____ -_itis:_ inflammation
chondr/o	cartilage	**chondr**/itis (kŏn-DRĪ-tĭs): _____ -_itis:_ inflammation
fasci/o	band, fascia (fibrous membrane supporting and separating muscles)	**fasci/o**/plasty (FĂSH-ē-ō-plăs-tē): _____ -_plasty:_ surgical repair
fibr/o	fiber, fibrous tissue	**fibr**/oma (fĭ-BRŌ-mă): _____ -_oma:_ tumor
kyph/o	humpback	**kyph**/osis (kī-FŌ-sĭs): _____ -_osis:_ abnormal condition; increase (used primarily with blood cells)
lamin/o	lamina (part of vertebral arch)	**lamin**/ectomy (lăm-ĭ-NĔK-tō-mē): _____ -_ectomy:_ excision, removal _Laminectomy is usually performed to relieve compression of the spinal cord or remove a lesion or herniated disk._
lord/o	curve, swayback	**lord**/osis (lor-DŌ-sĭs): _____ -_osis:_ abnormal condition; increase (used primarily with blood cells)
myel/o	bone marrow; spinal cord	**myel/o**/cyte (MĪ-ĕl-ō-sīt): _____ -_cyte:_ cell
orth/o	straight	**orth/o**/ped/ist (or-thō-PĒ-dĭst): _____ _ped:_ foot; child -_ist:_ specialist _Historically, an orthopedist corrected deformities and straightened children's bones. In today's medical practice, however, the orthopedist treats musculoskeletal disorders and associated structures in persons of all ages._
oste/o	bone	**oste**/oma (ŏs-tē-Ō-mă): _____ -_oma:_ tumor _Osteomas are benign bony tumors._

Medical Word Elements—cont'd

Element	Meaning	Word Analysis and Meaning
ped/o	foot; child	**ped/o**/graph (PĔD-ō-grăf): _____ *-graph:* instrument for recording *A pedograph produces an imprint of the foot and studies the gait (manner of walking).*
ped/i		**ped/i**/cure** (PĔD-ĭ-kūr): _____
scoli/o	crooked, bent	**scoli**/osis (skō-lē-Ō-sĭs): _____ *-osis:* abnormal condition; increase (used primarily with blood cells) *Scoliosis is characterized by a lateral spinal curvature.*
synov/o	synovial membrane, synovial fluid	**synov**/ectomy (sĭn-ō-VĔK-tō-mē): _____ *-ectomy:* excision, removal
ten/o	tendon	**ten/o**/desis (tĕn-ŌD-ĕ-sĭs): _____ *-desis:* binding, fixation (of a bone or joint)
tend/o		**tend/o**/plasty (TĔN-dō-plăs-tē): _____ *-plasty:* surgical repair
tendin/o		**tendin**/itis (tĕn-dĭn-Ī-tĭs): _____ *-itis:* inflammation

Suffixes

Element	Meaning	Word Analysis and Meaning
-asthenia	weakness, debility	my/**asthenia** (mī-ăs-THĒ-nē-ă): _____ *my:* muscle
-clasia	to break; surgical fracture	oste/o/**clasia** (ŏs-tē-ō-KLĀ-zē-ă): _____ *oste/o:* bone *Osteoclasia is the intentional fracture of a bone to correct a deformity and is also called* **osteoclasis.**
-clast	to break; surgical fracture	oste/o/**clast** (ŎS-tē-ō-klăst): _____ *oste/o:* bone *An osteoclast is a cell that breaks down the matrix of bone. Osteoblasts and osteoclasts work together to maintain a constant bone size in adults. An osteoclast also refers to an instrument used to surgically fracture a bone (osteoclasis).*
-desis	binding, fixation (of a bone or joint)	arthr/o/**desis** (ăr-thrō-DĒ-sĭs): _____ *arthr/o:* joint *This procedure immobilizes a joint to relieve intractable pain.*

**The *i* in *ped/i/cure* is an exception to the rule of using the connecting vowel *o*.

(continued)

Medical Word Elements—cont'd

Element	Meaning	Word Analysis and Meaning
-malacia	softening	chondr/o/**malacia** (kŏn-drō-măl-Ā-shē-ă): _____ *chondr/o:* cartilage *Chondromalacia is a deterioration of the articular cartilage, usually involving the patella.*
-porosis	porous	oste/o/**porosis** (ŏs-tē-ō-pŏ-RŌ-sĭs): _____ *oste/o:* bone *Osteoporosis is a disorder characterized by loss of bone density. It may cause pain, especially in the lower back; pathological fractures; loss of stature; and hairline fractures.*
-sarcoma	malignant tumor of connective tissue	chondr/o/**sarcoma** (kŏn-drō-săr-KŌ-mă): _____ *chondr/o:* cartilage *Connective tissue is found in cartilage, fat, blood vessels, bone, nerves, and muscles.*
a-	without, not	**a**/trophy (ĂT-rō-fē): _____ *-trophy:* development, nourishment *Atrophy causes a wasting or decrease in size or physiological activity of a part of the body because of disease or other influences.*
dys-	bad; painful; difficult	**dys**/trophy (DĬS-trō-fē): _____ *-trophy:* development, nourishment
syn-	union, together, joined	**syn**/dactyl/ism (sĭn-DĂK-tĭl-ĭzm): _____ *dactyl:* fingers, toes *-ism:* condition *Syndactylism results in a fusion of two or more fingers or toes.*

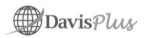 Visit the *Medical Terminology Systems* online resource center at Davis*Plus* for an audio exercise of the terms in this table. Other activities are also available to reinforce content.

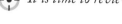 *It is time to review medical word elements by completing Learning Activities 10-1 and 10-2.*

Disease Focus

Musculoskeletal disorders include a variety of conditions that affect the muscles, bones, and joints found in neck, shoulders, wrists, back, hips, legs, knees, and feet. Pain and discomfort commonly associated with these disorders may interfere with everyday activities. These disorders are extremely common, and risk increases with age. Early diagnosis is the key to easing pain while potentially decreasing further bodily damage.

Given the different areas of the body that make up the musculoskeletal system, several other diseases can produce significant musculoskeletal signs and symptoms. These disorders include but are not limited to lower back pain, fibromyalgia, gout, osteoarthritis, rheumatoid arthritis, and tendinitis. Some of these disorders can cause mild discomfort to debilitating pain. Low back pain is the most common musculoskeletal disorder.

For diagnosis, treatment, and management of musculoskeletal disorders, the medical services of a specialist may be warranted. **Orthopedics** is the branch of medicine concerned with the prevention, diagnosis, care, and treatment of musculoskeletal disorders. The physician who specializes in the diagnoses and treatment of musculoskeletal disorders is known as an **orthopedist.** These physicians use medical, physical, and surgical methods to restore function that has been lost as a result of musculoskeletal injury or disease. Another physician who specializes in treating joint disease is a **rheumatologist.** Still another physician, a **Doctor of Osteopathy (DO),** maintains that good health requires proper alignment of bones, muscles, ligaments, and nerves. Like medical doctors, osteopathic physicians combine manipulative procedures with state-of-the-art methods of medical treatment, including prescribing drugs and performing surgeries. The osteopathic physician has the same rights, privileges, and responsibilities as the Doctor of Medicine (MD).

Fractures

A **fracture** is a break or crack in a bone. Fractures can range in severity from a simple hairline crack to the most serious type, where the end of the broken bone pierces through the flesh **(open fracture, compound fracture).** Fractures usually result from trauma but may also be caused by disease **(pathological fracture).** Imaging procedures confirm and determine the severity of fractures. Figure 10-8 on page 330 illustrates some common types of fractures.

Treatment of fractures involves restoring the bone to its normal position **(reduction).** In a **closed reduction,** the practitioner repairs the fracture without a surgical incision of the area by aligning the bone through manual manipulation or traction. Once the practitioner reduces the fracture, the bone is immobilized using a cast or sling to maintain the position of the bone until healing occurs. In an **open reduction,** realignment of the two broken ends of the bone takes place under direct observation by exposing the fracture using surgery. It is required when a bone pierces through the skin **(compound fracture),** when the practitioner cannot align the bone through closed reduction, or when the fracture extends into a joint. **Internal fixation devices,** such as screws, pins, wires, and nails, stabilize the bone to maintain alignment while healing takes place.

If the bone has a hairline or minor fracture, no repair may be necessary, except rest and refraining from doing activities that aggravate the area until it is healed. For larger fractures and pain that persists, the practitioner will immobilize the area.

Arthritis

Arthritis, a general term for many joint diseases, is an inflammation of a joint, usually accompanied by pain, swelling, and deformity. Because of their location and constant use, joints are prone to stress injuries and inflammation. The main types of arthritis are rheumatoid arthritis and osteoarthritis.

Rheumatoid arthritis (RA), a systemic disease characterized by inflammatory changes in joints and their related structures, results in crippling deformities. (See Fig. 10-9, on page 331.) This form of arthritis is caused by an autoimmune disease that destroys joint tissue. It occurs most commonly in women between ages 23 and 35 but can affect people of any age group. Flare-ups **(exacerbations)** of this disease are commonly associated with periods of increased physical or emotional stress. In addition to joint changes, adjacent muscles, bones, and skin atrophy. There is no specific cure, but **NSAIDs,** physical therapy, and orthopedic measures help treat less severe cases.

Osteoarthritis, also known as **degenerative joint disease (DJD),** is by far the most common form of arthritis. It is a progressive, degenerative disease that occurs when the protective cartilage at the end of the bones wears down. Pain and stiffness in the joints are the most common symptoms. The pain is commonly worse after exercise and when putting weight or pressure on the joint. Over time, the joints become stiffer and harder to move. There may also be a rubbing, grating, or crackling sound **(crepitation)** with movement of the joint. Nevertheless, some persons are asymptomatic, even though x-rays show the changes of osteoarthritis. Almost everyone has some symptoms by age 70, but these symptoms may be minor. The joints most commonly affected include the hands, knees, hips, and spine. There is a higher risk of DJD in younger athletes and overweight individuals of all ages. Playing sports that involve direct impact on the joint (such as tennis or football), twisting (such as basketball or soccer), and throwing also increase the risk of osteoarthritis. In osteoarthritis, new bone growth **(bone spur,** or **osteophyte)** commonly occurs

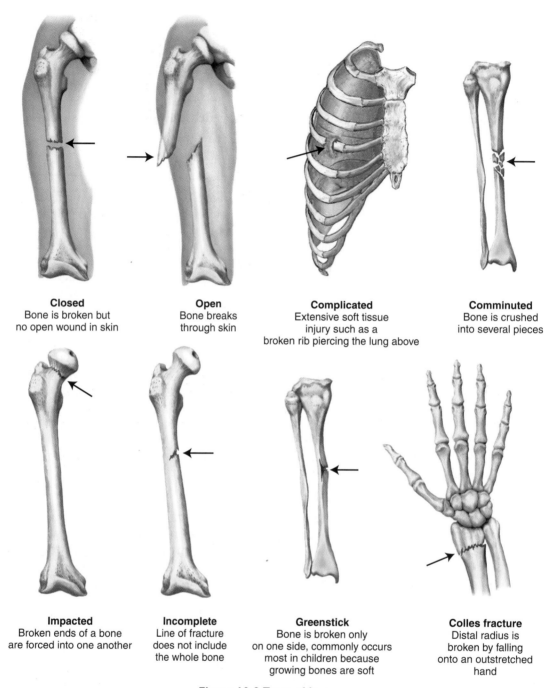

Closed
Bone is broken but
no open wound in skin

Open
Bone breaks
through skin

Complicated
Extensive soft tissue
injury such as a
broken rib piercing the lung above

Comminuted
Bone is crushed
into several pieces

Impacted
Broken ends of a bone
are forced into one another

Incomplete
Line of fracture
does not include
the whole bone

Greenstick
Bone is broken only
on one side, commonly occurs
most in children because
growing bones are soft

Colles fracture
Distal radius is
broken by falling
onto an outstretched
hand

Figure 10-8 Types of fracture.

at articular surfaces. The smallest joints at the ends of the fingers are commonly affected by spur formation that leads to the classic bony enlargement referred to as **Heberden nodes,** also known as *generalized osteoarthrosis of hand.* NSAIDs, physical therapy, and orthopedic measures are common treatments for osteoarthritis.

Muscular Dystrophy

Muscular dystrophy is a group of more than 30 inherited diseases that cause progressive weakness of skeletal muscles and loss of muscle mass. Some forms of muscular dystrophy also affect the heart muscle.

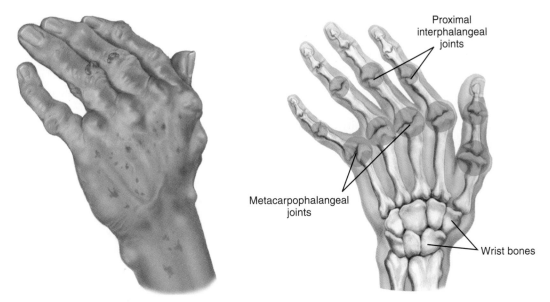

Proximal
interphalangeal
joints

Metacarpophalangeal
joints

Wrist bones

Figure 10-9 Rheumatoid arthritis.

Symptoms of the most common variety, Duchenne muscular dystrophy, begin in childhood, usually between ages 3 and 5. These symptoms occur primarily in boys and develop rapidly. By about 12 years of age, those afflicted are unable to walk. As the disease progresses, swallowing and breathing become difficult, and a respirator is required. With other types of muscular dystrophy, symptoms may not surface until adulthood.

There is no cure for muscular dystrophy. However, medications and therapy can help manage symptoms and slow the course of the disease.

Oncology

Two major types of malignancies that affect bone are those that arise directly from bone, called **primary bone cancer,** and those that arise in another region of the body and spread **(metastasize)** to bone, called **secondary bone cancer.** Primary bone cancers are rare, but secondary bone cancers are quite prevalent. They are usually caused by malignant cells that have metastasized to the bone from the lungs, breast, or prostate.

Malignancies that originate from bone, fat, muscle, cartilage, bone marrow, and cells of the lymphatic system are called **sarcomas.** Three major types of sarcomas are fibrosarcoma, osteosarcoma, and Ewing sarcoma. **Fibrosarcoma** develops in cartilage and generally affects the pelvis, upper legs, and shoulders. Patients with fibrosarcoma are usually between ages 50 and 60. **Osteosarcoma** develops from bone tissue and generally affects the knees, upper arms, and upper legs. Patients with osteosarcoma are usually between ages 20 and 25. **Ewing sarcoma** develops from primitive nerve cells in bone marrow. It usually affects the shaft of long bones but may occur in the pelvis or other bones of the arms or legs. This disease usually affects boys between ages 10 and 20.

Signs and symptoms of sarcoma include swelling and tenderness, with a tendency toward fractures in the affected area. Magnetic resonance imaging (MRI), bone scan, and a computed tomography (CT) scan are diagnostic tests that assist in identifying bone malignancies. All malignancies, including Ewing sarcoma, are staged and graded to determine the extent and degree of malignancy. This staging helps the physician determine an appropriate treatment modality. Generally, the practitioner will use combination therapy to treat sarcomas, including chemotherapy for management of metastasis and radiation when the tumor is radiosensitive. In some cases, amputation is required.

Diseases and Conditions

This section introduces diseases and conditions of the musculoskeletal system with their meanings and pronunciations. Word analyses for selected terms are also provided.

Term	Definition
bunion (hallux valgus) BŬN-yŭn (HĂL-ŭks VĂL-gŭs)	Deformity in which the great toe is angled laterally toward the other toes *A bunion may cause the tissues surrounding the joint to become swollen and tender. It is a common deformity seen in women who wear pointed-toe shoes. (See Fig. 10-10.)* **Figure 10-10** Bunion. (A) Preoperative. (B) Postoperative.
carpal tunnel syndrome (CTS) KĂR-păl	Painful condition resulting from compression of the median nerve within the carpal tunnel (wrist canal through which the flexor tendons and the median nerve pass)
claudication klăw-dĭ-KĀ-shŭn	Lameness, limping
contracture kŏn-TRĂK-chūr	Fibrosis of connective tissue in the skin, fascia, muscle, or joint capsule that prevents normal mobility of the related tissue or joint
crepitation krĕp-ĭ-TĀ-shŭn	Dry, grating sound or sensation caused by bone ends rubbing together, indicating a fracture or joint destruction
ganglion cyst GĂNG-lē-ŏn SĬST	Fluid-filled tumor that commonly develops along the tendons or joint of the wrists or hands but may also appear in the feet *In most instances, ganglion cysts cause no pain, require no treatment, and usually resolve spontaneously. Reasons for treatment are cosmetic or when the cyst causes pain or interferes with joint movement. Treatment involves removing the fluid or excising the cyst. (See Fig. 10-11.)*

Diseases and Conditions—cont'd

Term	Definition

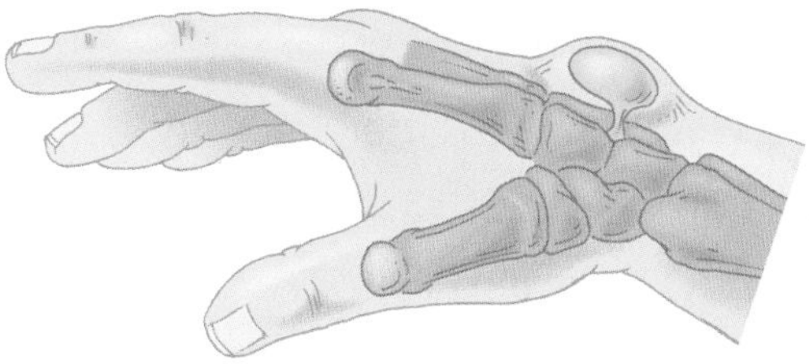

Figure 10-11 Ganglion cyst of the wrist.

gout
GOWT

Joint inflammation caused by uric acid crystal deposits in the joint space

Gout causes painful swelling and inflammation. Although the joint chiefly affected is the big toe, any joint may be involved.

herniated disk
HĔR-nē-āt-ĕd

Rupture of a vertebral disk's center (nucleus pulposus) through its outer edge, causing pain, numbness, or weakness in one or both legs; also called *slipped disc* or *herniated nucleus pulposus (HNP)* (See Fig. 10-12.)

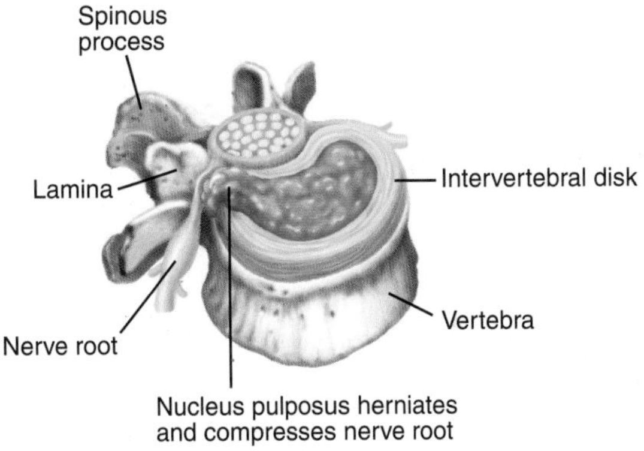

Figure 10-12 Herniated disk.

hypotonia
hī-pō-TŌ-nē-ă
hypo-: under, below, deficient
ton: tension
-ia: condition

Loss of muscle tone or a diminished resistance to passive stretching

Causes of hypotonia include genetic disorders, brain damage, muscular dystrophy, and disorders that affect nerves that supply muscles.

myasthenia gravis
mī-ăs-THĒ-nē-ă GRĂV-ĭs

Chronic, progressive disorder characterized by muscle weakness and droopiness, especially in the eyes, face, throat, and limbs

A loss of neurotransmitter receptors produces increasingly severe muscular weakness.

osteomyelitis
ŏs-tē-ō-mī-ĕ-LĪ-tĭs
oste/o: bone
myel: bone marrow, spinal cord
-itis: inflammation

Inflammation of the bone and bone marrow and the soft tissue that surrounds the bone

Osteomyelitis is generally caused by pyogenic (pus-producing) bacteria but may be the result of a viral or fungal infections. It most commonly occurs in the long bones especially, the tibia, femur, and fibula. (See Fig. 10-13.)

(continued)

Diseases and Conditions—cont'd

Term	Definition

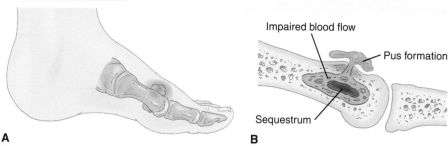

Figure 10-13 Osteomyelitis. (A) Bone infection in the toe. (B) Blocked blood flow in the area of infection, with sequestrum (bone death) and pus formation at the infection site.

osteoporosis
ŏs-tē-ō-por-Ō-sĭs
oste/o: bone
-porosis: porous

Loss of calcium and bone tissue, causing the bones to become porous, brittle, and easily fractured; most commonly seen in postmenopausal women

Prevention and treatment include calcium and vitamin D supplements, exercise, and osteoporosis medications.

Paget disease

Chronic inflammation of bones, resulting in thickening and softening of bones, that can occur in any bone but most commonly affects the long bones of the legs, the lower spine, the pelvis, and the skull

Paget disease is most common in middle-aged and elderly adults and is also called osteitis deformans.

phantom limb
FĂN-tŭm

Perceived sensation, following amputation of a limb, that the limb still exists

The sensation that pain exists in the removed part is known as phantom limb pain.

rickets
RĬK-ĕts

Form of osteomalacia in children caused by vitamin D deficiency; also called *rachitis*

spinal curvatures

Any persistent, abnormal deviation of the vertebral column from its normal position that causes an abnormal spinal curvature (See Fig. 10-14.)

scoliosis
skō-lē-Ō-sĭs
scoli/o: crooked, bent
-osis: abnormal condition, increase (used primarily with blood cells)

Abnormal lateral curvature of the spine, either to the right or left; also called *C-shaped curvature*

Scoliosis may be congenital, caused by chronic poor posture during childhood, or the result of one leg being longer than the other. Untreated scoliosis may result in pulmonary insufficiency, back pain, sciatica, disk disease, or degenerative arthritis.

kyphosis
kī-FŌ-sĭs
kyph/o: humpback
-osis: abnormal condition, increase (used primarily with blood cells)

Abnormal curvature of the upper portion of the spine; also known as *humpback* or *hunchback*

Kyphosis may be caused by rheumatoid arthritis, rickets, poor posture, or chronic respiratory disease. Treatment consists of spine-stretching exercises and wearing a brace to straighten the kyphotic curve.

lordosis
lor-DŌ-sĭs
lord/o: curve, swayback
-osis: abnormal condition, increase (used primarily with blood cells)

Abnormal, inward curvature of a portion of the lower part of the spine; also known as *swayback*

Lordosis may be caused by obesity or excessive weight gain during pregnancy. Kyphosis and lordosis can also occur in combination with scoliosis.

Diseases and Conditions—cont'd

Term	Definition

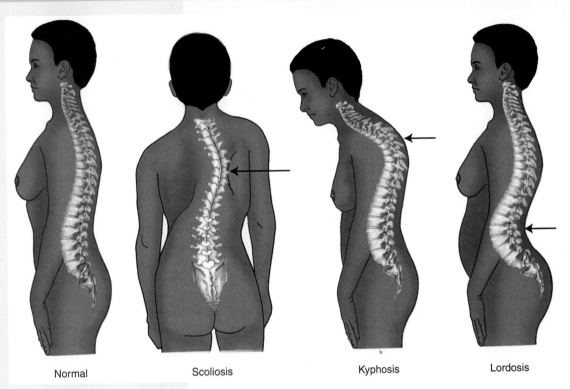

Normal   Scoliosis   Kyphosis   Lordosis

Figure 10-14 Spinal curvatures.

spondylolisthesis
spŏn-dĭ-lō-lĭs-THĒ-sĭs
spondyl/o: vertebrae (backbone)
-listhesis: slipping

Any slipping (subluxation) of a vertebra from its normal position in relationship to the one beneath it

spondylosis
spŏn-dĭ-LŌ-sĭs
spondyl: vertebrae (backbone)
-osis: abnormal condition; increase (used primarily with blood cells)

Degeneration of the cervical, thoracic, and lumbar vertebrae and related tissues

Spondylosis may cause pressure on nerve roots with subsequent pain or paresthesia in the extremities.

sprain and strain

Overstretching or tearing of ligaments (sprain) or muscle or tendon (strain)

The most common site of sprain is the ankles. The most common sites of strain are the lower back and the hamstring muscle in the back of the thigh. Initial treatment for sprains and strains includes rest, ice, compression, and elevation. Successful treatment for mild sprains and strains can occur at home. Severe sprains and strains sometimes require surgery to repair torn ligaments, muscles, or tendons.

(continued)

Diseases and Conditions—cont'd

Term	Definition
subluxation sŭb-lŭk-SĀ-shŭn	Partial or incomplete dislocation of one or more vertebrae
talipes equinovarus TĂL-ĭ-pēz ē-kwī-nō-VĀ-rŭs	Congenital deformity of one or both feet in which the foot is pulled downward and laterally to the side; also called *clubfoot* (See Fig. 10-15.) *In talipes, the heel never rests on the ground. Treatment consists of applying casts to progressively straighten the foot and surgical correction for severe cases.*

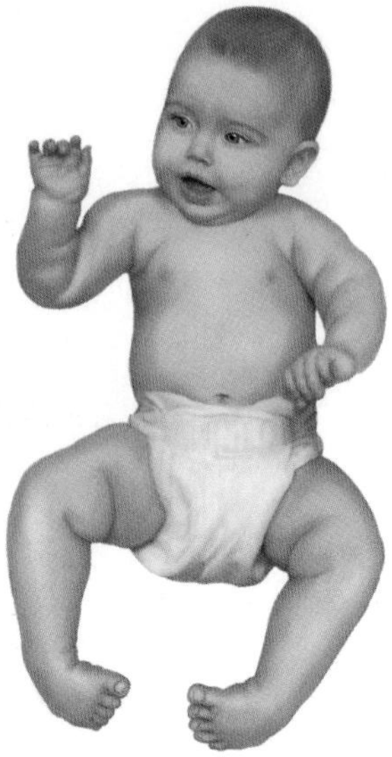

Figure 10-15 Talipes equinovarus.

It is time to review pathology, diseases, and conditions by completing Learning Activity 10-3.

Diagnostic, Surgical, and Therapeutic Procedures

This section introduces diagnostic, surgical, and therapeutic procedures used to diagnose and treat musculoskeletal disorders. Descriptions are provided, along with pronunciations and word analyses for selected terms.

Procedure	Description
Diagnostic	
Imaging	
arthrography ăr-THRŎG-ră-fē *arthr/o:* joint *-graphy:* process of recording	Series of radiographs taken after injection of contrast material into a joint cavity, especially the knee or shoulder, to outline the contour of the joint
bone density test (bone densitometry)	Noninvasive procedure that uses low-energy x-ray absorption to measure bone mineral density (BMD) and usually measures bones of the spine, hip, and forearm; also called *dual-energy x-ray absorptiometry (DEXA)* *Areas of decreased density indicate osteopenia and osteoporosis.*
discography dĭs-KŎG-ră-fē	Radiological examination of the intervertebral disk structures with injection of a contrast medium *Discography helps diagnose suspected cases of herniated disk.*
lumbosacral spinal radiography LŬM-bō-sā-krăl SPĪ-năl rā-dē-ŎG-ră-fē *lumb/o:* loins (lower back) *sacr:* sacrum *-al:* pertaining to, relating to *radi/o:* radiation, x-ray; radius (lower arm bone on thumb side) *-graphy:* process of recording	Radiography of the five lumbar vertebrae and the fused sacral vertebrae, including anteroposterior, lateral, and oblique views of the lower spine *The most common indication for lumbosacral (LS) spinal radiography is lower back pain. It helps identify or differentiate traumatic fractures, spondylosis, spondylolisthesis, and metastatic tumor.*
myelography mī-ĕ-LŎG-ră-fē *myel/o:* bone marrow; spinal cord *-graphy:* process of recording	Radiography of the spinal cord after injection of a contrast medium to identify and study spinal distortions caused by tumors, cysts, herniated intervertebral disks, or other lesions
bone scintigraphy sĭn-TĬG-ră-fē	Nuclear medicine procedure that involves intravenous injection of a radionuclide taken up into the bone *Bone scintigraphy helps detect bone disorders, especially arthritis, fractures, osteomyelitis, bone cancers, or areas of bony metastases.*
Surgical	
amputation ăm-pŭ-TĀ-shŭn	Partial or complete removal of an extremity as a result of disease, trauma, or a circulatory disorder *After removal of the extremity, the surgeon cuts a shaped flap from muscle and cutaneous tissue to cover the end of the bone and provide cushion and support for a prosthesis.*

(continued)

Diagnostic, Surgical, and Therapeutic Procedures—cont'd

Procedure	Description
arthrocentesis ăr-thrō-sĕn-TĒ-sĭs *arthr/o:* joint *-centesis:* surgical puncture	Puncture of a joint space using a needle to remove accumulated fluid or inject medications
arthroclasia ăr-thrō-KLĀ-zē-ă *arthr/o:* joint *-clasia:* to break; surgical fracture	Surgical breaking of an ankylosed joint to provide movement
arthroscopy ăr-THRŎS-kō-pē *arthr/o:* joint *-scopy:* visual examination	Visual examination of the interior of a joint and its structures using a thin, flexible fiberoptic scope called an *arthroscope* (See Fig. 10-16.) *The surgeon may insert other instruments through the arthroscope to scrape or cut damaged cartilage, excise tumors, remove fluid, and obtain biopsies.*

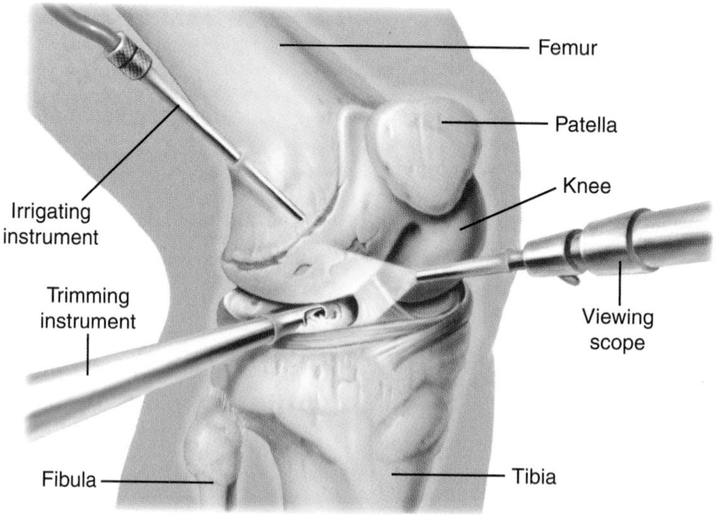

Figure 10-16 Arthroscopy (lateral view).

Procedure	Description
bone grafting GRĂFT-ĭng	Implantation or transplantation of bone tissue from another part of the body or from another person to serve as replacement for damaged or missing bone tissue
bursectomy bĕr-SĔK-tō-mē	Excision of a bursa (padlike sac or cavity found in connective tissue, usually in the vicinity of joints) *Bursectomy is commonly performed to treat chronic bursitis.*
laminectomy lăm-ĭ-NĔK-tō-mē *lamin:* lamina (part of vertebral arch) *-ectomy:* excision, removal	Excision of the posterior arch of a vertebra *Laminectomy is most commonly performed to relieve the symptoms of a ruptured (slipped) intervertebral disk.*
sequestrectomy sē-kwĕs-TRĔK-tō-mē *sequester:* separation *-ectomy:* excision, removal	Excision of a sequestrum (segment of necrosed bone)

Diagnostic, Surgical, and Therapeutic Procedures—cont'd

Procedure	Description
total hip replacement (THR)	Surgical procedure to replace a hip joint damaged by a degenerative disease, commonly arthritis (See Fig. 10-17.)
	In THR, the femoral head and the acetabulum are replaced with a metal ball and stem (prosthesis). The stem is anchored into the central core of the femur to achieve a secure fit.

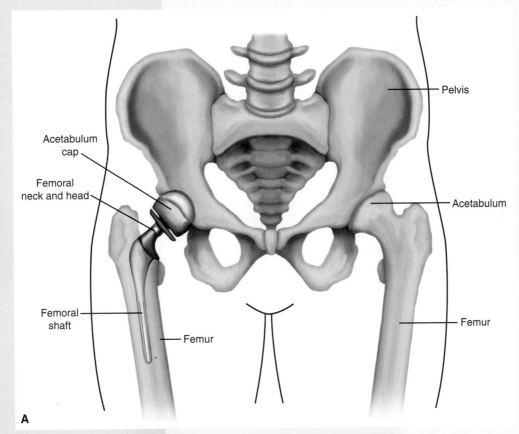

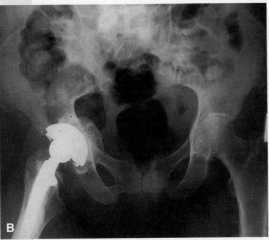

Figure 10-17 Total hip replacement. (A) Right total hip replacement. (B) Radiograph showing total hip replacement of an arthritic hip. From McKinnis: *Fundamentals of Musculoskeletal Imaging,* 2nd ed. F.A. Davis, Philadelphia, 2005, p. 314, with permission.

(continued)

Diagnostic, Surgical, and Therapeutic Procedures—cont'd

Procedure	Description
Therapeutic	
bone immobilization	Procedure used to restrict movement, stabilize and protect a fracture, and facilitate the healing process
casting	Bone immobilization by application of a solid, stiff dressing formed with plaster of Paris or similar material
splinting	Bone immobilization by application of an orthopedic device to the injured body part
	A splint is constructed from wood, metal, or plaster of Paris and may be moveable or immovable.
traction	Set of mechanisms for straightening broken bones or relieving pressure on the spine and skeletal system

Pharmacology

Unlike other medications that treat specific diseases, most pharmacological agents for musculoskeletal disorders treat symptoms. (See Table 10-3.) Analgesics and antiinflammatory drugs help treat acute musculoskeletal conditions, such as strains and sprains. NSAIDs, salicylates, muscle relaxants, opioid analgesics, and narcotics commonly treat pain by anesthetizing (numbing) the area or decreasing the inflammation. NSAIDs, gold salts, and salicylates treat arthritis. Calcium supplements treat hypocalcemia.

Table 10-3 Drugs Used to Treat Musculoskeletal Disorders

This table lists common drug classifications used to treat musculoskeletal disorders, their therapeutic actions, and selected generic and trade names.

Classification	Therapeutic Action	Generic and *Trade* Names
bone resorption inhibitors	Prevent bone loss and strengthen bone affected by osteoporosis by inhibiting bone resorption and prevent fractures associated with osteoporosis	**alendronate** ăh-LĔN-drō-nāt *Fosamax* **risedronate** rīz-ĔD-rō-nāt *Actonel*
calcium supplements KĂL-sē-ŭm	Treat and prevent hypocalcemia *Over-the-counter calcium supplements are numerous and contained in many antacids to provide a secondary therapeutic effect. They help prevent osteoporosis when the normal diet is lacking adequate amounts of calcium.*	**calcium carbonate** KĂL-sē-ŭm KĂR-bŏn-āt *Calci-Mix, Tums* **calcium citrate** KĂL-sē-ŭm SĬT-rāt *Cal-Citrate 250, Citracal*
disease modifying antirheumatic drugs (DMARDs)	Slow progression of joint destruction in arthritis by inhibiting a substance that triggers inflammation *DMARDs help treat rheumatoid arthritis, psoriatic arthritis, and inflammatory diseases of the bowel, such as Crohn disease and ulcerative colitis.*	**adalimumab** ā-dăh-LĬM-yū-măb *Humira* **methotrexate** mĕth-ōh-TRĔKS-āt
muscle relaxants	Relieve muscle spasms and stiffness *Muscle relaxants also help treat muscle spasms resulting from multiple sclerosis, spinal cord injury, cerebral palsy, and stroke.*	**cyclobenzaprine** sī-klō-BĔN-ză-prēn *Flexeril* **methocarbamol and aspirin** mĕth-ō-KĂR-bă-mōl *Robaxin*
nonsteroidal antiinflammatory drugs (NSAIDs) nŏn-STĒR-oyd-ăl ăn-tē-ĭn-FLĂM-ă-tō-rē	Decrease pain and suppress inflammation *NSAIDs help treat acute musculoskeletal conditions, such as sprains and strains, and inflammatory disorders, including rheumatoid arthritis, osteoarthritis, bursitis, gout, and tendinitis.*	**ibuprofen** ī-bū-PRŌ-fĕn *Advil, Motrin* **naproxen** nă-PRŎK-sĕn *Aleve, Naprosyn*
salicylates săl-ĬS-ĭl-ātz	Relieve mild to moderate pain and reduce inflammation *Salicylates have antiinflammatory abilities and alleviate pain. Aspirin (acetylsalicylic acid) is the oldest drug in this classification that is used to treat arthritis.*	**aspirin** ĂS-pĕr-ĭn *Acuprin, Aspergum, Bayer Aspirin* **magnesium salicylate** măg-NĒ-zē-ŭm să-LĬS-ĭ-lāt *Magan, Mobidin*
vitamin D analogs	Fat-soluble vitamins that facilitate the absorption and utilization of calcium to improve bone strength and structure. *Vitamin D is commonly found in combination with calcium.*	**cholecalciferol (vitamin D3)** kōl-ĕ-kăl-SĬ-fĕr-ōl *Maximum D3* **ergocalciferol (vitamin D$_2$)** ĕr-gō-kăl SĬ-fĕr-ōl *Drisdol*

Abbreviations

This section introduces musculoskeletal-related abbreviations and their meanings.

Abbreviation	Meaning	Abbreviation	Meaning
ACL	anterior cruciate ligament	IV	intravenous
BMD	bone mineral density	L1, L2, and so on	first lumbar vertebra, second lumbar vertebra, and so on
C1, C2, and so on	first cervical vertebra, second cervical vertebra, and so on	MD	Doctor of Medicine
CTS	carpal tunnel syndrome	MRI	magnetic resonance imaging
DEXA, DXA	dual-energy x-ray absorptiometry	NSAIDs	nonsteroidal antiinflammatory drugs
DJD	degenerative joint disease	PCL	posterior cruciate ligament
DMARDs	disease modifying antirheumatic drugs	RA	rheumatoid arthritis; right atrium
DO, D. O.	Doctor of Osteopathy	THR	total hip replacement
HNP	herniated nucleus pulposus (herniated disk)	TRAM	transverse rectus abdominis muscle

It is time to review procedures, pharmacology, and abbreviations by completing Learning Activity 10-5.

LEARNING ACTIVITIES

The activities that follow provide a review of the musculoskeletal system terms introduced in this chapter. Complete each activity and review your answers to evaluate your understanding of the chapter.

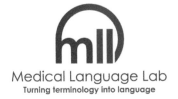

Medical Language Lab
Turning terminology into language

Visit the Medical Language Lab at *medicallanguagelab.com*. Use it to enhance your study and reinforcement of this chapter with the flash-card activity. We recommend that you complete the flash-card activity before starting Learning Activities 10-1 and 10-2.

Learning Activity 10-1
Medical Word Elements

Use the listed elements to build medical words. You may use elements more than once.

Combining Forms		Suffixes		Prefixes
ankyl/o	fasci/o	-algia	-osis	a-
arthr/o	leiomy/o	-ar	-pathy	
cephal/o	oste/o	-clast	-plasty	
chondr/o	patell/o	-desis	-tome	
crani/o		-itis	-tomy	
dactyl/o		-malacia	-trophy	
		-oma		

 1. without nourishment or development _____

 2. tumor of smooth muscle _____

 3. inflammation of bone _____

 4. pertaining to the patella (knee cap) _____

 5. softening of cartilage _____

 6. binding or fixation of a joint _____

 7. abnormal condition of (being) bent or crooked _____

 8. instrument to incise (cut) the skull _____

 9. incision of bone _____

10. inflammation of a joint _____

11. inflammation of fingers or toes _____

12. cell that breaks down bone _____

13. headache _____

14. tumor of cartilage _____

15. surgical repair of the fascia _____

Check your answers in Appendix A. Review any material that you did not answer correctly.

Correct Answers _____ X 6.67 = _____ % Score

Learning Activity 10-2
Building Medical Words

Use *oste/o* (bone) to build words that mean

1. bone cells _____
2. pain in bones _____
3. disease of bones and joints _____
4. beginning or formation of bones _____

Use *cervic/o* (neck) to build words that mean

5. pertaining to the neck _____
6. pertaining to the neck and arm _____
7. pertaining to the neck and face _____

Use *myel/o* (bone marrow; spinal cord) to build words that mean

8. tumor of bone marrow _____
9. sarcoma of bone marrow (cells) _____
10. bone marrow cell _____
11. resembling bone marrow _____

Use *stern/o* (sternum) to build words that mean

12. pertaining to above the sternum _____
13. resembling the breastbone _____

Use *arthr/o* (joint) or *chondr/o* (cartilage) to build words that mean

14. embryonic cell that forms cartilage _____
15. inflammation of a joint _____
16. inflammation of bones and joints _____

Use *pelv/i* (pelvis) to build a word that means

17. instrument for measuring the pelvis _____

Use *my/o* (muscle) to build words that mean

18. twitching of a muscle _____
19. any disease of muscle _____
20. rupture of a muscle _____

Build surgical words that mean

21. excision of one or more of the phalanges (bones of a finger or toe) _____

22. incision of the thorax (chest wall) _____

23. excision of a vertebra _____

24. binding of a joint _____

25. repair of muscle (tissue) _____

✓ *Check your answers in Appendix A. Review material that you did not answer correctly.*

Correct Answers _____ X 4 = _____ % Score

Learning Activity 10-3

Diseases and Conditions

Match the terms with the definitions in the numbered list.

ankylosis	ganglion cyst	myasthenia gravis	scoliosis
bunion	gout	necrosis	sequestrum
carpal tunnel	greenstick fracture	osteoporosis	spondylitis
chondrosarcoma	hypotonia	phantom limb	spondylolisthesis
claudication	kyphosis	pyogenic	subluxation
comminuted fracture	muscular dystrophy	rickets	talipes
Ewing			

1. incomplete or partial dislocation _____
2. softening of the bones caused by vitamin D deficiency _____
3. slipped vertebrae _____
4. limping _____
5. disease causing degeneration of muscles _____
6. congenital deformity of the foot, which is twisted out of shape or position _____
7. part of necrosed bone that has become separated from surrounding tissue _____
8. neuromuscular disorder characterized by weakness _____
9. painful condition caused by compression of the median nerve within the wrist canal _____
10. joint capsule tumor, commonly found in the wrist _____
11. loss of muscular tonicity; diminished resistance of muscles to passive stretching _____
12. type of sarcoma that attacks the shafts rather than the ends of long bones _____
13. bone that is partially bent and partially broken and occurs in children _____
14. exaggeration of the thoracic curve of the vertebral column; humpback _____
15. disease caused by a decrease in bone density that occurs in the elderly _____
16. deviation of the spine to the right or left _____
17. cartilaginous sarcoma _____
18. describes a bone that has splintered into pieces _____
19. inflammation of the vertebrae _____
20. accumulation of uric acid, usually in the big toe _____
21. lateral deviation of the great toe as it turns in toward the second toe (angulation), which may cause the surrounding joint to become swollen _____
22. pertaining to formation of pus _____
23. death of cells, tissues, or organs _____
24. stiffening and immobility of a joint _____
25. perceived sensation, following amputation, that the limb still exists _____

✔ *Check your answers in Appendix A. Review material that you did not answer correctly.*

Correct Answers _____ X 4 = _____ % Score

Learning Activity 10-4

Procedures, Pharmacology, and Abbreviations

Match the terms with the definitions in the numbered list.

amputation	closed reduction	myelography
arthrodesis	CTS	open reduction
arthrography	discography	relaxants
arthroscopy	HNP	salicylates
bone scintigraphy	laminectomy	sequestrectomy

1. imaging of the spinal cord after injection of a contrast medium _____
2. surgery to place fractured bones in normal position _____
3. imaging of intervertebral disk(s) after injection of a contrast medium _____
4. painful disorder of the wrist due to compression of the median nerve _____
5. excision of the posterior arch of a vertebra _____
6. imaging of a joint after injection of a radiopaque substance or air cavity _____
7. surgical binding or immobilizing of a joint _____
8. partial or complete removal of a limb _____
9. herniated nucleus pulposus _____
10. relieve mild to moderate pain and reduce inflammation _____
11. visual examination of a joint's interior, especially the knee _____
12. excising a segment of necrosed bone _____
13. nuclear procedure in which the radionuclide is injected intravenously to detect arthritis _____
14. relieve muscle spasms and stiffness _____
15. manipulative treatment to realign bone fractures _____

✓ *Check your answers in Appendix A. Review material that you did not answer correctly.*

Correct Answers _____ X 6.67 = _____ % Score

DOCUMENTING HEALTH-CARE ACTIVITIES

This section provides practical application activities in the form of exercises to help students develop skills in documenting patient care. First, read the medical report. Then complete the activities and exercises that follow.

Documenting Health-Care Activity 10-1

Operative Report: Right Knee Arthroscopy and Medial Meniscectomy

---

General Hospital

1511 Ninth Avenue ■ ■ Sun City, USA 12345 ■ ■ (555) 802–1887

OPERATIVE REPORT

Date: August 14, 20xx   Physician: Robert L. Mead, MD
Patient: Jay, Elizabeth   Patient ID#: 20798

PREOPERATIVE DIAGNOSIS: Tear, medial meniscus, right knee

POSTOPERATIVE DIAGNOSIS: Tear, medial meniscus, right knee.

CLINICAL HISTORY: This 42-year-old woman has jogged an average of 25 miles each week for the past 10 years. She has persistent posteromedial right knee pain with occasional effusions. The patient has an MRI-documented medial meniscal tear.

PROCEDURE: Right knee arthroscopy and medial meniscectomy

ANESTHESIA: General

COMPLICATIONS: None

OPERATIVE SUMMARY: Examination of the knee under anesthesia showed a full range of motion, no effusion, no instability, and negative Lachman and negative McMurray sign tests. Arthroscopic evaluation showed a normal patellofemoral groove and normal intracondylar notch with normal ACL and PCL, some anterior synovitis, and a normal lateral meniscus and lateral compartment to the knee. The medial compartment of the knee showed an inferior surface, posterior and midmedial meniscal tear that was flipped up on top of itself. This was resected, and then the remaining meniscus was contoured back to a stable rim. A sterile dressing was applied.

Patient was taken to the postanesthesia care unit in stable condition.

Robert L. Mead, MD
Robert L. Mead, MD

rlm:bg

D: 8–14–20xx; T: 8–14–20xx

Terminology

The terms listed in the table that follows are taken from *Operative Report: Right Knee Arthroscopy and Medial Meniscectomy.* Use a medical dictionary such as *Taber's Cyclopedic Medical Dictionary,* the appendices of this book, or other resources to define each term. Then review the pronunciation for each term and practice by reading the medical record aloud.

Term	Definition
ACL	
arthroscopy ăr-THRŎS-kō-pē	
effusions ĕ-FŪ-zh ŭnz	
intracondylar ĭn-tră-KŎN-dĭ-lăr	
Lachman test	
McMurray sign test	
meniscectomy mĕn-ĭ-SĔK-tō-mē	
MRI	
PCL	
synovitis sĭn-ō-VĪ-tĭs	

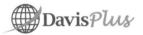

Visit the *Medical Terminology Systems* online resource center at Davis*Plus* to practice pronunciation and reinforce the meanings of the terms in this medical report.

Critical Thinking

Review *Operative Report: Right Knee Arthroscopy and Medial Meniscectomy* to answer the questions.

1. Describe the meniscus and identify its location.

_____

_____

_____

_____

2. What is the probable cause of the tear in the patient's meniscus?

_____

_____

_____

_____

3. What does normal ACL and PCL refer to in the report?

_____

_____

_____

_____

4. Explain the McMurray sign test.

_____

_____

_____

_____

5. Why was the surgery performed even though the Lachman and McMurray tests were negative (normal)?

_____

_____

_____

_____

Radiographic Consultation: Tibial Diaphysis Nuclear Scan

Physician Center

2422 Rodeo Drive ■ ■ **Sun City, USA 12345** ■ ■ **(555)333–2427**

September 3, 20xx

Grant Hammuda, MD
1115 Forest Ave
Sun City, USA 12345

Dear Doctor Hammuda:

We are pleased to provide the following in response to your request for consultation.

This is an 18-year-old male cross-country runner. He complains of pain of more than 1 month's duration with persistent symptoms over the middle one-third of his left tibia with resting. He finds no relief with NSAIDs.

Findings: Nuclear scan reveals the following: There is focal increased blood flow, blood pool, and delayed radiotracer accumulation within the left mid posterior tibial diaphysis. The delayed spot planar images demonstrate focal fusiform uptake involving 50%–75% of the tibial diaphysis width.

It is our opinion that with continued excessive, repetitive stress, the rate of resorption will exceed the rate of bone replacement. This will lead to weakened cortical bone with buttressing by periosteal and endosteal new bone deposition. If resorption continues to exceed replacement, a stress fracture will occur.

Please let me know if I can be of any further assistance.

Sincerely yours,

Adrian Jones, MD
Adrian Jones, MD

aj:bg

Terminology

The terms listed in the table that follows are taken from *Radiographic Consultation: Tibial Diaphysis Nuclear Scan.* Use a medical dictionary such as *Taber's Cyclopedic Medical Dictionary,* the appendices of this book, or other resources to define each term. Then review the pronunciation for each term and practice by reading the medical record aloud.

Term	Definition
buttressing BŬ-trĕs-ĭng	
cortical KOR-tĭ-kăl	
diaphysis dī-ĂF-ĭ-sĭs	
endosteal ĕn-DŎS-tē-ăl	
focal FŌ-kăl	
fusiform FŬ-zĭ-form	
NSAIDs	
nuclear scan NŪ-klē-ăr	
periosteal pĕr-ē-ŎS-tē-ăl	
resorption rē-SORP-shŭn	
tibial TĬB-ē-ăl	

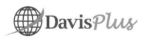 Visit the *Medical Terminology Systems* online resource center at Davis*Plus* to practice pronunciation and reinforce the meanings of the terms in this medical report.

Critical Thinking

Review the medical record *Radiographic Consultation: Tibial Diaphysis Nuclear Scan* to answer the questions.

1. Where was the pain located?

2. What medication was the patient taking for pain, and did it provide relief?

3. How was the blood flow to the affected area described by the radiologist?

4. How was the radiotracer accumulation described?

5. What will be the probable outcome with continued excessive and repetitive stress?

6. What will happen if resorption continues to exceed replacement?

_____

_____

_____

_____

Constructing Chart Notes

To construct chart notes, replace the italicized and boldfaced terms in each of the two scenarios with one of the listed medical terms.

clavicle	*open fracture*	*osteoporosis*
comminuted	*orthopedist*	*pathological fractures*
femur	*osteopenia*	*spondylalgia*
kyphosis		

Mr. L., a 30-year-old male, was brought to the ED following a head-on car collision. X-rays revealed a minor (1) *splintered* fracture of the right (2) *collarbone*. The more serious injury was a (3) *broken bone protruding through the skin surface* with laceration of the surrounding soft tissue of the right thigh. Mr. L. was immediately prepped for a surgical reduction of the right (4) *thigh bone*. Dr. Michaels, the (5) *specialist in treating bone disorders*, will undertake management of this patient.

1. _____
2. _____
3. _____
4. _____
5. _____

Mrs. P.'s previous surgical history shows an appendectomy at age 10 and a hysterectomy with the removal of the ovaries and fallopian tubes at age 35. She has a history of (6) *a decrease in bone minerals*. She is stooped over with a prominent (7) *humpback* and complains of (8) *pain in the vertebrae*. The results of her DEXA scan show (9) *porous bones*. She is at risk for (10) *bone fractures related to disease*.

6. _____
7. _____
8. _____
9. _____
10. _____

Check your answers in Appendix A. Review any material that you did not answer correctly.

Correct Answers _____ X 10 = _____ % Score

Urinary System

Objectives

Upon completion of this chapter, you will be able to:

- Locate and describe urinary structures.
- Describe the functional relationship between the urinary system and other body systems.
- Pronounce, spell, and build words related to the urinary system.
- Describe diseases, conditions, and procedures related to the urinary system.
- Explain pharmacology related to the treatment of urinary disorders.
- Demonstrate your knowledge of this chapter by completing the learning and documenting health-care activities.

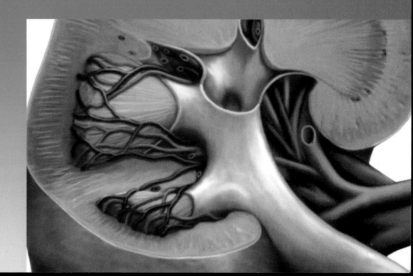

Anatomy and Physiology

The urinary system consists of two kidneys, two ureters, the urinary bladder, and the urethra. The kidneys carry out the major work of the urinary system, and the other structures are mainly passageways and storage areas. The primary function of the urinary system is regulation of the extracellular fluids of the body (primarily plasma and tissue fluid). The kidneys remove waste products from plasma as they form urine. Urine, containing waste products, passes from the kidneys via the ureters to the urinary bladder for temporary storage before it is excreted from the body through the urethra.

Anatomy and Physiology Key Terms

This section introduces important urinary system terms and their definitions. The key terms are highlighted in color in the Anatomy and Physiology section. Word analyses for selected terms are also provided. Pronounce the term, and place a check mark in the box after you do so.

Term	Definition
electrolyte ē-LĔK-trō-līt ☐	Mineral salt of the body that carries an electrical charge and regulates nerve impulses, muscle contraction, hydration, and blood pH *The major electrolytes of the body include sodium, chloride, potassium, magnesium, calcium, phosphate, and bicarbonate.*
filtrate FĬL-trāt ☐	Fluid that passes from the blood through the capillary walls of the glomeruli into Bowman capsule *Filtrate is similar to plasma but with less protein. Urine is formed from filtrate.*
nitrogenous waste nī-TRŎJ-ĕn-ŭs ☐	Product of protein metabolism that includes urea, uric acid, creatine, creatinine, and ammonia
peristaltic wave pĕr-ĭ-STĂL-tĭk ☐	Sequence of rhythmic contraction of smooth muscles of a hollow organ to force material forward and prevent backflow
peritoneum pĕr-ĭ-tō-NĒ-ŭm ☐	Serous membrane that lines the abdominopelvic cavity and covers most of the organs within the cavity
pH	Symbol that expresses the alkalinity or acidity of a solution *A solution with a pH of 7.0 is neutral, greater than 7.0 is alkaline, and less than 7.0 is acidic.*
plasma PLĂZ-mă ☐	Liquid portion of blood that is filtered by the nephrons to remove dissolved wastes

Pronunciation Help	Long Sound	ā — rate	ē — rebirth	ī — isle	ō — over	ū — unite
	Short Sound	ă — apple	ĕ — ever	ĭ — it	ŏ — not	ŭ — cut

Macroscopic Structures

The macroscopic structures that make up the urinary system include two kidneys, two ureters, a bladder, and a urethra. (See Fig. 11-1.) They regulate the composition of extracellular fluids (blood and tissue fluid) by removing harmful products from the body—especially **nitrogenous wastes** and excess **electrolytes**—while retaining beneficial products required by the body.

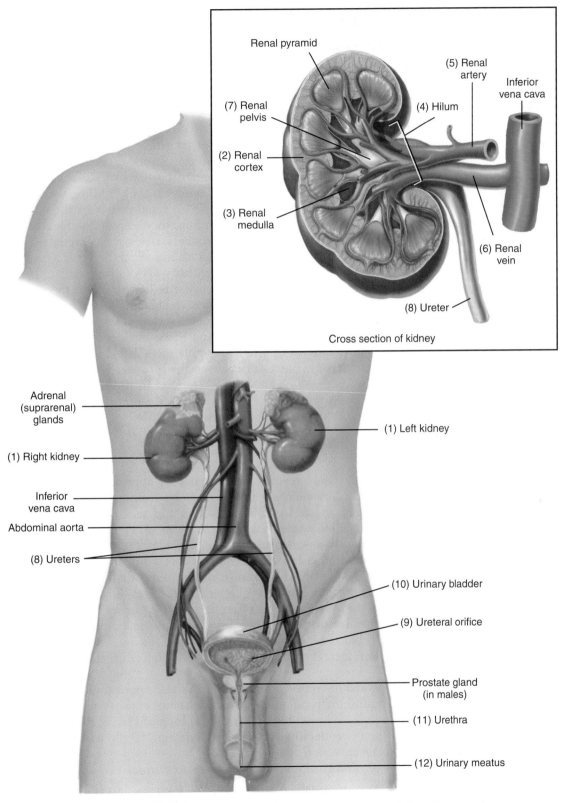

Renal pyramid

(5) Renal artery

Inferior vena cava

(7) Renal pelvis

(4) Hilum

(2) Renal cortex

(3) Renal medulla

(6) Renal vein

(8) Ureter

Cross section of kidney

Adrenal (suprarenal) glands

(1) Left kidney

(1) Right kidney

Inferior vena cava

Abdominal aorta

(8) Ureters

(10) Urinary bladder

(9) Ureteral orifice

Prostate gland (in males)

(11) Urethra

(12) Urinary meatus

Figure 11-1 Urinary structures, including a cross section of the kidney.

Nitrogenous products are toxic, and the kidneys must continuously eliminate them, or death will occur within a few days. Equally important is the proper balance of electrolytes, which are crucial to operation of the brain, nerves, and muscles and essential for tissue repair. Along with regulating the composition of extracellular fluids, the kidneys also secrete the hormone **erythropoietin.** This hormone acts on bone marrow to stimulate production of red blood cells when blood oxygen levels are low.

The (1) **left and right kidneys,** each about the size of a fist, are located in the abdominal cavity slightly above the waistline. The location of the kidneys is **retroperitoneal** because they are located outside of the **peritoneum.** A concave medial border gives the kidney its beanlike shape. In the cross section, two distinct areas are visible: an outer area, the (2) **renal cortex,** and a middle area, the (3) **renal medulla.** These structures contain portions of the microscopic filtering units of the kidney, the **nephrons.** Near the medial border is the (4) **hilum** (or **hilus**), an opening through which the (5) **renal artery** enters and the (6) **renal vein** exits the kidney. After the kidneys remove waste products during urine formation, the filtered blood leaves the kidney by way of the renal vein. Urine, now carrying waste products, enters the (7) **renal pelvis,** a hollow cavity formed where the (8) **ureter** merges with the kidney. Each ureter is a slender tube approximately 10″ to 12″ long. They carry urine in **peristaltic waves** to the bladder. These waves keep urine flowing toward the bladder, rather than regurgitating back into the kidney during urination when bladder pressure increases. Urine enters the bladder at the (9) **ureteral orifice.** The (10) **urinary bladder,** an expandable hollow organ, acts as a temporary reservoir for urine. The bladder has small folds called **rugae** that expand as the bladder fills. At its base, the two openings of the ureters and the urethra form a triangular area called the **trigone** that leads into the (11) **urethra,** a tube that discharges urine from the bladder. The length of the urethra is approximately 1.5″ in women and about 7″ to 8″ in men. In the male, the urethra passes through the prostate gland and the penis. During urination **(micturition),** the body expels urine through an opening in the urethra, the (12) **urinary meatus.**

Microscopic Structures

Microscopic examination of kidney tissue reveals the presence of approximately 1 million **nephrons.** These microscopic structures maintain homeostasis by continually adjusting and regulating the composition, volume, and **pH** of blood **plasma** and tissue fluid. Substances removed by nephrons include nitrogenous wastes, excess electrolytes, and many other products that exceed the amount tolerated by the body. Each nephron includes a renal corpuscle and a renal tubule. (See Fig. 11-2.) The **renal corpuscle** is composed of a tuft of capillaries called the (1) **glomerulus** and a modified, enlarged extension of the renal tubule known as the (2) **Bowman (glomerular) capsule** that surrounds the glomerulus. A larger (3) **afferent arteriole** carries blood to the glomerulus, and a smaller (4) **efferent arteriole** carries blood from the glomerulus. The difference in the size of these vessels provides the needed pressure to force fluids and soluble material from blood plasma into the Bowman capsule. These substances, now called **filtrate**, resemble plasma except that the amount of protein in filtrate is less than that found in plasma.

The efferent arteriole passes behind the renal corpuscle to form the (5) **peritubular capillaries,** a network of capillaries that surround the renal tubule. The renal tubule consists of four sections: the (6) **proximal convoluted tubule,** followed by the narrow (7) **loop of Henle,** then the larger (8) **distal tubule** and, finally, the (9) **collecting tubule.** The collecting tubule transports newly formed urine to the renal pelvis for excretion by the kidneys.

The nephron performs three physiological functions as it produces urine:

1. **Filtration** occurs in the renal corpuscle as water, electrolytes, sugar, and other small molecules in blood plasma in the afferent tubule pass into the Bowman capsule to form filtrate.

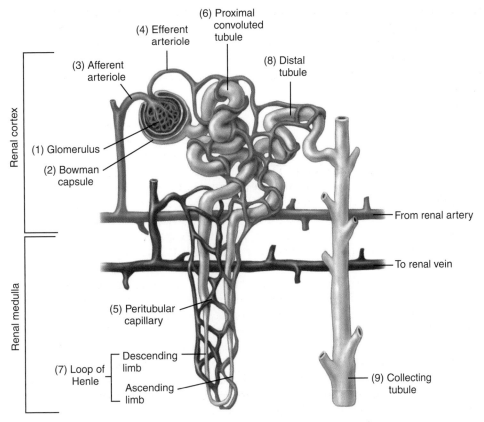

Figure 11-2 Nephron with its associated blood vessels.

2. **Reabsorption** begins as filtrate travels through the long, twisted pathway of the tubule. Most of the water and some of the electrolytes and amino acids from the tubule reenter the circulating blood through the peritubular capillaries.

3. **Secretion** is the final stage of urine formation. The peritubular capillaries actively secrete waste products, such as ammonia, uric acid, and metabolic products of medications, into the renal tubules for removal in urine.

Urine leaves the collecting tubule and enters the renal pelvis. From there, urine passes to the bladder for temporary storage until urination takes place.

Anatomy Review: Urinary Structures

Label the illustration using the listed terms.

hilum   *renal medulla*   *right kidney*   *urethra*
left kidney   *renal pelvis*   *ureteral orifice*   *urinary bladder*
renal artery   *renal vein*   *ureters*   *urinary meatus*
renal cortex

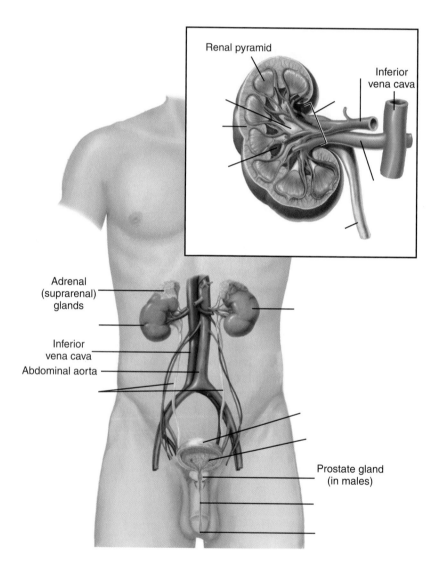

 Check your answers by referring to Figure 11-1 on page 359. Review material that you did not answer correctly.

Anatomy Review: Nephron

Label the illustration using the listed terms.

afferent arteriole   *distal tubule*   *loop of Henle*

Bowman capsule   *efferent arteriole*   *peritubular capillary*

collecting tubule   *glomerulus*   *proximal convoluted tubule*

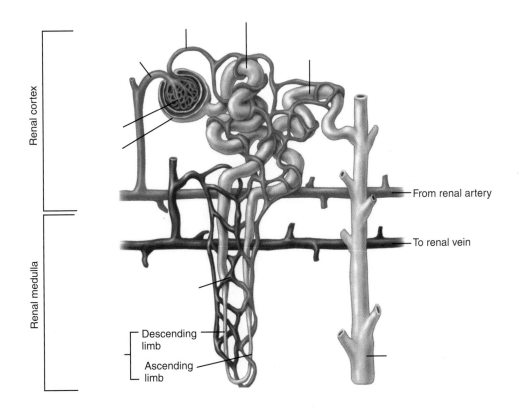

 Check your answers by referring to Figure 11-2 on page 361. Review material that you did not answer correctly.

CONNECTING BODY SYSTEMS—URINARY SYSTEM

The main function of the urinary system is to regulate extracellular fluids of the body. Specific functional relationships between the urinary system and other body systems are summarized here.

Blood, Lymphatic, and Immune

- The urinary system filters plasma, thereby regulating the composition, quantity, and quality of blood plasma and lymph.
- The urinary system retains needed products and integrates them back into plasma as it removes products that are excessive or toxic to the body.

Cardiovascular

- The urinary system helps regulate essential electrolytes needed for contraction of the heart.

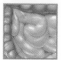

Digestive

- The urinary system aids in removing glucose from the blood when excessive amounts are consumed.
- The urinary system removes excessive fluids absorbed from the gastrointestinal (GI) tract.

Endocrine

- The urinary system regulates electrolyte and fluid balance, which is essential for hormone transport in the blood.
- The urinary system produces erythropoietin, a hormone synthesized mainly in the kidneys to stimulate bone marrow production of blood cells.

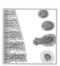

Female Reproductive

- The urinary system aids in removing waste products produced by the fetus in the pregnant woman.

Integumentary

- The urinary system compensates for extracellular fluid loss resulting from hyperhidrosis by regulating fluid loss during urine production.
- The urinary system adjusts electrolytes, especially potassium and sodium, in response to their loss through sweating.

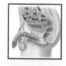

Male Reproductive

- The urinary system shares the urethra with the male reproductive system for delivery of semen to the female.

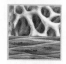

Musculoskeletal

- The urinary system works in conjunction with bone tissue to maintain a constant calcium level.

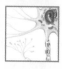

Nervous

- The urinary system regulates sodium, potassium, and calcium, which are the electrolytes responsible for the transmission of nervous stimuli.

Respiratory

- The urinary system assists the lungs in regulating the acid–base balance of the body.

Medical Word Elements

This section introduces combining forms, suffixes, and prefixes related to the urinary system. Word analyses are also provided. From the information provided, complete the meaning of the medical words in the right-hand column. The first one is completed for you.

Element	Meaning	Word Analysis
Combining Forms		
albumin/o	albumin, protein	**albumin**/oid (ăl-BBŪ-mĭ-noyd): *resembling albumin* *-oid:* resembling
azot/o	nitrogenous compounds	**azot**/emia (ăz-ō-TĒ-mē-ă): _____ *-emia:* blood condition *Azotemia results when the kidneys fail to excrete nitrogenous compounds, such as urea, creatinine, and other waste compounds containing nitrogen.*
bacteri/o	bacteria (singular, bacterium)	**bacteri**/uria (băk-tē-rē-Ū-rē-ă): _____ *-uria:* urine
cyst/o	bladder	**cyst/o**/scope (SĬST-ō-skōp): _____ *-scope:* instrument for examining
vesic/o		**vesic/o**/cele (VĔS-ĭ-kō-sēl): _____ *-cele:* hernia, swelling *With a vesicocele, also called cystocele, the bladder herniates into the vaginal wall, causing incomplete emptying of the bladder.*
glomerul/o	glomerulus	**glomerul/o**/pathy (glō-měr-ū-LŎP-ă-thē): _____ *-pathy:* disease
kal/i*	potassium (an electrolyte)	**kal/i**/ur/esis (kă-lē-ū-RĒ-sĭs): _____ *ur:* urine *-esis:* condition
keton/o	ketone bodies (acids and acetones)	**keton**/uria (kē-tō-NŪ-rē-ă): _____ *-uria:* urine *Ketonuria is commonly found in diabetes mellitus, starvation, and excessive dieting.*
lith/o	stone, calculus	**lith/o**/tripsy (LĬTH-ō-trĭp-sē): _____ *-tripsy:* crushing
meat/o	opening, meatus	**meat/o**/tomy (mē-ă-TŎT-ō-mē): _____ *-tomy:* incision *A meatotomy relieves stenosis of the urethra by enlarging the urethral opening, which may be inhibiting the proper passage of urine or semen.*

*The *i* in *kal/i* is an exception to the rule of using the connecting vowel *o*.

(continued)

Medical Word Elements—cont'd

Element	Meaning	Word Analysis
nephr/o	kidney	**nephr/o**/pexy (NĔF-rō-pĕks-ē): _____ *-pexy:* fixation (of an organ)
ren/o		**ren**/al (RĒ-năl): _____ *-al:* pertaining to
noct/o	night	**noct**/uria (nok-TŪ-rē-ă): _____ *-uria:* urine *Nocturia is associated with prostate disease, urinary tract infection, and uncontrolled diabetes.*
olig/o	scanty	**olig**/uria (ŏl-ĭg-Ū-rē-ă): _____ *-uria:* urine *Oliguria is usually caused by fluid and electrolyte imbalances, renal lesions, or urinary tract obstruction.*
py/o	pus	**py**/uria (pī-Ū-rē-ă): _____ *-uria:* urine *Pyuria is associated with bacterial infections of the urinary tract.*
pyel/o	renal pelvis	**pyel/o**/plasty (PĪ-ĕ-lō-plăs-tē): _____ *-plasty:* surgical repair
ur/o	urine, urinary tract	**ur/o**/lith (Ū-rō-lĭth): _____ *-lith:* stone, calculus
ureter/o	ureter	**ureter**/ectasis (ū-rē-tĕr-ĔK-tă-sĭs): _____ *-ectasis:* dilation, expansion
urethr/o	urethra	**urethr/o**/stenosis (ū-rē-thrō-stĕn-Ō-sĭs): _____ *-stenosis:* narrowing, stricture
Suffixes		
-genesis	forming; producing; origin	lith/o/**genesis** (lĭth-ō-JĔN-ĕ-sĭs): _____ *lith/o:* stone, calculus
-iasis	abnormal condition (produced by something specified)	lith/**iasis** (lĭth-Ī-ă-sĭs): _____ *lith/o:* stone, calculus
-uria	urine	poly/**uria** (pŏl-ē-Ū-rē-ă): _____ *poly:* many, much *Polyuria is generally considered the excretion of over 2.5 L in 24 hours.*

Medical Word Elements—cont'd

Element	Meaning	Word Analysis

Prefixes

dia- — through, across

dia/lysis (dī-ĂL-ĭ-sĭs): _____
   -lysis: separation; destruction; loosening
   Renal dialysis is a procedure that uses a membrane to separate and selectively remove waste products from the blood when the kidneys are unable to complete this function.

retro- — backward, behind

retro/peritone/al (rĕt-rō-pĕr-ĭ-tō-NĒ-ăl): _____
   peritone: peritoneum
   -al: pertaining to

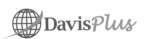 Visit the *Medical Terminology Systems* online resource center at Davis*Plus* for an audio exercise of the terms in this table. Other activities are also available to reinforce content.

 It is time to review medical word elements by completing Learning Activities 11-1 and 11-2.

Disease Focus

Causes of urinary system disorders include congenital anomalies, infectious diseases, trauma, and conditions that secondarily involve the urinary structures. Asymptomatic urinary diseases are commonly found when a routine urinalysis identifies abnormalities. When symptoms are present, they usually include changes in urination pattern, changes in output, or pain during urination **(dysuria).** Endoscopic tests, radiological evaluations, and laboratory tests that evaluate renal function typically identify disorders of the urinary system.

For diagnosis, treatment, and management of urinary disorders, the medical services of a specialist may be warranted. **Urology** is the branch of medicine concerned with urinary disorders and diseases of the male reproductive system. The physician who specializes in diagnosis and treatment of genitourinary disorders is known as a **urologist.** However, the branch of medicine concerned specifically with diseases of the kidney, electrolyte imbalance, renal transplantation, and dialysis therapy is a **nephrology.** Physicians who practice in this specialty are called **nephrologists.**

Glomerulonephritis

Glomerulonephritis is an inflammation of the glomerular membrane in the nephrons, causing it to become "leaky" **(permeable).** Red blood cells and protein, which normally remain in blood, pass through the inflamed glomerular membrane and enter the tubule. Urinalysis reveals protein in the urine **(proteinuria),** blood in the urine **(hematuria),** and bacteria in the urine **(bacteruria),** indicators of infection or inflammation. Other signs and symptoms include high blood pressure **(hypertension),** edema, and impaired renal function.

Causes of glomerulonephritis include bacterial endocarditis, viral infections, and autoimmune diseases. Another cause of glomerular inflammation is a reaction to the toxins produced by pathogenic bacteria, especially streptococci that have recently infected another part of the body, usually "strep throat." Most patients with acute glomerulonephritis associated with a streptococcal infection recover with no lasting kidney damage. Because most forms of glomerulonephritis are a consequence of another disorder, treatment of the underlying cause is important in the management of this disease.

Nephrolithiasis

Stones **(calculi)** may form in any part of the urinary tract **(urolithiasis),** but most arise in the kidney **(nephrolithiasis).** (See Fig. 11-3, page 368.) They commonly form when dissolved urine

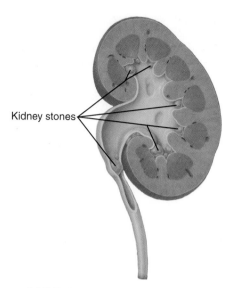

Kidney stones

Figure 11-3 Kidney stones in the calices and ureter.

salts begin to solidify. As the stones become larger, they commonly lodge in the ureters **(ureterolithiasis),** causing an intense, throbbing pain **(colic).** Because urine has difficulty passing into the bladder, it flows backward **(refluxes)** into the renal pelvis, causing it to dilate.

Treatment includes pulverizing the stone using concentrated ultrasound shock waves, generated from a machine outside the body **(extracorporeal shock-wave lithotripsy [ESWL]).** (See Fig. 11-4.) For patients who have contraindication to ESWL, an alternative minimally invasive surgery is available. In this procedure, the surgeon makes a small incision through the skin to create an opening into the kidney to remove the stone **(percutaneous nephrolithotomy [PCNL]).** If the stone is large, the surgeon breaks it into smaller fragments using an ultrasonic or electrohydraulic probe **(lithotriptor)** to remove the smaller fragments more easily. The surgeon may also insert a **nephrostomy** tube to drain urine from the kidney during the healing process.

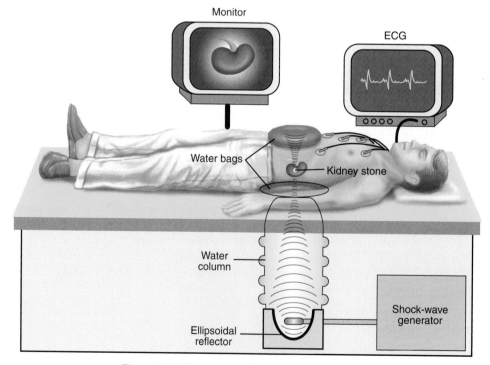

Monitor

ECG

Water bags

Kidney stone

Water column

Shock-wave generator

Ellipsoidal reflector

Figure 11-4 Extracorporeal shock-wave lithotripsy.

Acute Tubular Necrosis

In **acute tubular necrosis (ATN),** the tubular portion of the nephron is injured after the ingestion of toxic drugs **(nephrotoxic ATN)** or by a decrease in blood supply **(ischemic ATN).** Circulatory collapse, severe hypotension, hemorrhage, dehydration, or other disorders that affect blood supply are the common causes of ischemic ATN. Because specific signs and symptoms are not associated with ATN, the diagnosis relies on a positive history of risk factors. Nonspecific signs and symptoms of ATN commonly include scanty urine production **(oliguria),** fluid retention, mental apathy, nausea, vomiting, and increased blood levels of calcium **(hypercalcemia).** When tubular damage is not severe, the disorder is usually reversible.

Oncology

Bladder cancer is the fourth most common cancer in men and the eighth most common cancer in women. Two types of bladder cancer are transitional cell carcinoma and adenocarcinoma. Transitional cell carcinoma accounts for 95% of bladder cancers in the United States. Transitional cells line the bladder and the inside of the ureters and urethra. They are able to expand when the bladder is full and contract when it is empty. As bladder cancer progresses, malignant tumors invade the bladder, ureters, and urethra.

Adenocarcinoma, a less common type of bladder cancer, accounts for only 1% of bladder cancers in the United States. This malignancy arises from mucus-secreting glands in the bladder and generally tends to be invasive.

Signs and symptoms of bladder cancer include hematuria, frequency, dysuria, and abdominal or back pain. Diagnostic tests include cystoscopy with biopsy of suspicious lesions and urine cytology, in which malignant cells appear in a urine sample.

Treatment depends on the type, stage, and grade of the malignancy. In the early stages when the malignancy is confined to the bladder lining, the practitioner employs an electric current or high-energy laser using a device passed through the urethra **(transurethral resection of bladder tumor [TURBT])** to destroy malignant tissue. Advanced cancers require the removal of the bladder **(cystectomy).** Surgery combined with treatments that stimulate the immune response **(biological therapy; immunotherapy),** chemotherapy delivered intravenously or directly into the bladder **(intravesical),** and radiation therapy are other treatment options.

Diseases and Conditions

This section introduces diseases and conditions of the urinary system, along with their meanings and pronunciations. Word analyses for selected terms are also provided.

Term	Definition
anuria ăn-Ū-rē-ă *an-:* without, not *uria:* urine	Absence of urine production or output *Anuria may be obstructive, in which there is blockage proximal to the bladder, or unobstructive, which is caused by severe damage to the nephrons of the kidneys.*
bladder neck obstruction (BNO)	Blockage at the base of the bladder that reduces or prevents urine from passing into the urethra *Causes of BNO include an enlarged prostate, bladder stones, bladder tumors, and tumors in the pelvic cavity.*

(continued)

Diseases and Conditions—cont'd

Term	Definition

cystocele
SĬS-tō-sēl
cyst/o: bladder
-cele: hernia, swelling

Prolapsing or downward displacement of the bladder due to weakening of the supporting tissues between the bladder and vagina (See Fig. 11-5.)

Cystocele is commonly the result of vaginal childbirth, frequent straining with constipation, or lifting of heavy objects.

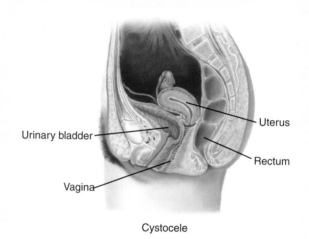

Cystocele

Figure 11-5 Cystocele.

end-stage renal disease (ESRD)
RĒ-năl
ren: kidney
-al: pertaining to

Any type of kidney disease in which there is little or no remaining kidney function, requiring the patient to undergo dialysis or kidney transplant for survival

The two most common causes of ESRD are diabetes and hypertension.

enuresis
ĕn-ū-RĒ-sĭs
en-: in, within
ur: urine
-esis: condition

Involuntary discharge of urine; also called *incontinence*

Enuresis that occurs during the night is called nocturnal enuresis; *during the day,* diurnal enuresis.

fistula
FĬS-tū-lă

Abnormal passage from a hollow organ to the surface or from one organ to another

The most common type of urinary fistula is vesicovaginal fistula, in which a passage forms between the bladder and vagina. Its causes include previous pelvic surgery, such as hysterectomy; difficult, prolonged labor; and reduced blood supply to the area.

Diseases and Conditions—cont'd

Term	Definition

hydronephrosis
hī-drō-nĕf-RŌ-sĭs
hydr/o: water
nephr: kidney
-osis: abnormal condition; increase (used primarily with blood cells)

Abnormal dilation of the renal pelvis and the calyces of one or both kidneys caused by pressure from accumulated urine that cannot flow past an obstruction in the urinary tract

The causes of hydronephrosis are enlargement of the prostate, urethral strictures, and calculi that lodge in the ureter. When dilation affects the ureter, it is called hydroureter. (See Fig. 11-6.)

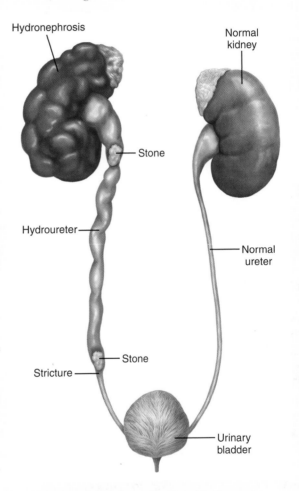

Figure 11-6 Hydronephrosis and hydroureter.

interstitial cystitis (IC)
ĭn-tĕr-STĬSH-ăl sĭs-TĪ-tĭs
cyst: bladder
-itis: inflammation

Chronic inflammation of the bladder wall that is not caused by bacterial infection and is not responsive to conventional antibiotic therapy; also called *painful bladder syndrome*

Two common symptoms include urinary frequency and bladder or pelvic pain ranging from mild to severe. Medications and physical therapy may help some patients, but other patients are unresponsive to treatment.

(continued)

Diseases and Conditions—cont'd

Term	Definition
nephrotic syndrome ně-FRŎT-ĭk SĬN-drŏm *nephr/o:* kidney *-tic:* pertaining to	Loss of large amounts of plasma protein, usually albumin, through urine due to an increased permeability of the glomerular membrane *Hypoproteinemia, edema, and hyperlipidemia are commonly associated with nephrotic syndrome.*
neurogenic bladder nū-rō-JĔN-ĭk *neur/o:* nerve *gen:* forming, producing, origin *-ic:* pertaining to	Impairment of bladder control as a result of brain, spinal cord, or nerve damage *Because the nervous system controls how the bladder stores and empties urine, neurogenic bladder leads to incontinence, difficulty in urinating, or the inability to urinate.*
polycystic kidney disease (PKD) pŏl-ē-SĬS-tĭk *poly-:* many, much *cyst:* bladder *-ic:* pertaining to	Inherited disease in which sacs of fluid called *cysts* develop in the kidneys *If cysts increase in number or size or if they become infected, kidney failure may result. Dialysis or kidney transplant may be necessary for renal failure caused by PKD.*
pyelonephritis pī-ě-lō-ně-FRĪ-tĭs *pyel/o:* renal pelvis *nephr:* kidney *-itis:* inflammation	Infection of the kidney, usually the result of an infection that begins in the urethra or bladder and ascends the ureters to the kidney *Pyelonephritis requires prompt attention to avoid permanent damage to the kidneys or from spreading to the bloodstream.*
urgency ĔR-jĕn-sē	Sensation of the need to void immediately *Urinary urgency commonly occurs in urinary tract infection (UTI).*
urinary tract infection (UTI) Ū-rĭ-nār-ē *urin:* urine; urinary tract *-ary:* pertaining to	An infection, typically of bacterial origin, in any part of the urinary tract, including the kidneys (acute pyelonephritis), bladder (cystitis), or urethra (urethritis) *Dysuria, although a symptom associated with numerous conditions, is commonly associated with UTI, especially cystitis and urethritis.*
vesicoureteral reflux (VUR) vĕs-ĭ-kō-ū-RĒ-tĕr-ăl RĒ-flŭks *vesic/o:* bladder *ureter:* ureter *-al:* pertaining to	Disorder caused by the failure of urine to pass through the ureters to the bladder, usually as a result of impairment of the valve between the ureter and bladder or obstruction in the ureter *VUR may result in hydronephrosis if the obstruction is in the proximal portion of the ureter or hydroureter and hydronephrosis if the obstruction is in the distal portion of the ureter.*
Wilms tumor VĬLMZ	Rapidly developing malignant tumor of the kidney that usually occurs in children; also called *nephroblastoma* *Diagnosis of Wilms tumor is established by an excretory urogram with tomography. The tumor is well encapsulated in the early stage but may metastasize to other sites, such as the lymph nodes and lungs, at later stages.*

 It is time to review pathology, diseases, and conditions by completing Learning Activity 11-3.

Diagnostic, Surgical, and Therapeutic Procedures

This section introduces diagnostic, surgical, and therapeutic procedures used to diagnose and treat urinary disorders. Descriptions are provided, along with pronunciations and word analyses for selected terms.

Procedure	Description
Diagnostic	

Clinical

| **electromyography (EMG)**
ē-lĕk-trō-mī-ŎG-ră-fē
   electr/o: electricity
   my/o: muscle
   -graphy: process of recording | Measures the contraction of muscles that control urination using electrodes placed in the rectum and urethra
EMG determines whether incontinence results from weak muscles or other causes. |

Endoscopic

| **cystoscopy (cysto)**
sĭs-TŎS-kō-pē
   cyst/o: bladder
   -scopy: examination | Examination of the urinary bladder for evidence of pathology, to obtain biopsies of tumors or other growths, or to remove polyps
In cystoscopy, the practitioner inserts a catheter into the hollow channel in the cystoscope to collect tissue samples or introduce contrast media during radiography. (See Fig. 11-7.) |

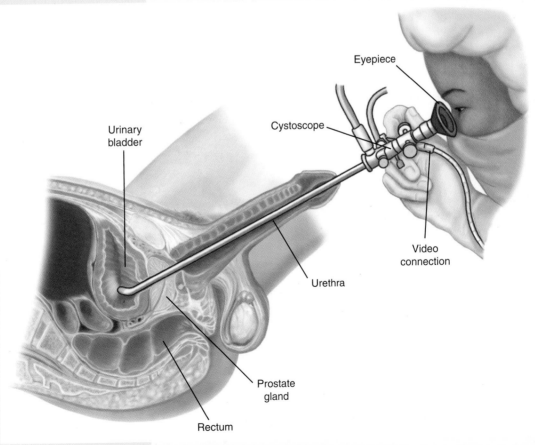

Urinary bladder

Eyepiece

Cystoscope

Video connection

Urethra

Prostate gland

Rectum

Figure 11-7 Cystoscopy.

(continued)

Diagnostic, Surgical, and Therapeutic Procedures—cont'd

Procedure	Description
Laboratory	
blood urea nitrogen (BUN) ū-RĒ-ă NĪ-trō-jĕn	Test that determines the amount of nitrogen in blood that comes from urea, a waste product of protein metabolism *Because the kidneys clear urea from the bloodstream, the BUN test helps evaluate kidney function.*
culture and sensitivity (C&S)	Test that determines the causative organism of an infection and identifies how the organism responds to various antibiotics *The practitioner may order a urine C&S test when a patient has chronic bladder infections or one that is unresponsive to treatment.*
urinalysis (UA) ū-rĭ-NĂL-ĭ-sĭs	Urine screening test that includes physical observation, chemical tests, and microscopic evaluation *UA not only provides information on the urinary structures but may also be the first indicator of such system disorders as diabetes and liver and gallbladder disease.*
Imaging	
bladder ultrasound	A noninvasive painless test that uses high-frequency soundwaves to produce images of the bladder before and after urination to check for urinary retention *During the examination, the practitioner directs sound waves into the bladder area and records images on a computer. (See Fig. 11-8.)*

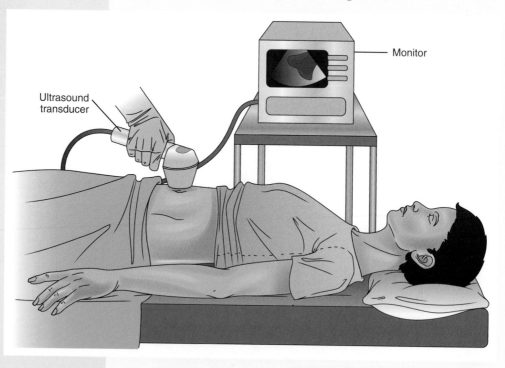

Monitor

Ultrasound
transducer

Figure 11-8 Bladder ultrasonography.

Diagnostic, Surgical, and Therapeutic Procedures—cont'd

Procedure	Description
intravenous pyelography (IVP) ĭn-tră-VĒ-nŭs pī-ĕ-LŎG-ră-fē *intra-:* in, within *ven:* vein *-ous:* pertaining to *pyel/o:* renal pelvis *-graphy:* process of recording	Imaging of the urinary tract after IV injection of a contrast medium; also called *excretory urography* *IVP detects kidney stones, enlarged prostate, internal injuries after an accident or trauma, and tumors in the kidneys, ureters, and bladder.*
renal nuclear scan RĒ-năl *ren:* kidney *-al:* pertaining to	Nuclear imaging test using a radioactive substance (tracer) injected intravenously to produce images of the kidneys *Renal nuclear scan evaluates the structure and function of the kidneys. It determines the size, shape, and position of the kidneys. It also determines the amount of blood filtered through the kidneys and evaluates kidney transplant to identify signs of rejection.*
voiding cystourethrography (VCUG) sĭs-tō-ū-rē-THRŎG-ră-fē *cyst/o:* bladder *urethr/o:* urethra *-graphy:* process of recording	X-ray of the bladder and urethra performed before, during, and after voiding using a contrast medium to enhance imaging *VCUG helps determine the cause of repeated bladder infections or stress incontinence and identify congenital or acquired structural abnormalities of the bladder and urethra.*

(continued)

Diagnostic, Surgical, and Therapeutic Procedures—cont'd

Procedure	Description
Surgical	
kidney transplant	Replacement of a diseased kidney with one that is supplied by a compatible donor (usually a family member or a cadaver who has donated the kidney before death)
	The surgeon usually places the new kidney below the diseased one for ease in attaching it to existing blood vessels. The diseased kidney usually remains in place unless there is concern that it will cause infection, uncontrolled hypertension, or reflux to the kidneys. (See Fig. 11-9.)

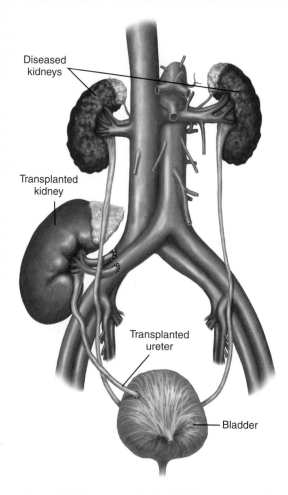

Figure 11-9 Kidney transplant with typical positioning of the new kidney beneath the diseased kidney.

Diagnostic, Surgical, and Therapeutic Procedures—cont'd

Procedure	Description
nephrostomy nĕ-FRŎS-tō-mē *nephr/o:* kidney *-stomy:* forming an opening (mouth)	Opening created between the skin and kidney to drain urine through a tube to a collecting receptacle outside the body when the ureters are unable to do so *Besides providing for urine drainage, nephrostomy may help access the kidney, evaluate kidney function, or deliver medications. (See Fig. 11-10.)*

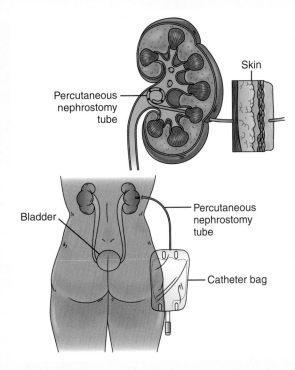

Figure 11-10 Percutaneous nephrostomy with a nephrostomy tube exiting through the skin.

(continued)

Diagnostic, Surgical, and Therapeutic Procedures—cont'd

Procedure	Description

ureteral stent placement
ū-RĒ-tĕr-ăl
   ureter: ureter
   -al: pertaining to

Insertion of a thin, narrow tube into the ureter to prevent or treat obstruction of urine flow from the kidney

Indwelling stents require constant monitoring because they may lead to infections, blockages, or stone formation. To avoid complications, they must be removed or changed periodically. (See Fig. 11-11.)

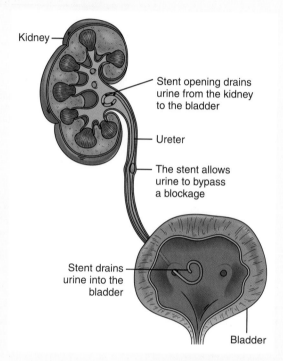

Kidney

Stent opening drains urine from the kidney to the bladder

Ureter

The stent allows urine to bypass a blockage

Stent drains urine into the bladder

Bladder

Figure 11-11 Ureteral stent placement.

Therapeutic

dialysis
dī-ĂL-ĭ-sĭs
   dia-: through, across
   -lysis: separation; destruction; loosening

Filtering procedure used to remove fluid and waste products from the blood and correct for electrolyte imbalances

Dialysis allows patients with kidney failure a chance to live productive lives.

hemodialysis
hē-mō-dī-ĂL-ĭ-sĭs
   hem/o: blood
   dia-: through, across
   -lysis: separation; destruction; loosening

Dialysis in which an artificial kidney machine receives waste-filled blood, filters it using a solution called a *dialysate*, and then returns the dialyzed (clean) blood to the patient's bloodstream (See Fig. 11-12.)

Diagnostic, Surgical, and Therapeutic Procedures—cont'd

Procedure	Description

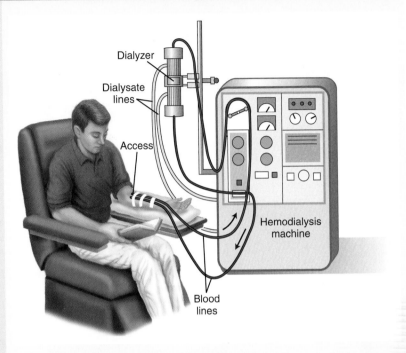

Figure 11-12 Hemodialysis.

peritoneal dialysis

pĕr-ĭ-tō-NĒ-ăl

peritone: peritoneum
-al: pertaining to
dia-: through, across
-lysis: separation; destruction;
loosening

Dialysis in which toxic substances are removed from the body by using the peritoneal membrane as the filter by perfusing (flushing) the peritoneal cavity with a warm, sterile chemical solution (See Fig. 11-13.)

Peritoneal dialysis is less restrictive on the patient than hemodialysis because it allows for self-treatment at home or while on trips.

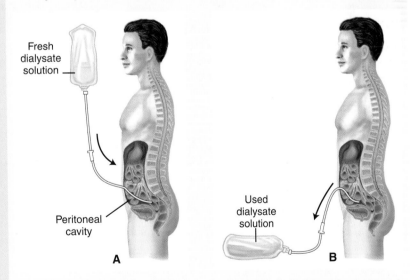

Figure 11-13 Peritoneal dialysis. (A) Introducing dialysis fluid into the peritoneal cavity. (B) Draining dialysate with waste products from the peritoneal cavity.

Pharmacology

Pharmacological agents used to treat urinary tract disorders include antibiotics, diuretics, antidiuretics, urinary antispasmodics, and potassium supplements, which are commonly taken concurrently with diuretics to counteract potassium depletion. (See Table 11-1.)

Table 11-1	**Drugs Used to Treat Urinary Disorders**

This table lists common drug classifications used to treat urinary disorders, their therapeutic actions, and selected generic and trade names.

Classification	Therapeutic Action	Generic and *Trade* Names
antibiotics ăn-tĭ-bī-ŎT-ĭks	Treat bacterial infections of the urinary tract by acting on the bacterial membrane or one of its metabolic processes *The type of antibiotic prescribed depends on the infecting organism and the type and extent of infection.*	**ciprofloxacin** sĭp-rō-FLŎX-ă-sĭn *Cipro* **sulfamethoxazole/trimethoprim** sŭl-fă-mĕth-ŎX-ă-zol trī-MĔTH-ō-prĭm *Bactrim*
antispasmodics ăn-tĭ-spăz-MŎT-ĭks	Decrease spasms in the urethra and bladder by relaxing the smooth muscles lining their walls, thus allowing normal emptying of the bladder *Bladder spasms can result from such conditions as urinary tract infections and catheterization.*	**tolterodine** tōl-TĔR-ō-dēn *Detrol LA* **solifenacin** sōl-ĭ-FĔN-ă-sĭn *Vesicare*
diuretics dī-ū-RĔT-ĭks	Promote and increase the excretion of urine *Diuretics are grouped by their action and are used to treat edema, hypertension, heart failure, and various renal and hepatic diseases.*	**furosemide** fū-RŌ-sĕ-mīd *Lasix* **spironolactone** spī-rō-nō-LĂK-tōn *Aldactone*
potassium supplements pō-TĂS-ē-ŭm	Replace potassium after depletion caused by diuretics *Dietary sources of potassium are usually not sufficient to replace potassium loss caused by diuretics.*	**potassium chloride** pō-TĂS-ē-ŭm KLŌ-rīd *K-Tab, Kaon Cl*

Abbreviations

This section introduces urinary-related abbreviations and their meanings.

Abbreviation	Meaning	Abbreviation	Meaning
ATN	acute tubular necrosis	pH	symbol for degree of acidity or alkalinity
BNO	bladder neck obstruction	PCNL	percutaneous nephrolithotomy
BUN	blood urea nitrogen	PKD	polycystic kidney disease
C&S	culture and sensitivity	TURBT	transurethral resection of bladder tumor
cysto	cystoscopy	UA	urinalysis
EMG	electromyogram, electromyography	US	ultrasound; ultrasonography
ESRD	end-stage renal disease	UTI	urinary tract infection
ESWL	extracorporeal shock-wave lithotripsy	VCUG	voiding cystourethrography
IC	interstitial cystitis	VUR	vesicoureteral reflux
IVP	intravenous pyelogram; intravenous pyelography		

It is time to review procedures, pharmacology, and abbreviations by completing Learning Activity 11–4.

LEARNING ACTIVITIES

The activities that follow provide a review of the urinary system terms introduced in this chapter. Complete each activity and review your answers to evaluate your understanding of the chapter.

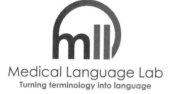

Medical Language Lab
Turning terminology into language

Visit the Medical Language Lab at *medicallanguagelab.com*. Use it to enhance your study and reinforcement of this chapter with the flash-card activity. We recommend that you complete the flash-card activity before starting Learning Activities 11-1 and 11-2.

Learning Activity 11-1
Medical Word Elements

Use the listed elements to build medical words. You may use the elements more than once.

Combining Forms		Suffixes		Prefixes
azot/o	pyel/o	-cele	-plasty	an-
cyst/o	ureter/o	-ectasis	-sclerosis	dia-
glomerul/o		-emia	-scopy	poly-
hemat/o		-genesis	-tome	
lith/o		-gram	-tripsy	
meat/o		-lysis	-uria	
nephr/o		-pathy		

1. disease of the kidney _____
2. forming (producing) stones _____
3. surgical repair of the renal pelvis _____
4. without (producing) urine _____
5. hardening of the glomerulus _____
6. process of examining the bladder _____
7. separation across (a membrane) _____
8. blood in the urine _____
9. (producing) much urine _____
10. dilation of the ureters _____
11. instrument to cut (enlarge) the meatus _____
12. nitrogenous compounds in the blood _____
13. hernia of the kidney _____
14. crushing of a stone _____
15. (x-ray) record of the bladder _____

✓ *Check your answers in Appendix A. Review any material that you did not answer correctly.*

Correct Answers _____ X 6.67 = _____ % Score

Learning Activity 11-2

Building Medical Words

Use *nephr/o* (kidney) to build words that mean

1. stone in the kidney _____
2. abnormal condition of pus in the kidney _____
3. abnormal condition of water in the kidney _____

Use *pyel/o* (renal pelvis) to build words that mean

4. process of recording the renal pelvis _____
5. disease of the renal pelvis _____

Use *ureter/o* (ureter) to build words that mean

6. dilation of a ureter _____
7. calculus in a ureter _____
8. pain in the ureters _____

Use *cyst/o* (bladder) to build words that mean

9. inflammation of the bladder _____
10. instrument to view the bladder _____
11. paralysis of the bladder _____

Use *vesic/o* (bladder) to build words that mean

12. herniation of the bladder _____
13. pertaining to the bladder and urethra _____

Use *urethr/o* (urethra) to build words that mean

14. narrowing or stricture of the urethra _____
15. instrument used to incise the urethra _____

Use *ur/o* (urine, urinary tract) to build words that mean

16. study of the urinary tract _____
17. disease of the urinary tract _____

Use the suffix *-uria* (urine) to build words that mean

18. difficult or painful urination _____
19. scanty urination _____
20. pus in the urine _____

Build surgical words that mean

21. surgical repair of the ureters _____

22. excision of the bladder _____

23. suture of the urethra _____

24. forming a mouth in the renal pelvis _____

25. fixation of the bladder _____

✓ *Check your answers in Appendix A. Review material that you did not answer correctly.*

Correct Answers _____ X 4 = _____ % Score

Learning Activity 11-3

Diseases and Conditions

Match the terms with the definitions in the numbered list.

anuria	fistula	neurogenic bladder	pyuria
azotemia	hydronephrosis	nocturia	reflux
cystocele	interstitial cystitis	oliguria	urgency
dysuria	nephrolithiasis	polycystic	urolithiasis
enuresis	nephrotic syndrome	pyelonephritis	Wilms tumor

1. need to void immediately _____
2. abnormal passage from a hollow organ to the surface or between organs _____
3. painful urination, usually a burning sensation _____
4. absence of urine production _____
5. nitrogenous wastes in the blood _____
6. abnormal condition of the kidneys due to water (urine reflux) _____
7. abnormal condition of a stone in any part of the urinary tract _____
8. chronic inflammation of the bladder wall _____
9. scanty urine production _____
10. inflammation of the kidney and renal pelvis _____
11. herniation of the bladder _____
12. involuntary discharge of urine _____
13. kidney disease characterized by the presence of fluid-filled sacs _____
14. impairment of bladder control due to brain or nerve conduction _____
15. pus in the urine _____
16. loss of plasma protein due to increased permeability of the glomerulus _____
17. excessive urination at night _____
18. backflow of urine into the kidney _____
19. rapidly developing malignant neoplasm of the kidney _____
20. abnormal condition of stones in the kidneys _____

✓ *Check your answers in Appendix A. Review any material that you did not answer correctly.*

Correct Answers _____ X 5 = _____ % Score

Learning Activity 11-4

Procedures, Pharmacology, and Abbreviations

Match the terms with the definitions in the numbered list.

antibiotics	electromyography	peritoneal
bladder US	ESWL	potassium
C&S	hemodialysis	renal nuclear scan
cystoscopy	IVP	stent placement
diuretics	nephrostomy	UA

1. imaging of urinary tract using contrast medium injected into the vein _____
2. measures the contraction of urinary muscles _____
3. visual examination of the urinary bladder _____
4. drugs that inhibit or kill bacterial microorganisms _____
5. laboratory test that identifies and evaluates the effect of an antibiotic on an organism _____
6. drugs used to promote the excretion of urine_____
7. positioning of a tube in the ureter to treat obstruction of urine flow _____
8. noninvasive procedure used to pulverize urinary or bile stones _____
9. dialysis of toxic substances by perfusing the abdominopelvic cavity _____
10. imaging that uses a tracer to produce images of the kidney _____
11. dialysis of toxic products by shunting blood from the body _____
12. opening created in the kidney to drain urine to an outside receptacle _____
13. imaging that uses sound waves to evaluate urine retention _____
14. supplement used to treat or prevent the hypokalemia commonly associated with the use of diuretics _____
15. test that includes physical observation as well as chemical and microscopic evaluation of urine _____

✓ *Check your answers in Appendix A. Review material that you did not answer correctly.*

Correct Answers _____ X 6.67 = _____ % Score

DOCUMENTING HEALTH-CARE ACTIVITIES

This section provides practical application activities in the form of exercises to help students develop skills in documenting patient care. First, read the medical report. Then complete the activities and exercises that follow.

Documenting Health-Care Activity 11-1

Operative Report: Ureterocele and Ureterocele Calculus

General Hospital

1511 Ninth Avenue ■ ■ Sun City, USA 12345 ■ ■ (555) 802–1887

OPERATIVE REPORT

Date: May 14, 20xx   Physician: Elmer Augustino, MD
Patient: Motch, Edwin   Patient: ID#: 48778

PREOPERATIVE DIAGNOSIS: Hematuria with left ureterocele and ureterocele calculus

POSTOPERATIVE DIAGNOSIS: Hematuria with left ureterocele and ureterocele calculus

OPERATION: Cystoscopy, transurethral incision of ureterocele, extraction of stone, and cystolithotripsy

ANESTHESIA: General

COMPLICATIONS: None

PROCEDURE: Patient was prepped and draped and placed in the lithotomy position. The urethra was calibrated with ease using a #26 French Van Buren urethral sound. A #24 resectoscope was inserted with ease. The prostate and bladder appeared normal, except for the presence of a left ureterocele, which was incised longitudinally; a large calculus was extracted from the ureterocele. There was minimal bleeding and no need for fulguration. The stone was crushed with the Storz stone-crushing instrument, and the fragments were evacuated. The bladder was emptied and the procedure terminated.

Patient tolerated the procedure well and was transferred to the postanesthesia care unit.

Elmer Augustino, MD
Elmer Augustino, MD

ea:bg

D: 5–14–20xx
T: 5–14–20xx

Terminology

The terms listed in the table that follows are taken from *Operative Report: Ureterocele and Ureterocele Calculus.* Use a medical dictionary such as *Taber's Cyclopedic Medical Dictionary,* the appendices of this book, or other resources to define each term. Then review the pronunciation for each term and practice by reading the medical record aloud.

Term	Definition
calculus KĂL-kū-lŭs	
cystolithotripsy sĭs-tō-LĬTH-ō-trĭp-sē	
cystoscope SĬST-ō-skōp	
fulguration fŭl-gŭ-RĀ-shŭn	
hematuria hē-mă-TŪ-rē-ă	
resectoscope rē-SĔK-tō-skōp	
transurethral trăns-ū-RĒ-thrăl	
ureterocele ū-RĒ-tĕr-ō-sēl	
urethral sound ū-RĒ-thrăl	

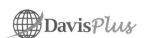

Visit the *Medical Terminology Systems* online resource center at Davis*Plus* to practice pronunciation and reinforce the meanings of the terms in this medical report.

Critical Thinking

Review *Operative Report: Ureterocele and Ureterocele Calculus* to answer the questions.

1. What were the findings from the resectoscopy?

_____

_____

_____

_____

2. What were the name and size of the urethral sound used in the procedure?

_____

_____

_____

_____

3. What is the function of the urethral sound?

_____

_____

_____

_____

4. In what direction was the ureterocele incised?

_____

_____

_____

_____

5. Was fulguration required? Why or why not?

_____

_____

_____

_____

Documenting Health-Care Activity II-2

Operative Report: Extracorporeal Shock-Wave Lithotripsy

General Hospital

1511 Ninth Avenue ■ ■ Sun City, USA 12345 ■ ■ (555) 802–1887

OPERATIVE REPORT

Date: April 1, 20xx   Physician: Elmer Augustino, MD
Patient: Marino, Julius   Room: 7201

PREOPERATIVE DIAGNOSIS: Left renal calculus

POSTOPERATIVE DIAGNOSIS: Left renal calculus

PROCEDURE: Extracorporeal shock-wave lithotripsy, cystoscopy with double-J stent removal

INDICATION FOR PROCEDURE: This 69-year-old male had undergone ESWL on 5/15/xx, with double-J stent placement to allow stone fragments to pass from the calyx to the bladder. At that time, approximately 50% of a partial staghorn calculus was fragmented. He now presents for the fragmenting of the remainder of the calculus and removal of the double-J stent.

ANESTHESIA: General

COMPLICATIONS: None

OPERATIVE TECHNIQUE: Patient was brought to the Lithotripsy Unit and placed in the supine position on the lithotripsy table. After induction of anesthesia, fluoroscopy was used to position the patient in the focal point of the shock waves. Being well positioned, he was given a total of 4,000 shocks with a maximum power setting of 3.0. After confirming complete fragmentation via fluoroscopy, the patient was transferred to the cystoscopy suite.

Patient was placed in the dorsal lithotomy position and draped and prepped in the usual manner. A cystoscope was inserted into the bladder through the urethra. Once the stent was visualized, it was grasped with the grasping forceps and removed as the scope was withdrawn.

Patient tolerated the procedure well and was transferred to recovery.

Elmer Augustino, MD
Elmer Augustino, MD

ea:bg

D: 4–1–20xx;
T: 4–1–20xx

Terminology

The terms listed in the table that follows are taken from *Operative Report: Extracorporeal Shock-Wave Lithotripsy.* Use a medical dictionary such as *Taber's Cyclopedic Medical Dictionary,* the appendices of this book, or other resources to define each term. Then review the pronunciation for each term and practice by reading the medical record aloud.

Term	Definition
calculus KĂL-kū-lŭs	
calyx KĀ-lĭx	
cystoscope SĬST-ō-skōp	
cystoscopy sĭs-TŎS-kō-pē	
dorsal lithotomy DOR-săl lĭth-ŎT-ō-mē	
ESWL	
extracorporeal ĕks-tră-kor- POR-ē-ăl	
fluoroscopy floo-or-ŎS-kō-pē	
lithotripsy LĬTH-ō-trĭp-sē	
shock-wave	
staghorn calculus STĂG-horn KĂL-kū-lŭs	
stent STĔNT	

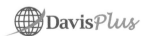

Visit the *Medical Terminology Systems* online resource center at Davis*Plus* to practice pronunciation and reinforce the meanings of the terms in this medical report.

Critical Thinking

Review *Operative Report: Extracorporeal Shock-Wave Lithotripsy* to answer the questions.

1. What previous procedures were performed on the patient?

\
\
\
\

2. Why is the current procedure being performed?

\
\
\
\

3. What imaging technique was used for positioning the patient to ensure that the shock waves would strike the calculus?

\
\
\
\

4. In what position was the patient placed in the cystoscopy suite?

\
\
\
\

5. How was the double-J stent removed?

\
\
\
\

Constructing Chart Notes

To construct chart notes, replace the italicized and boldfaced terms in each of the two case studies with one of the listed medical terms.

glomerulonephritis	oliguria	pyuria
hematuria	prognosis	pyelectasis
hypertension	proteinuria	ureterolithiasis
lithotripsy		

Mr. J. complains of intense pain in the abdomen and the side of the back with fever and chills. Urinalysis reveals (1) ***blood in the urine,*** uric acid crystals, and (2) ***pus in the urine.*** Radiology examination shows (3) ***the presence of a stone in the ureter.*** Because of its size, urine is unable to pass to the bladder, causing (4) ***dilation of the renal pelvis.*** It appears unlikely that the stone will pass through his urinary system. Because of its size and location, an ultrasound procedure will be used to (5) ***crush the stone.***

1. _____
2. _____
3. _____
4. _____
5. _____

Mr. K. was diagnosed with strep throat. Although he is on antibiotics, the infection is still present. Mr. K. now presents with (6) ***diminished urine output,*** (7) ***elevated blood pressure,*** and (8) ***protein in the urine.*** The physician explained that the toxins from the strep infection caused (9) ***inflammation of the glomerulus,*** impairing kidney function. The doctor's (10) ***anticipated outcome of this disease*** is full recovery once the strep infection is addressed and resolved.

6. _____
7. _____
8. _____
9. _____
10. _____

Check your answers in Appendix A. Review any material that you did not answer correctly.

Correct Answers _____ X 10 = _____ % Score

Female Reproductive System

Chapter Outline

Objectives

Upon completion of this chapter, you will be able to:

- Locate and describe the structures of the female reproductive system.
- Describe the functional relationship between the female reproductive system and other body systems.
- Pronounce, spell, and build words related to the female reproductive system.
- Describe diseases, conditions, and procedures related to the female reproductive system.
- Explain pharmacology related to the treatment of female reproductive disorders.
- Demonstrate your knowledge of this chapter by completing the learning and documenting health-care activities.

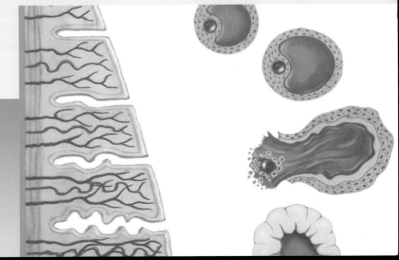

Anatomy and Physiology

The female reproductive system is designed to produce and transport ova (female sex cells), discharge ova from the body if fertilization does not occur, and nourish and provide a place for the developing fetus throughout pregnancy if fertilization occurs. The female reproductive system also produces the female sex hormones estrogen and progesterone, which play an important role in the reproductive process. These hormones are responsible for the development of secondary sex characteristics, such as breast development and regulation of the menstrual cycle.

Anatomy and Physiology Key Terms

This section introduces important terms, along with their definitions and pronunciations. The key terms are highlighted in color in the Anatomy and Physiology section. Word analyses for selected terms are also provided. Pronounce the term, and place a check mark in the box after you do so.

Term	Definition
external genitalia jĕn-ĭ-TĀL-ē-ă ☐	Sex, or reproductive, organs visible on the outside of the body; also called *genitals* *The external female genitalia are also called the* vulva. *Male genitalia include the penis, scrotum, and testicles.*
gestation jĕs-TĀ-shŭn ☐ *gest:* pregnancy *-ation:* process (of)	Length of time from conception to birth *The human gestational period typically extends approximately 280 days from the last menstrual period. Gestation (pregnancy) of less than 36 weeks is considered premature.*
lactation lăk-TĀ-shŭn ☐ *lact:* milk *-ation:* process (of)	Production and release of milk by mammary glands
orifice OR-ĭ-fĭs ☐	Mouth; entrance, or outlet of any anatomical structure

Pronunciation Help	Long Sound	ā — rate	ē — rebirth	ī — isle	ō — over	ū — unite
	Short Sound	ă — apple	ĕ — ever	ĭ — it	ŏ — not	ŭ — cut

Female Reproductive Structures

The female reproductive system is composed of the internal organs of reproduction and the **external genitalia.** (See Fig. 12-1.) The internal organs include the (1) **ovaries,** (2) **fallopian tubes,** (3) **uterus,** and (4) **vagina.** The **external genitalia** are collectively known as the **vulva.** Included in these structures are the (5) **labia minora,** (6) **labia majora,** (7) **clitoris,** (8) **Bartholin glands,** and **mons pubis,** an elevation of adipose tissue covered by skin and coarse pubic hair that cushions the **pubis (pubic bone).** The area between the vaginal **orifice** and the anus is known as the **perineum.**

Female Reproductive Organs

The female reproductive organs include the ovaries, fallopian tubes, uterus, and vagina. They are designed to produce female reproductive cells **(ova),** transport the cells to the site of fertilization, provide a favorable environment for a developing fetus through pregnancy and childbirth, and produce female sex hormones. Hormones play an important role in the reproductive process, providing their influence at critical times during preconception, fertilization, and **gestation.** (See Fig. 12-2, page 398.)

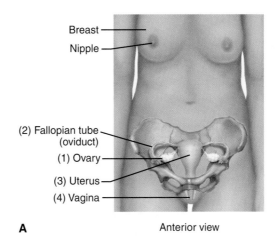

Breast
Nipple

(2) Fallopian tube (oviduct)
(1) Ovary
(3) Uterus
(4) Vagina

A   Anterior view

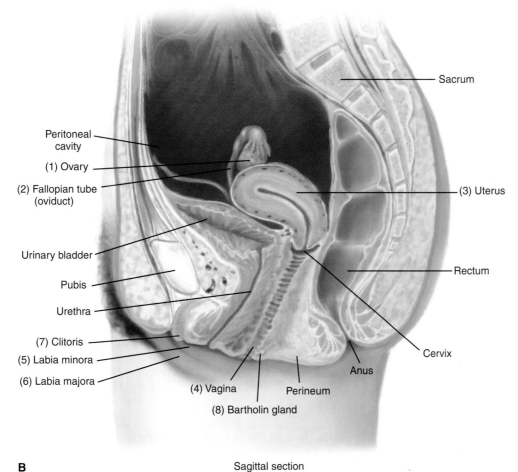

Sacrum

Peritoneal cavity
(1) Ovary
(2) Fallopian tube (oviduct)

(3) Uterus

Urinary bladder

Pubis

Urethra

Rectum

(7) Clitoris
(5) Labia minora
(6) Labia majora

Cervix

Anus

(4) Vagina   Perineum

(8) Bartholin gland

B   Sagittal section

Figure 12-1 Female reproductive system. (A) Anterior view. (B) Lateral view showing the organs within the pelvic cavity.

Ovaries

The (1) **ovaries** are almond-shaped glands located in the pelvic cavity, one on each side of the uterus. Each ovary contains thousands of tiny, saclike structures called (2) **graafian follicles,** each containing an ovum. When an ovum ripens, the (3) **mature follicle** moves to the surface of the ovary, ruptures, and releases the ovum in a process called **ovulation.** After ovulation, the empty follicle transforms into a structure called the (4) **corpus luteum,** a small yellow mass that secretes estrogen and progesterone. The corpus luteum degenerates at the end of a nonfertile

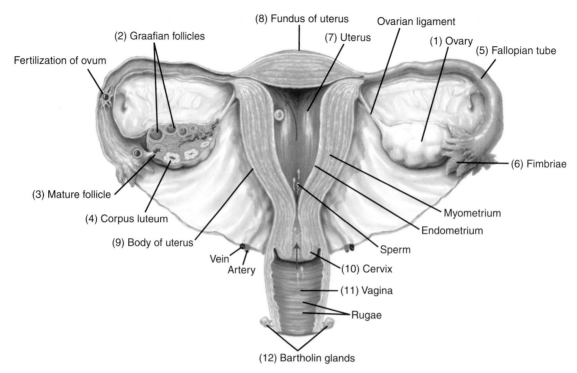

Figure 12-2 Anterior view of the female reproductive system with the developing follicles shown in the cross section of the right ovary.

cycle. Estrogen and progesterone influence the menstrual cycle and menopause. They also prepare the uterus for implantation of the fertilized egg, help maintain pregnancy, promote growth of the placenta, and play an important role in development of secondary sex characteristics. (See Chapter 14, Endocrine System.)

Fallopian Tubes

Two (5) **fallopian tubes (oviducts, uterine tubes)** extend laterally from superior angles of the uterus. The (6) **fimbriae** are fingerlike projections that create wavelike currents in fluid surrounding the ovary to move the ovum into the uterine tube. If the egg unites with a spermatozoon, the male reproductive cell, fertilization (or conception) takes place. The fertilized egg then continues its journey to the uterus, where it implants on the uterine wall. If conception does not occur, the ovum disintegrates within 48 hours and is discharged through the vagina.

Uterus and Vagina

The (7) **uterus** contains and nourishes the embryo from the time the fertilized egg is implanted until the fetus is born. It is a muscular, hollow structure shaped like an inverted pear and is located in the pelvic area between the bladder and rectum. The uterus normally tilts forward **(anteflexion)** in the pelvic cavity and consists of three parts: the (8) **fundus,** the upper, rounded part; the (9) **body,** the central part; and the (10) **cervix,** also called the **neck of the uterus** or **cervix uteri,** the inferior constricted portion that opens into the vagina.

The (11) **vagina** is a muscular tube that extends from the cervix to the exterior of the body. Its lining consists of folds of mucous membrane that give the organ an elastic quality. During sexual excitement, the vaginal orifice is lubricated by secretions from (12) **Bartholin glands.** In addition to serving as the organ of sexual intercourse and receptor of semen, the vagina discharges menstrual flow. It also acts as a passageway for the delivery of the fetus. The **clitoris,** located anterior to the vaginal orifice, is composed of erectile tissue that is richly innervated with sensory endings. The clitoris is similar in structure to the penis in the male, but it is smaller and has no urethra. The area between the vaginal orifice and the anus is known as the

perineum. During childbirth, this area may be surgically incised **(episiotomy)** to enlarge the vaginal opening for delivery.

Mammary Glands

Although mammary glands (breasts) are present in both sexes, they function only in females. (See Fig. 12-3.) The breasts are not directly involved in reproduction but become important after delivery. Their biological role is to secrete milk for the nourishment of the newborn, a process

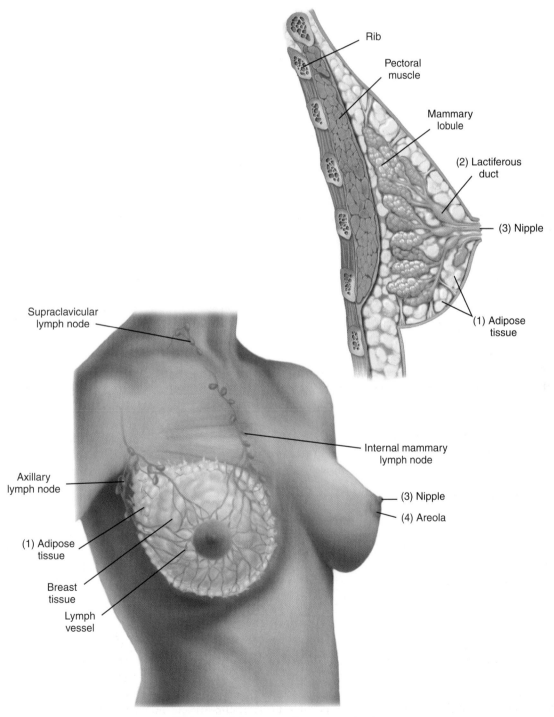

Figure 12-3 Structure of mammary glands.

called **lactation**. Breasts begin to develop during puberty as a result of periodic stimulation of the ovarian hormones estrogen and progesterone and are fully developed by age 16. Estrogen is responsible for the development of (1) **adipose tissue,** which enlarges the size of the breasts until they reach full maturity. Breast size is primarily determined by the amount of fat around the glandular tissue but is not indicative of functional ability. Each breast is composed of 15 to 20 lobules of milk-producing glands that are drained by a (2) **lactiferous duct,** which opens on the tip of the raised (3) **nipple.** Circling the nipple is a border of slightly darker skin called the (4) **areola.** During pregnancy, the breasts enlarge and remain so until lactation ceases. At menopause, breast tissue begins to atrophy.

Menstrual Cycle

Menarche, the initial menstrual period, occurs at puberty (about age 12), and menstruation continues for approximately 40 years, except during pregnancy. The menstrual cycle consists of a series of phases, during which the uterine endometrium changes as it responds to changing levels of ovarian hormones. (See Table 12-1.) The duration of the menstrual cycle is approximately 28 days. (See Fig. 12-4.)

Pregnancy

During pregnancy, the uterus changes its shape, size, and consistency. It increases greatly in size and muscle mass; houses the growing placenta, which nourishes the embryo-fetus; and expels the fetus after gestation. To prepare to serve as the birth canal at the end of pregnancy, the vaginal canal elongates as the uterus rises in the pelvis. The mucosa thickens, secretions increase, and the vascularity and elasticity of the cervix and vagina become more pronounced.

The average pregnancy (gestation) lasts approximately 9 months and is followed by childbirth (parturition). Up to the third month of pregnancy, the product of conception is referred to as the *embryo*. From the third month to the time of birth, the unborn offspring is referred to as the *fetus*.

Pregnancy also causes enlargement of the breasts, sometimes to the point of pain. Many other changes occur throughout the body to accommodate the development and birth of the

Table 12-1	**Phases of the Menstrual Cycle**	
This table outlines the changes involved during the typical 28-day menstrual cycle.		
Phase	**Description**	
Menstrual Days 1–5	Uterine endometrium sloughs off because of hormonal stimulation, a process accompanied by bleeding. The detached tissue and blood are discharged through the vagina as menstrual flow.	
Ovulatory Days 6–14	When menstruation ceases, the endometrium begins to thicken as new tissue is rebuilt. As the estrogen level rises, several ova begin to mature in the graafian follicles, usually with only one ovum reaching full maturity. At about the 14th day of the cycle, the graafian follicle ruptures, releasing the egg, a process called ovulation. The egg then leaves the ovary and travels down the fallopian tube toward the uterus.	
Postovulatory Days 15–28	The empty graafian follicle fills with a yellow material and is now called the *corpus luteum*. Secretions of estrogen and progesterone by the corpus luteum stimulate the building of the endometrium in preparation for implantation of an embryo. If fertilization does not occur, the corpus luteum begins to degenerate as estrogen and progesterone levels decrease.* With decreased hormone levels, the uterine lining begins to shed, the menstrual cycle starts over again, and the first day of menstruation begins.	

*Some women experience a loose grouping of symptoms called **premenstrual syndrome (PMS).** These symptoms usually occur about 5 days after the decrease in hormone levels and include nervous tension, irritability, headaches, breast tenderness, and a feeling of depression.

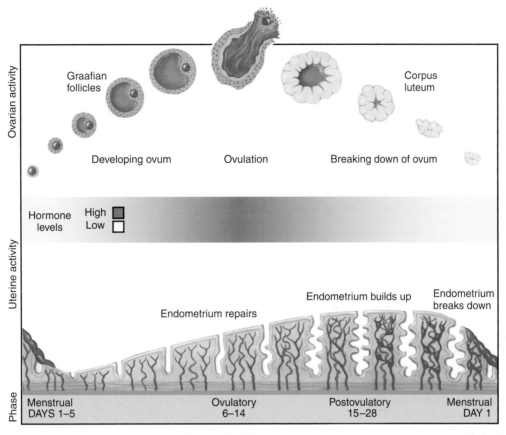

Ovarian activity

Graafian follicles

Developing ovum

Ovulation

Corpus luteum

Breaking down of ovum

Hormone levels — High / Low

Uterine activity

Endometrium repairs

Endometrium builds up

Endometrium breaks down

Phase

| Menstrual DAYS 1–5 | Ovulatory 6–14 | Postovulatory 15–28 | Menstrual DAY 1 |

Figure 12-4 Menstrual cycle.

fetus. Toward the end of gestation, the myometrium begins to contract weakly at irregular intervals. At this time, the full-term fetus is usually positioned head down within the uterus.

Labor and Childbirth

Labor is the physiological process by which the fetus is expelled from the uterus. Labor occurs in three stages. The first is the **stage of dilation,** which begins with uterine contractions and terminates when there is complete dilation of the cervix (10 cm). The second is the **stage of expulsion,** the time from complete cervical dilation to birth of the baby. The last stage is the **placental stage,** or **afterbirth.** This stage begins shortly after childbirth when the uterine contractions discharge the placenta from the uterus. (See Fig. 12-5, page 402.)

Menopause

Menopause is the cessation of ovarian activity and diminished hormone production that occurs at about age 50. Menopause is usually diagnosed if absence of menses **(amenorrhea)** has persisted for 1 year. The period in which symptoms of approaching menopause occur is known as the **change of life** or the **climacteric.**

Many women experience hot flashes and vaginal drying and thinning **(vaginal atrophy)** as estrogen levels fall. Although **hormone replacement therapy (HRT)** has become more controversial, it is still used to treat vaginal atrophy and porous bones **(osteoporosis),** and it is believed to play a role in heart attack prevention. Restraint in prescribing estrogens for long periods in all menopausal women arises from concern that there is an increased risk that long-term usage will induce neoplastic changes in estrogen-sensitive aging tissue.

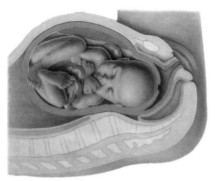

(1) Labor begins, membranes intact

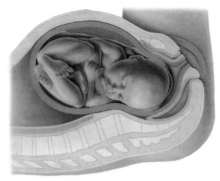

(2) Effacement of cervix,
which is now partially dilated

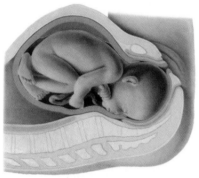

(3) When head reaches floor
of pelvis, it rotates

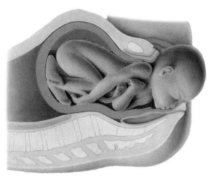

(4) Extension of the cervix allows head
to pass through

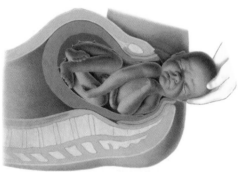

(5) Delivery of head, head rotates to
realign itself with body

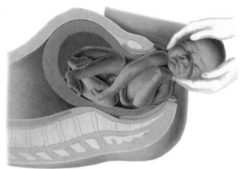

(6) Delivery of shoulders

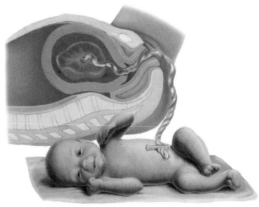

(7) Delivery of infant is complete,
uterus begins to contract

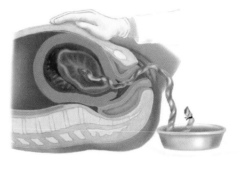

(8) Umbilical cord is cut, external massage
to uterus continues to stimulate
contractions, and placenta is delivered

Figure 12-5 Sequence of labor and childbirth.

Anatomy Review: Female Reproductive Structures (Lateral View)

To review the anatomy of the female reproductive system, label the illustration using the listed terms.

Bartholin gland

cervix

clitoris

fallopian tube

labia majora

labia minora

ovary

perineum

uterus

vagina

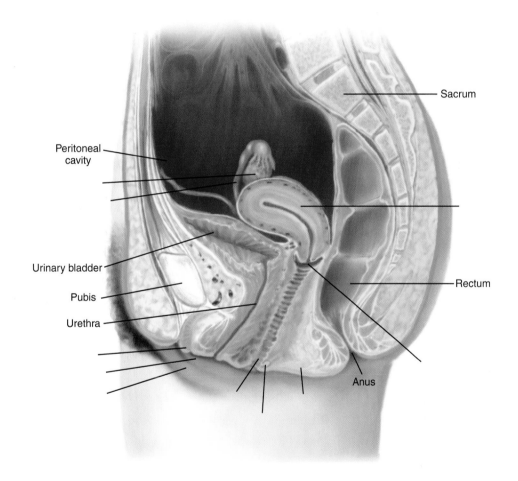

 Check your answers by referring to Fig. 12–1 on page 397. Review material that you did not answer correctly.

Anatomy Review: Female Reproductive Structures (Anterior View)

To review the anatomy of the female reproductive system, label the illustration using the listed terms.

Bartholin glands

body of the uterus

cervix

corpus luteum

fallopian tube

fertilization of ovum

fimbriae

fundus of uterus

graafian follicles

mature follicle

ovarian ligament

ovary

uterus

vagina

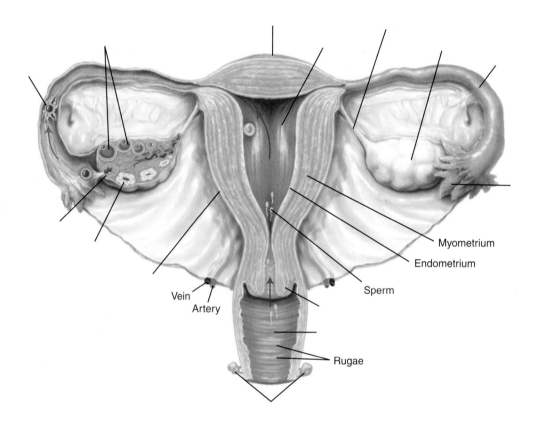

Myometrium

Endometrium

Sperm

Vein

Artery

Rugae

Check your answers by referring to Fig. 12-2 on page 398. Review material that you did not answer correctly.

CONNECTING BODY SYSTEMS—FEMALE REPRODUCTIVE SYSTEM

The main function of the female reproductive system is to produce hormones and to provide structures that support fertilization and development of a developing fetus. It also provides very limited support to the functions of other body systems. These limited functional relationships are summarized here.

Blood, Lymphatic, and Immune
• The female immune system has special mechanisms that inhibit destruction of sperm cells.
• The female reproductive tract secretes enzymes and other substances that inhibit entry of pathogens into the internal reproductive structures.

Cardiovascular
• Estrogens lower blood cholesterol levels and promote cardiovascular health in premenopausal women.

Digestive
• Estrogens have an effect on the metabolic rate.

Endocrine
• Estrogens provide a feedback mechanism that influences pituitary function.
• Estrogens assist in the production of human chorionic gonadotropin (HCG) hormone.

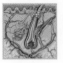

Integumentary
• Female hormones affect growth and distribution of body hair.
• Female hormones influence the activity of sebaceous glands.
• Female hormones influence skin texture and fat distribution.

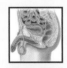

Male Reproductive
• The female reproductive system provides the ovum needed to make fertilization by sperm possible.

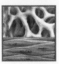

Musculoskeletal
• Estrogen influences muscle development and size.
• Estrogen influences bone growth, maintenance, and closure of epiphyseal plates.

Nervous
• Estrogen affects central nervous system development and sexual behavior.
• Estrogen provides antioxidants that have a neuroprotective function.

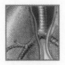

Respiratory
• Sexual arousal and pregnancy produce changes in the rate and depth of breathing.
• Estrogen is believed to provide a beneficial effect on the alveoli of the lungs.

Urinary
• Kidneys dispose of nitrogenous wastes and maintain the homeostatic mechanisms of the mother and fetus.

Medical Word Elements

This section introduces combining forms, suffixes, and prefixes related to the female reproductive system. From the information provided, complete the meaning of the medical words in the right-hand column. The first one is completed for you.

Element	Meaning	Analysis
Combining Forms		
amni/o	amnion (amniotic sac)	**amni/o**/centesis (ăm-nē-ō-sĕn-TĒ-sĭs): *surgical puncture of the amniotic sac* *-centesis:* surgical puncture *Amniocentesis is performed under ultrasound guidance using a needle and syringe to remove amniotic fluid.*
cervic/o	neck; cervix uteri (neck of the uterus)	**cervic/**itis (sĕr-vĭ-SĪ-tĭs): _____ *-itis:* inflammation
colp/o	vagina	**colp/o**/scopy (kŏl-PŎS-kō-pē): _____ *-scopy:* visual examination
vagin/o		**vagin/**itis (văj-ĭn-Ī-tĭs): _____ *-cele:* hernia, swelling *Vaginitis is usually caused by infection.*
galact/o	milk	**galact/o**/poiesis (gă-lăk-tō-poy-Ē-sĭs): _____ *-poiesis:* formation, production
lact/o		**lact/o**/gen (LĂK-tō-jĕn): _____ *-gen:* forming, producing, origin *The term* lactogen *refers to any substance that stimulates milk production, such as a hormone.*
gynec/o	woman, female	**gynec/o**/logist (gī-nĕ-KŎL-ō-jĭst): _____ *-logist:* specialist in the study of
hyster/o	uterus (womb)	**hyster/**ectomy (hĭs-tĕr-ĔK-tō-mē): _____ *-ectomy:* excision, removal
metri/o		endo/**metri/**al (ĕn-dō-MĒ-trē-ăl): _____ *endo-:* in, within *-al:* pertaining to
uter/o		**uter/o**/vagin/al (ū-tĕr-ō-VĂJ-ĭ-năl): _____ *vagin/o:* vagina *-al:* pertaining to
mamm/o	breast	**mamm/o**/gram (MĂM-ō-grăm): _____ *-gram:* record, writing
mast/o		**mast/o**/pexy (MĂS-tō-pĕks-ē): _____ *-pexy:* fixation (of an organ) *Mastopexy is reconstructive cosmetic surgery performed to affix sagging breasts in a more elevated position, commonly improving their shape.*

Medical Word Elements—cont'd

Element	Meaning	Analysis
men/o	menses, menstruation	**men/o**/rrhagia (mĕn-ō-RĀ-jē-ă): _____ *-rrhagia:* bursting forth (of) *Menorrhagia refers to an excessive amount of menstrual bleeding that lasts longer than seven days.*
metr/o	uterus (womb); measure	**metr/o**/ptosis (mē-trō-TŌ-sĭs): _____ *-ptosis:* prolapse, downward displacement

nat/o	birth	pre/**nat**/al (prē-NĀ-tăl): _____
		   pre-: before, in front
		   -al: pertaining to

oophor/o	ovary	**oophor**/oma (ō-ŏf-ō-RŌ-mă): _____ *-oma:* tumor
ovari/o		**ovari/o**/rrhexis (ō-vā-rē-ō-RĔK-sĭs): _____ *-rrhexis:* rupture
perine/o	perineum (area between the scrotum [or vulva in the female] and anus)	**perine/o**/rrhaphy (pĕr-ĭ-nē-OR-ă-fē): _____ *-rrhaphy:* suture *Perineorrhaphy repairs an episiotomy or a laceration that occurs during delivery of the fetus.*
salping/o	tube (usually fallopian or eustachian [auditory] tubes)	**salping/o**/plasty (săl-PĬNG-gō-plăs-tē): _____ *-plasty:* surgical repair
Suffixes		
-arche	beginning	men/**arche** (mĕn-ĂR-kē): _____ *men:* menses, menstruation
-cyesis	pregnancy	pseudo/**cyesis** (soo-dō-sī-Ē-sĭs): _____ *pseudo-:* false *Pseudocyesis is a condition in which a woman develops bodily changes consistent with pregnancy when she is not pregnant.*
-gravida	pregnant woman	multi/**gravida** (mŭl-tĭ-GRĂV-ĭ-dă): _____ *multi-:* many, much *The term* gravida *may be followed by numbers that indicate the number of pregnancies, such as* gravida 1 *and* gravida 2 *or* gravida I, gravida II, *and so forth.*

(continued)

Medical Word Elements—cont'd

Element	Meaning	Analysis
-para	to bear (offspring)	nulli/**para** (nŭl-ĬP-ă-ră): _____ *nulli-:* none *The term* para *followed by a Roman numeral or preceded by a Latin prefix (such as* primi-, quadri-, *and so forth) designates the number of times a pregnancy has culminated in a single or multiple birth. For example,* para I *and* primipara *refer to a woman who has given birth for the first time. Whether the births were multiple (twins, triplets) is irrelevant.*
-salpinx	tube (usually fallopian or eustachian [auditory] tubes)	hem/o/**salpinx** (hē-mŌ-SĂL-pĭnks): _____ *hem/o:* blood *Hemosalpinx is also called* **hematosalpinx.**
-tocia	childbirth, labor	dys/**tocia** (dĭs-TŌ-sē-ă): _____ *dys-:* bad; painful; difficult
-version	turning	retro/**version** (rĕt-rō-VĔR-shŭn): _____ *retro-:* backward, behind *Retroversion of the uterus occurs in one of every four otherwise healthy women.*
Prefixes		
ante-	before, in front of	**ante**/version (ăn-tē-VĔR-zhŭn): _____ *-version:* turning
dys-	bad; painful; difficult	**dys**/men/o/rrhea (dĭs-mĕn-ō-RĒ-ă): _____ *men/o:* menses, menstruation *-rrhea:* discharge, flow
endo-	in, within	**endo**/metr/itis (ĕn-dō-mē-TRĪ-tĭs): _____ *metr:* uterus (womb); measure *-itis:* inflammation
multi-	many, much	**multi**/para (mŭl-TĬP-ă-ră): _____ *-para:* to bear (offspring)
post-	after	**post**/nat/al (pōst-NĀ-tăl): _____ *nat:* birth *-al:* pertaining to
primi-	first	**primi**/gravida (prī-mĭ-GRĂV-ĭ-dă): _____ *-gravida:* pregnant woman

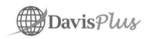

Visit the *Medical Terminology Systems* online resource center at Davis*Plus* for an audio exercise of the terms in this table. Other activities are also available to reinforce content.

⊙ *It is time to review medical word elements by completing Learning Activities 12-1 and 12-2.*

Disease Focus

Female reproductive disorders may be caused by infection, injury, or hormonal dysfunction. Although some disorders may be mild and correct themselves over time, others, such as those caused by infection, may require medical attention. Pain, itching, lesions, and discharge are signs and symptoms commonly associated with sexually transmitted diseases and must not be ignored. Other common problems of the female reproductive system are related to hormonal dysfunction that may cause menstrual disorders.

As a preventive measure, a woman should undergo pelvic examination regularly throughout life. This diagnostic procedure helps identify many pelvic abnormalities and diseases. Cytological and bacteriological specimens are usually obtained at the time of examination.

Gynecology (GYN) is the branch of medicine concerned with diseases of the female reproductive organs and breasts. **Obstetrics (OB)** is the branch of medicine that manages the health of a woman and her fetus during pregnancy and childbirth. It also includes the **puerperium,** which is the period of adjustment after childbirth during which the reproductive organs of the mother return to their normal, nonpregnant state. Generally, this period lasts 6 to 8 weeks and ends with the first ovulation and the return of normal menstruation. Because of the obvious overlap between gynecology and obstetrics, many practices include both specialties. The physician who simultaneously practices these specialties is called an **obstetrician/gynecologist (OB/GYN).**

Endometriosis

Endometriosis is the presence of functional endometrial tissue in areas outside the uterus. (See Fig. 12-6.) The endometrial tissue develops into what are called **implants, lesions,** or **growths** and can cause pain, infertility, and other problems. The ectopic tissue is usually confined to the pelvic area but may appear anywhere in the abdominopelvic cavity. Like normal endometrial tissue, the ectopic endometrium responds to the hormonal fluctuations of the menstrual cycle.

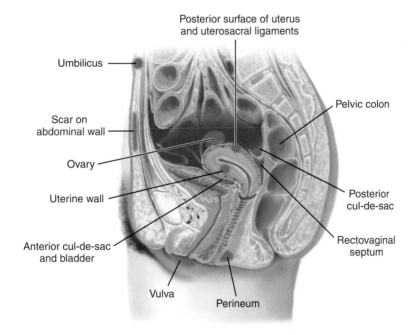

Figure 12-6 Endometriosis.

Pelvic Inflammatory Disease

Pelvic inflammatory disease (PID) is a general term for inflammation of the uterus, fallopian tubes, ovaries, and adjacent pelvic structures. It is usually caused by bacterial infection, but other organisms may be implicated. These disease-producing organisms **(pathogens)** generally enter through the vagina during coitus, induced abortion, childbirth, or the postpartum period. As an ascending infection, the pathogens spread from the vagina and cervix to the upper structures of the female reproductive tract. Untreated gonorrhea and chlamydia cause about 90% of all cases of PID. Other causes include abortion, childbirth, and pelvic procedures.

The symptoms of PID can vary and may include lower abdominal pain, vaginal discharge, fever, nausea, and vomiting. If diagnosed at an early stage, PID can be treated easily and effectively with antibiotics. If left untreated, it can lead to more serious, long-term complications.

Oncology

The two most common forms of cancer (CA) involving the female reproductive system are breast cancer and cervical cancer.

Breast Cancer

Breast cancer, also called **carcinoma of the breast,** is the most common malignancy of women in the United States. This disease appears to be associated with ovarian hormonal function. In addition, a diet high in fats appears to increase the incidence of breast cancer. Other contributing factors include a family history of the disease and, possibly, the use of hormone replacement therapy (HRT). Women who have never had children **(nulliparous)** or those who have had an early onset of the first menstrual period **(menarche)** or late onset of menopause are also more likely to develop breast cancer. Because this type of malignancy is highly responsive to treatment when detected early, women are urged to practice breast self-examination monthly and to receive periodic mammograms after age 40. Many breast malignancies are detected by the patient.

Cervical Cancer

Cancer of the cervix most commonly affects women between ages 40 and 49. Statistics indicate that infection associated with sexual activity has some relationship to the incidence of cervical cancer. First coitus at a young age, a large number of sex partners, infection with certain sexually transmitted viruses, and frequent intercourse with men whose previous partners had cervical cancer are all associated with increased risk of developing cervical cancer.

The Pap test, a cytological examination, can detect cervical cancer before the disease becomes clinically evident. Abnormal cervical cytology routinely calls for colposcopy, which can detect the presence and extent of preclinical lesions requiring biopsy and histological examination. Treatment of cervical cancer consists of surgery, radiation, and chemotherapy. If left untreated, the cancer will eventually metastasize and lead to death.

Diseases and Conditions

This section introduces diseases and conditions of the female reproductive system, along with their meanings and pronunciations. Word analyses for selected terms are also provided.

Term	Definition
Female Reproductive System	
atresia ă-TRĒ-zē-ă	Congenital absence or closure of a normal body opening, such as the vagina
choriocarcinoma kō-rē-ō-kăr-sĭ-NŌ-mă *chori/o:* chorion *carcin:* cancer *-oma:* tumor	Malignant neoplasm of the uterus or at the site of an ectopic pregnancy *Although its actual cause is unknown, choriocarcinoma is a rare tumor that may occur after pregnancy or abortion.*
dyspareunia dĭs-pă-RŪ-nē-ă	Occurrence of pain during sexual intercourse

Diseases and Conditions—cont'd

Term	Definition

endocervicitis
ĕn-dō-sĕr-vĭ-SĪ-tĭs
  endo-: in, within
  cervic: neck; cervix uteri (neck of the uterus)
  -itis: inflammation

Inflammation of the mucous lining of the cervix uteri

Endocervicitis is usually chronic, commonly as a result of infection, and accompanied by cervical erosion.

---

menstrual disorders
MĔN-stroo-ăl
  menstru/o: monthly discharge of blood
  -al: pertaining to

Abnormal condition in the menstrual cycle; also called *dysfunctional uterine bleeding (DUB)*

Menstrual irregularities can be caused by a variety of conditions, including pregnancy, hormonal imbalances, infections, malignancies, diseases, trauma, and certain medications.

amenorrhea
ă-mĕn-ō-RĒ-ă
  a-: without, not
  men/o: menses; menstruation
  -rrhea: discharge, flow

Absence of a menstrual period in a woman of reproductive age

Normal causes of amenorrhea include pregnancy and lactation (breastfeeding). Outside of reproductive years, absence of menses occurs during childhood and after menopause.

dysmenorrhea
dĭs-mĕn-ō-RĒ-ă
  dys-: bad; painful; difficult
  men/o: menses; menstruation
  -rrhea: discharge, flow

Cramps or painful menstruation

Dysmenorrhea includes menstrual periods that are accompanied by sharp, intermittent pain or dull, aching pain—usually in the pelvis or lower abdomen.

menorrhagia
mĕn-ō-RĀ-jē-ă
  men/o: menses; menstruation
  -rrhagia: bursting forth (of)

Abnormally heavy, prolonged menstrual period

In early life, menorrhagia may be caused by endocrine disturbances; in later life, it is usually a result of inflammatory diseases, fibroids, tumors, or emotional disturbances.

metrorrhagia
mē-trō-RĀ-jē-ă
  metr/o: uterus (uterus); measure
  -rrhagia: bursting forth (of)

Irregular uterine bleeding between menstrual periods or after menopause

Metrorrhagia is usually symptomatic of disease, including benign or malignant uterine tumors. It is considered one of the most serious menstrual disorders. Thus, early diagnosis and treatment are warranted.

oligomenorrhea
ŏl-ĭ-gō-mĕn-ō-RĒ-ă
  olig/o: scanty
  men/o: menses, menstruation
  -rrhea: discharge, flow

Abnormally light or infrequent menstrual periods

Causes of oligomenorrhea include a side effect of birth control pills, hormonal imbalances, excessive exercise, and ovarian cysts.

premenstrual syndrome (PMS)
prē-MĔN-stroo-ăl SĬN-drōm

Symptoms that occur between ovulation and the onset of menstruation

PMS symptoms include such physical symptoms as breast tenderness, back pain, abdominal cramps, headache, and changes in appetite and the psychological symptoms of anxiety, depression, and unrest.

---

sterility
stĕr-ĬL-ĭ-tē

Inability of the female to become pregnant or the male to impregnate the female

---

uterine fibroids
Ū-tĕr-ĭn FĪ-broyds
  fibr: fiber, fibrous tissue
  -oids: resembling

Benign tumors composed of muscle and fibrous tissue that develop in the uterus; also called *leiomyomas, myomas,* or *fibroids*

Myomectomy or hysterectomy may be indicated if the fibroids grow too large, causing such symptoms as metrorrhagia, pelvic pain, and menorrhagia.

(continued)

Diseases and Conditions—cont'd

Term	Definition

Obstetrics

abortion (AB)
ă-BOR-shŭn

Termination of pregnancy before the embryo or fetus is capable of surviving on its own

Abortions are spontaneous or induced (deliberate). A spontaneous abortion occurs without any apparent cause and is also called a miscarriage. A woman undergoes an induced abortion when she elects to end pregnancy because her health is endangered (therapeutic abortion) or for some other personal reason.

abruptio placentae
ă-BRŪP-shē-ō plă-SĔN-tē

Premature separation of the placenta from the uterine wall before the third stage of labor; also called *placental abruption*

Abruptio placentae results in uterine hemorrhage and threatens the life of the mother. It also disrupts blood flow and oxygen through the umbilical cord and threatens the life of the fetus.

breech presentation

Common abnormality of delivery in which the fetal buttocks or feet present first rather than the head

Down syndrome
DOWN SĬN-drōm

Genetic condition in which there is an extra copy of chromosome 21 (trisomy), altering physical and mental development of the child; also called *trisomy 21*

Symptoms vary and can range from mild to severe. However, children with Down syndrome have a widely recognized appearance.

eclampsia
ĕ-KLĂMP-sē-ă

Most serious form of toxemia during pregnancy

Signs of eclampsia include high blood pressure, edema, convulsions, renal dysfunction, proteinuria, and in severe cases, coma.

ectopic pregnancy
ĕk-TŎP-ĭk PRĔG-năn-sē

Pregnancy in which the fertilized ovum becomes implanted on any tissue other than the lining of the uterine cavity

Types of ectopic pregnancy include abdominal pregnancy, ovarian pregnancy, and tubal pregnancy. (See Fig. 12–7.)

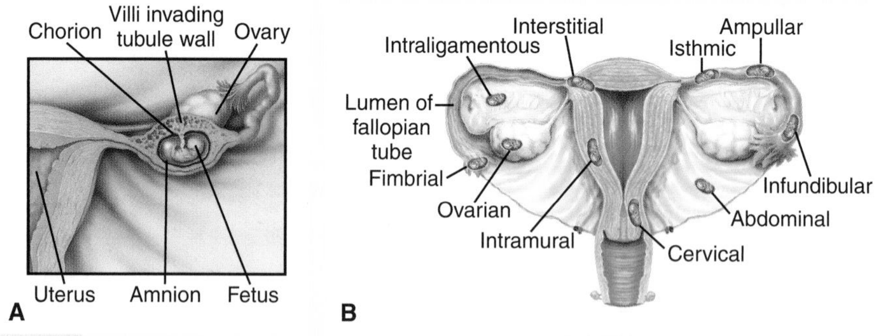

Figure 12-7 (A) Tubal pregnancy. (B) Other sites of ectopic pregnancy.

placenta previa
plă-SĔN-tă PRĒ-vē-ă

Obstetric complication in which the placenta is attached close to or covers the cervical canal and that results in bleeding during labor when the cervix dilates

Placenta previa is a leading cause of vaginal bleeding (spotting) that may lead to other complications. It may also necessitate a cesarean delivery.

It is time to review pathology, diseases, and conditions by completing Learning Activity 12-3.

Diagnostic, Surgical, and Therapeutic Procedures

This section introduces diagnostic, surgical, and therapeutic procedures used to diagnose and treat female reproductive disorders. Descriptions are provided, along with pronunciations and word analyses for selected terms.

Procedure	Description
Diagnostic	
amniocentesis ăm-nē-ō-sĔn-TĒ-sĭs *amni/o:* amnion (amniotic sac) *-centesis:* surgical puncture	Transabdominal puncture of the amniotic sac under ultrasound guidance using a needle (with the needle's position verified by US on a monitor screen) and syringe to remove amniotic fluid (See Fig. 12-8.) *Chemical and cytological studies of the sample obtained in amniocentesis detect genetic and biochemical disorders and fetal maturity. The procedure also enables transfusion of blood to the fetus and instillation of drugs for treating the fetus.* **Figure 12-8** Amniocentesis.
chorionic villus sampling (CVS) kor-ē-ŎN-ĭk VĬL-ŭs SĂM-plĭng	Sampling of placental tissues for prenatal diagnosis of potential genetic defects *CVS involves insertion of a catheter into the uterus to obtain the sample. The advantage of CVS over amniocentesis is that it can be undertaken in the first trimester of pregnancy.*
colposcopy kŏl-PŎS-kō-pē *colp/o:* vagina *-scopy:* visual examination	Visual examination of the vagina and cervix with an optical magnifying instrument (colposcope) *Colposcopy is used chiefly to identify areas of cervical dysplasia in women with abnormal Papanicolaou tests and as an aid in biopsy or excision procedures, including cautery, cryotherapy, and loop electrosurgical excision.*
cordocentesis kor-dō-sĕn-TĒ-sĭs	Diagnostic prenatal test in which a sample of the baby's blood is removed from the umbilical cord for testing; also called *percutaneous umbilical blood sampling (PUBS)* *Cord blood is evaluated in the laboratory to identify hemolytic diseases or genetic abnormalities.*

(continued)

Diagnostic, Surgical, and Therapeutic Procedures—cont'd

Procedure	Description
endometrial biopsy ĕn-dō-MĒ-trē-ăl BĪ-ŏp-sē *endo-:* in, within *metri:* uterus (womb); measure *-al:* pertaining to	Removal of a sample of uterine endometrium for microscopic study *Endometrial biopsy is commonly used in fertility assessment to confirm ovulation and as a diagnostic tool to determine the cause of dysfunctional and postmenopausal bleeding.*
insufflation ĭn-sŭ-FLĀ-shŭn	Delivery of pressurized air or gas into a cavity, chamber, or organ to allow visual examination, remove an obstruction, or apply medication *Insufflation increases the distance between structures so that the physician can see more clearly and better diagnose possible disorders.*
Papanicolaou (Pap) test pă-pă-NĪ-kō-lŏw	An exfoliative cytology test to detect abnormal cells that are scraped from the cervix, usually obtained during routine pelvic examination (See Fig. 12-9.) *A Pap test is commonly used to screen for and diagnose cervical cancer. It may also be used to evaluate cells from any organ, such as the pleura and peritoneum, to detect changes that indicate malignancy.* **Figure 12-9** Papanicolaou (Pap) test. (A) Insertion of speculum to expand the vaginal walls and reveal the cervix. (B) Cervix is exposed to obtain cells for Pap test. From Dillon, *Nursing Health Assessment,* 2nd ed. F.A. Davis, Philadelphia, 2007, pp. 634–635, with permission.
pelvimetry pĕl-VĬM-ĕ-trē *pelv/i:* pelvis *-metry:* act of measuring	Measurement of pelvic dimensions to determine whether the head of the fetus will be able to pass through the bony pelvis to allow vaginal delivery *Pelvimetry is performed manually, by x-ray, or by ultrasound, depending on the stage of the pregnancy. The size of the pelvic outlet determines whether or not the baby is delivered vaginally or by cesarean section.*

Diagnostic, Surgical, and Therapeutic Procedures—cont'd

Procedure	Description
Imaging	
hysterosalpingography (HSG) hĭs-tĕr-ō-săl-pĭn-GŎG-ră-fē *hyster/o:* uterus (womb) *salping/o:* tube (usually fallopian or eustachian [auditory] tube) *-graphy:* process of recording	Radiography and, usually, fluoroscopy of the uterus and uterine tubes (oviducts) following injection of a contrast medium *Hysterosalpingography helps determine pathology in the uterine cavity, evaluate tubal patency, and determine the cause of infertility.*
mammography măm-ŎG-ră-fē *mamm/o:* breast *-graphy:* process of recording	Radiographic examination of the breast to screen for breast cancer *Mammography detects tumors, cysts, and microcalcifications and may help locate a malignant lesion.*
transvaginal ultrasonography (TVUS) trănz-VĂJ-ĭ-năl ŭl-tră-sōn-ŎG-ră-fē *trans-:* through, across *vagin:* vagina *-al:* pertaining to	Ultrasonography of the pelvic area performed with a probe inserted into the vagina, which provides sharper images of pathological and normal structures within the pelvis
Surgical	
cerclage sĕr-KLĂZH	Suturing of the cervix to prevent it from dilating prematurely during pregnancy, thus decreasing the chance of a spontaneous abortion or preterm birth *Cerclage is sometimes referred to as the purse-string procedure. The sutures are removed before delivery.*
cesarean section (C-section) sē-SĀR-ē-ăn	Incision of the abdomen and uterus to remove the fetus; also called *C-section* *C-section is most commonly used in the event of cephalopelvic disproportion, presence of sexually transmitted disease, fetal distress, and breech presentation.*
colpocleisis kŏl-pō-KLĪ-sĭs *colp/o:* vagina *-cleisis:* closure	Surgical closure of the vaginal canal *Colpocleisis is used in elderly women who are no longer sexually active to reduce prolapse of the vagina.*
conization kŏn-ĭ-ZĀ-shŭn	Excision of a cone-shaped piece of tissue, such as mucosa of the cervix, for histological examination
cryosurgery krī-ō-SĔR-jer-ē	Process of freezing tissue to destroy cells; also called *cryocautery* *Cryosurgery is used for chronic cervical infections and erosions because offending organisms may be entrenched in cervical cells and glands. The process destroys these infected areas; in the healing process, normal cells are replenished.*

(continued)

Diagnostic, Surgical, and Therapeutic Procedures—cont'd

Procedure	Description

dilation and curettage (D&C)
dī-LĂ-sh ŭn, kū-r ĕ-TĂZH

Widening of the cervical canal with a dilator and scraping of the uterine endometrium with a curette

D&C obtains a sample for cytological examination of tissue, controls abnormal uterine bleeding, and treats incomplete abortion. (See Fig. 12-10.)

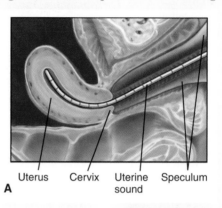

Uterus   Cervix   Uterine   Speculum
sound
A

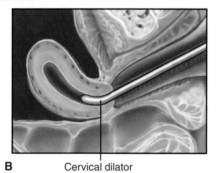 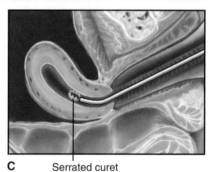

B   Cervical dilator   **C**   Serrated curet

Figure 12-10 Dilation and curettage. (A) Examination of the uterine cavity with a uterine sound. (B) Dilation of the cervix with a series of cervical dilators. (C) Curettage (scraping) of the uterine lining with a serrated uterine curet.

hysterectomy
hĭs-tĕr-ĔK-tō-mē
  hyster: uterus (womb)
  -ectomy: excision, removal

Excision of the uterus (See Fig. 12-11.)

Indications for hysterectomy include abnormalities of the uterus and cervix (cancer, severe dysfunctional bleeding, large or bleeding fibroid tumors, prolapse of the uterus, or severe endometriosis). The surgical approach may be abdominal or vaginal.

  subtotal

Hysterectomy in which the cervix, ovaries, and fallopian tubes remain

  total

Hysterectomy in which the cervix is removed but the ovaries and fallopian tubes remain; also called *complete hysterectomy*

  total plus bilateral
  salpingo-oophorectomy
    bī-LĂT-ĕr-ăl săl-pĭng-gō-ō-ŏf-ō-
    RĔK-tō-mē
      bi-: two
      later: side, to one side
      -al: pertaining to
      salping/o: tube (usually the fallopian
      or eustachian [auditory] tube)
      oophor: ovary
      -ectomy: excision, removal

Total (complete) hysterectomy, including removal of the uterus, cervix, fallopian tubes, and ovaries

Diagnostic, Surgical, and Therapeutic Procedures—cont'd

Procedure	Description

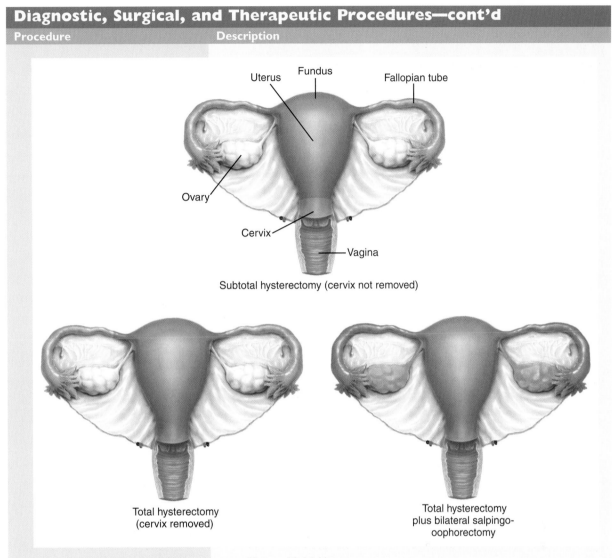

Subtotal hysterectomy (cervix not removed)

Uterus · Fundus · Fallopian tube · Ovary · Cervix · Vagina

Total hysterectomy (cervix removed)

Total hysterectomy plus bilateral salpingo-oophorectomy

Figure 12-11 Hysterectomy.

laparoscopy lăp-ăr-ŎS-kō-pē *lapar/o:* abdomen *-scopy:* visual examination	Visual examination of the abdominal cavity with a laparoscope through one or more small incisions in the abdominal wall, usually at the umbilicus (See Fig. 12-12, page 418.) *Laparoscopy has become a standard technique for many routine surgical procedures, including gynecological sterilization by fulguration of the oviducts and tubal ligation.*

(continued)

Diagnostic, Surgical, and Therapeutic Procedures—cont'd

Procedure	Description

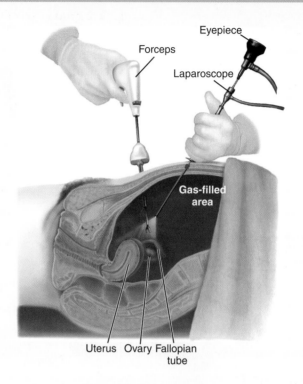

Figure 12-12 Laparoscopy.

lumpectomy
lŭm-PĔK-tō-mē

Excision of a small primary breast tumor (or "lump") and some of the normal tissue that surrounds it (See Fig. 12-13.)

In lumpectomy, lymph nodes may also be removed because they are located within the breast tissue taken during surgery. Typically, the patient will undergo radiation therapy after lumpectomy.

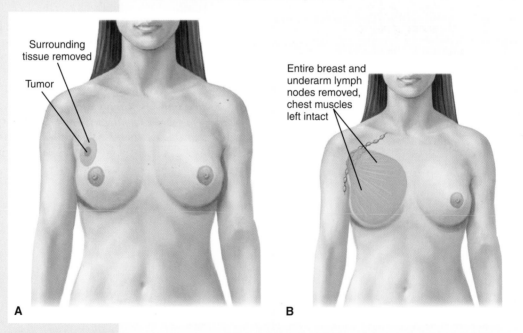

Figure 12-13 Lumpectomy and mastectomy. (A) Lumpectomy with the primary tumor in red and the surrounding tissue removed in pink. (B) Modified radical mastectomy.

Diagnostic, Surgical, and Therapeutic Procedures—cont'd

Procedure	Description
mammoplasty MĂM-ō-plăs-tē *mamm/o:* breast *-plasty:* surgical repair	Surgical reconstruction of the breast(s) to change the size, shape, or position
augmentation	Insertion of a breast prosthesis (filled with silicone gel or saline) beneath the skin or beneath the pectoralis major muscle *Augmentation surgery increases breast size or replaces a breast that has been surgically removed.*
reduction	Breast reduction to reduce the size of a large, pendulous breast *Breast reduction may be performed in conjunction with mastopexy, a surgery to uplift a sagging breast.*
mastectomy măs-TĔK-tō-mē *mast:* breast *-ectomy:* excision, removal	Removal of the breast
total (simple)	Excision of the entire breast, nipple, areola, and the involved overlying skin *In total mastectomy, lymph nodes are removed only if they are included in the breast tissue being removed.*
modified radical	Excision of the entire breast, including the lymph nodes in the underarm (axillary dissection) but with the chest muscles left intact (See Fig. 12-13B.) *Most women who have mastectomies today have modified radical mastectomies.*
radical	Excision of the entire breast, all underarm lymph nodes, and the chest wall muscles under the breast
reconstructive breast surgery	Creation of a breast-shaped mound to replace a breast that has been removed as a result of cancer or other disease *Reconstruction is commonly possible immediately following mastectomy so that the patient awakens from anesthesia with a breast mound already in place.*
tissue (skin) expansion	Common breast reconstruction technique in which a balloon expander is inserted beneath the skin and chest muscle, saline solution is gradually injected to increase size, and the expander is then replaced with a more permanent implant (See Fig. 12-14, page 420.)

(continued)

Diagnostic, Surgical, and Therapeutic Procedures—cont'd

Procedure	Description

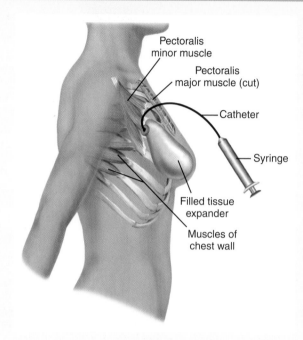

Figure 12-14 Tissue expander for breast reconstruction.

transverse rectus abdominis muscle (TRAM) flap

Surgical creation of a skin flap using skin and fat from the lower half of the abdomen, which is passed under the skin to the breast area; the abdominal tissue (flap) is then shaped into a natural-looking breast and sutured into place (See Fig. 12-15.)

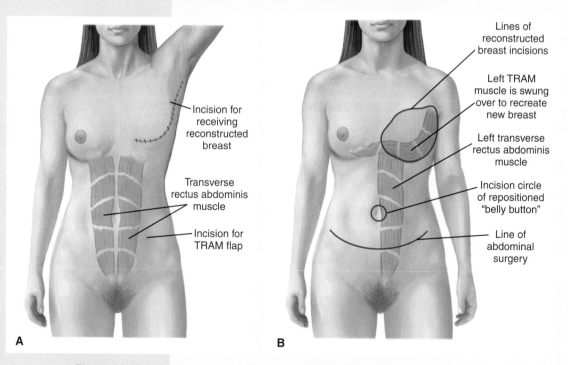

Figure 12-15 TRAM flap. (A) After mastectomy. (B) Process of TRAM reconstruction.

Diagnostic, Surgical, and Therapeutic Procedures—cont'd

Procedure	Description
tubal ligation TŪ-băl lī-GĀ-shŭn	Procedure that ties (ligates) the fallopian tubes to prevent pregnancy *Tubal ligation is a form of sterilization surgery usually performed during laparoscopy.*
Therapeutic	
intrauterine device (IUD) ĭn-tră-Ū-tĕr-ĭn	Small, T-shaped device inserted by a physician inside the uterus to prevent pregnancy *Two types of modern IUDs are available: a copper IUD, which releases copper particles to prevent pregnancy, and a hormonal IUD, which releases the hormone progestin to prevent pregnancy.*

Pharmacology

Hormone replacement therapy (HRT) is the use of synthetic or natural estrogens or a combination of estrogen and progestin to replace the decline or lack of natural hormones, a condition that accompanies hysterectomy and menopause. (See Table 12-2.) Estrogen may be administered orally, transdermally, by injection, or as a topical cream (to treat vaginal symptoms only). Other hormones, including oxytocics and prostaglandins, are used for obstetrical applications. In addition, pharmacological agents are available for birth control and family planning. These agents include oral contraceptives, implants, and spermicides.

Table 12-2	**Drugs Used to Treat Obstetrical and Gynecological Disorders**	

This table lists common drug classifications used to treat obstetric and gynecological disorders, along with their therapeutic actions and selected generic and trade names.

Classification	Therapeutic Action	Generic and *Trade* Names
antifungals ăn-tĭ-FŬNG-găls	Treat vaginal yeast infection by altering the yeast cell membrane or interfering with a metabolic process *Most antifungals used to treat vaginal yeast infections are applied topically as ointments, suppositories, or vaginal tablets. Fluconazole is used orally.*	**fluconazole** flū-KŎN-ă-zōl *Diflucan* **miconazole** mī-KŎN-ă-zōl *Monistat*
estrogens ĔS-trō-jĕns	Treat symptoms of menopause (hot flashes, vaginal dryness, fatigue) through hormone replacement therapy (HRT); may be given orally or topically; topical use may decrease risks *Long-term use of estrogen has been linked with an increased risk of thrombophlebitis and breast and endometrial cancers.*	**conjugated estrogens (oral only)** KŎN-jū-gā-tĕd ĔS-trō-jĕnz *Cenestin, Premarin* **estradiol** ĕs-tră-DĪ-ŏl *Estrace (oral), Climara (topical)*
oral contraceptives kŏn-tră-SĔP-tĭvs	Synthetic hormones used to prevent pregnancy and treat menstrual disorders *Oral contraceptives, or birth control pills, contain a combination of estrogen and progestin and are highly effective in preventing pregnancy if taken as directed.*	**desogestrel/ethinyl estradiol** dĕz-ō-JĔS-trăl, ĔTH-ĭ-nĭl ĕs-tră-DĪ-ŏl *Desogen, Ortho-Cept* **ethinyl estradiol/norgestrel** ĔTH-ĭ-nĭl ĕs-tră-DĪ-ŏl, nor-JĔS-trĕl *Lo/Ovral-28*
oxytocics ŏk-sē-TŌ-sĭks	Induce labor at term by increasing the strength and frequency of uterine contractions *Oxytocics are also used during the postpartum period to control bleeding after the expulsion of the placenta.*	**oxytocin** ŏk-sē-TŌ-sĭn *Pitocin*
prostaglandins PRŎS-tă-glănd-ĭns	Terminate pregnancy *Large doses of certain prostaglandins can cause the uterus to contract strongly enough to spontaneously abort a fetus.*	**dinoprostone** dī-nō-PRŎS-tōn *Prostin E2, Cervidil* **mifepristone** mī-fĕ-PRĬS-tōn *Mifeprex*
spermicides SPĔR-mĭ-sīds	Chemically destroy sperm by creating a highly acidic environment in the uterus *Spermicides are available in foam, gel, and suppository forms. They are used within the female vagina for contraception. When used alone, spermicides have a higher failure rate than other methods of birth control.*	**nonoxynol 9, octoxynol 9** nŏn-ŎK-sĭ-nŏl, ŏk-TŎKS-ĭ-nŏl *Semicid, Koromex, Ortho-Gynol*

Abbreviations

This section introduces female reproductive-related abbreviations and their meanings.

Abbreviation	Meaning	Abbreviation	Meaning
AUB	abnormal uterine bleeding	OB	obstetrics
C-section, CS	cesarean section	OCPs	oral contraceptive pills
CVS	chorionic villus sampling	Pap	Papanicolaou (test)
D&C	dilatation (dilation) and curettage	para 1, 2, 3 and so on	unipara, bipara, tripara (number of viable births)
DUB	dysfunctional uterine bleeding	PUBS	percutaneous umbilical blood sampling
GYN	gynecology	PID	pelvic inflammatory disease
HRT	hormone replacement therapy	STI	sexually transmitted infection
IUD	intrauterine device	TRAM	transverse rectus abdominis muscle (flap)
LMP	last menstrual period	TVUS	transvaginal ultrasonography

It is time to review procedures, pharmacology, and abbreviations by completing Learning Activity 12-4.

LEARNING ACTIVITIES

The activities that follow provide a review of the female reproductive system terms introduced in this chapter. Complete each activity and review your answers to evaluate your understanding of the chapter.

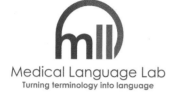

Medical Language Lab
Turning terminology into language

Visit the Medical Language Lab at *medicallanguagelab.com*. Use it to enhance your study and reinforcement of this chapter with the flash-card activity. We recommend that you complete the flash-card activity before starting Learning Activities 12-1 and 12-2.

Learning Activity 12-1
Medical Word Elements

Use the listed elements to build medical words. You may use the elements more than once.

Combining Forms		Suffixes		Prefixes
amni/o	oophor/o	-al	-plasty	dys-
cervic/o	perine/o	-arche	-poiesis	multi-
colp/o	salping/o	-centesis	-rrhaphy	pre-
galact/o		-cyesis	-rrhexis	primi-
hem/o		-gravida	-salpinx	pseudo-
hyster/o		-itis	-scopy	
men/o		-oma	-tocia	
nat/o		-para		

1. visual examination of the vagina _____
2. pertaining to (the time) before birth _____
3. difficult childbirth _____
4. rupture of the uterus _____
5. tumor of the ovary _____
6. inflammation of the cervix uteri (neck of the uterus) _____
7. surgical puncture of the amnion (amniotic sac) _____
8. suture of the perineum _____
9. surgical repair of a fallopian tube _____
10. pregnant woman (for the) first (time) _____
11. false pregnancy _____
12. blood in a fallopian tube _____
13. to bear many (offspring) _____
14. beginning of menses or menstruation _____
15. formation or production of milk _____

✓ *Check your answers in Appendix A. Review any material that you did not answer correctly.*

Correct Answers _____ X 6.67 = _____ % Score

Learning Activity 12-2
Building Medical Words

Use *gynec/o* (woman, female) to build words that mean

 1. disease (specific to) women _____
 2. physician who specializes in diseases of the female _____

Use *cervic/o* (neck; cervix uteri) to build words that mean

 3. inflammation of the cervix uteri and vagina _____
 4. pertaining to the cervix uteri and bladder _____

Use *colp/o* (vagina) to build words that mean

 5. instrument used to examine the vagina _____
 6. visual examination of the vagina _____

Use *vagin/o* (vagina) to build words that mean

 7. inflammation of the vagina _____
 8. herniation of the vagina _____

Use *hyster/o* (uterus) to build words that mean

 9. myoma of the uterus _____
10. disease of the uterus _____
11. radiography of the uterus and oviducts _____

Use *metr/o* (uterus) to build words that mean

12. hemorrhage from the uterus _____
13. inflammation around the uterus _____

Use *uter/o* (uterus) to build words that mean

14. herniation of the uterus _____
15. relating to the uterus and cervix _____
16. pertaining to the uterus and bladder _____

Use *oophor/o* (ovary) to build words that mean

17. inflammation of an ovary _____
18. inflammation of an ovary and oviduct _____

Use *salping/o* (fallopian tube) to build words that mean

19. herniation of a fallopian tube _____

20. radiography of uterine tubes _____

Build surgical words that mean

21. fixation of (a displaced) ovary _____

22. excision of the uterus and ovaries _____

23. suturing the perineum _____

24. excision of the uterus, oviducts, and ovaries _____

25. puncture of the amnion (amniotic sac) _____

✓ *Check your answers in Appendix A. Review any material that you did not answer correctly.*

Correct Answers _____ X 4 = _____ % Score

Learning Activity 12-3
Diseases and Conditions

Match the terms with the definitions in the numbered list.

atresia	*dystocia*	*menarche*	*primipara*
breech	*eclampsia*	*metrorrhagia*	*pyosalpinx*
choriocarcinoma	*endocervicitis*	*oligomenorrhea*	*retroversion*
Down syndrome	*fibroids*	*pathogen*	*sterility*
dyspareunia	*gestation*	*primigravida*	*septicemia*

1. accumulation of pus in a uterine tube _____
2. woman who has had one pregnancy that has resulted in a viable offspring _____
3. average pregnancy; approximately 9 months _____
4. inability of the female to become pregnant _____
5. uterus that is tipped backward from its normal position _____
6. inflammation of the mucous lining of the cervix uteri _____
7. difficult labor or childbirth _____
8. congenital absence of a normal body opening, such as the vagina _____
9. trisomy 21 _____
10. bacteria in the blood that commonly occurs with severe infection _____
11. occurrence of pain during sexual intercourse _____
12. irregular uterine bleeding between menstrual periods _____
13. beginning of menstrual function _____
14. benign uterine tumor composed of muscle and fibrous tissue _____
15. infrequent menstrual flow _____
16. abnormal delivery in which fetal buttocks or feet present first rather than the head _____
17. most serious form of toxemia during pregnancy _____
18. malignant neoplasm of the uterus or at the site of an ectopic pregnancy _____
19. disease-producing organism _____
20. woman during her first pregnancy _____

✓ *Check your answers in Appendix A. Review any material that you did not answer correctly.*

Correct Answers _____ X 5 = _____ % Score

Learning Activity 12-4

Procedures, Pharmacology, and Abbreviations

Match the terms with the definitions in the numbered list.

amniocentesis	cordocentesis	hysterosalpingography	oxytocins
antifungals	cryosurgery	IUD	Pap test
cerclage	episiotomy	laparoscopy	PID
chorionic villus sampling	estrogens	lumpectomy	prostaglandins
colpocleisis	hysterectomy	OCPs	tubal ligation

1. cytological study of tissue to detect cancer cells _____

2. radiography of the uterus and oviducts after injection of a contrast medium _____

3. puncture of the amniotic sac to remove amniotic fluid for biochemical and cytological study _____

4. drugs used to treat vaginal yeast infections _____

5. surgical closure of the vaginal canal _____

6. diagnostic test in which a sample of baby's blood is removed from the umbilical cord for testing _____

7. suturing the cervix to prevent it from dilating prematurely during pregnancy _____

8. tying uterine tubes to prevent pregnancy _____

9. birth control pills taken orally _____

10. examination of the abdominal cavity using an endoscope _____

11. incision of the perineum to facilitate childbirth _____

12. inflammation of the uterus, fallopian tubes, ovaries, and adjacent pelvic structures, usually caused by bacterial infection _____

13. test to detect chromosomal abnormalities that can be done earlier than amniocentesis _____

14. hormone replacement to reduce adverse symptoms of menopause _____

15. agents used to induce labor and rid the uterus of an unexpelled placenta or a fetus that has died _____

16. freezing tissue to destroy cells _____

17. birth control method in which an object is placed inside the uterus to prevent pregnancy _____

18. excision of the uterus _____

19. excision of a small primary breast tumor _____

20. agents used to terminate pregnancy _____

✓ *Check your answers in Appendix A. Review material that you did not answer correctly.*

Correct Answers _____ X 5 = _____ % Score

DOCUMENTING HEALTH-CARE ACTIVITIES

This section provides practical application activities in the form of exercises to help students develop skills in documenting patient care. First, read the medical report. Then complete the activities and exercises that follow.

Documenting Health-Care Activity 12-1
SOAP Note: Primary Herpes 1 Infection

Progress Notes

O'Malley, Roberta   09/01/xx

S: This 24-year-old patient started having some sore areas around the labia, both rt and lt side. She stated that the last few days she started having a brownish discharge. She has pruritus and pain of her vulvar area with adenopathy, p.m. fever, and blisters. Apparently, her partner had a cold sore and they had oral-genital sex. Patient has been using condoms since last seen in April. She has not missed any OCPs. LMP 5/15/xx.

O: Patient has what looks like herpes lesions and ulcers all over vulva and introitus area. Rt labia appears as an ulcerlike lesion; it appears to be almost like an infected follicle. Speculum inserted, a brown discharge noted. GC screen, chlamydia screen, and genital culture obtained. Wet prep revealed monilial forms. Viral culture obtained from the ulcerlike lesion on the right labia.

A: Primary herpes 1 infection; will rule out other infectious etiologies.

P: Patient advised to return next week for consultation with Dr. Abdu.

Joanna Masters, MD
Joanna Masters, MD

JM:st

Terminology

The terms listed in the table that follows are taken from *SOAP Note: Primary Herpes 1 Infection.* Use a medical dictionary such as *Taber's Cyclopedic Medical Dictionary,* the appendices of this book, or other resources to define each term. Then review the pronunciation for each term and practice by reading the medical record aloud.

Term	Definition
adenopathy ăd-ĕ-NŎP-ă-thē	
chlamydia klă-MĬD-ē-ă	
GC screen	
herpes lesions HĔR-pēz LĒ-zhŭnz	
introitus ĭn-TRŌ-ĭ-tŭs	
labia LĀ-bē-ă	
LMP	
monilial mō-NĬL-ē-ăl	
OCPs	
pruritus proo-RĪ-tŭs	
R/O	
vulvar VŬL-văr	
wet prep	

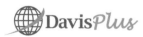

Visit the *Medical Terminology Systems* online resource center at Davis*Plus* to practice pronunciation and reinforce the meanings of the terms in this medical report.

Critical Thinking

Review *SOAP Note: Primary Herpes 1 Infection* to answer the questions.

1. Did the patient have any discharge? If so, describe it.

   _____

   _____

   _____

   _____

2. What type of discomfort did the patient experience around the vulvar area?

   _____

   _____

   _____

   _____

3. Has the patient been taking her oral contraceptive pills regularly?

   _____

   _____

   _____

   _____

4. Where was the viral culture obtained?

   _____

   _____

   _____

   _____

5. Even though the patient's partner used a condom, how do you think the patient became infected with herpes?

   _____

   _____

   _____

   _____

Documenting Health-Care Activity 12-2

Preoperative Consultation: Menometrorrhagia

Physician Center

2422 Rodeo Drive ▪ ▪ Sun City, USA 12345 ▪ ▪ (555)788–2427

Preoperative Consultation

Mazza, Rosemary   July 2, 20xx

CHIEF COMPLAINT: Dysmenorrhea and night sweats

HISTORY OF PRESENT ILLNESS: Patient is a 43-year-old gravida 2, para 1 with multiple small uterine fibroids, irregular menses twice a month, family history of ovarian cancer, benign endometrial biopsy, normal Pap, normal mammogram, and normal thyroid function tests. Negative cervical cultures. She has completed childbearing and desires definitive treatment of endometrial ablation, hormonal regulation.

SURGICAL HISTORY: Cesarean section, therapeutic abortion, and cholecystectomy

ASSESSMENT: This is a patient with menometrorrhagia who declines palliative treatment and desires definitive treatment in the form of a hysterectomy.

PLAN: The plan is to perform a laparoscopic-assisted vaginal hysterectomy because the patient has essentially no uterine prolapse and desires her ovaries to be taken out. She desires to be started on Premarin in the postoperative period. She has been counseled concerning the risks of surgery, including injury to bowel or bladder, infection, and bleeding. She voices understanding and agrees to the plan to perform a laparoscopic-assisted vaginal hysterectomy and bilateral salpingo-oophorectomy.

Julia Masters, MD
Julia Masters, MD

JM:st

Terminology

The terms listed in the table that follows are taken from *Preoperative Consultation: Menometrorrhagia.*
Use a medical dictionary such as *Taber's Cyclopedic Medical Dictionary,* the appendices of this book,
or other resources to define each term. Then review the pronunciation for each term and practice by
reading the medical record aloud.

Term	Definition
ablation ăb-LĀ-shŭn	
benign bē-NĪN	
cesarean section sĕ-SĀR-ē-ăn	
cholecystectomy kō-lē-sĭs- TĔK-tō-mē	
dysmenorrhea dĭs-mĕn-ō-RĒ-ă	
endometrial biopsy ĕn-dō-MĒ-trē-ăl BĪ-ŏp-sē	
fibroids FĪ-broyds	
gravida 2 GRĂV-ĭ-dă	
hysterectomy hĭs-tĕr-ĔK-tō-mē	
laparoscopic lăp-ă-rō-SKŎP-ĭk	
mammogram MĂM-ō-grăm	
menometrorrhagia mĕn-ō-mĕt-rō- RĀ-jē-ă	
palliative PĂL-ē-ā-tĭv	

(continued)

Term	Definition
para I PĂR-ă	
postoperative pōst-ŎP-ĕr-ă-tĭv	
Premarin PRĔM-ă-rĭn	
salpingo- oophorectomy săl-pĭng-gō-ō-ŏf-ō- RĔK-tō-mē	
therapeutic abortion thĕr-ă-PŪ-tĭk ă-BOR-shŭn	
thyroid function test THĪ-royd	

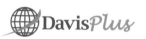

Visit the *Medical Terminology Systems* online resource center at Davis*Plus* to practice pronunciation and reinforce the meanings of the terms in this medical report.

Critical Thinking

Review the medical record *Preoperative Consultation: Menometrorrhagia* to answer the questions.

1. How many pregnancies did this patient have? How many viable infants did she deliver?

_____

_____

_____

_____

2. What is a therapeutic abortion?

_____

_____

_____

_____

3. Why did the physician propose to perform a hysterectomy?

_____

_____

_____

_____

4. What is a vaginal hysterectomy?

_____

_____

_____

_____

5. Does the surgeon plan to remove one or both ovaries and fallopian tubes?

_____

_____

_____

_____

6. Why do you think the physician will use the laparoscope to perform the hysterectomy?

_____

_____

_____

_____

Constructing Chart Notes

To construct chart notes, replace the italicized and boldfaced terms in each of the two case studies with one of the listed medical terms.

dysmenorrhea	menopause	needle biopsy
gravida 3, para 3	menorrhagia	nullipara
mammography	metrorrhagia	uterine fibroids
menarche		

Ms. T. is a 32-year-old female who presents at our office with complaints of bleeding. Her past reproductive history includes (1) *3 pregnancies resulting in 3 live births.* She is now experiencing (2) *midcycle bleeding* and complains of (3) *excessively heavy periods*, commonly with blood clots. The patient further complains of (4) *severe cramps, headache, and tension* during her period. She is scheduled for a complete pelvic examination and a transvaginal ultrasound to establish the diagnosis of (5) *benign tumors of the uterus.*

1. _____
2. _____
3. _____
4. _____
5. _____

Mrs. D. presents with a complaint of a small lump in her right breast and is concerned that this may be cancer. Her mother and sister are both cancer survivors. Besides a family history of the disease, she has several risk factors, including (6) *never giving birth* and early (7) *onset of menstruation.* She admits that she went through the (8) *change of life* 3 years ago at age 53. She is scheduled for (9) *breast x-ray* and (10) *an examination of a small piece of tissue obtained using a needle*, which will be performed under ultrasound guidance.

6. _____
7. _____
8. _____
9. _____
10. _____

✓ *Check your answers in Appendix A. Review any material that you did not answer correctly.*

Correct Answers _____ X 10 = _____ % Score

CHAPTER

Male Reproductive System

13

Chapter Outline

Objectives

Upon completion of this chapter, you will be able to:

- Locate and describe the structures of the male reproductive system.

- Describe the functional relationship between the male reproductive system and other body systems.

- Pronounce, spell, and build words related to the male reproductive system.

- Describe diseases, conditions, and procedures related to the male reproductive system.

- Explain pharmacology related to the treatment of male reproductive disorders.

- Demonstrate your knowledge of this chapter by completing the learning and documenting health-care activities.

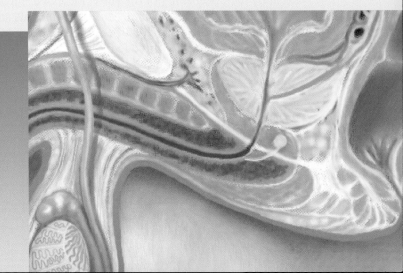

Anatomy and Physiology

The male reproductive system produces, maintains, and transports sperm, the male sex cell required for fertilization of the female egg. It is also responsible for developing and maintaining male secondary sex characteristics. (See Fig. 13-1.)

Anatomy and Physiology Key Terms

This section introduces important terms, along with their definitions and pronunciations. The key terms are highlighted in color in the Anatomy and Physiology section. Word analyses for selected terms are also provided. Pronounce the term, and place a check mark in the box after you do so.

Term	Definition
gamete GĂM-ēt ☐	Reproductive cell (ovum or sperm) that contains one-half of the chromosomes required to produce an offspring of the species
libido lĭ-BĒ-dō ☐	Psychological and physical drive for sexual activity
semen SĒ-mĕn ☐	Fluid containing sperm and secretions from the prostate and other structures of the male reproductive system; also called *seminal fluid*
sphincter SFĬNGK-tĕr ☐	Ringlike muscle that opens and closes a body opening to allow or restrict passage through the structure
testosterone tĕs-TŎS-tĕr-ōn ☐	Androgenic hormone responsible for the development of the male sex organs, including the penis, testicles, scrotum, and prostate *Testosterone is also responsible for the development of secondary sex characteristics (musculature, hair patterns, thickened vocal cords, and so forth.).*

Pronunciation Help	Long Sound	ā — rate	ē — rebirth	ī — isle	ō — over	ū — unite
	Short Sound	ă — apple	ĕ — ever	ĭ — it	ŏ — not	ŭ — cut

Male Reproductive Structures

The primary male reproductive organ consists of two (1) **testes** (singular, **testis**) located in the (2) **scrotum,** an external sac lying behind and below the penis. The muscular wall of the scrotum allows for the control of temperature of the testes. It moves the testes closer to the body for warmth and farther from the body for cooling. The testes produce the hormone **testosterone,** which enables development of secondary sex characteristics, including the growth of facial and body hair, deepening of the voice, increased muscle mass, and so forth. It also plays an important role in **libido.** Within the testes are numerous small tubes that twist and coil to form (3) **seminiferous tubules,** which produce sperm, the male **gamete.** Lying over the superior surface of each testis is a single, tightly coiled tube called the (4) **epididymis.** This structure stores sperm after it leaves the seminiferous tubules. The epididymis is the first duct through which sperm passes after its production in the testes. During ejaculation, the epididymis contracts, expelling sperm into the

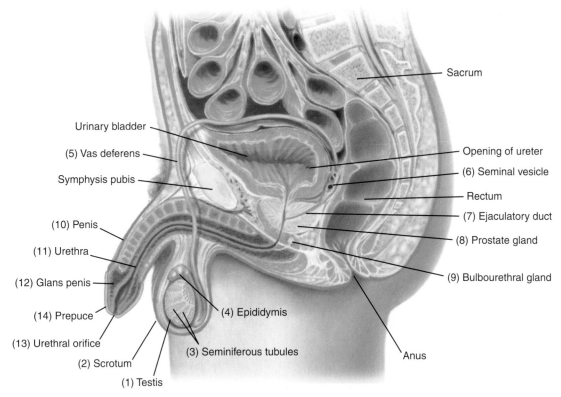

Sacrum

Urinary bladder

(5) Vas deferens

Symphysis pubis

Opening of ureter

(6) Seminal vesicle

Rectum

(7) Ejaculatory duct

(8) Prostate gland

(10) Penis

(11) Urethra

(12) Glans penis

(14) Prepuce

(13) Urethral orifice

(9) Bulbourethral gland

(4) Epididymis

(2) Scrotum

(3) Seminiferous tubules

Anus

(1) Testis

Figure 13-1 Midsagittal section of the male reproductive structures shown through the pelvic cavity.

(5) **vas deferens (seminal duct** or **ductus deferens),** a narrow tube that passes through the inguinal canal into the abdominal cavity. The vas deferens extends over the top and down the posterior surface of the bladder, where it joins the (6) **seminal vesicle.** The seminal vesicle contains nutrients that support sperm viability and produces approximately 60% of the **semen** (seminal fluid) that is ultimately ejaculated during sexual intercourse **(coitus).** The union of the vas deferens with the duct from the seminal vesicle forms the (7) **ejaculatory duct.** The ejaculatory duct joins to the urethra as it passes at an angle through the (8) **prostate gland,** a triple-lobed organ fused to the base of the bladder. The prostate gland secretes a thin, alkaline substance that accounts for about 30% of seminal fluid. Its alkalinity helps protect sperm from the acidic environments of the male urethra and the female vagina. Two pea-shaped structures, the (9) **bulbourethral (Cowper) glands,** are located below the prostate and are connected by a small duct to the urethra. The bulbourethral glands provide additional alkaline fluid that neutralizes any residual acidity in the male urethra to further assist in sperm viability. The (10) **penis** is the male organ of copulation. It is cylindrical and composed of erectile tissue that becomes rigid and erect upon sexual arousal. The penis encloses the (11) **urethra** that expels both **semen** and urine from the body. During ejaculation, the **sphincter** at the base of the bladder closes, stopping urine from being expelled with semen while also preventing semen from entering the bladder. The enlarged tip of the penis, the (12) **glans penis,** contains the (13) **urethral orifice (meatus)** through which urine and semen exit the body. The glans penis contains a number of highly sensitive nerve endings. A movable hood of skin, the (14) **prepuce (foreskin),** covers the glans penis.

Anatomy Review: Male Reproductive System

To review the anatomy of the male reproductive system, label the illustration using the listed terms.

bulbourethral gland   prepuce   testis

ejaculatory duct   prostate gland   urethra

epididymis   scrotum   urethral orifice

glans penis   seminal vesicle   vas deferens

penis   seminiferous tubules

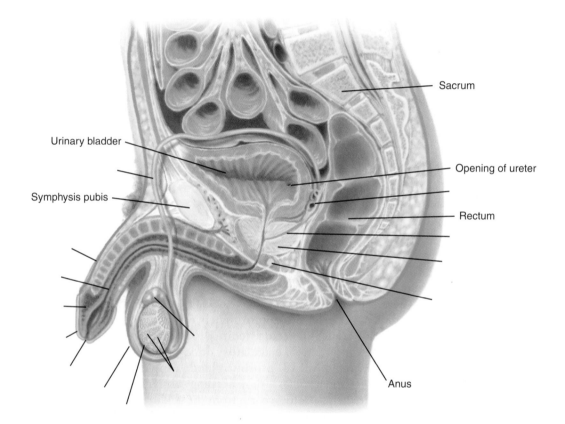

Sacrum

Urinary bladder

Opening of ureter

Symphysis pubis

Rectum

Anus

 Check your answers by referring to Figure 13-1 on page 441. Review material that you did not answer correctly.

CONNECTING BODY SYSTEMS—MALE REPRODUCTIVE SYSTEM

The main function of the male reproductive systems is to enable sexual reproduction. Specific functional relationships between the male reproductive system and other body systems are discussed here.

Blood, Lymphatic, and Immune
- The male reproductive system secretes testosterone into the extracellular fluids of the blood, lymphatic, and immune system for delivery throughout the body.
- The male reproductive system relies on increased blood supply to support the erectile tissue needed for copulation.

Cardiovascular
- Male hormones are transported through-out the body by the vascular system.
- Increased heart rate maintains the sexual excitement needed for ejaculation.

Digestive
- The male reproductive structures rely on a continuous supply of food and nourish-ment for proper functioning of the organs of reproduction.
- Male reproductive activities require food and nourishment for sexual behavior.

Endocrine
- The gonads produce hormones that provide feedback to influence pituitary function.
- Hormones produce and regulate the de-velopment of secondary sex characteristics.

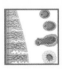

Female Reproductive
- The male reproductive structures pro-duce and deliver sperm, the cell that pro-vides one-half of the genetic complement required for the development of a fetus.
- The male organs of reproduction work in conjunction with the female reproductive system to enable fertilization of the ovum.

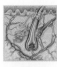

Integumentary
- Male hormones produce facial and body hair growth consistent with maleness.

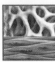

Musculoskeletal
- Male hormones produce skeletal and muscular structures consistent with a larger body frame than that normally found in females.

Nervous
- The male reproductive structures rely on the nervous system to innervate the organs responsible for copulation.
- Mature male reproductive activities are regulated by the emotional aspects of the nervous system, especially the brain.

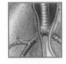

Respiratory
- The male reproductive system relies on the increased respiratory activity required for sexual activity.
- The male organs of reproduction require a constant supply of oxygen and the removal of waste gases for healthy functioning.
- The male reproductive system causes laryngeal changes, resulting in a deepening of the voice.

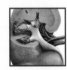

Urinary
- The male reproductive system and the urinary system share common structures.
- Waste substances produced by the male reproductive organs are removed by the urinary system.

Medical Word Elements

This section introduces combining forms, suffixes, and prefixes related to the male reproductive system. Word analyses are also provided. From the information provided, complete the meaning of the medical words in the right-hand column. The first one is completed for you.

Element	Meaning	Word Analysis
Combining Forms		
andr/o	male	**andr/o**/gen/ic (ăn-drō-JĔN-ĭk): *pertaining to maleness* *gen:* forming, producing, origin *-ic:* pertaining to *Androgenic hormones include all natural or synthetic compounds that stimulate or maintain male characteristics. The most common androgenic hormone is testosterone.*
balan/o	glans penis	**balan/o**/plasty (BĂL-ă-nō-plăs-tē): _____ *-plasty:* surgical repair
crypt/o	hidden	**crypt**/orchid/ism (krĭpt-OR-kĭd-ĭzm): _____ *orchid:* testis (plural, testes) *-ism:* condition *Cryptorchidism, also called cryptorchism, is the failure of the testes to descend into the scrotum and is usually a congenital disorder.*
epididym/o	epididymis	**epididym/o**/tomy (ĕp-ĭ-dĭd-ĭ-MŎT-ō-mē): _____ *-tomy:* incision
genit/o	genitalia	**genit/o**/urin/ary (jĕn-ĭ-tō-ŪR-ĭ-nār-ē): _____ *-urin:* urine, urinary tract *-ary:* pertaining to
gonad/o	gonads, sex glands	**gonad/o**/pathy (gŏn-ă-DŎP-ă-thē): _____ *-pathy:* disease
gon/o	seed (ovum or spermatozoon)	**gon/o**/rrhea (gŏn-ō-RĒ-ă): _____ *-rrhea:* discharge, flow *Characteristic of gonorrhea is a discharge of pus, mistakenly believed to be sperm in the early days of medicine.*
olig/o	scanty	**olig/o**/sperm/ia (ŏl-ĭ-gō-SPĔR-mē-ă): _____ *sperm:* spermatozoa, sperm cells *-ia:* condition *Oligospermia is a low concentration of sperm in the semen and may be a cause of male infertility.*
orch/o	testis (plural, testes)	**orch**/itis (or-KĪ-tĭs): _____ *-itis:* inflammation *A common cause of orchitis in young males is a mumps infection.*
orchi/o		**orchi**/algia (or-kē-ĂL-jē-ă): _____ *-algia:* pain
orchid/o		**orchid/o**/rrhaphy (or-kĭ-DOR-ă-fē): _____ *-rrhaphy:* suture

Medical Word Elements—cont'd

Element	Meaning	Analysis
test/o		**test**/algia (tĕs-TĂL-jē-ă): _____ _-algia:_ pain
perine/o	perineum (area between scrotum [or vulva in the female] and anus)	**perine**/al (pĕr-ĭ-NĒ-ăl): _____ _-al:_ pertaining to
prostat/o	prostate gland	**prostat/o**/megaly (prŏs-tă-tō-MĔG-ă-lē): _____ _-megaly:_ enlargement
spermat/o	spermatozoa, sperm cells	**spermat/o**/cele (spĕr-MĂT-ō-sēl): _____ _-cele:_ hernia, swelling *A spermatocele is usually an epididymal cyst, commonly containing sperm.*
sperm/o		**sperm**/ic (SPĔR-mĭk): _____ _-ic:_ pertaining to
varic/o	dilated vein	**varic/o**/cele (VĂR-ĭ-kō-sēl): _____ _-cele:_ hernia, swelling *Varicocele is a dilation of the veins of the spermatic cord, the structure that supports the testicles.*
vas/o	vessel; vas deferens; duct	**vas**/ectomy (văs-ĔK-tō-mē): _____ _-ectomy:_ excision, removal *Bilateral vasectomy is a surgical procedure to produce sterility in the male.*
vesicul/o	seminal vesicle	**vesicul**/itis (vĕ-sĭk-ū-LĪ-tĭs): _____ _-itis:_ inflammation
Suffixes		
-cide	killing	sperm/i/**cide** (SPĔR-mĭ-sīd): _____ *sperm/i:* spermatozoa, sperm cells *Spermicide is also called spermaticide.*
-genesis	forming, producing, origin	spermat/o/**genesis** (spĕr-măt-ō-JĔN-ĕ-sĭs): _____ *spermat/o:* sperm
-ism	condition	an/orch/**ism** (ăn-OR-kĭzm): _____ *an-:* without, not *orch:* testis (plural, testes) *Anorchism is the congenital or acquired absence of one or both testes.*
-spadias	slit, fissure	hypo/**spadias** (hī-pō-SPĀ-dē-ăs): _____ *hypo-:* under, below *Hypospadias is a congenital defect in which the urethra opens on the underside of the glans penis instead of the tip.*

(continued)

Medical Word Elements—cont'd

Element	Meaning	Analysis
Prefixes		
brachy-	short	**brachy**/therapy (brăk-ē-THĔR-ă-pē): _____ –*therapy:* treatment *In brachytherapy, radioactive seeds are implanted directly into the malignant tissue.*
epi-	above, upon	**epi**/spadias (ĕp-ĭ-SPĀ-dē-ăs): _____ –*spadias:* slit, fissure

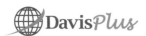 Visit the *Medical Terminology Systems* online resource center at Davis*Plus* for an audio exercise of the terms in this table. Other activities are also available to reinforce content.

 It is time to review medical word elements by completing Learning Activities 13-1 and 13-2.

Disease Focus

Diseases of the male reproductive system include reproductive disorders, congenital abnormalities, diseases and infections, and various types of cancers. Signs and symptoms commonly include pain, especially during urination; erectile dysfunction; and loss of libido. Performance of a complete evaluation of the genitalia, reproductive history, and past and present genitourinary infections and disorders is necessary to identify disorders associated with male reproductive structures.

For diagnosis, treatment, and management of male reproductive disorders, the medical services of a specialist may be warranted. **Urology** is the branch of medicine concerned with the male reproductive system and urinary disorders in males and females. The physician who specializes in diagnosis and treatment of genitourinary disorders is known as a **urologist.**

Sexually Transmitted Infections

Sexually transmitted infections (STIs), also called **sexually transmitted diseases (STDs),** include any contagious disease acquired during sexual activity with an infected partner. In the United States, the widespread occurrence of STIs is regarded as epidemic. The Centers for Disease Control estimates that there are nearly 20 million new STIs annually, and half of these are among young adults between 15 and 24 years old. Because genital warts, genital herpes, and trichomonas infections are not routinely reported, the current statistics of STIs captures only a fraction of the actual number of these cases. Many STIs can lead to severe reproductive problems, including sterility and infertility in males and females and ectopic pregnancy, preterm delivery, and infection transmitted to the newborn during delivery in females. In addition, many STIs increase the risk of acquiring HIV infection. (See Chapter 9 for a discussion of HIV infection.)

Gonorrhea

Gonorrhea is caused by the bacterium *Neisseria gonorrheae.* It involves the mucosal surface of the genitourinary tract and can also involve the rectum and pharynx. This disease spreads through sexual intercourse and through orogenital and anogenital contact. The most common symptoms of gonorrhea include pain on urination **(dysuria)** and a white discharge **(leukorrhea).** Left untreated, the disease may infect the bladder **(cystitis)** and inflame joints **(arthritis).** In males, gonorrhea can cause epididymitis that leads to infertility or scarring inside the urethra, making urination difficult. Many women are asymptomatic; however, when symptoms are present, they include a vaginal discharge or pelvic pain. Scars may develop in the reproductive tubes and cause infertility. The organism can infect the eyes of the newborn during vaginal delivery, leading to blindness. As a precaution, physicians instill silver nitrate in the eyes of all newborns immediately after delivery as a preventive measure to ensure that this infection does not occur. Both sex partners require treatment for gonorrhea because the infection can recur. The usual treatment is antibiotics.

Chlamydia

Chlamydia, caused by infection with the bacterium ***Chlamydia trachomatis,*** is the most prevalent and one of the most damaging STIs in the United States. It is called the "silent disease" because symptoms are commonly absent or mild, and the disease remains untreated until there is irreversible damage to the reproductive structures. If symptoms are present, males produce a whitish discharge from the penis. Inflammation of epididymis **(epididymitis)** can cause pain and swelling in the scrotum. In women, there is a mucopurulent discharge and inflammation of the cervix uteri **(cervicitis).** During the birth process, chlamydia may spread to the newborn baby and cause conjunctivitis or pneumonia. Antibiotics are effective in treating chlamydia infections. Screening for other STIs is important because chlamydia places the individual at higher risk of having other STIs, including gonorrhea and HIV.

Syphilis

Although less common than gonorrhea, syphilis is the more serious of the two diseases. It is caused by the bacterium ***Treponema pallidum.*** If left untreated, syphilis may become a chronic, infectious, multisystemic disease.

Syphilis manifests in three distinct stages. In primary syphilis, a painless sore, called a **chancre** appears 3 to 90 days after exposure. In secondary syphilis, a body rash that that commonly occurs on the palms of the hands and soles of the feet appears 4 to 10 weeks after exposure. A latency period of several years usually follows when sign and symptoms are absent or very mild; however, the individual is still infectious. Tertiary syphilis develops 3 to 15 years after exposure when the disease spreads throughout the body, especially in the nervous and cardiovascular systems. Early treatment is very effective, sometimes with just a single injection. Without treatment, the disease becomes life-threatening, causing blindness, stroke, mental disorders, and eventually, death.

Genital Herpes

Genital herpes causes red, blisterlike, painful lesions in the genital area that closely resemble fever blisters or cold sores that appear on the lips and around the mouth. Although genital herpes and oral herpes are caused by the herpes simplex virus (HSV), genital herpes is associated with type 2 (HSV-2), and oral herpes is associated with type 1 (HSV-1). Regardless, both forms can cause oral and genital infections through oral-genital sexual activity. Fluid in the blisters in genital herpes is highly infectious and contains the active virus. However, this disease is communicable even when the blisters are not present, through a phenomenon called *viral shedding.* In men, lesions appear on the glans, foreskin, or penile shaft. In females, lesions appear in the vaginal area, buttocks, and thighs. Individuals with a herpes infection may have only one episode or may have repeated attacks that usually lessen in severity over the years. The disease may spread to a baby during the birth process and, although rare, may lead to death of the infant. Antiviral medication can relieve pain and discomfort during an outbreak by healing the sores more quickly. However, there is no cure available for this disease.

Genital Warts

Genital warts **(condylomata, condylomas)** are caused by one or more of the many different human papillomavirus (HPV) strains. The warts may be very small and barely visible or may be large and appear in clusters. HPV can spread from one person to another during skin-to-skin contact and does not require sexual activity. The warts can also spread from one part of the body to another. In males, the lesions commonly appear on the penis or around the rectum. In females, the lesions commonly appear on the vulva, in the vagina, or on the cervix.

Some high-risk strains of HPV are associated with anal and penile cancer in males and vaginal and cervical cancer in females. Females diagnosed with high-risk strains of HPV require regular Pap smears. HPV vaccines are available and protect against the high-risk strains. To be effective, young adults require vaccination before they begin engaging in sexual activity.

Many warts disappear without treatment, but there is no way to determine which ones will resolve. When treatment is required, the usual method is surgical excision or freezing the wart.

Trichomoniasis

Trichomoniasis, caused by the protozoan *Trichomonas vaginalis,* affects males and females but symptoms are more common in females. When symptoms are present in males, they include irritation inside the penis, mild discharge, or slight burning during urination **(dysuria)** or ejaculation. In women, trichomonas causes vaginitis, urethritis, and cystitis with discomfort during urination or intercourse. Often there is a frothy, yellow-green vaginal discharge with a strong odor and irritation or itching of the vulva. Both sexual partners require treatment because reinfection is possible.

Oncology

Prostate cancer is one of the most common forms of cancer among men, second only to skin cancer. With early diagnosis and treatment, the prognosis for long-term survival is excellent.

In the United States, men younger than age 50 rarely develop prostate cancer. However, the incidence dramatically increases with age. Early presymptomatic tests include a blood test for prostate-specific antigen (PSA) and periodic digital rectal examination (DRE). In early stages of prostate cancer, symptoms include dysuria, frequency, loss of bladder control, and hematuria. As prostate cancer progresses, symptoms include blood in the semen, erectile dysfunction, and numbness or pain in the pelvis.

Once diagnosed, oncologists stage and grade prostate cancer to determine appropriate forms of therapy. Very early stages of prostate cancer may not require medical intervention, and many men may never need any further treatment. Nevertheless, active surveillance with blood tests, digital rectal examinations, and possibly biopsies with follow-up is required.

Surgery and radiation therapy are common treatments for prostate cancer. For malignancy confined only to the prostate, surgery that removes the entire prostate, seminal vesicles, and surrounding lymph nodes **(radical prostatectomy)** provides the best treatment option. Because testosterone fuels the growth of prostate cancer, hormone therapy, called **androgen-deprivation therapy (ADT),** is important in the management of the disease. Removal of both testes **(bilateral orchiectomy, castration)** blocks testosterone but is permanent and irreversible, and many men opt for drug therapy. Drug therapy that includes antiandrogenic agents and hormones that deplete the body of testicular hormones **(combined hormonal therapy)** is part of this form of treatment.

Diseases and Conditions

This section introduces diseases and conditions of the male reproductive system with their meanings and pronunciations. Word analyses for selected terms are also provided.

Term	Definition
benign prostatic hyperplasia (BHP) bē-NĪN prŏs-TĂT-ĭk hī-pĕr-PLĀ-zē-ă *prostat:* prostate *-ic:* pertaining to *hyper-:* excessive, above normal *-plasia:* formation, growth	Enlargement of the prostate, usually as part of the aging process that constricts the urethra, causing urinary symptoms including frequency, hesitancy, nocturia, and urinary retention (See Fig. 13-2.) *Urine that remains in the bladder commonly becomes a breeding ground for bacteria, causing cystitis and, ultimately, nephritis.*

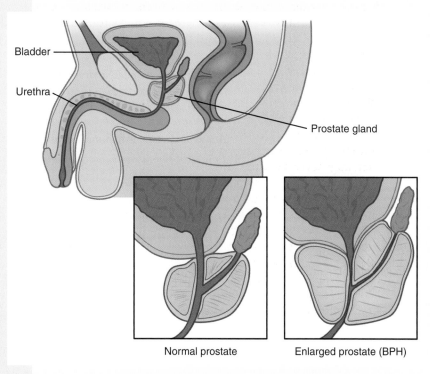

Bladder

Urethra

Prostate gland

Normal prostate   Enlarged prostate (BPH)

Figure 13-2 Benign prostatic hyperplasia.

Term	Definition
balanitis băl-ă-NĪ-tĭs *balan:* glans penis *-itis:* inflammation	Inflammation of the skin covering the glans penis, caused by bacteria, fungi, or a virus *Uncircumcised men with poor personal hygiene are prone to this disorder.*
erectile dysfunction (ED) ĕ-RĔK-tĭl	Repeated inability to initiate or maintain an erection sufficient for sexual intercourse *Any disorder that causes injury to the nerves or impairs blood flow in the penis has the potential to cause ED.*
hypogonadism hī-pō-GŌ-năd-ĭzm *hypo-:* under, below, deficient *gonad:* gonads, sex glands *-ism:* condition	Decrease or lack of hormones normally produced by the gonads *Hypogonadism involves a lack of testosterone, which plays a key role in masculinization and development during puberty.*

(continued)

Diseases and Conditions—cont'd

Term	Definition
hypospadias hī-pō-SPĀ-dē-ăs *hypo-:* under, below, deficient *-spadias:* slit, fissure	Congenital abnormality in which the opening of the male urethra is on the undersurface of the penis, instead of at its tip
phimosis fĭ-MŌ-sĭs *phim:* muzzle *-osis:* abnormal condition; increase (used primarily with blood cells)	Stenosis or narrowing of foreskin so that it cannot be retracted over the glans penis
priapism PRĪ-ă-pĭzm	Prolonged, commonly painful erection of the penis, which occurs without sexual stimulation *Priapism is associated with sickle cell disease, leukemia, spinal cord injury, and as an adverse effect of drugs used to treat erectile dysfunction. Prompt treatment is necessary to prevent permanent tissue damage that could result in the erectile dysfunction or disfigurement of the penis.*
prostatitis prŏs-tă-TĪ-tĭs *prostat:* prostate *-itis:* inflammation	Acute or chronic inflammation of the prostate *Prostatitis is commonly caused by a urinary tract infection or a sexually transmitted infection.*
sterility stĕr-ĬL-ĭ-tē	Inability to produce offspring *In the male, sterility is the inability to fertilize the ovum.*
testicular abnormalities tĕs-TĬK-ū-lăr	Any of the various disorders that affect the testes (See Fig. 13-3.)

anorchism
   ăn-OR-kĭzm
 	
   an-: without, not
   orch: testis (plural, testes)
   -ism: condition
	Absence of one or both testicles; also called *anorchia* or *anorchidism*
	
	Treatment includes androgen (male hormone) supplementation, testicular prosthetic implantation, and psychological support.

epididymitis
   ĕp-ĭ-dĭd-ĭ-MĪ-tĭs
 	
   epididym: epididymis
   -itis: inflammation
	Inflammation of the epididymis (See Fig. 13-3A.)
	
	Epididymitis is most common in males between ages 14 and 35 and is usually associated with STIs, especially gonorrhea and chlamydia.

hydrocele
   HĪ-drō-sēl
 	
   hydr/o: water
   -cele: hernia, swelling
	Swelling of the sac surrounding the testes that is typically harmless (See Fig. 13-3B.)
	
	Hydrocele in a neonate usually resolves without treatment within a year. In men and young males, it is commonly caused by inflammation or injury to the scrotum.

orchitis
   or-KĪ-tĭs
 	
   orch: testis (plural, testes)
   -itis: inflammation
	Painful swelling of one or both testes commonly associated with mumps that develop after puberty (See Fig. 13-3C.)
	
	Other causes of orchitis include infection of the epididymis or STIs.

Diseases and Conditions—cont'd

Term	Definition
spermatocele spĕr-MĂT-ō-sēl *spermat/o:* spermatozoa, sperm cells *-cele:* hernia, swelling	Abnormal, fluid-filled sac that develops in the epididymis and may or may not contain sperm; also called *spermatic cyst* (See Fig. 13-3D.)
testicular mass tĕs-TĬK-ū-lăr	New tissue growth that appears on one or both testes and may be malignant or benign (See Fig. 13-3E.)
testicular torsion tĕs-TĬK-ū-lăr TOR-shŭn	Spontaneous twisting of a testicle within the scrotum, leading to a decrease in blood flow to the affected testicle (See Fig. 13-3F.) *Testicular torsion is a medical emergency because interruption of blood supply may permanently damage the testicle.*
testicular cancer tĕs-TĬK-ū-lăr	Malignancy that develops in one or both testes, commonly presenting as a small lump or tenderness on the testicle, swelling in the scrotum and, occasionally, enlargement of breast tissue (gynecomastia) *Because most forms of testicular cancer are responsive to treatment when found in the early stages, physicians encourage testicular self-examination (TSE) on a monthly basis.*
varicocele VĂR-ĭ-kō-sēl *varic/o:* dilated vein *-cele:* hernia, swelling	Swelling and distention of veins of the spermatic cord, somewhat resembling varicose veins of the legs (See Fig. 13-3G.) *Some varicoceles cause sterility as a result of low sperm production or poor sperm quality. Varicoceles can be treated surgically.*

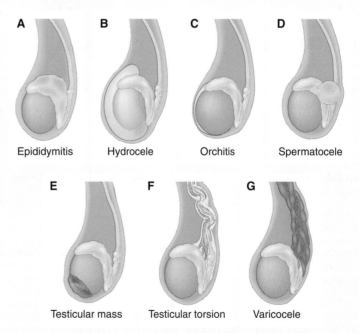

Figure 13-3 Testicular abnormalities. (A) Epididymitis. (B) Hydrocele. (C) Orchitis. (D) Spermatocele. (E) Testicular mass. (F) Testicular torsion. (G) Varicocele.

 It is time to review pathology, diseases, and conditions by completing Learning Activity 13-3.

Diagnostic, Surgical, and Therapeutic Procedures

This section introduces diagnostic, surgical, and therapeutic procedures used to treat and diagnose male reproductive disorders. Descriptions are provided, along with pronunciations and word analyses for selected terms.

Procedure	Description
Diagnostic	

Clinical

digital rectal examination (DRE) DĬJ-ĭt-ăl RĔK-tăl	Screening test in males that evaluates the size and consistency of the prostate (See Fig. 13-4.) *In males and females, DRE helps assess the rectal wall surface for lesions or evaluate abnormalities of the pelvic area.*

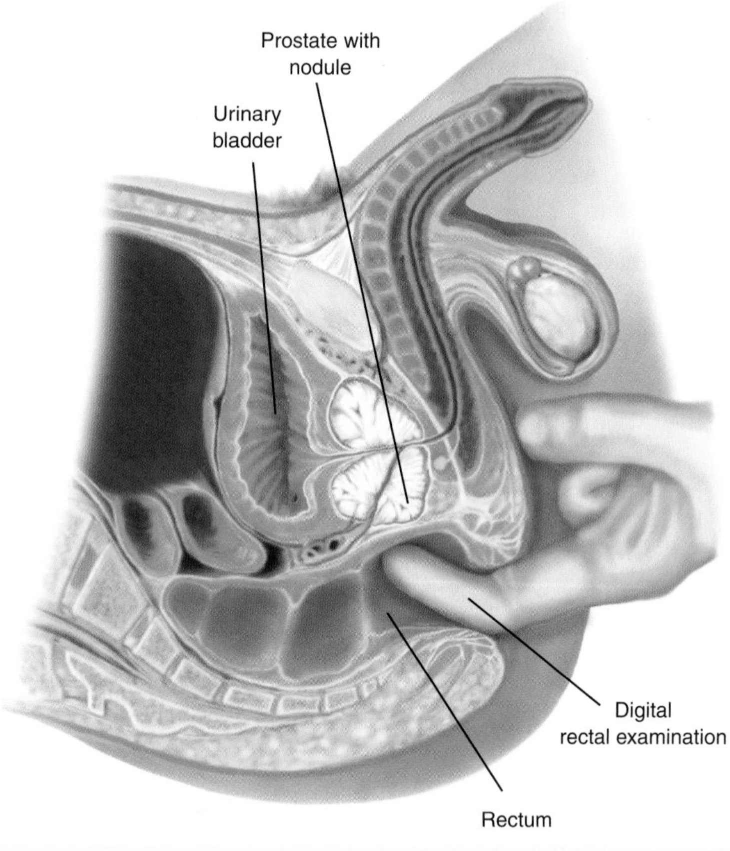

Figure 13-4 Digital rectal examination.

Laboratory

prostate-specific antigen (PSA) PRŎS-tāt spĕ-SĬF-ĭk ĂN-tĭ-jĕn	Blood test used to detect prostatic disorders, especially prostate cancer; also called *tumor marker test* *PSA is a substance produced by the prostate, and found in small quantities in blood. The blood level is elevated in prostatitis, benign prostatic hyperplasia, and tumors of the prostate.*

Diagnostic, Surgical, and Therapeutic Procedures—cont'd

Procedure	Description
semen analysis SĒ-mĕn ă-NĂL-ĭ-sĭs	Test that analyzes a semen sample for volume, sperm count, motility, and morphology to evaluate fertility or verify sterilization after a vasectomy

Imaging

Procedure	Description
scrotal ultrasound (US) SKRŌ-tăl ŬL-tră-sownd	Imaging procedure using sound waves to assess the contents of the scrotum, including the testicles, epididymis, and vas deferens; also called *testicular ultrasound*

transrectal ultrasound (TRUS)
biopsy of the prostate
trăns-RĔK-tăl ŬL-tră-sownd
BĪ-ŏp-sē PRŎS-tāt
  trans: across, through
  rect: rectum
  -al: pertaining to
	Imaging procedure using soundwaves emitted by a probe inserted through the rectum to serve as a guide for biopsy of the prostate when PSA and DRE are abnormal (See Fig. 13-5.)

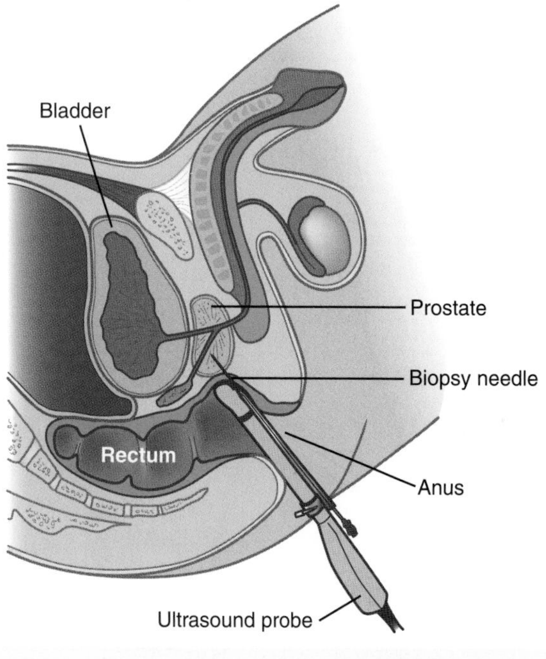

Figure 13-5 Transrectal ultrasound and needle biopsy of the prostate.

Surgical

Procedure	Description
circumcision sĕr-kŭm-SĬ-zhŭn	Removal of the foreskin, or fold of skin covering the tip (glans) of the penis *Circumcision is usually performed on infant males for religious or social reasons.*

orchiopexy
or-kē-ō-PĔK-sē
  orchi/o: testis (plural, testes)
  -pexy: fixation (of an organ)
	Fixation of the testes in the scrotum
	Orchiopexy is performed for undescended testicles (cryptorchidism), usually before age 2, or for correction of testicular torsion.

(continued)

Diagnostic, Surgical, and Therapeutic Procedures—cont'd

Procedure	Description
prostatectomy prŏs-tă-TĔK-tō-mē *prostat:* prostate *-ectomy:* excision, removal	Removal of all or part of the prostate *Several prostatectomy procedures are possible, depending on the extent and reason for removal; however, transurethral resection of the prostate (TURP) is one of the most common.*
transurethral resection of the prostate (TURP) trăns-ū-RĒ-thrăl rē-SĔK-shŭn, PRŎS-tāt *trans:* across, through *urethr:* urethra *-al:* pertaining to	Excision of prostate tissue by inserting a special endoscope (resectoscope) through the urethra and into the bladder to remove small pieces of tissue from the prostate gland (See Fig. 13-6.) *The resectoscope is fitted with an electrically activated wire loop that removes tissue when dragged over the site and cauterizes it to minimize bleeding.*

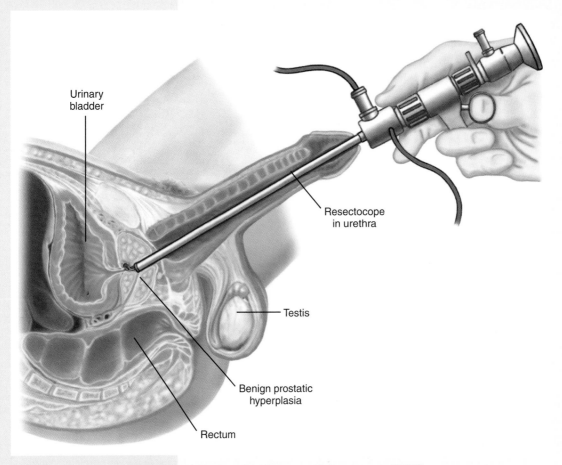

Urinary bladder

Resectocope in urethra

Testis

Benign prostatic hyperplasia

Rectum

Figure 13-6 Transurethral resection of the prostate (TURP).

urethroplasty ū-RĒ-thrō-plăs-tē *urethr/o:* urethra *-plasty:* surgical repair	Reconstruction of the urethra to relieve stricture or narrowing *Urethroplasty relieves pain and discomfort experienced during voiding and reduces the risk of contracting orchitis, prostatitis, and urinary tract infections.*

Diagnostic, Surgical, and Therapeutic Procedures—cont'd

Procedure	Description
vasectomy văs-ĔK-tō-mē *vas:* vessel; vas deferens; duct *-ectomy:* excision, removal	Removal of all or a segment of the vas deferens for male sterilization *Vasectomy reversal (vasovasostomy) rejoins the two segments of the vas deferens. The reversal has the greatest chance of producing a pregnancy if performed within 3 years of the vasectomy. After 10 years, the success rate for producing pregnancy is less than 30%. (See Fig. 13-7.)*

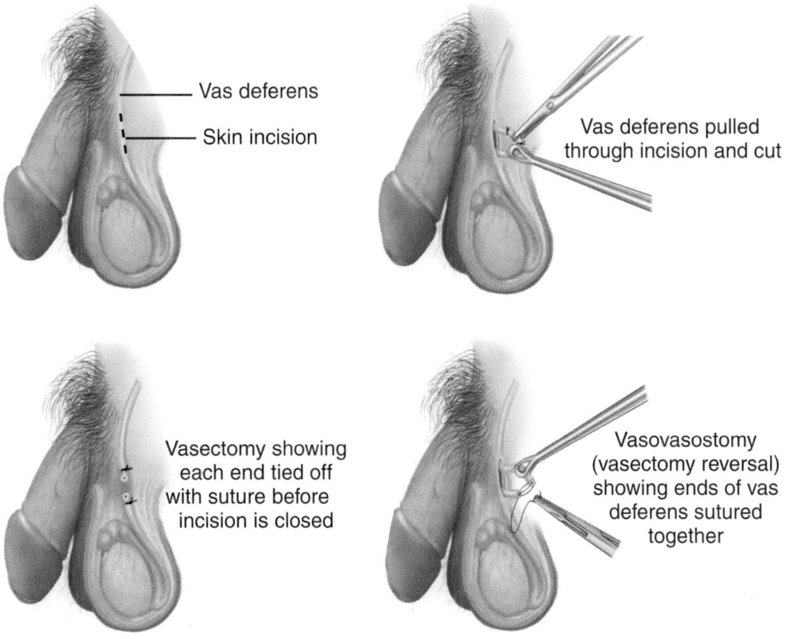

— Vas deferens

— Skin incision

Vas deferens pulled through incision and cut

Vasectomy showing each end tied off with suture before incision is closed

Vasovasostomy (vasectomy reversal) showing ends of vas deferens sutured together

Figure 13-7 Vasectomy and vasovasostomy.

(continued)

Diagnostic, Surgical, and Therapeutic Procedures—cont'd

Procedure	Description

Therapeutic

brachytherapy of the prostate
brăk-ē-THĔR-ă-pē
brachy: short (distance)
-therapy: treatment

Radiation oncology procedure where radioactive "seeds" are placed directly within or near a tumor in the prostate to destroy malignant cells (See Fig. 13-8.)

Brachytherapy reduces radiation exposure of surrounding healthy tissue in the region of the tumor.

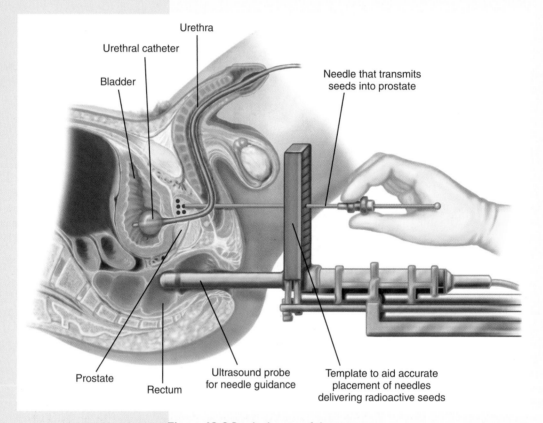

Urethra
Urethral catheter
Bladder
Needle that transmits seeds into prostate
Prostate
Rectum
Ultrasound probe for needle guidance
Template to aid accurate placement of needles delivering radioactive seeds

Figure 13-8 Brachytherapy of the prostate.

Diagnostic, Surgical, and Therapeutic Procedures—cont'd

Procedure	Description

cryotherapy of the prostate
krī-ō-THĔR-ă-pē PRŎS-tāt

  cry/o: cold

  -therapy: treatment

Freezing of the prostate, causing cancer cells to die (See Fig. 13-9.)

Cryotherapy is used in early stages of prostate cancer or when prostate cancer has returned after other types of treatments failed.

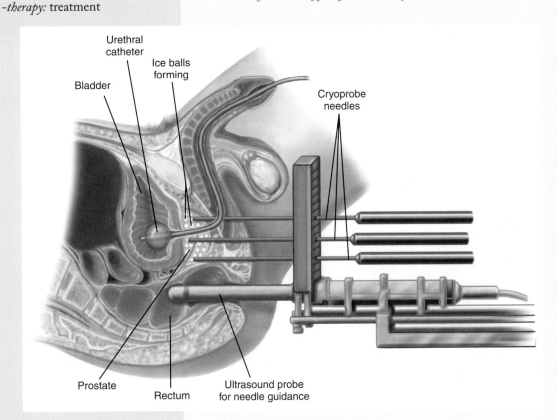

Figure 13-9 Cryosurgery of the prostate.

external beam radiation therapy (EBRT)

Procedure in which the patient is positioned at a distance from the radiation source, which is then directed at the prostate; also called *external beam radiation (EBT)* or *teletherapy*

EBRT may also be performed before surgery to reduce the size of the tumor or after surgery to prevent recurrence of the tumor.

Pharmacology

Several classes of drugs are used to treat conditions of the male reproductive system, including antiviral and antibiotic agents to treat diseases and infections. In addition, hormones help treat hypogonadism and some reproductive disorders. (See Table 13-1.)

Table 13-1 Drugs Used to Treat Disorders of the Male Reproductive System

This table lists common drug classifications used to treat male reproductive disorders, their therapeutic actions, and selected generic and trade names.

Classification	Therapeutic Action	Generic and *Trade* Names
alpha-1 blockers ĂL-fă	Block alpha-1 receptors in the prostate and bladder, relaxing muscles and improving urine flow in benign prostatic hyperplasia (BPH)	**tamsulosin** tăm-SŪ-lō-sĭn *Flomax* **terazosin** tĕr-Ā-zō-sĭn *Hytrin*
androgens ĂN-drō-jĕnz	Increase testosterone levels *Androgens, administered topically or intramuscularly, help correct hormone deficiency in hypogonadism and treat delayed puberty in males.*	**testosterone base** tĕs-TŎS-tĕr-ōn *Androderm, Testim* **testosterone cypionate** tĕs-TŎS-tĕr-ōn SĬP-ē-ō-nāt *Depo-testosterone*
antiandrogens ăn-tĭ-ĂN-drō-jĕnz	Suppress the production of androgen *Antiandrogens may stop the growth of certain types of cancer cells and may help treat prostate cancer. Some antiandrogens in combination with alpha-1 blockers help treat BPH.*	**dutasteride** doo-TĂS-tĭr-īd *Avodart* **flutamide** FLOO-tă-mīd *Eulexin*
anti-impotence agents ăn-tĭ-ĬM-pō-tĕnts	Treat erectile dysfunction (impotence) by increasing blood flow to the penis, resulting in an erection *Anti-impotence drugs should not be used by patients with coronary artery disease or hypertension.*	**sildenafil citrate** sĭl-DĔN-ă-fĭl SĬT-răt *Viagra* **vardenafil** văr-DĔN-ă-fĭl *Levitra*
antivirals ăn-tĭ-VĪ-rălz	Treat viral disorders by inhibiting the development of the offending virus *Antivirals do not have the ability to destroy a virus. They are used to treat recurrent herpes in adults and lesions associated with chickenpox and shingles.*	**acyclovir** ā-SĪ-klō-vēr *Zovirax* **famciclovir** făm-SĪ-klō-vēr *Famvir*

Abbreviations

This section introduces abbreviations related to the male reproductive system, along with their meanings.

Abbreviation	Meaning	Abbreviation	Meaning
ADT	androgen deprivation therapy	HSV	herpes simplex virus
BPH	benign prostatic hyperplasia; benign prostatic hypertrophy	PSA	prostate-specific antigen
DRE	digital rectal examination	STD	sexually transmitted disease
EBRT	external beam radiation therapy	STI	sexually transmitted infection
EBT	external beam therapy	TRUS	transrectal ultrasound
ED	erectile dysfunction; emergency department	TSE	testicular self-examination
HIV	human immunodeficiency virus	TURP	transurethral resection of the prostate
HPV	human papillomavirus	US	ultrasound; ultrasonography

It is time to review procedures, pharmacology, and abbreviations by completing Learning Activity 13–4.

LEARNING ACTIVITIES

The activities that follow provide a review of the male reproductive system terms introduced in this chapter. Complete each activity and review your answers to evaluate your understanding of the chapter.

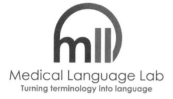

Visit the Medical Language Lab at *medicallanguagelab.com*. Use it to enhance your study and reinforcement of this chapter with the flash-card activity. We recommend that you complete the flash-card activity before starting Learning Activities 13-1 and 13-2.

Learning Activity 13-1
Medical Word Elements

Use the listed elements to build medical words. You may use these elements more than once.

Combining Forms		Suffixes		Prefixes
andr/o	prostat/o	-ary	-itis	an-
balan/o	scrot/o	-cele	-megaly	epi-
epididym/o	sperm/i	-cide	-plasty	hypo-
genit/o	urin/o	-ectomy	-rrhaphy	
gonad/o	varic/o	-gen	-spadias	
orch/o	vas/o	-graphy		
perine/o	vesicul/o	-ism		

1. killing sperm _____
2. swelling of a dilated vein _____
3. surgical repair of the scrotum _____
4. enlargement of the prostate _____
5. condition without testes _____
6. excision of a gonad _____
7. pertaining to genitals and the urinary tract _____
8. excision of the epididymis _____
9. fissure on the dorsum (of the penis) _____
10. condition of deficiency (in hormones) of the sex glands _____
11. inflammation of the glans penis _____
12. forming or producing a male _____
13. suture of the perineum _____
14. excision of the vas deferens _____
15. process of recording the seminal vesicle _____

 Check your answers in Appendix A. Review any material that you did not answer correctly.

Correct Answers _____ X 6.67 = _____ % Score

Building Medical Words

Use *orchid/o* (testis [plural, testes]) to build words that mean

1. inflammation of the testes _____
2. prolapse or downward displacement of the testes _____

Use *balan/o* (glans penis) to build words that mean

3. flow or discharge of the glans penis _____
4. hernia, swelling of the glans penis _____

Use *spermat/o* to build words that mean

5. sperm cell _____
6. embryonic sperm (cell) _____
7. swelling or hernia (containing) sperm _____

Use *prostat/o* to build words that mean

8. pain of the prostate _____
9. discharge of the prostate _____
10. enlargement of the prostate _____
11. stone or calculus of the prostate _____

Use the suffix *-spadias* (slit, fissure) to build words that mean

12. fissure under (ventrum of the penis) _____
13. fissure above (dorsum of the penis) _____

Use *vesicul/o* (seminal vesicle) to build words that mean

14. inflammation of the seminal vesicle _____
15. process of recording the seminal vesicle _____

Use *gonad/o* (gonads, sex glands) to build a word that means

16. disease of the gonads _____

Build surgical words that mean

17. surgical repair of glans penis _____
18. excision of (a segment of the) vas deferens _____
19. surgical repair of the scrotum _____
20. suture of the perineum _____

✔ *Check your answers in Appendix A. Review any material that you did not answer correctly.*

Correct Answers _____ X 5 = _____ % Score

Diseases and Conditions

Match the terms with the definitions in the numbered list.

anorchidism	cryptorchidism	hydrocele	priapism
balanitis	epididymitis	hypogonadism	prostatitis
chancre	epispadias	hypospadias	sterility
chlamydia	gynecomastia	leukorrhea	testicular torsion
condyloma	herpes	phimosis	varicocele

1. white discharge commonly associated with gonorrhea _____

2. STI that causes blisterlike lesions in the genital area _____

3. failure of the testicles to descend into the scrotum before birth _____

4. condition where the urethra opens on the underside of the penis _____

5. stenosis of the foreskin so that it cannot be drawn over the glans _____

6. swelling and distention of the spermatic cord veins _____

7. condition where the urethra opens on the dorsum of the penis _____

8. twisting of the testicle within the scrotum _____

9. wart located in the genital area _____

10. condition of the absence of (one or both) testicles _____

11. inflammation of the glans penis _____

12. persistent, painful erection lasting more than 4 hours _____

13. inflammation of the prostate _____

14. inflammation of the epididymis _____

15. inability to produce offspring _____

16. fluid in the sac surrounding the testes, causing swelling in the scrotum _____

17. common STI called "silent disease" because symptoms are mild or absent _____

18. syphilitic lesion found in primary syphilis _____

19. decrease in hormones produced by the sex glands _____

20. enlargement of breast tissue associated with testicular cancer _____

✓ *Check your answers in Appendix A. Review any material that you did not answer correctly.*

Correct Answers _____ X 5 = _____ % Score

Learning Activity 13-4

Procedures, Pharmacology, and Abbreviations

Match the terms with the definitions in the numbered list.

androgens	*cryosurgery*	*semen analysis*
antiandrogens	*HPV*	*TURP*
antivirals	*orchiopexy*	*urethroplasty*
BPH	*PSA*	*vasectomy*
circumcision	*scrotal*	*vasovasostomy*

1. test used to evaluate fertility or verify sterilization after vasectomy _____

2. agents used to increase testosterone levels _____

3. US procedure to assess the testicles, epididymis, and vas deferens for abnormalities _____

4. freezing technique used to destroy cancer _____

5. male sterilization procedure _____

6. surgical repair of the urethra to relieve a stricture or narrowing _____

7. reversal of a vasectomy _____

8. agents that suppress the production of an androgen _____

9. excision of the prostate through the urethra _____

10. blood test to detect prostate disorders, especially cancer _____

11. medications used to treat recurrent herpes _____

12. fixation of the testes in the scrotum _____

13. removal of the foreskin from the glans _____

14. virus causing genital warts _____

15. nonmalignant enlargement of the prostate that is usually associated with aging _____

✓ *Check your answers in Appendix A. Review any material that you did not answer correctly.*

Correct Answers _____ X 6.67 = _____ % Score

DOCUMENTING HEALTH-CARE ACTIVITIES

This section provides practical application activities in the form of exercises to help students develop skills in documenting patient care. First, read the medical report. Then complete the activities and exercises that follow.

Consultation Report: Benign Prostatic Hyperplasia

General Hospital

1511 Ninth Avenue ■ ■ Sun City, USA 12345 ■ ■ (555) 802–1887

Patient: Smith, Milton
Birthdate: 05/10/xx

Consulting Physician: Richard Apper, MD
Patient ID#: 23–3444

CONSULTATION

DATE: 03/04/xx

REASON FOR CONSULTATION: Benign prostatic hyperplasia.

HISTORY OF PRESENT ILLNESS: This 82-year-old white male was admitted 03/04/xx for left inguinal hernia repair and ventral hernia repair. The patient has been seen by me in the past and is currently on Proscar. He had a Foley catheter in place postoperatively, which was removed this a.m., and since then, the patient has complained of dysuria, frequency, and a feeling of incomplete emptying with weak stream. The patient has a history of hesitancy, weak stream, and voiding every 2–3 hours. He denies incontinence, nocturia, dysuria, and hematuria and only had microscopic hematuria and is being followed by me. History of urinary tract infection with catheter in the past. The patient recently voided 300 cc and then 250 cc again. He feels that he may have to void now. He has no history of any calculi or genitourinary malignancies.

PAST MEDICAL HISTORY: Benign prostatic hyperplasia and hyperlipidemia.

PAST SURGICAL HISTORY: Right inguinal hernia x3, lysis of adhesions, ventral hernia repair.

SOCIAL HISTORY: Plus tobacco.

MEDICATIONS: Lipitor, Proscar, Demerol, and Darvocet.

ALLERGIES: No known drug allergies.

PHYSICAL EXAMINATION: Afebrile, and vital signs are stable. Urine output is good. Abdomen is soft, and there is plus suprapubic tenderness. The incision overlies the bladder area, and it is difficult to assess for bladder distention. Rectal has a 4- to 5-cm prostate without nodules.

IMPRESSION: This is an 82-year-old white male with questionable urinary retention. Will hold on postvoid residual check because patient is voiding well. Send a urinalysis and culture and sensitivity. Will pass a catheter if he has any difficulty voiding.

Richard Apper, MD
Richard Apper, MD

RC:kan

D: 03/04/xx; T: 03/04/xx

Terminology

The terms listed in the table that follows are taken from *Consultation Report: Benign Prostatic Hyperplasia*. Use a medical dictionary such as *Taber's Cyclopedic Medical Dictionary*, the appendices of this book, or other resources to define each term. Then review the pronunciation for each term and practice by reading the medical record aloud.

Term	Definition
adhesions ăd-HĒ-zhŭnz	
benign bē-NĪN	
calculi KĂL-kū-lī	
catheter KĂTH-ĕ-tĕr	
culture and sensitivity KŬL-tūr, sĕn-sĭ-TĬV-ĭ-tē	
dysuria dīs-Ū-rē-ă	
hematuria hē-mă-TŪ-rē-ă	
hernia HĔR-nē-ă	
hesitancy HĔS-ĭ-tăn-sē	
hyperlipidemia hī-pĕr-lĭp-ĭ-DĒ-mē-ă	
hyperplasia hī-pĕr-PLĀ-zē-ă	
incontinence ĭn-KŎNT-ĭn-ĕns	

Term	Definition
lysis LĪ-sĭs	
malignancies mă-LĬG-năn-sēz	
nocturia nŏk-TŪ-rē-ă	
suprapubic soo-pră-PŪ-bĭk	

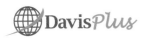 Visit the *Medical Terminology Systems* online resource center at Davis*Plus* to practice pronunciation and reinforce the meanings of the terms in this medical report.

Critical Thinking

Review *Consultation Report: Benign Prostatic Hyperplasia* to answer the questions.

1. What is the reason for the present admission?

_____

_____

_____

_____

2. What occurred when the physician removed the Foley catheter?

_____

_____

_____

_____

3. What did the patient's previous history indicate regarding these symptoms?

_____

_____

_____

_____

4. Why was it difficult to assess for bladder distention?

_____

_____

_____

_____

5. Was there a definitive diagnosis identified in the impression?

_____

_____

_____

_____

6. What procedure will the physician perform if the patient has difficulty voiding?

_____

_____

_____

_____

Chart Note: Acute Epididymitis

Homer, Aaron	**April 1, 20xx**
Age: 31	

HISTORY OF PRESENT ILLNESS: Patient presents with complaints of severe left-sided groin pain, scrotal pain, and urethritis with a clear urethral discharge. He says it has developed over the last 2 days. He is sexually active, heterosexual, and says he had two sexual partners within the last month, the most recent being 4 days ago.

PHYSICAL EXAMINATION: The patient is uncircumcised and the prepuce is easily retractable. There are no observable lesions on the glans or shaft, and there is no balanitis. The urethral meatus is normal. A clear discharge is expressed upon compression of the glans, and swabs are obtained for testing. The testes are descended bilaterally, smooth, and without masses. There is moderate pain and tenderness of the left testicle, which is alleviated with elevation of the testicles. There is no evidence of torsion of the spermatic cord. The scrotum is erythematous, and there is a left-sided hydrocele. The left epididymis is palpable, with significant induration and tenderness. The right epididymis is normal and nontender. No inguinal or femoral hernia is felt. There is enlargement of the left inguinal lymph nodes. Rectal examination reveals mild prostatic hyperplasia and tenderness. Urinalysis is positive for leukocytes and bacteria.

IMPRESSION: Acute epididymitis.

Plan: Laboratory tests for chlamydia, gonorrhea, and prostate-specific antigen. Administer intravenous antibiotics, prescribe oral antibiotics and analgesics.

Julia Halm, MD
Julia Halm, MD

D: 04–01–20xx; T: 04–01–20xx

bcg

Terminology

The terms listed in the table that follows are taken from *Chart Note: Acute Epididymitis*. Use a medical dictionary such as *Taber's Cyclopedic Medical Dictionary*, the appendices of this book, or other resources to define each term. Then review the pronunciation for each term and practice by reading the medical record aloud.

Term	Definition
balanitis băl-ă-NĪ-tĭs	
erythematous ěr-ĭ-THĔM-ă-tŭs	
hydrocele HĪ-drō-sēl	
hyperplasia hī-pěr-PLĀ-zē-ă	
induration ĬN-dū-rā-shŭn	
inguinal ĬNG-gwĭ-năl	
meatus mē-Ā-tŭs	
prepuce PRĒ-pūs	
prostate-specific antigen PRŎS-tāt, ĂN-tĭ-jěn	
scrotal SKRŌ-tăl	
torsion TOR-shŭn	

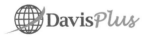 **DavisPlus**   Visit the *Medical Terminology Systems* online resource center at Davis*Plus* to practice pronunciation and reinforce the meanings of the terms in this medical report.

Critical Thinking

Review *Chart Note: Acute Epididymitis* to answer the questions.

1. What were the complaints of the patient?

_____

_____

_____

_____

2. What procedure did the physician perform regarding the urethral discharge?

_____

_____

_____

_____

3. What information does the chart note provide regarding the left testicle?

_____

_____

_____

_____

4. How does the chart note describe the left epididymis?

_____

_____

_____

5. What did the rectal examination reveal?

_____

_____

_____

_____

Constructing Chart Notes

To construct chart notes, replace the italicized and boldfaced terms in each of the two case studies with one of the listed medical terms.

asymptomatic	leukorrhea	prostatomegaly
benign	meatus	pruritus
digital rectal examination	orchialgia	PSA
dysuria		

Mr. R. is a sexually active junior at State College. For the last 6 weeks, he was aware of a slight (1) **white discharge** from the tip of the penis but ignored this symptom. He now complains of (2) **pain upon urination**, (3) **intense itching** around the tip of the penis, and (4) **pain in the testicles.** Suspecting chlamydia, the physician will confirm his diagnosis with a swab taken from the urethral (5) **opening** and a urine test for the presence of chlamydia. In the meantime, the patient will begin a regimen of oral antibiotics and will return for a retest in 2 weeks. He was instructed on the benefits of condom use and advised to refrain from sexual activity until his infection resolves.

1. _____
2. _____
3. _____
4. _____
5. _____

Mr. L. is a 68-year-old male who presents for his annual checkup. His blood test shows a slight elevation of the (6) **prostate tumor marker** test. During the (7) **manual examination of his lower rectum,** there was no evidence of nodules or lumps on the prostate gland. However, Dr. P. noted a slight (8) **enlargement of the prostate gland.** Because Mr. L. has (9) **no symptoms** related to the urinary system, his diagnosis is noted as a (9) **nonmalignant** enlargement of the prostate. The patient was advised to have a follow-up examination in 6 months.

6. _____
7. _____
8. _____
9. _____
10. _____

✓ *Check your answers in Appendix A. Review any material that you did not answer correctly.*

Correct Answers _____ X 10 = _____ % Score

Endocrine System

Chapter Outline

Objectives

Upon completion of this chapter, you will be able to:

- Locate and describe the structures of the endocrine system.

- Describe the functional relationship between the endocrine system and other body systems.

- Pronounce, spell, and build words related to the endocrine system.

- Describe diseases, conditions, and procedures related to the endocrine system.

- Explain pharmacology related to the treatment of endocrine disorders.

- Demonstrate your knowledge of this chapter by completing the learning and documenting health-care activities.

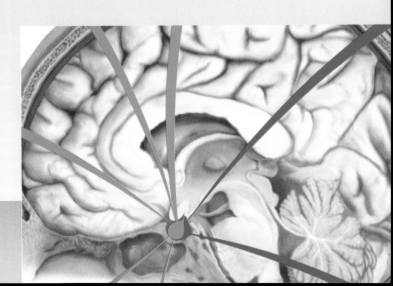

Anatomy and Physiology

The primary function of the endocrine system is to produce specialized chemicals called **hormones** that directly enter the bloodstream and travel to specific tissues or organs of the body called **targets.** Some hormonal actions cause short-term changes, such as a faster heartbeat or sweaty palms during a panic situation. Others control long-term changes, such as bone and muscle development. Still other hormones help maintain continuous body functions, such as a balance of body fluids and a normal metabolism. The endocrine system also maintains an internal state of equilibrium in the body **(homeostasis)** so that all body systems function effectively. The ductless glands of the endocrine system include the **pituitary, thyroid, parathyroid, adrenal, pancreatic, pineal, and thymus glands** and the **ovaries** and **testes.** (See Fig. 14-1.)

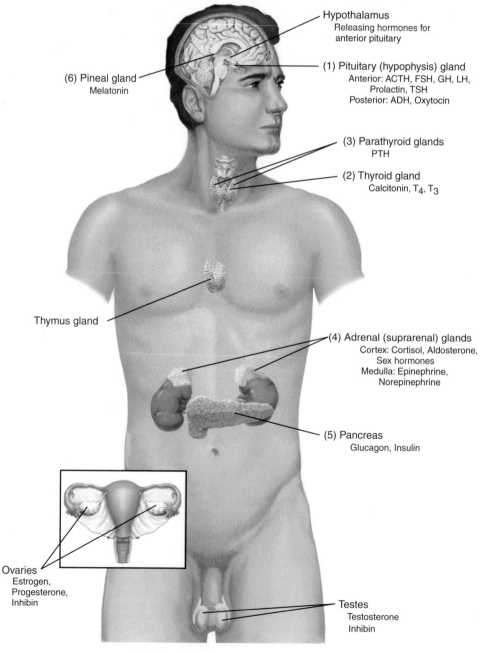

Hypothalamus
Releasing hormones for
anterior pituitary

(6) Pineal gland
Melatonin

(1) Pituitary (hypophysis) gland
Anterior: ACTH, FSH, GH, LH,
Prolactin, TSH
Posterior: ADH, Oxytocin

(3) Parathyroid glands
PTH

(2) Thyroid gland
Calcitonin, T_4, T_3

Thymus gland

(4) Adrenal (suprarenal) glands
Cortex: Cortisol, Aldosterone,
Sex hormones
Medulla: Epinephrine,
Norepinephrine

(5) Pancreas
Glucagon, Insulin

Ovaries
Estrogen,
Progesterone,
Inhibin

Testes
Testosterone
Inhibin

Figure 14-1 Locations of major endocrine glands.

Although hormones travel throughout the body in blood and lymph, they affect only the target tissues or organs that have specific receptors for the hormone. Once bound to the receptor, the hormone initiates a specific biological effect. For example, thyroid-stimulating hormone (TSH) binds to receptors on cells of the thyroid gland, causing it to secrete thyroxine. However, it does not bind to cells of the ovaries because ovarian cells do not have TSH receptors. Some hormones, such as insulin and thyroxine, have many target organs. Other hormones, such as calcitonin and some pituitary gland hormones, have only one or a few target organs. In general, hormones regulate growth, metabolism, reproduction, energy level, and sexual characteristics.

Anatomy and Physiology Key Terms

This section introduces important terms, along with their definitions and pronunciations. The key terms are highlighted in color in the Anatomy and Physiology section. Word analyses for selected terms are also provided. Pronounce the term, and place a check mark in the box after you do so.

Term	Definition
antagonistic ăn-TĂG-ō-nĭst-ĭk ☐	Acting in opposition; mutually opposing
electrolytes ē-LĔK-trō-līts ☐	Salts and minerals that conduct electrical impulses in the body *Electrolytes control the fluid balance of the body and are important in muscle contraction, energy generation, and almost every major biochemical reaction in the body. Common human electrolytes are sodium chloride, potassium, calcium, and sodium bicarbonate.*
glucagon GLOO-kă-gŏn ☐	Hormone produced by pancreatic alpha cells that stimulates the liver to change stored glycogen (a starch form of sugar) to glucose *Glucagon opposes the action of insulin. It is used to reverse hypoglycemic reactions in insulin shock.*
glucose GLOO-kōs ☐	Simple sugar that is the end product of carbohydrate digestion *Glucose is found in many foods, especially fruits, and is a major source of energy for living organisms. Analysis of blood glucose levels is an important diagnostic test in diabetes and other disorders.*
sympathomimetic sĭm-pă-thō-mĭm-ĔT-ĭk ☐	Agent that mimics the effects of the sympathetic nervous system, the division of the nervous system that increases the "fight or flight" response *Epinephrine and norepinephrine are sympathomimetic hormones because they produce effects that mimic those brought about by the sympathetic nervous system.*

Pronunciation Help	Long Sound	ā — rate	ē — rebirth	ī — isle	ō — over	ū — unite
	Short Sound	ă — apple	ĕ — ever	ĭ — it	ŏ — not	ŭ — cut

Pituitary Gland

The (1) **pituitary gland,** or **hypophysis,** is a pea-sized organ located at the base of the brain. It is known as the **master gland** because it regulates many body activities and stimulates other glands to secrete their own specific hormones. (See Fig. 14-2.) The pituitary gland consists of two distinct portions, an anterior lobe **(adenohypophysis)** and a posterior lobe **(neurohypophysis).** The anterior lobe, triggered by the action of the hypothalamus, produces at least six hormones. The posterior lobe stores and secretes two hormones produced by the hypothalamus: antidiuretic hormone (ADH) and oxytocin. These hormones are released into the bloodstream as needed. (See Table 14-1.)

Thyroid Gland

The (2) **thyroid gland** is the largest gland of the endocrine system. An H-shaped organ located in the neck just below the larynx, this gland is composed of two large lobes that are separated by a strip of tissue called an **isthmus.** Thyroid hormone (TH) is the body's major metabolic hormone.

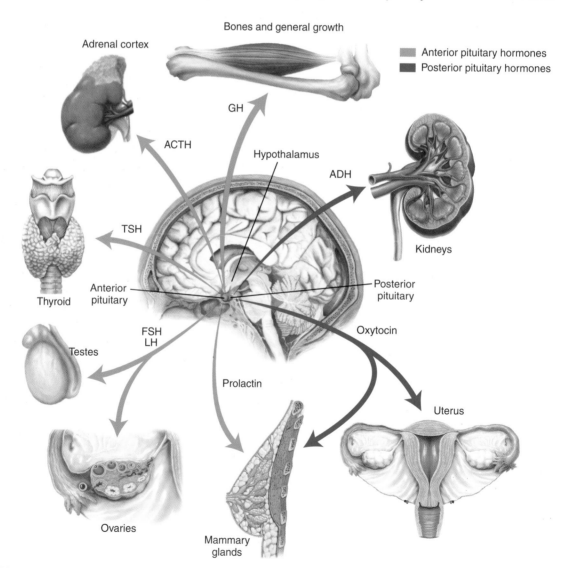

Figure 14-2 Hormones secreted by the anterior and posterior pituitary gland, along with target organs.

Table 14-1 **Pituitary Hormones**

This table identifies pituitary hormones, their target organs and functions, and associated disorders.

Hormone	Target Organ and Functions	Disorders
Anterior Pituitary Hormones (Adenohypophysis)		
Adrenocorticotropic hormone (ACTH)	• Adrenal cortex—promotes secretion of corticosteroids, especially cortisol	• Hyposecretion is rare. • Hypersecretion causes Cushing disease.
Follicle-stimulating hormone (FSH)	• Ovaries—in females, stimulates egg (ova) production; increases secretion of estrogen • Testes—in males, stimulates sperm production	• Hyposecretion causes failure of sexual maturation. • Hypersecretion has no known significant effects.
Growth hormone (GH) or somatotropin	• Regulates growth of bone, muscle, and other body tissues • Increases use of fats for energy	• Hyposecretion during childhood and puberty causes pituitary dwarfism. • Hypersecretion during childhood and puberty causes gigantism; hypersecretion during adulthood causes acromegaly.
Luteinizing hormone (LH)	• Ovaries—in females, promotes ovulation; stimulates production of estrogen and progesterone • Testes—in males, promotes secretion of testosterone	• Hyposecretion in nursing mothers causes poor lactation. • Hyposecretion causes failure of sexual maturation. • Hypersecretion has no known significant effects.
Prolactin (PRL)	• Breast—in conjunction with other hormones, promotes lactation	• Hypersecretion in nursing mothers causes excessive secretion of milk (galactorrhea).
Thyroid-stimulating hormone (TSH) or thyrotropin	• Thyroid gland—stimulates secretion of thyroid hormones	• Hyposecretion in infants causes cretinism; hyposecretion in adults causes myxedema. • Hypersecretion causes Graves disease, which results in exophthalmos.
Posterior Pituitary Hormones (Neurohypophysis)		
Antidiuretic hormone (ADH)	• Kidney—increases water reabsorption (water returns to the blood)	• Hyposecretion causes diabetes insipidus (DI). • Hypersecretion causes syndrome of inappropriate antidiuretic hormone (SIADH).
Oxytocin	• Uterus—stimulates uterine contractions; initiates labor • Breast—promotes milk secretion from the mammary glands	• Unknown

TH increases the rate of oxygen consumption and, thus, the rate at which carbohydrates, proteins, and fats are metabolized. TH is actually two active iodine-containing hormones: **thyroxine (T_4)** and **triiodothyronine (T_3).** T_4 is the major hormone secreted by the thyroid; most T_3 is formed at the target tissues by conversion of T_4 to T_3. Except for the adult brain, spleen, testes, uterus, and the thyroid gland itself, thyroid hormone affects virtually every cell in the body. TH also influences growth hormone and plays an important role in maintaining blood pressure. (See Table 14-2.)

Table 14-2	**Thyroid Hormones**	
This table identifies thyroid hormones, their functions, and associated disorders.		
Hormone	**Target Organs and Functions**	**Disorders**
Calcitonin	• Regulates calcium levels in the blood in conjunction with parathyroid hormone • Decreases the reabsorption of calcium and phosphate from bones to blood	• The most significant effects are exerted in childhood when bones are growing and changing dramatically in mass, size, and shape. • At best, calcitonin is a weak hypocalcemic agent in adults.
Thyroxine (T4) and triiodothyronine (T3)	• Increases energy production from all food types • Increases rate of protein synthesis	• Hyposecretion in infants causes cretinism; hyposecretion in adults causes myxedema. • Hypersecretion causes Graves disease, which results in exophthalmos.

Parathyroid Glands

The (3) **parathyroid glands** consist of at least four separate glands located on the posterior surface of the lobes of the thyroid gland. The only hormone known to be secreted by the parathyroid glands is parathyroid hormone (PTH). PTH helps to regulate calcium balance by stimulating three target organs: bones, kidneys, and intestines. (See Table 14-3.) Because of PTH stimulation, calcium and phosphates are released from bones, increasing concentration of these substances in blood. Thus, calcium that is necessary for the proper functioning of body tissues is available in the bloodstream. At the same time, PTH enhances the absorption of calcium and phosphates from foods in the intestine, causing a rise in blood levels of calcium and phosphates. PTH causes the kidneys to conserve blood calcium and increase the excretion of phosphates in urine.

Table 14-3	**Parathyroid Hormones**	
This table identifies the target organs and functions of parathyroid hormone and associated disorders.		
Hormone	**Target Organ and Functions**	**Disorders**
Parathyroid hormone (PTH)	• Bones—increases the reabsorption of calcium and phosphate from bone to blood • Kidneys—increases calcium absorption and phosphate excretion • Small intestine—increases absorption of calcium and phosphate	• Hyposecretion causes tetany. • Hypersecretion causes osteitis fibrosa cystica.

Adrenal Glands

The (4) **adrenal glands** are paired organs covering the superior surface of the kidneys. Because of their location, the adrenal glands are also known as **suprarenal glands**. Each adrenal gland is divided into two sections, each having its own structure and function. The outer adrenal cortex makes up the bulk of the gland, and the adrenal medulla makes up the inner portion. Although these regions are not sharply divided, they represent distinct glands that secrete different hormones.

Adrenal Cortex

The adrenal cortex secretes three types of steroid hormones:

1. **Mineralocorticoids,** mainly aldosterone, are essential to life. These hormones act mainly through the kidneys to maintain the balance of **electrolytes** (sodium and potassium) in the body. More specifically, aldosterone causes the kidneys to conserve sodium and excrete potassium (K). At the same time, it promotes water conservation by reducing urine output.
2. **Glucocorticoids,** mainly cortisol, influence the metabolism of carbohydrates, fats, and proteins. The glucocorticoid with the greatest activity is cortisol. It helps regulate the concentration of **glucose** in the blood, protecting against low blood glucose levels between meals. Cortisol also stimulates the breakdown of fats in adipose tissue and releases fatty acids into the blood. The increase in fatty acids causes many cells to use relatively less glucose.
3. **Sex hormones,** including androgens, estrogens, and progestins, help maintain secondary sex characteristics, such as development of the breasts in females and distribution of body hair in adults.

Adrenal Medulla

The cells of the adrenal medulla secrete two closely related hormones: epinephrine **(adrenaline)** and norepinephrine **(noradrenaline).** Both hormones are activated when the body responds to crisis situations, and they are considered **sympathomimetic** agents because they produce effects that mimic those brought about by the sympathetic nervous system. Because hormones of the adrenal medulla merely intensify activities set into motion by the sympathetic nervous system, their deficiency does not cause dysfunction.

Of the two hormones, epinephrine is secreted in larger amounts. In the physiological response to stress, epinephrine is responsible for maintaining blood pressure and cardiac output, dilating airways, and raising blood glucose levels. All of these functions are useful for frightened, traumatized, injured, or sick persons. Norepinephrine reduces the diameter of blood vessels in the periphery (vasoconstriction), thereby raising blood pressure. (See Table 14-4, page 482.)

Table 14-4	**Adrenal Hormones**	

This table identifies adrenal hormones, their target organs and functions, and associated disorders.

Hormone	Target Organ and Functions	Disorders
Adrenal Cortex Hormones		
Glucocorticoids (mainly cortisol)	• Body cells—promote gluconeogenesis; regulate metabolism of carbohydrates, proteins, and fats; and help depress inflammatory and immune responses	• Hyposecretion causes Addison disease. • Hypersecretion causes Cushing syndrome.
Mineralocorticoids (mainly aldosterone)	• Kidneys—increase blood levels of sodium and decrease blood levels of potassium in the kidneys	• Hyposecretion causes Addison disease. • Hypersecretion causes aldosteronism.
Sex hormones (any of the androgens, estrogens, or related steroid hormones produced by the ovaries, testes, and adrenal cortices)	• In females, possibly responsible for female libido and source of estrogen after menopause (otherwise, insignificant effects in adults)	• Hypersecretion of adrenal androgen in females leads to virilism (development of male secondary sex characteristics). • Hypersecretion of adrenal estrogen and progestin secretion in males leads to feminization (development of female secondary sex characteristics). • Hyposecretion has no known significant effect.
Adrenal Medullary Hormones		
Epinephrine and norepinephrine	• Sympathetic nervous system target organs—hormone effects mimic sympathetic nervous system activation (sympathomimetic), increase metabolic rate and heart rate, and raise blood pressure by promoting vasoconstriction	• Hyposecretion has no known significant effect. • Hypersecretion causes prolonged "fight-or-flight" reaction and hypertension.

Pancreas

The **pancreas** lies inferior to the stomach in a bend of the duodenum. It functions as an exocrine and endocrine gland. In its exocrine role, it carries digestive secretions from the pancreas to the small intestine through a large pancreatic duct. The digestive secretions assist in the breakdown of proteins, starches, and fats in the small intestine. In its endocrine role, the pancreas secretes two other hormones through the **islets of Langerhans: glucagon,** which is produced by the alpha cells, and **insulin,** which is produced by the beta cells. Both hormones play important roles in regulating blood glucose (sugar) levels:

- **Glucagon** stimulates the release of glucose from storage sites in the liver when blood glucose levels are low **(hypoglycemia),** thereby raising the blood glucose level.

- **Insulin** clears glucose molecules from the blood by promoting their storage in tissues as carbohydrates when blood glucose levels are high **(hyperglycemia),** thereby lowering the blood glucose level and enabling the cells to use glucose for energy.

Insulin and glucagon function **antagonistically,** so that normal secretion of both hormones ensures a blood glucose level that fluctuates within normal limits. (See Table 14-5.)

Table 14-5	Pancreatic Hormones	
This table identifies pancreatic hormones, their target organs and functions, and associated disorders.		
Hormone	**Target Organ and Functions**	**Disorders**
Glucagon	• Liver and blood—raises the blood glucose level by accelerating conversion of glycogen into glucose in the liver (glycogenolysis) and other nutrients into glucose in the liver (gluconeogenesis) and releasing glucose into blood (glycogen to glucose)	• A deficiency in glucagon may cause persistently low blood glucose levels (hypoglycemia).
Insulin	• Tissue cells—lowers blood glucose level by accelerating glucose transport into cells and the use of that glucose for energy production (glucose to glycogen)	• Hyposecretion of insulin causes diabetes mellitus. • Hypersecretion of insulin causes hyperinsulinism.

Pineal Gland

The (6) **pineal gland** is a small organ shaped like pine cone and located deep within the brain, just behind the thalamus. Although the exact functions of this gland have not been established, there is evidence that it secretes the hormone melatonin. It is believed that melatonin may inhibit the activities of the ovaries. When melatonin production is high, ovulation is blocked, and there may be a delay in puberty.

Thymus Gland

The (7) **thymus gland** is a butterfly-shaped gland that lies at the base of the neck and is formed mostly of lymphatic tissue. The thymus functions as part of the body's immune system (discussed in Chapter 9, Blood, Lymphatic, and Immune Systems) and part of the endocrine system. As an endocrine gland, the thymus secretes **thymosin,** which plays a role in the development of the immune response in newborns. After puberty, the lymphatic tissue gradually degenerates.

Anatomy Review: Endocrine System

To review the anatomy of the endocrine system, label the illustration using the listed terms.

adrenal (suprarenal) glands   parathyroid glands   testes

ovaries   pineal gland   thymus gland

pancreas   pituitary (hypophysis) gland   thyroid gland

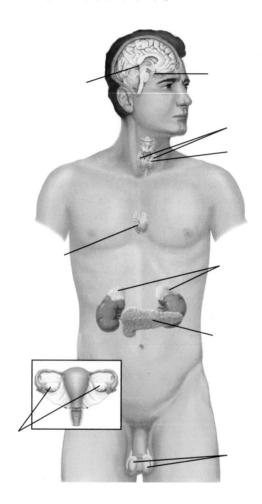

 Check your answers by referring to Figure 14–1 on page 476. Review material that you did not answer correctly.

CONNECTING BODY SYSTEMS—ENDOCRINE SYSTEM

The main function of the endocrine system is to secrete hormones that have a diverse effect on cells, tissues, organs, and organ systems. Specific functional relationships between the endocrine system and other body systems are summarized here.

Blood, Lymphatic, and Immune
- Hormones from the thymus stimulate lymphocyte production.
- Glucocorticoids depress the immune response and inflammation.

Cardiovascular
- Hormones influence heart rate, contraction strength, blood volume, and blood pressure.
- Estrogen helps maintain vascular health in women.

Digestive
- Hormones help control digestive system activity.
- Hormones influence the motility and glandular activity of the digestive tract, gallbladder secretion, and secretion of enzymes from the pancreas.
- Insulin and glucagon adjust glucose metabolism in the liver.

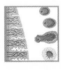

Female Reproductive
- Hormones play a major role in the development and function of the reproductive organs.
- Hormones influence the menstrual cycle, pregnancy, parturition, and lactation.
- Sex hormones play a major role in the development of secondary sex characteristics.
- The hormone oxytocin triggers contraction of the pregnant uterus and later stimulates the release of breast milk.

Integumentary
- Hormones regulate the activity of the sebaceous glands, the distribution of subcutaneous tissue, and hair growth.
- Hormones stimulate melanocytes to produce skin pigment.
- The hormone estrogen increases skin hydration.

Male Reproductive
- Hormones play a major role in the development and function of the reproductive organs.
- Sex hormones play a major role in the development of secondary sex characteristics.
- Hormones play a role in sexual development, sex drive, and sperm production.

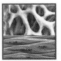

Musculoskeletal
- Hormone secretions influence blood flow to muscles during exercise.
- Hormones influence muscle metabolism, mass, and strength.
- Hormones from the pituitary and thyroid glands and the gonads stimulate bone growth.
- Hormones govern blood calcium balance.

Nervous
- Several hormones play an important role in the normal maturation and function of the nervous system.

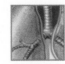

Respiratory
- Hormones stimulate red blood cell production when the body experiences a decrease in oxygen.
- Epinephrine influences ventilation by dilating the bronchioles; epinephrine and thyroxine stimulate cell respiration.

Urinary
- Hormones regulate water and electrolyte balance in the kidneys.

Medical Word Elements

This section introduces combining forms, suffixes, and prefixes related to the endocrine system. Word analyses are also provided. From the information provided, complete the meaning of the medical words in the right-hand column. The first one is completed for you.

Element	Meaning	Word Analysis
Combining Forms		
adren/o	adrenal glands	**adren/o**/megaly (ăd-rēn-ō-MĔG-ă-lē): enlargement of adrenal glands *-megaly:* enlargement
adrenal/o		**adrenal**/ectomy (ăd-rē-năl-ĔK-tō-mē): _____ *-ectomy:* excision, removal
calc/o	calcium	hyper/**calc**/emia (hī-pĕr-kăl-SĒ-mē-ă): _____ *hyper-:* excessive, above normal *-emia:* blood condition
crin/o	secrete	endo/**crin/o**/logy (ĕn-dō-krĭn-ŎL-ō-jē): _____ *endo-:* in, within *-logy:* study of *Endocrinology is the branch of medicine concerned with endocrine glands and hormones.*
gluc/o	sugar, sweetness	**gluc/o**/genesis (gloo-kō-JĔN-ĕ-sĭs): _____ *-genesis:* forming, producing, origin
glyc/o		hypo/**glyc**/emia (hī-pō-glī-SĒ-mē-ă): _____ *hypo-:* under, below *-emia:* blood condition *Common causes of hypoglycemia include too much insulin, excessive secretion of insulin by the islet cells of the pancreas, and dietary deficiency.*
glycos/o		**glycos**/uria (glī-kō-SŪ-rē-ă): _____ *-uria:* urine
home/o	same, alike	**home/o**/stasis (hō-mē-ō-STĀ-sĭs): _____ *-stasis:* standing still
kal/i	potassium (an electrolyte)	**kal**/emia (kă-LĒ-mē-ă): _____ *-emia:* blood condition
pancreat/o	pancreas	**pancreat/o**/tomy (păn-krē-ă-TŎT-ō-mē): _____ *-tomy:* incision
parathyroid/o	parathyroid glands	**parathyroid**/ectomy (păr-ă-thī-royd-ĔK-tō-mē): _____ *-ectomy:* excision, removal
thym/o	thymus gland	**thym**/oma (thī-MŌ-mă): _____ *-oma:* tumor *A thymoma is a rare neoplasm of the thymus gland. Treatment includes surgical removal, radiation therapy, and chemotherapy.*

Medical Word Elements—cont'd

Element	Meaning	Analysis
thyr/o	thyroid gland	**thyr/o**/megaly (thī-rō-MĔG-ă-lē): _____ -_megaly:_ enlargement

thyroid/o		hyper/**thyroid/i**sm (hī-pĕr-THĪ-royd-ĭzm): _____
		  hyper-: excessive, above normal
		  -_ism:_ condition

toxic/o	poison	**toxic/o**/logist (tŏks-ĭ-KŎL-ō-jĭst): _____
		  -_logist:_ specialist in the study of
		  Toxicologists study the effects of toxins and antidotes used for treatment of toxic disorders.

Suffixes

Element	Meaning	Analysis
-crine	secrete	endo/**crine** (ĔN-dō-krĭn): _____ _endo-:_ in, within

-dipsia	thirst	poly/**dipsia** (pŏl-ē-DĬP-sē-ă): _____
		  poly: many, much
		  Polydipsia is one of the three "polys" (along with polyphagia and polyuria) associated with diabetes.

-gen	forming, producing, origin	andr/o/**gen** (ĂN-drō-jĕn): _____ _andr/o:_ male
-toxic	pertaining to poison	thyr/o/**toxic** (thī-rō-TŎKS-ĭk): _____ _thyr/o:_ thyroid gland
-uria	urine	glycos/**uria** (glī-kō-SŪ-rē-ă): _____ _glycos:_ sugar, sweetness

Prefixes

Element	Meaning	Analysis

eu-	good	**eu**/thyr/oid (ū-THĪ-royd): _____
		  thyr/o: thyroid gland
		  -_oid:_ resembling

exo-	outside	**exo**/crine (ĔKS-ō-krĭn): _____
		  -_crine:_ secrete
		  Exocrine glands (sweat and oil glands) secrete their products outwardly through excretory ducts.

poly	many	**poly**/uria (pŏl-ē-Ū-rē-ă): _____
		  -_uria:_ urine
		  Some causes of polyuria are diabetes, use of diuretics, excessive fluid intake, and hypercalcemia.

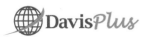 Visit the _Medical Terminology Systems_ online resource center at DavisPlus for an audio exercise of the terms in this table. Other activities are also available to reinforce content.

It is time to review medical word elements by completing Learning Activities 14-1 and 14-2.

Disease Focus

Disorders of the endocrine system are caused by underproduction **(hyposecretion)** or overproduction **(hypersecretion)** of hormones. In general, hyposecretion is treated with drug therapy in the form of hormone replacement. Hypersecretion is generally treated with surgery. Most hormone deficiencies result from genetic defects in the glands, surgical removal of the glands, or production of poor-quality hormones.

For diagnosis, treatment, and management of endocrine disorders, the medical services of a specialist may be warranted. **Endocrinology** is the branch of medicine concerned with endocrine glands and hormones. The physician who specializes in the diagnosis and treatment of endocrine disorders is known as an **endocrinologist.**

Thyroid Disorders

Thyroid gland disorders are common and may occur at any time during life. They may be the result of a developmental problem, injury, disease, or dietary deficiency.

Deficiency of thyroid hormone **(hypothyroidism)** that develops in infants is called **cretinism.** If not treated, this disorder leads to mental retardation, impaired growth, low body temperatures, and abnormal bone formation. Usually these symptoms do not appear at birth because the infant has received thyroid hormones from the mother's blood during fetal development. When hypothyroidism develops during adulthood, it is known as **myxedema.** The signs and symptoms of this disease include edema, low blood levels of T_3 and T_4, weight gain, cold intolerance, fatigue, depression, muscle or joint pain, and sluggishness.

Hyperthyroidism is a condition in which the thyroid gland produces excessive amounts of thyroid hormone. The most common form is **Graves disease,** also known as **thyrotoxicosis/autoimmune hyperthyroidism,** an autoimmune disorder in which the immune system produces autoantibodies that stimulate the production of excessive thyroid hormone. Another cause of hyperthyroidism is the formation of nodules or lumps on the thyroid gland **(toxic nodular** or **multinodular hyperthyroidism),** causing the excess production of thyroid hormone.

Signs and symptoms of hyperthyroidism include an elevated metabolic rate, abnormal weight loss, excessive perspiration, muscle weakness, and emotional instability. Also, the eyes are likely to protrude **(exophthalmos)** because of edematous swelling in the tissues behind them. (See Fig. 14-3.) At the same time, the thyroid gland is likely to enlarge, producing **goiter.** (See Fig. 14-4.)

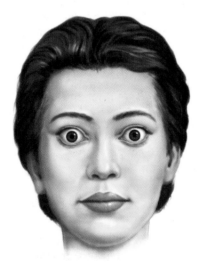

Figure 14-3 Exophthalmos caused by Graves disease.

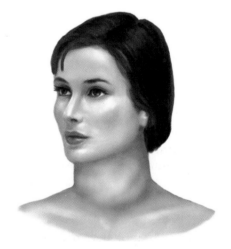

Figure 14-4 Enlargement of the thyroid gland in goiter.

Treatment for **hyperthyroidism** may involve drug therapy to block the production of thyroid hormones or surgical removal of all or part of the thyroid gland. Another method for treating this disorder is to administer a sufficient amount of radioactive iodine to destroy the thyroid secretory cells.

Parathyroid Disorders

As with the thyroid gland, dysfunction of the parathyroids is usually characterized by inadequate or excessive hormone secretion. Insufficient production of parathyroid hormone (PTH), called **hypoparathyroidism,** may be caused by primary parathyroid dysfunction or elevated blood calcium levels. This condition can result from an injury or from surgical removal of the glands, sometimes in conjunction with thyroid surgery. The primary effect of hypoparathyroidism is a decreased blood calcium level **(hypocalcemia).** Decreased calcium causes muscle twitches and spasms **(tetany).**

Excessive production of PTH, called **hyperparathyroidism,** is commonly caused by a benign tumor. The increase in PTH secretion leads to demineralization of bones **(osteitis fibrosa cystica),** making them porous **(osteoporosis)** and highly susceptible to fracture and deformity. When this condition is the result of a benign glandular tumor **(adenoma)** of the parathyroid, the tumor is removed. Excess PTH also causes calcium deposits in the kidneys.

Adrenal Gland Disorders

The adrenal cortex and adrenal medulla have their own structures and functions and their own sets of associated disorders.

Adrenal Cortex

The adrenal cortex is mainly associated with Addison disease and Cushing syndrome.

Addison Disease

Addison disease, also called **corticoadrenal insufficiency,** is a relatively uncommon chronic disorder caused by a deficiency of cortical hormones. It commonly results from damage to or atrophy of the adrenal cortex. Hypofunction of the adrenal cortex interferes with the body's ability to handle internal and external stress. Other clinical manifestations include muscle weakness, anorexia, gastrointestinal symptoms, fatigue, hypoglycemia, hypotension, low blood sodium **(hyponatremia),** and high serum potassium **(hyperkalemia).** If treatment for this condition begins early (usually with adrenocortical hormone therapy), the prognosis is excellent. If untreated, the disease will continue a chronic course with progressive but relatively slow deterioration. In some patients, the deterioration may be rapid.

Cushing Syndrome

Cushing syndrome is a cluster of symptoms produced by excessive amounts of cortisol, adrenocorticotropic hormone (ACTH), or both circulating in the blood. (See Fig. 14-5, page 490.)

Causes of this excess secretion include the following:

* Long-term administration of steroid drugs (glucocorticoids) in treating such diseases as rheumatoid arthritis, lupus erythematosus, and asthma
* Adrenal tumor, resulting in excessive production of cortisol
* Cushing disease, a pituitary disorder caused by hypersecretion of ACTH from an adenoma in the anterior pituitary gland.

Regardless of the cause, Cushing syndrome alters carbohydrate and protein metabolism and electrolyte balance. Overproduction of mineralocorticoids and glucocorticoids causes blood glucose concentration to remain high, depleting tissue protein. In addition, sodium retention causes increased fluid in tissues, leading to edema. These metabolic changes produce weight

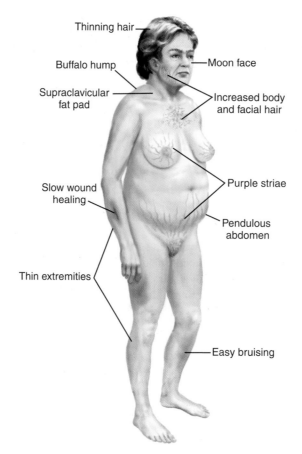

Thinning hair

Buffalo hump

Supraclavicular fat pad

Moon face

Increased body and facial hair

Slow wound healing

Purple striae

Pendulous abdomen

Thin extremities

Easy bruising

Figure 14-5 Physical manifestations of Cushing syndrome.

gain and may cause structural changes, such as a moon-shaped face, grossly exaggerated head and trunk, and pencil-thin arms and legs. Other symptoms include fatigue, high blood pressure, and excessive hair growth in unusual places **(hirsutism),** especially in women. The treatment goal for this disease is to restore serum cortisol to normal levels. Nevertheless, treatment varies with the cause and may necessitate radiation, drug therapy, surgery, or a combination of these methods.

Adrenal Medulla

No specific diseases can be traced directly to a deficiency of hormones from the adrenal medulla. However, medullary tumors sometimes cause excess secretions. The most common disorder is a neoplasm known as **pheochromocytoma,** which produces excessive amounts of epinephrine and norepinephrine. Most of these tumors are encapsulated and benign. These hypersecretions produce high blood pressure, rapid heart rate, stress, fear, palpitations, headaches, visual blurring, muscle spasms, and sweating. Typical treatment consists of antihypertensive drugs and surgery.

Pancreatic Disorders

By far, the most common pancreatic disorder is diabetes. **Diabetes** is a general term that, when used alone, refers to diabetes mellitus (DM). DM is a chronic metabolic disorder of impaired carbohydrate, protein, and fat metabolism resulting from insufficient production of insulin or the body's inability to use insulin properly. When body cells are deprived of glucose, their principal energy fuel, they begin to metabolize proteins and fats. Fat metabolism produces ketones, which enter the blood, causing a condition called **ketosis.** Hyperglycemia and ketosis are responsible for the host of troubling and, commonly, life-threatening symptoms of diabetes mellitus.

Although genetics and environmental factors, such as obesity and lack of exercise, seem significant in the development of this disease, the cause of diabetes is not always clear. Diabetes mellitus occurs in two primary forms: type 1 and type 2.

Type 1 Diabetes

Type 1 diabetes is an autoimmune disease. It is usually diagnosed in children and young adults. In type 1 diabetes, the body does not produce a sufficient amount of insulin. Like all autoimmune diseases, it requires constant monitoring and medicating. Blood glucose levels are monitored by the patient several times a day using a **glucometer** to determine the amount of insulin needed to control blood sugar levels. The patient administers insulin injections as needed. Insulin injections should be administered in a different subcutaneous site each time to avoid injury to the tissues. (See Fig. 14-6.)

Type 2 Diabetes

In **type 2 diabetes**, either the body's cells are resistant to insulin or the pancreas is deficient in producing insulin. In both cases, the body's cells do not absorb glucose, and it remains in the blood, causing **hyperglycemia.** Type 2 diabetes is the most common form and is distinctively different from type 1. Its onset is typically later in life; however, it has become more prevalent in children as the incidence of obesity has increased. Risk factors include a family history of diabetes and obesity. Treatment for type 2 diabetes includes exercise, diet, weight loss, and insulin or oral antidiabetic agents, if needed. (See Table 14-6.)

Oncology

Oncological disorders of the endocrine system vary based on the organ involved and include pancreatic cancer, pituitary tumors, and thyroid carcinoma.

Pancreatic Cancer

Most carcinomas of the pancreas arise as epithelial tumors **(adenocarcinomas)** and make their presence known by causing obstructions and local invasion. Because the pancreas is richly supplied with nerves, pain is a prominent feature of pancreatic cancer, whether it arises in the head, body, or tail of the organ.

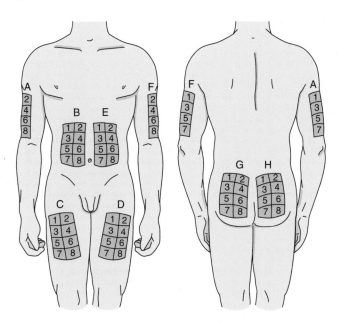

Rotation sites for injection of insulin.

Figure 14-6 Rotation sites for injection of insulin. From Williams and Hopper: *Understanding Medical-Surgical Nursing,* 4th ed. F.A. Davis, Philadelphia, 2011, p. 922, with permission.

Table 14-6	Differences Between Type 1 and Type 2 Diabetes		
*This table summarizes the differences between type 1 and type 2 diabetes.**			
	Onset	**Low Blood Glucose**	**Prevention**
type 1 diabetes	• Symptoms usually start in childhood or young adulthood. • Patients commonly seek medical attention because they experience serious symptoms associated with a high blood glucose level.	• Episodes of low blood glucose level (hypoglycemia) are common.	• Prevention is not possible.
type 2 diabetes	• The disease is usually discovered during a routine checkup, commonly before symptoms occur. • It is commonly diagnosed in adulthood, but an increasing number of children are being diagnosed with the disease.	• There are no episodes of low blood glucose level, unless the person is taking excessive insulin or certain diabetes medicines.	• Healthy lifestyle measures to prevent or delay onset include maintaining a healthy weight, eating sensibly, and exercising regularly.

*Both types of diabetes greatly increase a person's risk for a range of serious complications. Although monitoring and managing the disease can prevent complications, diabetes remains the leading cause of blindness and kidney failure. It also continues to be a critical risk factor for heart disease, stroke, and foot or leg amputations.

The prognosis in pancreatic cancer is poor, with only a 2% survival rate in 5 years. Pancreatic cancer is the fourth leading cause of cancer death in the United States. The highest incidence is among people ages 60 to 70. The etiology is unknown, but cigarette smoking, exposure to occupational chemicals, a diet high in fats, and heavy coffee intake are associated with an increased incidence of pancreatic cancer.

Pituitary Tumors

Pituitary tumors are abnormal growths that develop in the pituitary gland. Some pituitary tumors cause excessive production of hormones that regulate important functions of the body. Other pituitary tumors can restrict normal function of the pituitary gland, causing it to produce lower levels of hormones. The vast majority of pituitary tumors are noncancerous **(benign)** growths known as **adenomas.** Adenomas remain confined to the pituitary gland or surrounding tissues and do not spread to other parts of the body. As the tumor grows, it can cause a variety of symptoms, including compression of nearby nerves, resulting in vision problems. Treatment involves removing the tumor, especially if it is pressing on the optic nerves, which could cause blindness. Removal of pituitary tumors commonly occurs through the nose and sphenoid sinuses **(transsphenoidal hypophysectomy).** Other treatment modalities include restoring normal hormone levels or radiation therapy to shrink the tumor. These treatments occur in combination with surgery or for patients who cannot tolerate surgery.

Thyroid Carcinoma

Cancer of the thyroid gland, or **thyroid carcinoma,** is classified according to the specific tissue that is affected. In general, however, all types share many predisposing factors, including radiation, prolonged TSH stimulation, familial disposition, and chronic goiter. The malignancy usually begins with a painless, commonly hard nodule or a nodule in the adjacent lymph nodes accompanied by an enlarged thyroid. When the tumor is large, it typically destroys thyroid tissue, which results in symptoms of hypothyroidism. Sometimes the tumor stimulates the production of thyroid hormone, resulting in symptoms of hyperthyroidism. Treatment includes surgical removal, radiation, or both.

Diseases and Conditions

This section introduces diseases and conditions of the endocrine system, along with their meanings and pronunciations. Word analyses for selected terms are also provided.

Term	Definition
diabetes insipidus (DI) dī-ă-BĒ-tēz ĭn-SĬP-ĭ-dŭs	Disorder characterized by excessive thirst (polydipsia) and excessive urination (polyuria) due to inadequate production of antidiuretic hormone (ADH)
diuresis dī-ū-RĒ-sĭs *di-:* double *ur:* urine *-esis:* condition	Increased formation and secretion of urine *Diuresis commonly occurs in diabetes mellitus. Alcohol and coffee are common diuretics that increase formation and secretion of urine.*
gestational diabetes jĕs-TĀ-shŭn-ăl dī-ă-BĒ-tēz	Diabetes that develops during pregnancy (gestation) *In gestational diabetes, blood glucose level usually returns to normal soon after delivery. However, it places the woman at risk for type 2 diabetes.*
growth hormone (GH) **disorders**	Pituitary gland disorder that generally involves a hypersecretion or hyposecretion of GH and commonly results from a pituitary tumor

acromegaly
  ăk-rō-MĔG-ă-lē
   acr/o: extremity
   -megaly: enlargement
	Hypersecretion of GH in adults, resulting in enlargement of bones in the extremities and head (See Fig. 14-7.)
	Treatment for acromegaly includes radiation, pharmacological agents, or surgery to remove a portion of the pituitary gland.

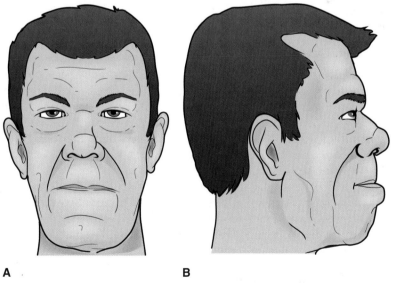

Figure 14-7 Acromegaly. (A) Frontal view. (B) Lateral view.

dwarfism	Hyposecretion of GH during childhood, resulting in extreme shortness in stature (final height of only 3′ to 4′) but normal body proportions *Treatment for dwarfism includes administration of GH during childhood, before skeletal growth is complete.*

(continued)

Diseases and Conditions—cont'd

Term	Definition
giantism	Hypersecretion of GH during childhood, resulting in abnormal increase in the length of long bones and extreme height (up to 8′ tall) but with body proportions remaining about normal (See Fig. 14-8.) *Removal of the pituitary tumor using radiation, surgery, or medications may lower GH hormone levels and control abnormal growth.* 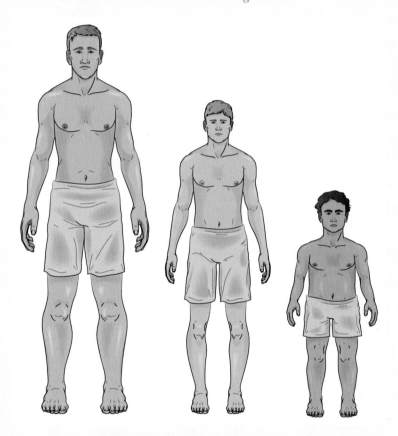 **Figure 14-8** Giantism and dwarfism.
hirsutism HĬR-sū-tĭzm	Excessive distribution of body hair, especially in women *Common causes of hirsutism include abnormalities of androgen production, medications, and tumors.*
hypercalcemia hī-pĕr-kăl-SĒ-mē-ă *hyper-:* excessive, above normal *calc:* calcium *-emia:* blood	Condition in which the calcium level in the blood is higher than normal *The main cause of hypercalcemia is overactivity in one or more parathyroid glands. Other causes include cancer, medications, and excessive use of calcium and vitamin D supplements.*
hyperkalemia hī-pĕr-kă-LĒ-mē-ă *hyper-:* excessive, above normal *kal:* potassium (an electrolyte) *-emia:* blood	Condition in which the potassium level in the blood is higher than normal *Potassium is a critical electrolyte in the proper functioning of nerve and muscle cells, including the heart. Severe hyperkalemia requires immediate treatment because it can lead to cardiac arrest and death.*

Diseases and Conditions—cont'd

Term	Definition
hypervolemia hī-pĕr-vŏl-Ē-mē-ă *hyper-:* excessive, above normal *vol:* volume *-emia:* blood	Abnormal increase in the volume of blood plasma (liquid part of the blood and lymphatic fluid) in the body *Hypervolemia commonly results from retention of large amounts of sodium and water by the kidneys.*
hyponatremia hī-pō-nă-TRĒ-mē-ă *hypo-:* under, below, deficient *natr:* sodium (an electrolyte) *-emia:* blood	Lower-than-normal level of sodium in the blood *Hyponatremia is commonly caused by drinking too much water when exercising (especially in the heat), thereby diluting the amount of sodium in the blood.*
insulinoma ĭn-sū-lĭn-Ō-mă *insulin:* insulin *-oma:* tumor	Tumor of the islets of Langerhans of the pancreas, causing the excessive production of insulin and leading to hypoglycemia; also called *pancreatic tumor*
neurofibromatosis (NF) nū-rō-fī-brō-mă-TŌ-sĭs	Genetic disorder with multiple benign fibrous tumors that grow anywhere in the nervous system including the brain, spinal cord, and peripheral nerves *Most tumors are benign but some may become cancerous.*
obesity ō-BĒ-sĭ-tē	Abnormal accumulation of body fat, usually 20% or more of an individual's ideal body weight *Obesity is associated with increased risk of illness, disability, and death. The branch of medicine that deals with the study and treatment of obesity is known as bariatrics and has become a separate medical and surgical specialty.*
panhypopituitarism păn-hī-pō-pĭ-TŪ-ĭ-tăr-ĭzm *pan-:* all *hyp/o:* under, below, deficient *pituitar:* pituitary gland *-ism:* condition	Total pituitary impairment that brings about a progressive and general loss of hormone activity *Panhypopituitarism can lead to symptoms associated primarily with insufficiency of gonadotropins, growth hormones, and thyroid hormones.*
thyroid storm THĪ-royd *thyr:* thyroid gland *-oid:* resembling	Crisis of uncontrolled hyperthyroidism caused by the release into the bloodstream of an increased amount of thyroid hormone; also called *thyroid crisis* or *thyrotoxic crisis* *Thyroid storm is a medical emergency and, if left untreated, may be fatal.*
virilism VĬR-ĭl-ĭzm	Masculinization or development of male secondary sex characteristics in a woman

It is time to review pathology, diseases, and conditions by completing Learning Activity 14-3.

Diagnostic, Surgical, and Therapeutic Procedures

This section introduces diagnostic, surgical, and therapeutic procedures used to diagnose and treat endocrine system disorders. Descriptions are provided, along with pronunciations and word analyses for selected terms.

Procedure	Description
Diagnostic	
Clinical	

exophthalmometry
ĕk-sŏf-thăl-MŎM-ĕ-trē
   ex-: out, out from
   ophthalm/o: eye
   -metry: act of measuring
	Measures the degree of forward displacement of the eyeball (exophthalmos) as seen in Graves disease

Laboratory	
A1c test	Blood test used to diagnose and manage type 1 and type 2 diabetes; also called *glycated hemoglobin, hemoglobin A1c,* and *HbA1c.* *The A1c test result reflects the average blood sugar level for the past two to three months by measuring the percentage of hemoglobin (a protein in red blood cells that carries oxygen) coated with sugar (glycated).*
fasting blood sugar (FBS)	Test that measures glucose levels in a blood sample following a fast of at least 8 hours *This test helps diagnose diabetes and monitor glucose levels in diabetic patients.*
glucose tolerance test (GTT) GLOO-kōs	Screening test in which a dose of glucose is administered and blood samples are taken at regular intervals following the dose to determine how quickly glucose is cleared from the blood *GTT is performed to diagnose prediabetes and gestational diabetes.*
insulin tolerance test (ITT) ĬN-sŭ-lĭn	Diagnostic test in which insulin is injected into the vein, causing severe hypoglycemia to assess growth hormone (GH) and cortisol reserve *The symptoms of low blood glucose will cause the release of growth hormone and cortisol. The test measures GH and cortisol at specified intervals.*
thyroid function test (TFT) THĪ-royd	Test that detects an increase or decrease in thyroid function *The TFT measures levels of thyroid-stimulating hormone (TSH), triiodothyronine (T_3), and thyroxine (T_4).*
total calcium test KĂL-sē-ŭm	Test that measures blood calcium levels to detect bone and parathyroid disorders, malabsorption, or an overactive thyroid *Hypercalcemia can indicate primary hyperparathyroidism; hypocalcemia can indicate hypoparathyroidism.*

Diagnostic, Surgical, and Therapeutic Procedures—cont'd

Procedure	Description

Imaging

radioactive iodine uptake (RAIU) and scan rā-dē-ō-ĂK-tĭv Ī-ō-dīn	Nuclear imaging procedure that combines a thyroid scan with an RAIU procedure to evaluate the structure and physiological functioning of the thyroid gland *The thyroid scan shows the size and shape of the thyroid gland and identifies areas of the thyroid gland that are underactive or overactive. A normal scan shows a uniform distribution of radioactive tracer throughout the thyroid gland. The RAIU measures how well the thyroid gland is able to absorb iodine from the blood (iodine uptake) and evaluates thyroid function and thyroid abnormalities, especially an overactive thyroid gland (hyperthyroidism).*

Surgical

parathyroidectomy păr-ă-thī-royd-ĔK-tō-mē *para-:* near, beside; beyond *thyroid:* thyroid gland *-ectomy:* excision, removal	Excision of one or more of the parathyroid glands, usually to control hyperparathyroidism
thyroidectomy thī-royd-ĔK-tō-mē *thyroid:* thyroid gland *-ectomy:* excision, removal	Excision of the entire thyroid gland (thyroidectomy), a part of it (subtotal thyroidectomy), or a single lobe (thyroid lobectomy) *Thyroidectomy is performed for goiter, tumors, or hyperthyroidism that does not respond to iodine therapy and antithyroid drugs.*
transsphenoidal hypophysectomy trăns-sfē-NOY-dăl hī-pŏf-ĭ-SĔK-tō-mē	Endoscopic surgery to remove a pituitary tumor through an incision in the sphenoid sinus (transsphenoidal) without disturbing brain tissue (See Fig. 14-9.) *Transsphenoidal hypophysectomy is a minimally invasive procedure that is commonly performed to remove abnormal pituitary gland tissue or pituitary tumors. It also treats Cushing syndrome resulting from a pituitary tumor.*

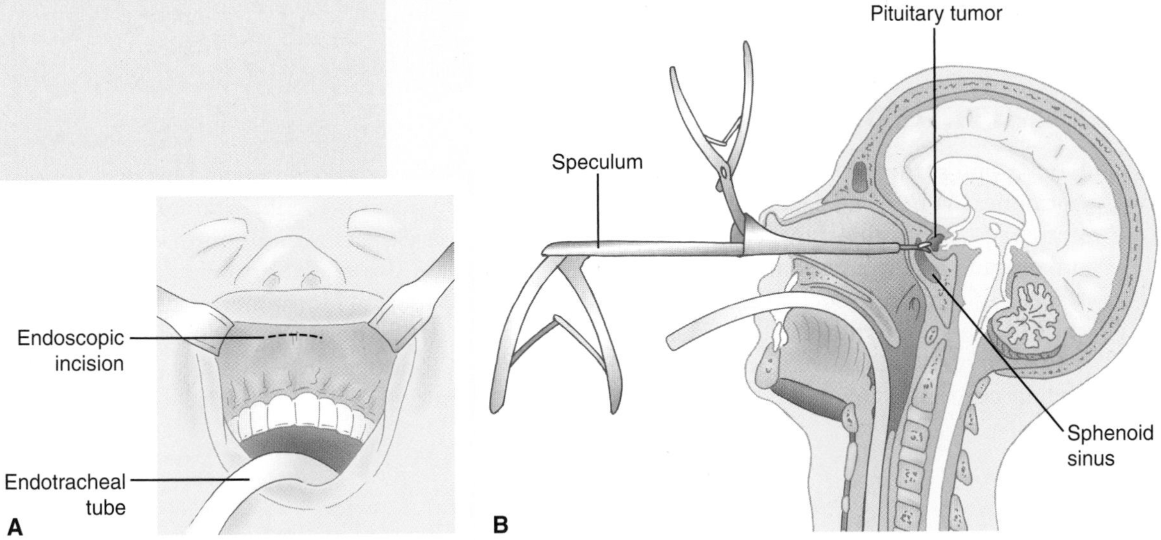

Figure 14-9 Hypophysectomy. (A) Incision made beneath the upper lip to enter the nasal cavity and gain access to the pituitary gland. (B). Insertion of a speculum and special forceps used to remove the pituitary tumor.

(continued)

Diagnostic, Surgical, and Therapeutic Procedures—cont'd

Procedure	Description
Therapeutic	
insulin injection therapy	Lifelong therapy using a fine needle and syringe to inject insulin for controlling type 1 diabetes *Treatment usually requires a mixture of insulin types or combinations, including long-acting and rapid-acting insulins, to keep blood glucose levels in a target range. The patient calculates insulin types and dosage by monitoring the blood glucose level throughout the day using a handheld monitor such as a glucometer.*
insulin pump therapy	Treatment for type 1 diabetes that uses a device that continuously delivers insulin through a catheter placed under the skin (See Fig. 14-10.) *The pump delivers a basal rate of insulin continuously over a 24-hour period. Buttons on the pump allow the patient to increase the insulin dose at mealtime (bolus dose) or to deliver correction and supplemental doses when glucose levels are out of target range.*

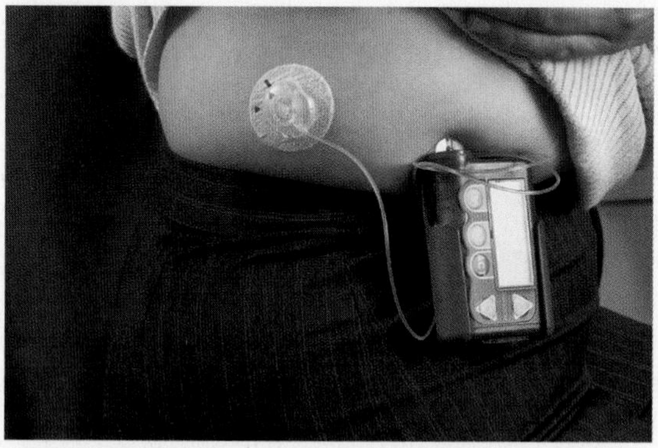

Figure 14-10 Insulin pump attached to the abdomen. From Williams and Hopper: *Understanding Medical-Surgical Nursing,* 4th ed. F.A. Davis, Philadelphia, 2011, p. 923, with permission.

Pharmacology

Common disorders associated with endocrine glands include hyposecretion and hypersecretion of hormones. When deficiencies of this type occur, the physician prescribes natural and synthetic hormones, such as insulin and thyroid agents. These agents normalize hormone levels to maintain proper functioning and homeostasis. Therapeutic agents are also available to regulate various substances in the body, such as glucose levels in diabetic patients. Hormone replacement therapy (HRT), such as synthetic thyroid and estrogen, treat these hormone deficiencies. Although this section does not cover specific chemotherapy drugs, hormone chemotherapy drugs help treat certain cancers, such as testicular, ovarian, breast, and endometrial cancer. (See Table 14-7.)

Table 14-7 Drugs Used to Treat Endocrine Disorders

This table lists common drug classifications used to treat endocrine disorders, their therapeutic actions, and selected generic and trade names.

Classification	Therapeutic Action	Generic and Trade Names
antithyroids ăn-tĭ-THĪ-roydz	Treat hyperthyroidism by impeding the formation of T_3 and T_4 hormone *Antithyroids are administered in preparation for a thyroidectomy, in thyrotoxic crisis, and for treatment of Graves disease.*	**methimazole** měth-ĬM-ă-zōl *Tapazole* **strong iodine solution** Ī-ō-dīn *Lugol's solution*
corticosteroids kor-tĭ-kō-STĔR-oydz	Replace hormones lost in adrenal insufficiency (Addison disease) *Corticosteroids are also widely used to suppress inflammation, control allergic reactions, reduce rejection in transplantation, and treat some cancers.*	**cortisone** KOR-tĭ-sōn *Cortisone acetate* **hydrocortisone** hī-drō-KOR-tĭ-sōn *A-Hydrocort, Cortef*
growth hormone replacements	Increase skeletal growth in children and growth hormone deficiencies in adults *Growth hormones increase spinal bone density and help manage growth failure in children.*	**somatropin (recombinant)** sō-mă-TRŌ-pĭn *Humatrope, Norditropin*
insulins* ĬN-sŭ-lĭns	Lower blood glucose levels by promoting its entrance into body cells and converting glucose to glycogen (a starch-storage form of glucose) *Type 1 diabetes must always be treated with insulin. Insulin can also be administered through an implanted pump, which infuses the drug continuously. Type 2 diabetes that cannot be controlled with oral antidiabetics may require insulin to maintain a normal level of glucose in the blood.*	**regular insulin** ĬN-sŭ-lĭn *Humulin R, Novolin R* **insulin aspart** ĬN-sŭ-lĭn *Novolog* **insulin glargine** ĬN-sŭ-lĭn GLĂR-jēn *Lantus*
oral antidiabetics ăn-tĭ-dī-ă-BĔT-ĭks	Treat type 2 diabetes mellitus by stimulating the pancreas to produce more insulin and decrease peripheral resistance to insulin *Antidiabetic drugs are not insulin, and they are not used in treating type 1 diabetes mellitus.*	**glipizide** GLĬP-ĭ-zīd *Glucotrol, Glucotrol XL* **metformin** mět-FOR-mĭn *Glucophage*
thyroid supplements	Replace or supplement thyroid hormones *Each thyroid supplement contains T_3, T_4, or a combination of both. Thyroid supplements are also used to treat some types of thyroid cancer.*	**levothyroxine** lē-vō-thī-RŎK-sēn *Levo-T, Levoxyl, Synthroid* **liothyronine** lī-ō-THĪ-rō-nēn *Cytomel, Triostat*

*Traditionally, insulin has been derived from beef or pork pancreas. Human insulin is genetically produced using recombinant DNA techniques to avoid the potential for allergic reaction.

Abbreviations

This section introduces endocrine-related abbreviations and their meanings.

Abbreviation	Meaning	Abbreviation	Meaning
ACTH	adrenocorticotropic stimulating hormone	PRL	prolactin
ADH	antidiuretic hormone	PTH	parathyroid hormone; also called *parathormone*
DI	diabetes insipidus	RAI	radioactive iodine
DKA	diabetic ketoacidosis	RAIU	radioactive iodine uptake
DM	diabetes mellitus	SIADH	syndrome of inappropriate antidiuretic hormone
FBS	fasting blood sugar	T_3	triiodothyronine (thyroid hormone)
FSH	follicle-stimulating hormone	T_4	thyroxine (thyroid hormone)
GH	growth hormone	TFT	thyroid function test
GTT	glucose tolerance test	TH	thyroid hormone
ITT	insulin tolerance test	TSH	thyroid-stimulating hormone
LH	luteinizing hormone	NF	neurofibromatosis

It is time to review procedures, pharmacology, and abbreviations by completing Learning Activity 14–4.

LEARNING ACTIVITIES

The activities that follow provide a review of the endocrine system terms introduced in this chapter. Complete each activity and review your answers to evaluate your understanding of the chapter.

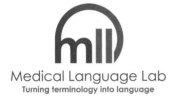

Visit the Medical Language Lab at *medicallanguagelab.com*. Use it to enhance your study and reinforcement of this chapter with the flash-card activity. We recommend that you complete the flash-card activity before starting Learning Activities 14-1 and 14-2.

Learning Activity 14-1
Medical Word Elements

Use the listed elements to build medical words. You may use elements more than once.

Combining Forms		Suffixes		Prefixes	
acr/o	pancreat/o	-crine	-logist	a-	poly-
adrenal/o	thym/o	-dipsia	-lysis	endo-	
calc/o	thyr/o	-emia	-megaly	exo-	
glyc/o	toxic/o	-genesis	-oma	hyper-	
kal/i		-itis		hypo-	

1. tumor of the thymus _____

2. inflammation of the pancreas _____

3. much thirst _____

4. forming or producing sugar _____

5. (glands that) secrete within (the blood) _____

6. without thirst _____

7. (glands that) secrete outward (through ducts) _____

8. blood condition of excessive sugar _____

9. destruction of the thymus _____

10. enlargement of the thyroid gland _____

11. inflammation of the adrenal glands _____

12. blood condition of below-normal calcium _____

13. blood condition of excessive potassium (an electrolyte) _____

14. enlargement of the extremities _____

15. specialist in the study of poison(s) _____

 Check your answers in Appendix A. Review any material that you did not answer correctly.

Correct Answers _____ X 6.67 = _____ % Score

Learning Activity 14-2

Building Medical Words

Use *glyc/o* (sugar) to build words that mean

1. blood condition of excessive glucose _____
2. blood condition of deficiency of glucose _____
3. forming or producing glycogen _____

Use *pancreat/o* (pancreas) to build words that mean

4. inflammation of the pancreas _____
5. destruction of the pancreas _____
6. disease of the pancreas _____

Use *thyr/o* or *thyroid/o* (thyroid gland) to build words that mean

7. inflammation of the thyroid gland _____
8. enlargement of the thyroid _____

Build surgical words that mean

9. excision of a parathyroid gland _____
10. removal of the adrenal gland _____

Check your answers in Appendix A. Review any material that you did not answer correctly.

Correct Answers _____ X 10 = _____ % Score

Diseases and Conditions

Match the terms with the definitions in the numbered list.

acromegaly	*exophthalmic goiter*	*myxedema*
Addison disease	*glycosuria*	*pheochromocytoma*
cretinism	*hirsutism*	*thyroid storm*
Cushing syndrome	*hyperkalemia*	*type 1*
diuresis	*hyponatremia*	*type 2*

1. abnormal enlargement of the extremities _____

2. hypothyroidism acquired in adulthood _____

3. increased excretion of urine _____

4. excessive growth of hair in unusual places, especially in women _____

5. congenital hypothyroidism _____

6. crisis of uncontrolled hyperthyroidism _____

7. caused by deficiency in the secretion of adrenocortical hormones _____

8. characterized by protrusion of the eyeballs, increased heart action, enlargement of the thyroid gland, weight loss, and nervousness _____

9. excessive amount of potassium in the blood _____

10. small chromaffin cell tumor usually located in the adrenal medulla _____

11. insulin-dependent diabetes mellitus; occurs most commonly in children and adolescents (juvenile onset) _____

12. decreased concentration of sodium in the blood _____

13. abnormal presence of glucose in the urine _____

14. metabolic disorder caused by hypersecretion of the adrenal cortex resulting in excessive production of glucocorticoids, mainly cortisol _____

15. noninsulin-dependent diabetes mellitus; occurs later in life (maturity onset) _____

✔ *Check your answers in Appendix A. Review any material that you did not answer correctly.*

Correct Answers _____ X 6.67 = _____ % Score

Learning Activity 14-4

Procedures, Pharmacology, and Abbreviations

Match the terms with the definitions in the numbered list.

antithyroids	GTT	T_4
corticosteroids	insulin	TFT
exophthalmometry	oral antidiabetics	thyroid scan
FBS	RAIU	total calcium test
growth hormone	T_3	transsphenoidal

1. measures circulating glucose level after a 12-hour fast _____

2. detects how quickly ingested iodine is taken into the thyroid gland _____

3. replacement hormones for adrenal insufficiency (Addison disease) _____

4. increases skeletal growth in children _____

5. nuclear imaging procedure that shows the size and shape of the thyroid gland _____

6. thyroxine _____

7. used to treat type 2 diabetes _____

8. test to determine how quickly glucose is cleared from the blood _____

9. used to treat hyperthyroidism by impeding the formation of T_3 and T_4 hormone

_____

10. type of hypophysectomy to remove a pituitary tumor without disturbing brain tissue

_____

11. triiodothyronine _____

12. abbreviation for a test that measures thyroid function _____

13. test that measures the degree of forward displacement of the eyeball as seen in Graves disease _____

14. used to detect bone and parathyroid disorders _____

15. hormone used to treat type 1 diabetes _____

Check your answers in Appendix A. Review any material that you did not answer correctly.

Correct Answers _____ X 6.67 = _____ % Score

DOCUMENTING HEALTH-CARE ACTIVITIES

This section provides practical application activities in the form of exercises to help students develop skills in documenting patient care. First, read the medical report. Then complete the activities and exercises that follow.

Documenting Health-Care Activity 14-1
Consultation Note: Hyperparathyroidism

Consultation Note

Day, Phyllis 5/25/xx   Med Record: P25882

HISTORY OF PRESENT ILLNESS: This 66-year-old former blackjack dealer is under evaluation for hyperparathyroidism. Surgery evidently has been recommended, but there is confusion as to how urgent this is. She has a 13-year history of type 1 diabetes mellitus, a history of shoulder pain, osteoarthritis of the spine, and peripheral vascular disease with claudication. She states her 548-pack/year smoking history ended 3-1/2 years ago. Her first knowledge of parathyroid disease was about 3 years ago when laboratory findings revealed an elevated calcium level. This subsequently led to the diagnosis of hyperparathyroidism. She was further evaluated by an endocrinologist in the Lake Tahoe area, who determined that she also had hypercalciuria, although there is nothing to suggest a history of kidney stones.

IMPRESSION: Hyperparathyroidism and hypercalciuria, probably a parathyroid adenoma

PLAN: Patient advised to make a follow-up appointment with her endocrinologist.

Juan Perez, MD
Juan Perez, MD

D: 05–25–xx
T: 05–25–xx

jp:lg

Terminology

The terms listed in the table that follows are taken from *Consultation Note: Hyperparathyroidism.* Use a medical dictionary such as *Taber's Cyclopedic Medical Dictionary,* the appendices of this book, or other resources to define each term. Then review the pronunciation for each term and practice by reading the medical record aloud.

Term	Definition
adenoma ăd-ĕ-NŌ-mă	
claudication klăw-dĭ-KĀ-shŭn	
diabetes mellitus dī-ă-BĒ-tēz MĔ-lĭ-tŭs	
endocrinologist ĕn-dō-krĭn- ŎL-ō-jĭst	
hypercalciuria hī-pĕr-kăl-sē-Ū-rē-ă	
hyperparathyroidism hī-pĕr-păr-ă- THĪ-roy-dĭzm	
impression ĭm-PRĔSH-ŭn	
osteoarthritis ŏs-tē-ō-ăr-THRĪ-tĭs	
peripheral vascular disease pĕr-ĬF-ĕr-ăl VĂS-kū-lăr	

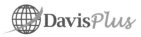

Visit the *Medical Terminology Systems* online resource center at Davis*Plus* to practice pronunciation and reinforce the meanings of the terms in this medical report.

Critical Thinking

Review *Consultation Note: Hyperparathyroidism* to answer the questions.

1. What is an adenoma?

_____

_____

_____

_____

2. What does the physician suspect caused the patient's hyperparathyroidism?

_____

_____

_____

_____

3. What type of laboratory findings revealed parathyroid disease?

_____

_____

_____

_____

4. What is hypercalciuria?

_____

_____

_____

_____

5. If the patient smoked 548 packs of cigarettes per year, how many packs did she smoke in an average day?

_____

_____

_____

SOAP Note: Diabetes Mellitus

Emergency Department Record

Date: 2/4/xx
Patient: Pleume, Roberta
Age: 68

Time Registered: 1445 hours
Physician: Samara Batichara, MD
Patient ID#: 22258

Chief Complaint: Frequent urination, increased hunger and thirst

S: This 200-pound patient was admitted to the hospital because of a 10-day history of polyuria, polydipsia, and polyphagia. She has been very nervous, irritable, and very sensitive emotionally and cries easily. During this period, she has had headaches and has become very sleepy and tired after eating. On admission, her Accu-Chek was 540 mg/dL. Family history is significant in that both parents and two sisters have type 1 diabetes.

O: Physical examination was essentially negative. The abdomen was difficult to evaluate because of morbid obesity.

A: Diabetes mellitus; obesity, exogenous

P: Patient admitted to the hospital for further evaluation.

Samara Batichara, MD
Samara Batichara, MD

D: 02–04-xx
T: 02–04-xx

sb:lb

Terminology

The terms listed in the table that follows are taken from *SOAP Note: Diabetes Mellitus.* Use a medical dictionary such as *Taber's Cyclopedic Medical Dictionary,* the appendices of this book, or other resources to define each term. Then review the pronunciation for each term and practice by reading the medical record aloud.

Term	Definition
Accu-chek ĂK-ū-ch ĕk	
morbid obesity MOR-bĭd ō-BĒ-sĭ-tē	
obesity, exogenous ō-BĒ-sĭ-tē, ĕks-ŎJ-ĕ-nŭs	
polydipsia pŏl-ē-DĬP-sē-ă	
polyphagia pŏl-ē-FĀ-jē-ă	
polyuria pŏl-ē-Ū-rē-ă	

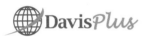 Visit the *Medical Terminology Systems* online resource center at Davis*Plus* to practice pronunciation and reinforce the meanings of the terms in this medical report.

Critical Thinking

Review *SOAP Note: Diabetes Mellitus* to answer the questions.

1. How long has this patient been experiencing voracious eating?

_____

_____

_____

_____

2. Was the patient's obesity a result of overeating or a metabolic imbalance?

_____

_____

_____

3. Why did the doctor experience difficulty in examining the patient's abdomen?

_____

_____

_____

_____

4. Was the patient's blood glucose above or below normal on admission?

_____

_____

_____

5. What is the reference range for fasting blood glucose?

_____

_____

_____

_____

Documenting Health-Care Activity 14-3

Constructing Chart Notes

To construct chart notes, replace the italicized and boldfaced terms in each of the scenarios with one of the listed medical terms.

bradycardia	hypopnea	polyphagia
constipation	lethargy	polyuria
glycosuria	polydipsia	triiodothyronine and thyroxine
hyperglycemia		

Ms. H., a 20-year-old nursing student, presents with complaints of (1) *excessive thirst*, (2) *excessive urination*, and (3) *excessive hunger*. She has headaches and occasional blurred vision. Because of her training as a health-care provider, she recognizes that these symptoms are associated with diabetes. She is further concerned because her mother and sister have diabetes. Her laboratory tests indicate (4) *high blood sugar* and (5) *sugar in the urine*. She will be seen by Dr. M. for a more complete workup, and he will begin management of her condition.

1. _____
2. _____
3. _____
4. _____
5. _____

Ms. C., a 56-year-old female, presents with complaints of (6) *lack of energy*, (7) *difficulty passing stool,* and "always feeling cold." Although she has decreased appetite, she has slowly gained 12 lb over the last 2 years. Her hair appears thin and brittle. Her physical examination was unremarkable except for a (8) *slow heart rate* and (9) *shallow breathing*. The physician schedules her for a CBC, metabolic blood panel, lipid panel, and (10) T_3 *and* T_4 tests.

6. _____
7. _____
8. _____
9. _____
10. _____

 Check your answers in Appendix A. Review any material that you did not answer correctly.

Nervous System

Chapter Outline

Objectives

Upon completion of this chapter, you will be able to:

- Locate and describe the structures of the nervous system.
- Describe the functional relationship between the nervous system and other body systems.
- Pronounce, spell, and build words related to the nervous system.
- Describe diseases, conditions, and procedures related to the nervous system.
- Explain pharmacology related to the treatment of nervous disorders.
- Demonstrate your knowledge of this chapter by completing the learning and documenting health-care activities.

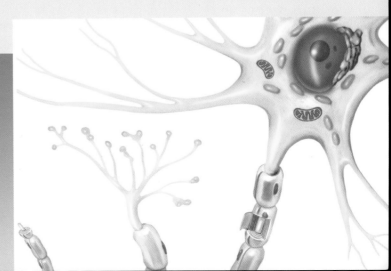

Anatomy and Physiology

The nervous system is one of the most complicated systems of the body in structure and function. It senses physical and chemical changes in the internal and external environments, processes them, and then responds to maintain homeostasis. The nervous system coordinates, regulates, and integrates voluntary activities, such as walking and talking, and involuntary activities, such as digestion and circulation. The entire neural network of the body relies on the transmission of electrochemical impulses that travel from one area of the body to another. The speed at which this transmission occurs is almost instantaneous, thus providing an immediate response to change.

Anatomy and Physiology Key Terms

This section introduces important terms, along with their definitions and pronunciations. The key terms are highlighted in color in the Anatomy and Physiology section. Word analyses for selected terms are also provided. Pronounce the term, and place a check mark in the box after you do so.

Term	Definition
afferent ĂF-ĕr-ĕnt ☐	Carry or move inward or toward a central structure *In the nervous system, afferent impulses travel toward the central nervous system.*
blood–brain barrier	Protective mechanism that blocks specific substances found in the bloodstream from entering delicate brain tissue
efferent ĔF-ĕ-rĕnt ☐	Carry or move away from a central structure *In the nervous system, efferent impulses travel away from the central nervous system.*
limbic system LĬM-bĭk ☐	Complex neural system located beneath the cerebrum that controls basic emotions and drives and plays an important role in memory *The limbic system is primarily related to survival and includes such emotions as fear, anger, and pleasure (food and sexual behavior).*
neurilemma nū-rĭ-LĔM-ă ☐	Additional external myelin sheath that is formed by Schwann cells and found only on axons in the peripheral nervous system *Because the neurilemma does not disintegrate after injury to the axon, its enclosed hollow tube provides an avenue for regeneration of injured axons.*
ventricle VĔN-trĭk-l ☐ *ventr:* belly, belly side *-icle:* minute, small	Organ chamber or cavity that receives or holds fluid *In the nervous system, cerebrospinal fluid flows through the ventricles of the brain into the spinal cavity and then returns to the brain, where it is absorbed into the blood.*

Pronunciation Help	Long Sound	ā — rate	ē — rebirth	ī — isle	ō — over	ū — unite
	Short Sound	ă — apple	ĕ — ever	ĭ — it	ŏ — not	ŭ — cut

Cellular Structure of the Nervous System

Despite its complexity, the nervous system is composed of only two principal cell types: neurons and neuroglia. Together, neurons and neuroglia constitute the nervous tissue of the body.

Neurons

Neurons transmit impulses. Depending on the direction in which they transmit information, neurons and nerves are classified as **afferent** (when the impulse moves toward the brain or spinal cord) or **efferent** (when the impulse moves away from the brain or spinal cord). The three major structures of the neuron are the cell body, axon, and dendrites. (See Fig. 15-1.) The (1) **cell body**

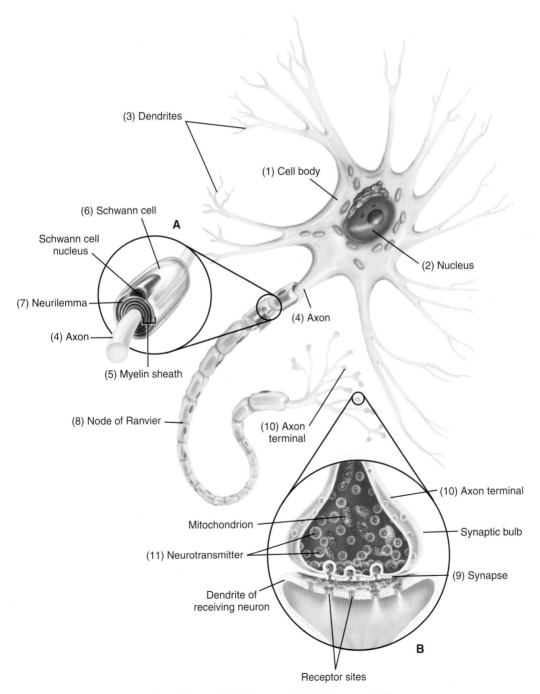

Figure 15-1 Neuron. (A) Schwann cell. (B) Axon terminal synapse.

is the enlarged structure of the neuron that contains the (2) **nucleus** of the cell and various organelles. Its branching cytoplasmic projections are (3) **dendrites** that carry impulses to the cell body and (4) **axons** that carry impulses from the cell body. Dendrites resemble tiny branches on a tree, providing additional surface area for receiving impulses from other neurons. Axons are threadlike extensions of nerve cells that transmit impulses to dendrites of other neurons and to muscles and glands.

Axons possess a white, lipoid covering called a (5) **myelin sheath.** This covering acts as an electrical insulator that reduces the possibility of an impulse stimulating adjacent nerves. It also accelerates impulse transmission through the axon. On nerves in the **peripheral nervous system,** the myelin sheath is formed by a neuroglial cell called a (6) **Schwann cell** that wraps tightly around the axon. Its exterior surface forms a thin tube called the (7) **neurilemma,** or **neurolemma.** The neurilemma acts as a protective coat for peripheral neurons. If the neurilemma covering remains intact after an injury to the nerve, it forms a tube that provides a pathway for possible neuron regeneration after injury.

Oligodendrocytes, rather than Schwann cells, form the myelin sheath that covers the axons in the central nervous system. Oligodendrocytes do not produce neurilemma, and thus injury or damage to neurons located in the central nervous system is irreparable. The short, unmyelinated spaces between adjacent segments of the myelin sheath are called (8) **nodes of Ranvier.** These nodes help speed the transmission of impulses down the axon.

The functional connection between two neurons or between a neuron and its effector organ (muscle or gland) is a gap or space called a (9) **synapse.** Impulses must travel from the (10) **axon terminal** of one neuron to the dendrite of the next neuron or to its effector organ by crossing this synapse. The impulse within the transmitting axon causes a chemical substance called a (11) **neurotransmitter** to be released at the end of its axon. The neurotransmitter diffuses across the synapse and attaches to the receiving neuron at specialized receptor sites. When sufficient receptor sites are occupied, it signals an acceptance "message" and the impulse passes to the receiving neuron. The receiving neuron immediately inactivates the neurotransmitter and prepares the site to receive another impulse.

Neuroglia

Neuroglia are cells that support neurons and bind them to other neurons or other tissues of the body. Although they do not transmit impulses, they provide a variety of activities essential to the proper functioning of neurons. The term **neuroglia** literally means "nerve glue" because these cells were originally believed to serve only to bind neurons to each other and to other structures. They are now known to supply nutrients and oxygen to neurons and assist in other metabolic activities. They also play an important role when the nervous system suffers injury or infection. The four major types of neuroglia are astrocytes, oligodendrocytes, microglia, and ependyma. (See Fig. 15-2.)

Astrocytes, as their name suggests, are star-shaped neuroglia. They provide three-dimensional mechanical support for neurons and form tight sheaths around the capillaries of the brain. These sheaths provide an obstruction called the **blood–brain barrier** that keeps large molecular substances from entering the delicate tissue of the brain. Even so, small molecules, such as water, carbon dioxide, oxygen, and alcohol, readily pass from blood vessels through the barrier and enter the interstitial spaces of the brain. Researchers must consider the blood–brain barrier when developing drugs that treat brain disorders. Astrocytes also perform mildly phagocytic functions in the brain and spinal cord. **Oligodendrocytes,** also called **oligodendroglia,** are responsible for developing myelin on the axons of neurons in the central nervous system. **Microglia,** the smallest of the neuroglia, possess phagocytic properties and become very active during times of infection. **Ependyma** are ciliated cells that line the fluid-filled cavities of the central nervous system, especially the **ventricles** of the brain. They assist in the circulation of cerebrospinal fluid (CSF).

Nervous System Divisions

The two major divisions of the nervous system are the central nervous system and the peripheral nervous system. The central nervous system consists of all nervous tissue located in the brain and spinal cord. The peripheral nervous system includes all nervous tissue located outside the central nervous system and consists of cranial and spinal nerves. (See Table 15-1.)

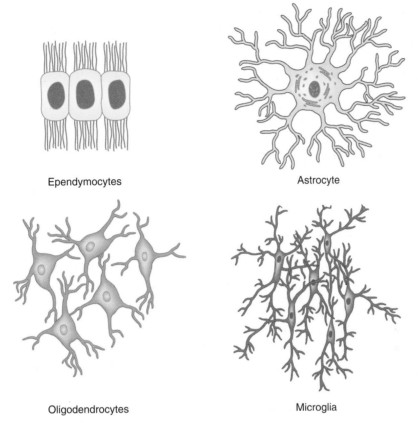

Ependymocytes

Astrocyte

Oligodendrocytes

Microglia

Figure 15-2 Four types of neuroglia.

Table 15-1	**Nervous System Structures and Functions**	
	This table lists the structures of the nervous system, along with their functions.	
	Structures	**Function**
	Central	
	Brain	Center for thought and emotion, interpretation of sensory stimuli, and coordination of body functions
	Spinal cord	Main pathway for transmission of information between the brain and body
	Peripheral	
	Cranial nerves	12 pairs of nerves that emerge from the base of the skull and may act in a motor capacity, sensory capacity, or both
	Spinal nerves	31 pairs of nerves that emerge from the spine and act in motor and sensory capacities

Central Nervous System

The **central nervous system (CNS)** consists of the brain and spinal cord. Its nervous tissue consists of **white matter** and **gray matter.** Bundles of axons and their white lipoid myelin sheaths constitute white matter. Unmyelinated fibers, dendrites, and nerve cell bodies make up the gray matter of the brain and spinal cord.

Brain

In addition to being one of the largest organs of the body, the brain is highly complex in structure and function. (See Fig. 15-3.) It integrates almost every physical and mental activity of the body and is the center for memory, emotion, thought, judgment, reasoning, and consciousness. The four major structures of the brain are the following:

- Cerebrum
- Cerebellum
- Diencephalon
- Brainstem

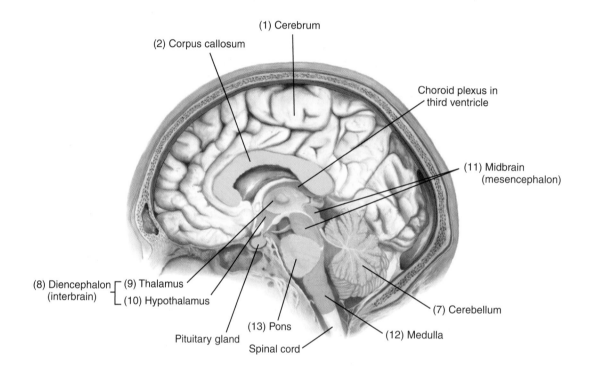

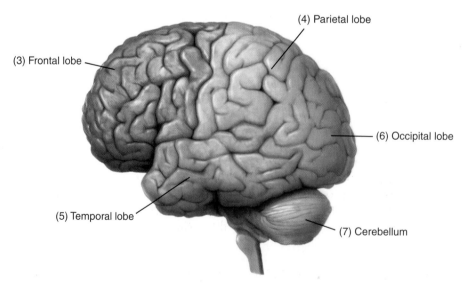

Figure 15-3 Brain structures.

Cerebrum

The (1) **cerebrum** is the largest, uppermost portion of the brain. It consists of two hemispheres divided by a deep longitudinal fissure, or groove. The fissure does not completely separate the hemispheres. A structure called the (2) **corpus callosum** joins these hemispheres, permitting communication between the right and left sides of the brain. Each hemisphere consists of five lobes. Four of these lobes are named for the bones that lie directly above them: (3) **frontal,** (4) **parietal,** (5) **temporal,** and (6) **occipital.** The fifth lobe, the **insula** (not shown in Fig. 15-3), is hidden from view and can be seen only upon dissection.

The cerebral surface consists of numerous folds, or convolutions, called **gyri.** The gyri are separated by furrows, or fissures, called **sulci.** A thin layer called the **cerebral cortex** covers the entire cerebrum and is composed of gray matter. Most information processing occurs in the cerebral cortex. The remainder of the cerebrum is primarily composed of white matter (myelinated axons).

Major functions of the cerebrum include sensory perception and interpretation, language, voluntary movement, and memory. Beneath the cerebrum is a primitive "emotional brain" called the **limbic system.** The limbic system is essential for survival and works in conjunction with the "thinking brain." It controls such behaviors as rage, fear, and anger and such emotional aspects as food enjoyment and sexual behavior. Mental and emotional illnesses are commonly the result of an imbalance in brain chemicals or electrical activity in the limbic system.

Cerebellum

The second largest structure of the brain, the (7) **cerebellum,** occupies the posterior portion of the skull. Most functions of the cerebellum involve movement, posture, or balance. When the cerebrum initiates muscular movement, the cerebellum coordinates and refines it.

Diencephalon

The (8) **diencephalon** (also called the **interbrain**) is composed of many smaller structures, including the thalamus and the hypothalamus. The (9) **thalamus** receives all sensory stimuli except olfactory stimuli and processes and transmits them to the appropriate centers in the cerebral cortex. In addition, the thalamus receives impulses from the cerebrum and relays them to efferent nerves. The (10) **hypothalamus** regulates involuntary activities, such as heart rate, body temperature, and fluid balance. It also controls many endocrine functions.

Brainstem

The brainstem is composed of three structures: the (11) **midbrain** (also called the **mesencephalon**), separating the cerebrum from the brainstem; the (12) **medulla,** which attaches to the spinal cord; and (13) the **pons,** or "bridge," connecting the midbrain to the medulla. In general, the brainstem is a pathway for impulse conduction between the brain and spinal cord. The brainstem is the origin of 10 of the 12 pairs of cranial nerves and controls respiration, blood pressure, and heart rate. The brainstem is the site that controls the beginning of life (initiation of the heartbeat in a fetus) and the end of life (cessation of respiration and heart activity).

Spinal Cord

The **spinal cord** transmits sensory impulses from the body to the brain and motor impulses from the brain to the muscles and organs of the body. The sensory nerve tracts are called **ascending tracts** because the direction of the impulse is upward. Conversely, motor nerve tracts are called **descending tracts** because they carry impulses in a downward direction to muscles and organs. A cross-sectional view of the spinal cord reveals an inner area of gray matter composed of cell bodies and dendrites and an outer area of white matter composed of myelinated tissue of the ascending and descending tracts.

The entire spinal cord is located within the spinal cavity of the vertebral column, with spinal nerves exiting between the intervertebral spaces throughout almost the entire length of the spinal column. Unlike the cranial nerves, which have specific names, the spinal nerves are identified by the region of the vertebral column from which they exit.

Meninges

The brain and spinal cord receive limited protection from three coverings called **meninges** (singular, **meninx**). These coverings are the dura mater, arachnoid, and pia mater.

The **dura mater** is the outermost covering of the brain and spinal cord. It is tough, fibrous, and dense and composed primarily of connective tissue. Because of its thickness, this membrane is also called the **pachymeninges.** Beneath the dura mater is a cavity called the **subdural space,** which is filled with serous fluid.

The **arachnoid** is the middle covering and, as its name suggests, has a spider-web appearance. It fits loosely over the underlying structures. A **subarachnoid space** contains **cerebrospinal fluid,** a colorless fluid that contains proteins, glucose, urea, salts, and some white blood cells. This fluid circulates around the spinal cord and brain and through ventricles located within the inner portion of the brain. It provides nutritive substances to the central nervous system and adds additional protection for the brain and spinal cord by acting as a shock absorber. Normally, cerebrospinal fluid is absorbed as rapidly as it is formed, maintaining a constant fluid volume. Any interference with its absorption results in a collection of fluid in the brain, a condition called **hydrocephalus.**

The **pia mater** is the innermost meninx. This membrane directly adheres to the brain and spinal cord. As it passes over the brain, it follows the contours of the gyri and sulci. It contains numerous blood vessels and lymphatics that nourish the underlying tissues. Because of the thinness and delicacy of the arachnoid and pia mater, these two meninges are collectively called the **leptomeninges.**

Peripheral Nervous System

The **peripheral nervous system (PNS)** is composed of all nervous tissue located outside the spinal column and skull. It consists of sensory neurons, which carry impulses from the body to the CNS **(afferent),** and motor neurons, which carry impulses from the brain and spinal cord to muscles and glands **(efferent).** The PNS is divided into the somatic nervous system and the autonomic nervous system. Some motor nerves in the peripheral nervous system innervate muscles under conscious control of the individual. They regulate such actions as walking and talking. The motor nerves that influence voluntary muscles comprise the **somatic nervous system.** Other motor nerves innervate involuntary muscles (muscles of the digestive or respiratory organs), glands, and cardiac muscles. The motor nerves that influence involuntary muscles, glands, and heart muscle make up the **autonomic nervous system.** (See Fig. 15-4.)

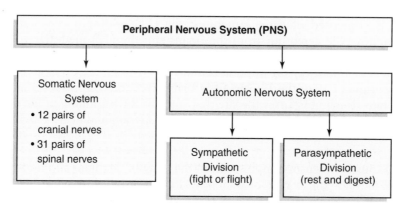

Figure 15-4 Divisions of the peripheral nervous system.

Somatic Nervous System

The somatic nervous system, the part of the peripheral nervous system associated with voluntary muscle control, is made up of the cranial nerves and the spinal nerves.

Cranial Nerves

The 12 pairs of cranial nerves originate in the brain and emerge through canals or openings in the base of the skull. Each cranial nerve is designated by name or number. (See Fig. 15-5.)

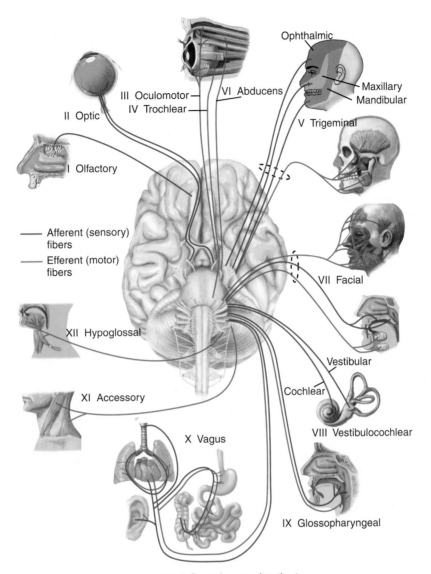

Figure 15-5 Cranial nerve distribution.

Cranial nerves may be sensory, motor, or a mixture of both types of neurons. **Sensory (afferent) nerves** receive impulses from the sense organs, the environment, and the visceral organs and transmit them to the CNS. **Motor (efferent) nerves** conduct impulses from the CNS to muscles and glands. **Mixed nerves** are composed of sensory (afferent) and motor (efferent) neurons. An example of a mixed nerve is the facial nerve. It acts in a motor capacity by transmitting impulses to the facial muscles for smiling or frowning. However, it also acts in a sensory capacity by transmitting taste impulses from the tongue to the brain.

Spinal Nerves

The spinal nerves emerge from the intervertebral spaces in the spinal column and extend to various locations of the body. All 31 pairs of spinal nerves are mixed nerves. (See Fig. 15-6, page 522.) Each pair is identified according to the vertebra from which it exits. All spinal nerves have two points of attachment to the spinal cord: an anterior (ventral) root and a posterior (dorsal) root. The **anterior root** contains motor fibers, and the **posterior root** contains sensory fibers. These two roots unite to form the spinal nerve, which has afferent and efferent qualities.

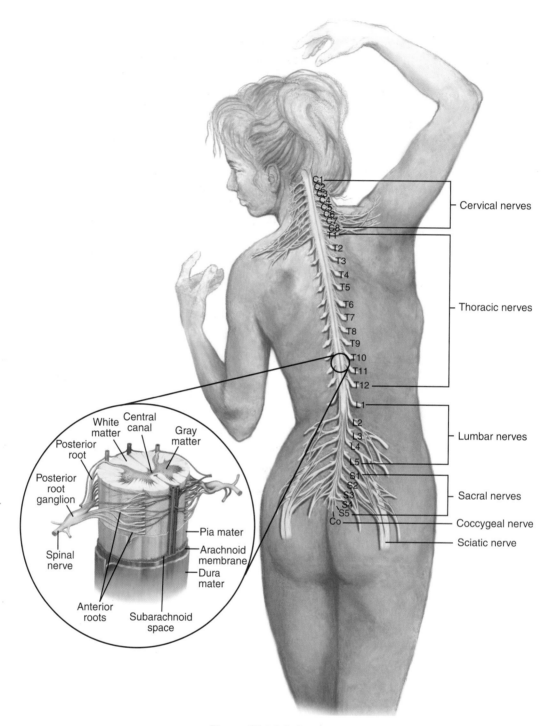

C1
C2
C3
C4
C5
C6
C7
C8
T1
T2
T3
T4
T5
T6
T7
T8
T9
T10
T11
T12
L1
L2
L3
L4
L5
S1
S2
S3
S4
S5
Co

— Cervical nerves

— Thoracic nerves

— Lumbar nerves

— Sacral nerves

— Coccygeal nerve

— Sciatic nerve

White matter
Central canal
Gray matter
Posterior root
Posterior root ganglion
Spinal nerve
Anterior roots
Subarachnoid space
Pia mater
Arachnoid membrane
Dura mater

Figure 15-6 Spinal nerves.

Autonomic Nervous System

Because the individual cannot control autonomic nervous system activities, a specialized system consisting of the **sympathetic** and **parasympathetic divisions** acts as the regulator of the autonomic nervous system. In general, the sympathetic division and the parasympathetic division bring about opposite effects on the activity of the same organs. In other words, the sympathetic and parasympathetic divisions act as "increase" and "decrease" switches for controlling the actions of the autonomic nervous system. Ordinarily, what one division stimulates, the other inhibits. The sympathetic division regulates body activities when an immediate action is required in stressful or threatening situations. It increases heart rate, depth of breathing, and muscle strength, preparing the body for a "fight-or-flight" response. Conversely, the parasympathetic division decreases the rate and intensity of these processes and exerts its influence when stressful or threatening situations resolve. It causes a decrease in heart rate, dilation of visceral blood vessels, and an increase in the activity of the digestive tract, preparing the body for "rest-and-digest" responses. (See Table 15-2.)

Table 15-2 Sympathetic and Parasympathetic Actions

This table shows the opposing actions of the sympathetic and the parasympathetic divisions of the autonomic nervous system.

Sympathetic Division	Parasympathetic Division
Dilates the pupils to increase the amount of light entering the eye to optimize vision	Decreases or increases the diameter of the pupils in response to changing levels of light
Decreases the flow of saliva	Increases the flow of saliva
Dilates the bronchi	Constricts the bronchi
Increases heart rate and metabolic rate	Decreases heart rate, blood pressure, and metabolic rate
Decreases digestive activities	Increases digestive activities
Constricts visceral blood vessels	Dilates visceral blood vessels

Anatomy Review: Brain Structures

To review the anatomy of the nervous system, label the illustration using the listed terms.

cerebellum

cerebrum

corpus callosum

diencephalon (interbrain)

frontal lobe

hypothalamus

medulla

midbrain (mesencephalon)

occipital lobe

parietal lobe

pons

temporal lobe

thalamus

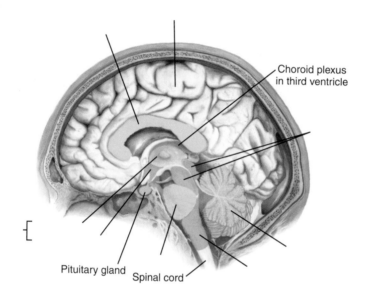

Choroid plexus in third ventricle

Pituitary gland   Spinal cord

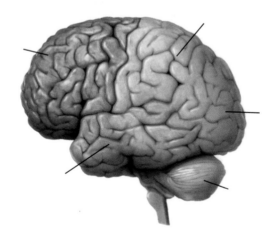

Check your answers by referring to Figure 15-3 on page 518. Review material that you did not answer correctly.

CONNECTING BODY SYSTEMS—NERVOUS SYSTEM

The main function of the nervous system is to identify and respond to internal and external changes in the environment to maintain homeostasis. Specific functional relationships between the nervous system and other body systems are discussed here.

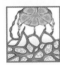
Blood, Lymphatic, and Immune
- The nervous system identifies changes in blood and lymph composition and provides the stimuli to maintain homeostasis.
- The nervous system identifies pathologically altered tissue and assists the immune system in containing injury and promoting healing.

Cardiovascular
- Nervous tissue, especially the conduction system of the heart, transmits a contraction impulse.
- The nervous system identifies pressure changes on vascular walls and responds to regulate blood pressure.

Digestive
- Nervous stimuli of digestive organs propel food by peristalsis.
- Nerve receptors in the lower colon identify the need to defecate.

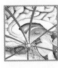
Endocrine
- The hypothalamus regulates hormone production.

Female Reproductive
- The nervous system transmits the contraction impulses needed for delivery of a fetus.
- The nervous system provides the stimuli needed for lactation.
- The nervous system regulates the hormones needed for the menstrual cycle.

Integumentary
- The sensory nervous system supplies receptors in the skin that respond to environmental stimuli.
- The autonomic nervous system regulates body temperature by controlling shivering and sweating.

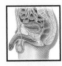
Male Reproductive
- The nervous system regulates sexual responses.
- Nervous tissue in reproductive organs provides pleasure responses.

Musculoskeletal
- The nervous system provides impulses for contraction, resulting in voluntary and involuntary movement of muscles.
- Autonomic nervous tissue responds to positional changes.

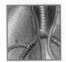
Respiratory
- The nervous system stimulates muscle contractions that create the pressure changes necessary for ventilation.
- The nervous system regulates the rate and depth of breathing.

Urinary
- The nervous system stimulates the thirst reflex when body fluid levels are low.
- The nervous system regulates all aspects of urine formation.

Medical Word Elements

This section introduces combining forms, suffixes, and prefixes related to the nervous system. Word analyses are also provided. From the information provided, complete the meaning of the medical words in the right-hand column. The first one is completed for you.

Element	Meaning	Word Analysis
Combining Forms		
cerebr/o	cerebrum	**cerebr/o**/tomy (sĕr-ĕ-BRŎT-ō-mē): *incision of the cerebrum* *-tomy:* incision
crani/o	cranium (skull)	**crani/o**/malacia (krā-nē-ō-mă-LĀ-shē-ă): _____ *-malacia:* softening
encephal/o	brain	**encephal/o**/cele (ĕn-SĔF-ă-lō-sēl): _____ *-cele:* hernia, swelling *Encephalocele is a condition in which portions of the brain and meninges protrude through a bony midline defect in the skull.*
gangli/o	ganglion (knot or knotlike mass)	**gangli**/ectomy (găng-glē-ĔK-tō-mē): _____ *-ectomy:* excision, removal *A ganglion is a mass of nerve cell bodies (gray matter) in the peripheral nervous system.*
gli/o	glue; neuroglial tissue	**gli**/oma (glī-Ō-mă): _____ *-oma:* tumor
kinesi/o	movement	brady/**kines**/ia (brăd-ē-kĭ-NĒ-sē-ă): _____ *brady-:* slow *-ia:* condition
lept/o	thin, slender	**lept/o**/mening/o/pathy (lĕp-tō-mĕn-ĭn-GŎP-ă-thē): _____ *-mening/o:* meninges (membranes covering the brain and spinal cord) *-pathy:* disease *The leptomeninges include the pia mater and arachnoid, both of which are thin and delicate in structure, as opposed to the dura mater.*
lex/o	word, phrase	dys/**lex**/ia (dĭs-LĔK-sē-ă): _____ *dys-:* bad; painful; difficult *-ia:* condition *Dyslexia is a difficulty with reading or an inability to read, including the tendency to reverse letters or words when reading or writing.*
mening/o	meninges (membranes covering the brain and spinal cord)	**mening/o**/cele (mĕn-ĬN-gō-sēl): _____ *-cele:* hernia, swelling
meningi/o		**meningi**/oma (mĕn-ĭn-jē-Ō-mă): _____ *-oma:* tumor

Medical Word Elements—cont'd

Element	Meaning	Word Analysis
myel/o	bone marrow; spinal cord	**poli/o**/myel/itis (pōl-ē-ō-mī-ĕl-Ī-tĭs): _____ *poli/o:* gray; gray matter (of the brain or spinal cord) *-itis:* inflammation
narc/o	stupor; numbness; sleep	**narc/o**/tic (năr-KŎT-ĭk): _____ *-tic:* pertaining to *Narcotics depress the central nervous system, thus relieving pain and producing sleep.*
neur/o	nerve	**neur/o**/lysis (nū-RŎL-ĭs-ĭs): _____ *-lysis:* separation; destruction; loosening *Neurolysis is sometimes performed using cryoablation or radiofrequency techniques to relieve intractable pain as a temporary or permanent measure.*
radicul/o	nerve root	**radicul**/algia (ră-dĭk-ū-LĂL-jē-ă): _____ *-algia:* pain
sthen/o	strength	hyper/**sthen**/ia (hī-pĕr-STHĒ-nē-ă): _____ *hyper-:* excessive, above normal *-ia:* condition *Hypersthenia is characterized by rigid muscles and muscle tension when resting; also called* hypertonia
thalam/o	thalamus	**thalam/o**/tomy (thăl-ă-MŎT-ō-mē): _____ *-tomy:* incision *Thalamotomy is performed to treat intractable pain or psychoses.*
thec/o	sheath (usually referring to the meninges)	intra/**thec**/al (ĭn-tră-THĒ-kăl): _____ *intra-:* in, within *-al:* pertaining to
ton/o	tension	dys/**ton**/ia (dĭs-TŌ-nē-ă): _____ *dys-:* bad; painful; difficult *-ia:* condition *Dystonia is characterized by sustained muscle contractions, causing twisting, repetitive movements, or an abnormal posture.*
ventricul/o	ventricle (of the heart or brain)	**ventricul**/itis (vĕn-trĭk-ū-LĪ-tĭs): _____ *-itis:* inflammation

Suffixes		
-algesia	pain	an/**algesia** (ăn-ăl-JĒ-zē-ă): _____ *an-:* without, not
-algia		syn/**algia** (sĭn-ĂL-jē-ă): _____ *syn-:* union, together, joined *Synalgia, commonly called referred pain, is pain experienced in a part of the body other than the place of pathology. For example, right shoulder pain is commonly associated with gallstones.*

(continued)

Medical Word Elements—cont'd

Element	Meaning	Word Analysis
-asthenia	weakness, debility	my/**asthenia** (mī-ăs-THĒ-nē-ă): _____ _my:_ muscle
-esthesia	feeling	hyper/**esthesia** (hī-pĕr-ĕs-THĒ-zē-ă): _____ _hyper-:_ excessive, above normal _Hyperesthesia involves a marked sensitivity to touch, pain, or other sensory stimuli._
-kinesia	movement	hyper/**kinesia** (hī-pĕr-kĭ-NĒ-zē-ă): _____ _hyper-:_ excessive, above normal
-lepsy	seizure	narc/o/**lepsy** (NĂR-kō-lĕp-sē): _____ _narc/o:_ sleep _In narcolepsy, the individual has a sudden and uncontrollable urge to sleep at an inappropriate time, such as when driving._
-paresis	partial paralysis	hemi/**paresis** (hĕm-ē-pă-RĒ-sĭs): _____ _hemi-:_ one-half _When used alone, the term paresis refers to partial paralysis or motor weakness._
-phasia	speech	a/**phasia** (ă-FĀ-zē-ă): _____ _a-:_ without, not
-plegia	paralysis	quadri/**plegia** (kwŏd-rĭ-PLĒ-jē-ă): _____ _quadri-:_ four
-taxia	order, coordination	a/**taxia** (ă-TĂK-sē-ă): _____ _a-:_ without, not _Ataxia refers to poor muscle coordination, especially when voluntary movements are attempted._
Prefixes		
pachy-	thick	**pachy**/mening/itis (păk-ē-mĕn-ĭn-JĪ-tĭs): _____ _mening:_ meninges (membranes covering the brain and spinal cord) _-itis:_ inflammation _The dura mater (pachymeninx) is a thick membrane that provides protection for the brain and spinal cord._
para-	near, beside; beyond	**para**/plegia (păr-ă-PLĒ-jē-ă): _____ _-plegia:_ paralysis
syn-	union, together, joined	**syn**/algia (sĭn-ĂL-jē-ă): _____ _-algia:_ pain _Pain in a deteriorated hip commonly causes referred pain in a healthy knee._

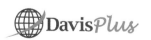 Visit the _Medical Terminology Systems_ online resource center at Davis_Plus_ for an audio exercise of the terms in this table. Other activities are also available to reinforce content.

⊙ _It is time to review medical word elements by completing Learning Activities 15-1 and 15-2._

Disease Focus

Damage to the brain and spinal cord invariably causes signs and symptoms in other parts of the body. Common signs and symptoms for many neurological disorders include headache, insomnia, back or neck pain, weakness, and involuntary movement (dyskinesia). Careful observation of the patient during the history and physical examination may provide valuable clues about mental status and cognitive and motor ability.

For diagnosis, treatment, and management of neurological disorders, the medical services of a specialist may be warranted. **Neurology** is the branch of medicine concerned with neurological diseases. The physician who specializes in the diagnosis and treatment of nervous system disorders is known as a **neurologist. Psychiatry** is the branch of medicine concerned with mental illnesses. The physician who specializes in diagnosing and treating mental illnesses is a **psychiatrist.**

Cerebrovascular Disease

Cerebrovascular disease is a group of disorders affecting the vessels that supply blood to the brain. Denied oxygen, brain tissue begins to die, a medical emergency called **stroke, cerebrovascular accident (CVA),** or **"brain attack."** The three major types of stroke are ischemic stroke, intracerebral hemorrhage, and subarachnoid hemorrhage. The causes of an **ischemic stroke** are similar to that of a heart attack and include emboli, thrombi, and atherosclerosis that limit blood flow to brain tissue. A common cause of ischemic stroke is atherosclerosis of the arteries of the brain or neck **(carotid).** An **intracerebral hemorrhage** occurs when there is a sudden rupture of an artery within the brain. After the rupture, released blood compresses brain structures and destroys them. In a **subarachnoid hemorrhage,** blood is released into the space between the brain and the tissues that surround the brain. This condition is commonly caused by a ruptured aneurysm and is usually fatal.

Depending on the area of the brain affected by the stroke, signs and symptoms include weakness or paralysis in one-half of the body **(hemiparesis, hemiplegia),** speech difficulty **(dysphasia),** lack of muscle coordination **(ataxia),** confusion, and loss of consciousness. A "mini stroke," also called a **transient ischemic attack (TIA),** is a type of stroke in which symptoms resolve within 24 hours and do not cause permanent damage. TIAs require immediate medical attention because they are often a precursor to a full-blown stroke.

Risk factors for stroke include family history, obesity, smoking, and excessive alcohol use. Because high blood pressure is a risk factor for strokes, antihypertensive medications are important in prevention.

Computed tomography (CT) helps determine the type of stroke and treatment options. For ischemic strokes, "clot-buster" **(thrombolytic)** medications administered within 3 hours of symptom onset can usually prevent permanent disability. Treatment for disabilities caused by stroke involves speech, physical, and occupational therapy and various medications, depending on the type of stroke.

Seizure Disorders

Seizure disorders include any medical condition characterized by sudden changes in behavior or consciousness caused by uncontrolled electrical activity in the brain. They include **epileptic seizures,** which have no known cause, are chronic, and occur repeatedly, and **nonepileptic seizures,** which are triggered by disorders or conditions that irritate the brain. These triggers commonly include brain injury, congenital anomalies, metabolic disorders, brain tumors, fever, vascular disturbances, and genetic disorders.

Whether epileptic or nonepileptic, seizures manifest in various forms. The two most common forms are **partial seizures** and **generalized seizures.** In **partial seizures,** only a portion of the brain is involved. There is a short alteration of consciousness of about 10 to 30 seconds with repetitive, unusual movements and confusion. In a **generalized seizure,** the entire brain is involved. The most common type of generalized seizure is the **tonic-clonic (grand mal) seizure.** In tonic-clonic seizures, the body alternates between excessive muscle tone and rigidity **(tonic)** and jerking muscle contractions **(clonic)** in the extremities. After the seizure, such neurological symptoms as weakness, confusion, headache, and nausea may occur. These symptoms are called a **postictal event,** which commonly lasts for 5 to 30 minutes but may last longer with a severe seizure.

Many patients experience a warning signal **(aura)** of an imminent seizure. Auras vary considerably and may include sensory phenomena without a precipitating stimulus, such as a strange taste in the mouth, the sound of a ringing bell, or an inability to react properly to usual situations. Auras provide time for preparation, such as lying down, avoiding staircases, and so forth, to minimize injuries should a grand mal seizure occur.

Diagnosis and evaluation of epilepsies commonly rely on electroencephalography and magnetic source imaging (MSI) to locate the affected area of the brain. Antiepileptic medications help control seizures.

Multiple Sclerosis

Multiple sclerosis (MS) is an autoimmune disease that targets the myelin sheath on the nerves of the central nervous system. MS causes inflammation, hardening **(sclerosing),** and, finally, loss of myelin **(demyelination)** throughout the spinal cord and brain. Myelin deterioration impedes the transmission of electrical impulses from one neuron to another. In effect, the pathway of nerve impulses develops "short circuits," producing a wide variety of symptoms.

Signs and symptoms of MS include tremors, muscle weakness, bradykinesia, and such visual disturbances as blurred vision, poor contrast, double vision, and eye pain. Other symptoms include bowel and bladder disorders, sexual disfunction, balance problems, cognitive difficulties, numbness, tingling, and pain. Many patients require a cane, walker, or wheelchair as the disease progresses. During remissions, symptoms temporarily disappear, but progressive hardening of myelinated areas leads to other attacks. MS generally affects a person's quality of life, rather than longevity. Medications and physical therapy can ease or control symptoms, but currently there is no cure for the disease.

Mental Illness

Mental illness includes an array of psychological disorders, syndromes, and behavioral patterns that cause alterations in mood, behavior, and thinking. Its forms range from mild to serious. Mental illness is a disease that affects mood, thought, behavior, or all three, with symptoms ranging from mild to severe. Signs and symptoms include excessive fears, strong feelings of anger, hallucinations, extreme highs and lows, confused thinking, and prolonged depression. Although many people may experience one or more of these problems from time to time, when any of them are ongoing and affect the person's ability to meet the demands of daily life, it is considered a mental illness. Causes of mental illness include genetic factors; prenatal environment, including exposure to drugs and alcohol; biochemical imbalances; and stress. Left untreated, mental illness can cause relationship difficulties, social isolation, poverty, and homelessness.

Diagnosis and treatment of serious mental disorders usually requires the skills of a medical specialist called a **psychiatrist.** In the capacity of a physician, the psychiatrist is licensed to prescribe medications and perform medical procedures not available to those who do not hold a medical license. Psychiatrists commonly work in association with **clinical psychologists,** individuals trained in evaluating human behavior, intelligence, and personality. (See Table 15-3.)

Research and education have removed much of the stigma attached to mental illness. Today, mental illness is becoming a more recognizable and treatable disorder. Family physicians, school psychologists, marriage and family counselors, and even such support groups as grief support and Alcoholics Anonymous can effectively help in managing psychological problems.

Table 15-3	**Common Terms Associated with Mental Illness**
Term	**Definition**
affective disorder	Psychological disorder in which the major characteristic is an abnormal mood, usually mania or depression
anorexia nervosa ăn-ō-RĔK-sē-ă nĕr-VŌS-ă	Eating disorder characterized by a refusal to maintain adequate weight for age and height and an all-consuming desire to remain thin
anxiety	Psychological "worry" disorder characterized by excessive pondering or thinking "what if…" *Feelings of worry, dread, lack of energy, and a loss of interest in life are common signs associated with anxiety.*
attention deficit-hyperactivity disorder (ADHD) hī-pĕr-ăk-TĬV-ĭ-tē	Disorder affecting children and adults and characterized by impulsiveness, overactivity, and the inability to remain focused on a task *Behavioral modification with or without medical management is commonly used in the treatment of ADHD.*
autism AW-tĭzm	Developmental disorder characterized by extreme withdrawal and an abnormal absorption in fantasy, usually accompanied by an inability to communicate even on a basic level *A person with autism may engage in repetitive behavior, such as rocking or repeating words.*
bipolar disorder bī-PŌL-ăr	Mental disorder that causes unusual shifts in mood, emotion, energy, and the ability to function; also called *manic-depressive illness*
bulimia nervosa bū-LĒM-ē-ă nĕr-VŌS-ă	Eating disorder characterized by binging (overeating) and purging (vomiting or use of laxatives)
depression dē-PRĔSH-ŭn	Mood disorder associated with sadness, despair, discouragement and, commonly, feelings of low self-esteem, guilt, and withdrawal
mania MĀ-nē-ă	Mood disorder characterized by mental and physical hyperactivity, disorganized behavior, and excessively elevated mood
neurosis nū-RŌ-sĭs	Nonpsychotic mental illness that triggers feelings of distress and anxiety and impairs normal behavior *A child who has consistently been warned of "germs" by an overprotective parent may later develop an irrational fear of such things as using public restrooms and touching doorknobs or phones.*
panic attack PĂN-ĭk	Sudden, intense feeling of fear that comes without warning and is not attributable to any immediate danger *A key symptom of a panic attack is the fear of its recurrence.*
psychosis sī-KŌ-sĭs	Major emotional disorder in which contact with reality is lost to the point that the individual is incapable of meeting the challenges of daily life

Oncology

Intracranial tumors that originate directly in brain tissue are called **primary intracranial tumors.** They are commonly classified according to histological type and include those that originate in neurons and those that develop in glial tissue. A major symptom of intracranial tumors is headache, especially upon arising in the morning, during coughing episodes, and upon bending or sudden movement. Occasionally, the optic disc in the back of the eyeball swells (**papilledema**) because of increased intracranial pressure. Personality changes are common and include depression, anxiety, and irritability.

Intracranial tumors can arise from any structure within the cranial cavity, including the pituitary and pineal glands, cranial nerves, and the arachnoid and pia mater (**leptomeninges**). In addition, all of these tissues may be the sites of metastatic spread from primary malignancies that occur outside the nervous system. Metastatic tumors of the cranial cavity tend to exhibit growth characteristics similar to those of the primary malignancy but tend to grow more slowly than the parent tumor. Metastatic tumors of the cranial cavity are usually easier to remove than primary intracranial tumors.

Computed tomography (CT) scans and magnetic resonance imaging (MRI) help establish a diagnosis but are not definitive. Surgical removal relieves pressure and confirms or rules out malignancy. Even after surgery, most intracranial tumors require radiation therapy as a second line of treatment. Chemotherapy combined with radiation therapy usually provides the best chance for survival and quality of life.

Diseases and Conditions

This section introduces diseases and conditions of the nervous system, along with their meanings and pronunciations. Word analyses for selected terms are also provided.

Term	Definition
agnosia ăg-NŌ-zē-ă *a-:* without, not *gnos:* knowing *-ia:* condition	Inability to comprehend auditory, visual, spatial, olfactory, or other sensations, even though the sensory sphere is intact *The type of agnosia is usually identified by the sense or senses affected, such as visual agnosia. Agnosia is common in parietal lobe tumors.*
Alzheimer disease (AD) ĂLTS-hī-mĕr	Type of age-associated dementia caused by small lesions called *plaques* that develop in the cerebral cortex and interrupt the passage of electro-chemical signals between cells; also called *cerebral degeneration* *Clinical manifestations include memory loss, emotional and behavioral changes, and a decline in cognitive and social skills eventually leading to death. There is no specific treatment, but medications may provide moderate relief.*
anencephaly ăn-ĕn-SĔF-ă-lē *an-:* without, not, loss *encephal:* brain *-y:* noun ending	Congenital deformity in which some or all of the fetal brain is missing *In anencephaly, the infant is usually stillborn or dies shortly after birth. This deformity can be detected through amniocentesis or ultrasonography early in pregnancy.*
closed head trauma TRAW-mă	Injury to the head in which the dura mater remains intact and brain tissue is not exposed *In closed head trauma, the injury site may occur at the impact site, where the brain hits the inside of the skull (coup), or at the rebound site, where the opposite side of the brain strikes the skull (contrecoup).*
coma KŌ-mă	Abnormally deep unconsciousness with an absence of voluntary response to stimuli
concussion kŏn-KŬSH-ŭn	Traumatic injury to the brain that causes unconsciousness and is commonly of a temporary nature *Symptoms of concussion may include headache, dizziness, nausea, vomiting, and blurred vision, but symptoms may not appear for days or weeks after the injury.*

Diseases and Conditions—cont'd

Term	Definition
convulsion kŏn-VŬL-shŭn	Any sudden and violent contraction of one or more voluntary muscles that is commonly associated with such brain disorders as epilepsy
dementia dĭ-MĔN-shē-ă *de-:* cessation *ment:* mind *-ia:* condition	Broad term that refers to cognitive deficit, including memory impairment
dyslexia dĭs-LĔK-sē-ă *dys-:* bad; painful; difficult *lex:* word, phrase *-ia:* condition	Inability to learn and process written language, despite adequate intelligence, sensory ability, and exposure
Guillain-Barré syndrome gē-YĂ băr-RĀ	Autoimmune condition that causes acute inflammation of the peripheral nerves damaging their myelin sheaths, resulting in decreased nerve impulses, loss of reflex response, and sudden muscle weakness; also called *infective or idiopathic polyneuritis* *Guillain-Barré syndrome usually follows a gastrointestinal or respiratory infection. In the acute phase, the patient may temporarily require respiratory support until the inflammation subsides.*
herpes zoster HĔR-pēz ZŎS-tĕr	Acute inflammatory eruption of highly painful vesicles on the trunk of the body or, occasionally, the face that is caused by the same virus that causes chickenpox; also called *shingles* (See Fig. 15-7.) *Vaccines can reduce the risk of contracting shingles. Early treatment can shorten the infection or reduce the chance of complications.*

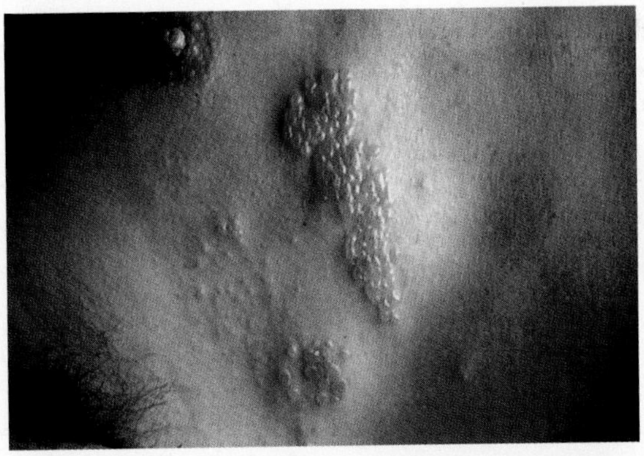

Figure 15-7 Herpes zoster (shingles). From Goldsmith, Lazuarus, and Tharp: *Adult and Pediatric Dermatology: A Color Guide to Diagnosis and Treatment,* F.A. Davis, Philadelphia, 1997, p. 307, with permission.

Term	Definition
Huntington chorea HŬNT-ĭng-tŭn kō-RĒ-ă	CNS disorder characterized by quick, involuntary movements, speech disturbances, and mental deterioration; also called *neurodegenerative genetic disorder* *Onset of Huntington chorea commonly occurs between ages 30 and 50.*

(continued)

Diseases and Conditions—cont'd

Term	Definition
hydrocephalus hī-drō-SĚF-ă-lŭs *hydr/o:* water *cephal:* head *-us:* condition; structure	Accumulation of fluid in the ventricles of the brain, causing increased intracranial pressure (ICP), thinning of brain tissue, and separation of cranial bones *The two forms of hydrocephalus are acquired hydrocephalus, which occurs after birth, and congenital hydrocephalus, which occurs during fetal development and is found at birth.*
lethargy LĚTH-ăr-jē	Abnormal inactivity or lack of response to normal stimuli
myasthenia gravis (MG) mī-ăs-THĒ-nē-ă GRĂV-ĭs *my:* muscle *-asthenia:* weakness, debility	Chronic, progressive disorder in which a loss of neurotransmitter receptors produces increasingly severe muscle weakness (See Fig. 15-8.)

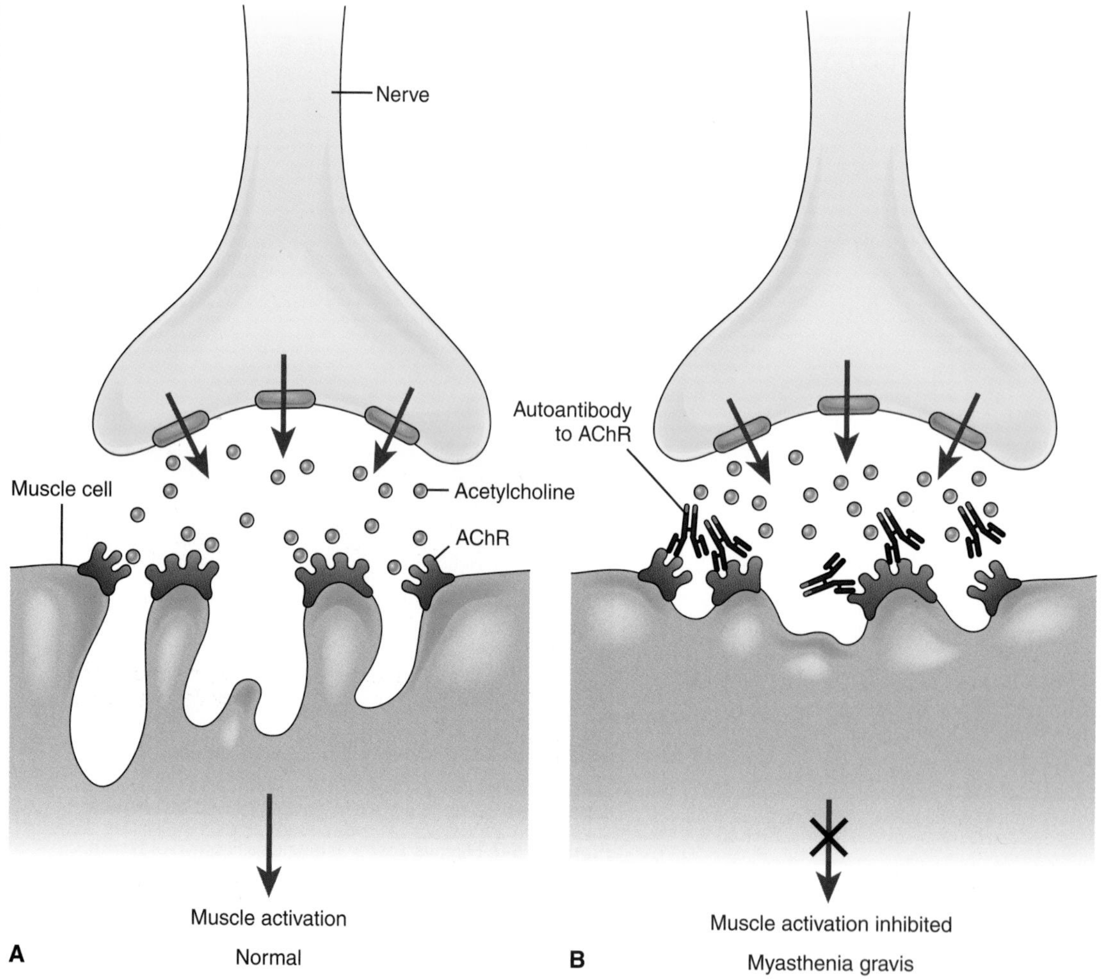

Figure 15-8 Myasthenia gravis. (A) Acetylcholine binding to acetylcholine receptor (AChR) sites on muscle to stimulate contraction. (B) Auto-antibodies destroying AChR binding sites and inhibiting the binding of acetylcholine required for muscle contraction.

Diseases and Conditions—cont'd

Term	Definition

spina bifida
SPĪ-nă BĬ-fĭ-dă

Congenital deformity of the neural tube (embryonic structure that becomes the fetal brain and spinal cord), which fails to close during fetal development; also called *neural tube defect*

The most common forms of spina bifida are meningocele, meningomyelocele, and occulta. (See Fig. 15-9.)

meningocele
měn-ĬN-gō-sēl
mening/o: meninges (membranes covering the brain and spinal cord)
-cele: hernia, swelling

Form of spina bifida in which the spinal cord develops properly but the meninges protrude through the spine

myelomeningocele
mī-ě-lō-měn-ĬN-gō-sēl
myel/o: bone marrow; spinal cord
mening/o: meninges (membranes covering the brain and spinal cord)
-cele: hernia, swelling

Most severe form of spina bifida in which the spinal cord and meninges protrude through the spine

occulta
ŏ-KŬL-tă

Form of spina bifida in which one or more vertebrae are malformed, and the spinal cord is covered with a layer of skin

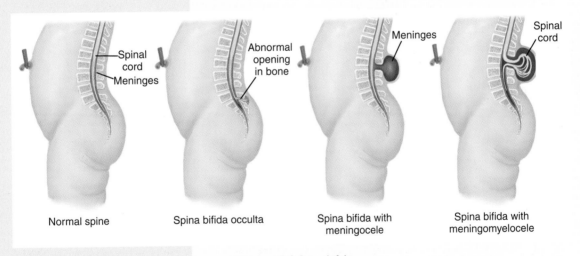

Figure 15-9 Spina bifida.

(continued)

Diseases and Conditions—cont'd

Term	Definition
palsy PAWL-zē	Paralysis, usually partial, and commonly characterized by weakness and shaking or uncontrolled tremor
Bell palsy	Facial paralysis caused by a functional disorder of the seventh cranial nerve; also called *facial nerve palsy* *Bell palsy is commonly associated with herpes virus, but other viruses may be implicated. It is self-limiting and usually resolves spontaneously in 3–5 weeks.*
cerebral palsy (CP) sĕ-RĒ-brăl *cerebr:* cerebrum *-al:* pertaining to	Type of paralysis that affects movement and muscle coordination and may affect gross and fine motor skills *CP commonly occurs because of trauma to the brain before or during the birthing process.*
paralysis pă-RĂL-ĭ-sĭs *para-:* near, beside; beyond *-lysis:* separation; destruction; loosening	Loss of voluntary motion in one or more muscle groups with or without loss of sensation *Strokes and spinal cord injuries are the most common causes of paralysis. Strokes usually affect only one side of the body. Spinal cord injuries result in paralysis below the site of the injury. (See Fig. 15-10.)*

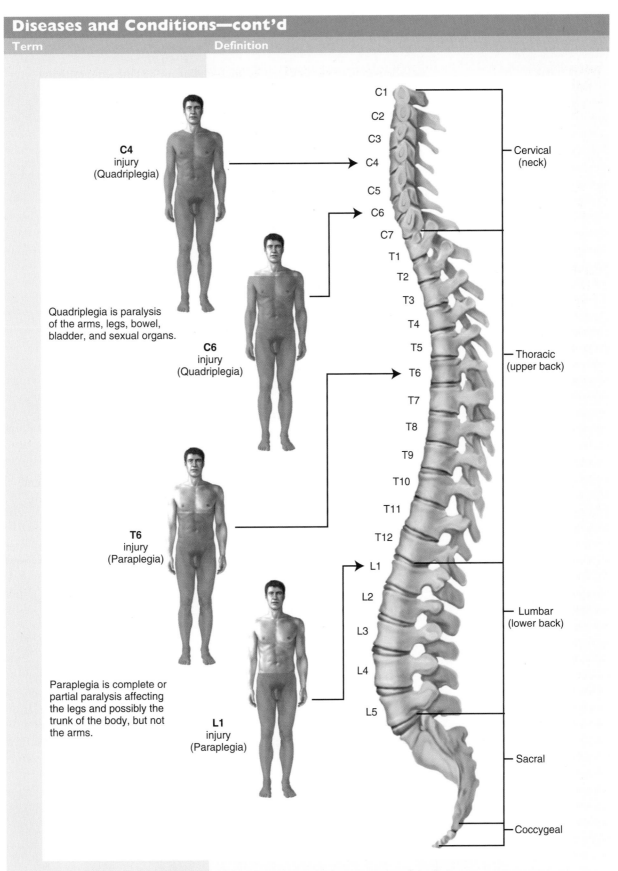

Quadriplegia is paralysis of the arms, legs, bowel, bladder, and sexual organs.

C4 injury (Quadriplegia)

C6 injury (Quadriplegia)

T6 injury (Paraplegia)

Paraplegia is complete or partial paralysis affecting the legs and possibly the trunk of the body, but not the arms.

L1 injury (Paraplegia)

C1
C2
C3
C4
C5
C6
C7
T1
T2
T3
T4
T5
T6
T7
T8
T9
T10
T11
T12
L1
L2
L3
L4
L5

Cervical (neck)

Thoracic (upper back)

Lumbar (lower back)

Sacral

Coccygeal

Figure 15-10 Spinal cord injuries showing extent of paralysis.

(continued)

Diseases and Conditions—cont'd

Term	Definition
paresthesia păr-ĕs-THĒ-zē-ă	Sensation of numbness, prickling, tingling, or heightened sensitivity *Paresthesia can be caused by disorders affecting the central nervous system, such as stroke, transient ischemic attack, multiple sclerosis, transverse myelitis, and encephalitis.*
Parkinson disease PĂR-kĭn-sŏn	Degenerative disorder in which the progressive loss of brain cells leads to impairment in motor function, including tremors, muscular rigidity, and a slowing of movement; also called *paralysis agitans* or *shaking palsy*
poliomyelitis pōl-ē-ō-mī-ĕl-Ī-tĭs *poli/o:* gray; gray matter (of the brain or spinal cord) *myel:* bone marrow; spinal cord *-itis:* inflammation	Inflammation of the gray matter of the spinal cord caused by a virus, commonly resulting in spinal and muscle deformity and paralysis *Polio is preventable with standard vaccinations administered to children.*
radiculopathy ră-dĭk-ū-LŎP-ă-thē *radicul/o:* nerve root *-pathy:* disease	Disorder affecting one or more nerves at the location where the nerve root exits the spine and commonly the result of a herniated or compressed disk, degenerative changes, arthritis, or bone spurs; also called *radiculitis* *The areas most commonly affected are the neck (cervical radiculopathy) and lower back (lumbar radiculopathy or sciatica). Rest and antiinflammatory medications are the usual method of treatment.*
Reye syndrome RĪ	Potentially fatal syndrome that commonly causes brain swelling and liver damage and is characterized by confusion, hyperventilation, violent behavior, seizures, and possibly coma; also called *acute noninflammatory encephalopathy* and *fatty degenerative liver failure* *Reye syndrome primarily affects children and teenagers recovering from a viral infection, most commonly flu or chickenpox, especially when aspirin products have been used.*
syncope SĬN-kō-pē	Brief loss of consciousness and posture caused by a temporary decrease of blood flow to the brain; also called *fainting* *Syncope may be associated with a sudden decrease in blood pressure, a decrease in heart rate, or changes in blood volume or distribution. The person usually regains consciousness and becomes alert right away but may experience a brief period of confusion.*

 It is time to review pathology, diseases, and conditions by completing Learning Activity 15-3.

Diagnostic, Surgical, and Therapeutic Procedures

This section introduces diagnostic, surgical, and therapeutic procedures used to diagnose and treat neurological disorders. Descriptions are provided, along with pronunciations and word analyses for selected terms.

Procedure	Description
Diagnostic Procedures	

Clinical

electroencephalography (EEG)
ē-lĕk-trō-ĕn-sĕf-ă-LŎG-ră-fē
  electr/o: electricity
  encephal/o: brain
  -graphy: process of recording
	Recording of electrical activity in the brain, whose cells emit distinct patterns of rhythmic electrical impulses (See Fig. 15-11, page 540.)
	
	Different wave patterns in the EEG are associated with normal and abnormal waking and sleeping states. They help diagnose such conditions as tumors and infections and help locate seizure focus or areas of inactivity.

(continued)

Diagnostic, Surgical, and Therapeutic Procedures—cont'd

Procedure	Description

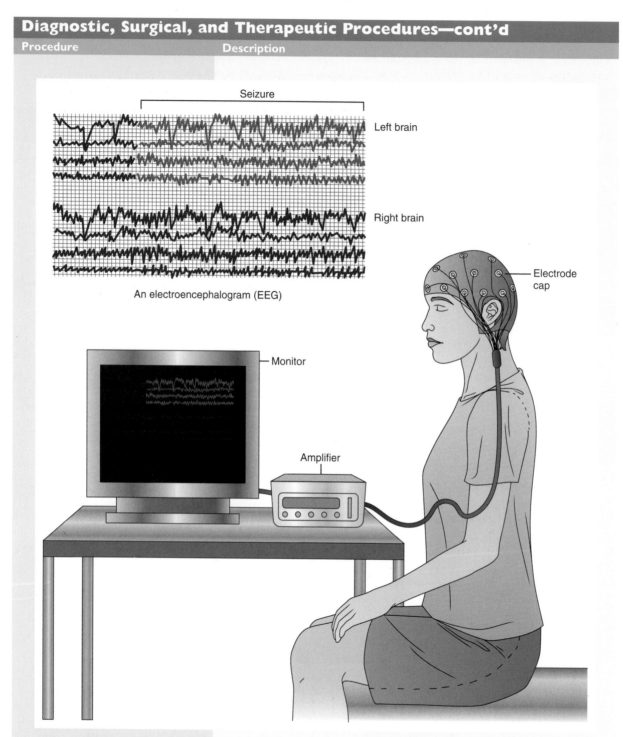

Figure 15-11 Electroencephalography. (A) Electrode cap recording electrical activity of the brain. (B) Amplifier receiving and enlarging the information and sending it to a computer. (C) Monitor displaying and recording the results.

electromyography (EMG) ē-lĕk-trō-mī-ŎG-ră-fē *electr/o:* electricity *my/o:* muscle *-graphy:* process of recording	Recording of electrical signals (action potentials) that occur in a muscle when it is at rest and during contraction to assess muscular disease or nerve damage *In an EMG, an electrode inserted into a muscle transmits electrical activity of the muscle and displays it on a monitor to assess the health of the muscle and the motor neurons that control it.*

Diagnostic, Surgical, and Therapeutic Procedures—cont'd

Procedure	Description
lumbar puncture (LP) LŬM-băr PŬNK-chūr	Needle puncture of the spinal cavity to extract spinal fluid for diagnostic purposes, introduce anesthetic agents into the spinal canal, or remove fluid to allow other fluids (such as radiopaque substances) to be injected; also called *spinal puncture* and *spinal tap* (See Fig. 15-12.)

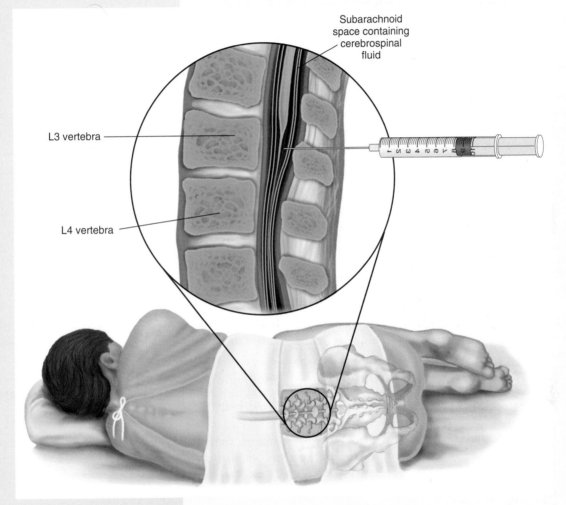

Subarachnoid space containing cerebrospinal fluid

L3 vertebra

L4 vertebra

Figure 15-12 Lumbar puncture.

Procedure	Description
nerve conduction velocity (NCV) NĔRV kŏn-DŬK-shŭn vĕ-LŎ-sĭ-tē	Test that measures the speed at which impulses travel through a nerve *In NCV, one electrode stimulates a nerve while other electrodes placed over different areas of the nerve record an electrical signal (action potential) as it travels through the nerve. This test helps diagnose muscular dystrophy and neurological disorders that destroy myelin.*

(continued)

Diagnostic, Surgical, and Therapeutic Procedures—cont'd

Procedure	Description

Laboratory

cerebrospinal fluid (CSF) analysis
sĕr-ē-brō-SPĪ-năl
  cerebr/o: cerebrum
  spin: spine
  -al: pertaining to
	Laboratory test to examine a sample of the fluid surrounding the brain and spinal cord that helps diagnose disorders of the central nervous system, including viral and bacterial infections, tumors, and hemorrhage

Imaging

computed tomography angiography (CTA, CT angiography)
kŏm-PŪ-tĕd tō-MŎG-ră-fē
ăn-jē-ŎG-ră-fē
  tom/o: to cut
  -graphy: process of recording
  angi/o: vessel (usually blood or lymph)
  -graphy: process of recording
	Radiographic image of the interior of a vessel in combination with a CT scan to produce high-resolution, three-dimensional images of blood vessels
	
	CTA identifies blocked blood vessels, aneurysms, and buildup of plaque in a blood vessel. It also aids in differentiating hemorrhagic stroke and ischemic stroke.

discography dĭs-KŎG-ră-fē	CT scan of the lumbar region after injection of a contrast medium to detect problems with the spine and spinal nerve roots

echoencephalography
ĕk-ō-ĕn-sĕf-ă-LŎG-ră-fē
  echo-: repeated sound
  encephal/o: brain
  -graphy: process of recording
	Ultrasound technique used to study intracranial structures of the brain and diagnose conditions that cause a shift in the midline structures of the brain
	
	Echoencephalography is a bedside procedure that is especially useful in detecting hemorrhage and hydrocephalus in children less than 2 years of age and infants in the neonatal unit but has largely been replaced by CT for older children and adults.

magnetic source imaging (MSI)	Noninvasive neuroimaging technique to pinpoint the specific location where seizure activity originates and enable custom surgical treatment for tumor and epileptic tissue resection; also called *magnetoencephalography* (MEG) *MSI is medically necessary for presurgical evaluation of persons with epilepsy to identify and localize areas of epileptic activity.*

myelography
mī-ĕ-LŎG-ră-fē
  myel/o: bone marrow; spinal cord
  -graphy: process of recording
	Radiographic examination to detect pathology of the spinal cord, including the location of a spinal cord injury, cysts, and tumors following injection of a contrast medium

positron emission tomography (PET) PŎZ-ĭ-trŏn ē-MĬSH-ŭn tō-MŎG-ră-fē	Computed tomography that records the positrons (positively charged particles) emitted from a radiopharmaceutical and produces a cross-sectional image of metabolic activity of body tissues to determine the presence of disease *PET is particularly useful in scanning the brain and nervous system to diagnose disorders that involve abnormal tissue metabolism, such as schizophrenia, brain tumors, epilepsy, stroke, and Alzheimer disease, in addition to cardiac and pulmonary disorders.*

Diagnostic, Surgical, and Therapeutic Procedures—cont'd

Procedure	Description
Surgical	

cryosurgery
krī-ō-SĔR-jĕr-ē

Technique that exposes abnormal tissue to extreme cold to destroy it

Cryosurgery is sometimes used to destroy malignant tumors of the brain.

thalamotomy
thăl-ă-MŎT-ō-mē
    thalam/o: thalamus
    -tomy: incision

Partial destruction of the thalamus to treat intractable pain; involuntary movements, including tremors in Parkinson disease; or emotional disturbances

Thalamotomy produces few neurological deficits or changes in personality.

tractotomy
trăk-TŎT-ō-mē

Transection of a nerve tract in the brainstem or spinal cord

Tractotomy is sometimes used to relieve intractable pain.

trephination
trĕf-ĭn-Ā-shŭn

Technique that cuts a circular opening into the skull to reveal brain tissue and decrease intracranial pressure

ventriculoperitoneal shunting
vĕn-trĭk-ū-lō-pĕr-ĭ-tō-NĒ-ăl
SHŬNT-ĭng
    ventricul/o: ventricle
    peritone: peritoneum
    -al: pertaining to

Relieves intracranial pressure due to hydrocephalus by diverting (shunting) excess cerebrospinal fluid from the ventricles into the peritoneal or thoracic cavity (See Fig. 15-13.)

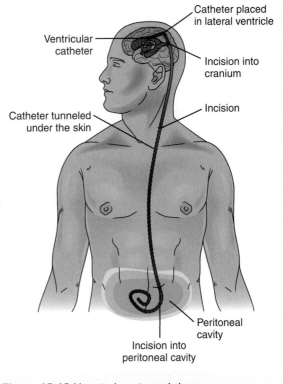

Ventricular catheter

Catheter placed in lateral ventricle

Incision into cranium

Incision

Catheter tunneled under the skin

Peritoneal cavity

Incision into peritoneal cavity

Figure 15-13 Ventriculoperitoneal shunt.

(continued)

Diagnostic, Surgical, and Therapeutic Procedures—cont'd

Procedure	Description
Therapeutic	
intravenous (IV) tissue plasminogen activator (tPA) *intra-:* in, within *ven:* vein *-ous:* pertaining to	Treatment for ischemic stroke using tissue plasminogen activator (tPA), a potent clot-busting drug, injected directly into a vein *IV tPA helps treat ischemic stroke but must be given within 4 hours of symptom onset. Knowing the symptoms of stroke and calling 911 are essential because there is a very narrow window for diagnosing and effectively treating the patient.*
plasmapheresis plăz-mă-fěr-Ē-sĭs	Extracorporeal procedure to treat patients with autoimmune diseases by removing their plasma containing the offending antibodies and replacing it with donor plasma or plasma substitutes *Plasmapheresis helps treat such autoimmune diseases as multiple sclerosis, Guillain-Barré syndrome, and myasthenia gravis.*
stereotactic radiosurgery (SRS) stěr-ē-ō-TĂK-tĭk rā-dē-ō-SŬR-jěr-ē	Procedure that uses three-dimensional imaging (stereotactic) along with high doses of highly focused radiation to destroy tumors and other abnormal growths in the brain, spinal column, and other body sites with minimal exposure to surrounding healthy tissue *Because of its accuracy and precision, the principles used in SRS are now being applied to treat various body tumors with a procedure called stereotactic body radiotherapy (SBRT).*

Pharmacology

Neurological agents help relieve or eliminate pain, suppress seizures, control tremors, and reduce muscle rigidity. (See Table 15-4.) Hypnotics, a class of drugs used as sedatives, depress CNS function to relieve agitation and induce sleep. Anesthetics are capable of producing a complete or partial loss of feeling and are used for surgery. Psychotherapeutic agents alter brain chemistry to treat mental illness. These drugs are used as mood stabilizers in various mental disorders. They also reduce symptoms of depression and treat ADHD and narcolepsy.

Table 15-4 Drugs Used to Treat Neurological and Psychiatric Disorders

This table lists common drug classifications used to treat neurological and psychiatric disorders, along with their therapeutic actions and selected generic and trade names.

Classification	Therapeutic Action	Generic and Trade Names
Neurological		
anesthetics ăn-ĕs-THĔT-ĭks	Produce partial or complete loss of sensation, with or without loss of consciousness *Forms of anesthetics include general, local, and nerve block.*	
general	Act upon the brain to produce complete loss of feeling with loss of consciousness *General anesthetics affect all areas of the body, including the brain. Because they suppress all reflexes, including coughing and swallowing, breathing tubes are usually required during their administration.*	**propofol** PRŎ-pō-fŏl *Diprivan*
local	Act upon nerves or nerve tracts to affect only a local area *Local anesthetics are injected directly into the area involved in the local surgery. Patients may remain fully alert unless additional medications to induce sleep are given.*	**procaine** PRŌ-kān *Novocain* **lidocaine** LĪ-dō-kān *Xylocaine*
nerve block	Blocks pain from the area supplied by that nerve *A nerve block is a type of regional anesthetic usually used for procedures on the arms, legs, hands, feet, and face.*	**levobupivacaine** lĕv-ō-bū-PĪ-vă-kān *Chirocaine*
anticonvulsants ăn-tĭ-kŏn-VŬL-sănts	Prevent uncontrolled neuron activity associated with seizures by altering electrical transmission along neurons or altering the chemical composition of neurotransmitters; also called antiepileptics *Many anticonvulsants are also used as mood stabilizers.*	**carbamazepine** kăr-bă-MĂZ-ĕ-pēn *Tegretol* **valproate** văl-PRŌ-āt *Depacon* **phenytoin** FĔN-ĭ-tō-ĭn *Dilantin*
antiparkinsonian agents ăn-tĭ-păr-kĭn-SŌN-ē-ăn	Control tremors and muscle rigidity associated with Parkinson disease by increasing dopamine in the brain	**levodopa** lē-vō-DŌ-pă *l-dopa, Larodopa* **levodopa/carbidopa** kăr-bĭ-DŌ-pă *Sinemet, Sinemet CR*

(continued)

Table 15-4   Drugs Used to Treat Neurological and Psychiatric Disorders—cont'd

Classification	Therapeutic Action	Generic and Trade Names
Psychiatric		
antianxiety agents ăn-tĭ-ăng-ZĪ-ĕ-tē	React at distinct receptor sites in the limbic and cortical system to decrease anxiety *Benzodiazepine drugs, such as alprazolam, may be used to treat panic disorder.*	**alprazolam** ăl-PRĀ-zō-lăm *Xanax* **buspirone** bū-SPĪ-rōn *Buspar*
antipsychotics ăn-tĭ-sī-KŎT-ĭks	Treat psychosis, paranoia, and schizophrenia by altering chemicals in the brain, including the limbic system, which controls emotions	**clozapine** CLŌ-ză-pēn *Clozaril* **risperidone** rĭs-PĔR-ĭ-dōn *Risperdal*
antidepressants ăn-tĭ-dē-PRĔS-săntz	Treat multiple symptoms of depression by increasing levels of specific neurotransmitters *Antidepressants fall under different classifications, and some are also used to treat anxiety and pain.*	**citalopram** sī-TĂL-ō-prăm *Celexa* **fluoxetine** floo-ŎK-sĕ-tēn *Prozac*
hypnotics hĭp-NŎT-ĭks	Depress central nervous system (CNS) functions, promote sedation and sleep, and relieve agitation, anxiousness, and restlessness *Historically, barbiturates were commonly used to induce sleep; however, because of the risk for addiction, these drugs have been replaced by drugs that affect benzodiazepine receptors.*	**temazepam** tĕ-MĂZ-ĕ-păm *Restoril* **zolpidem** ZŌL-pĭ-dĕm *Ambien*
psychostimulants sī-kō-STĬM-ū-lăntz	Reduce impulsive behavior by increasing the level of neurotransmitters *Psychostimulants have a calming effect on people with attention deficit-hyperactivity disorder (ADHD) and are also used to treat narcolepsy.*	**dextroamphetamine** dĕks-trō-ăm-FĔT-ă-mēn *Dexedrine* **methylphenidate** mĕth-ĭl-FĔN-ĭ-dāt *Ritalin*

Abbreviations

This section introduces abbreviations related to the nervous system, along with their meanings.

Abbreviation	Meaning	Abbreviation	Meaning
AD	Alzheimer disease	LP	lumbar puncture
AChR	acetylcholine receptor	MEG	magnetoencephalography
ADHD	attention deficit-hyperactivity disorder	MG	myasthenia gravis
CNS	central nervous system	MRI	magnetic resonance imaging
CP	cerebral palsy	MS	multiple sclerosis; mental status; musculoskeletal; mitral stenosis
CSF	cerebrospinal fluid	MSI	magnetic source imaging
CT	computed tomography	NCV	nerve conduction velocity
CTA	computed tomography angiography	PET	positron emission tomography
CVA	cerebrovascular accident	PNS	peripheral nervous system
EEG	electroencephalography	SRS	stereotactic radiosurgery
EMG	electromyography	TIA	transient ischemic attack
ICP	intracranial pressure	tPA	tissue plasminogen activator
IV	intravenous		

It is time to review procedures, pharmacology, and abbreviations by completing Learning Activity 15-4.

LEARNING ACTIVITIES

The activities that follow provide a review of the nervous system terms introduced in this chapter. Complete each activity and review your answers to evaluate your understanding of the chapter.

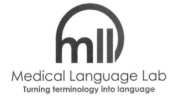

Medical Language Lab
Turning terminology into language

Visit the Medical Language Lab at *medicallanguagelab.com*. Use it to enhance your study and reinforcement of this chapter with the flash-card activity. We recommend that you complete the flash-card activity before starting Learning Activities 15-1 and 15-2.

Learning Activity 15-1
Medical Word Elements

Use the listed elements to build medical words. You may use elements more than once.

Combining Forms		Suffixes		Prefixes
cerebr/o	myel/o	-al	-lepsy	hyper-
encephal/o	narc/o	-algia	-oma	intra-
gangli/o	neur/o	-asthenia	-pathy	quadri-
kinesi/o	radicul/o	-cele	-plegia	uni-
later/o	thec/o	-ectomy	-rrhaphy	
mening/o	ventricul/o	-itis	-stomy	
my/o		-kinesia	-therapy	

1. forming an opening (mouth) in the ventricle _____

2. tumor of a nerve _____

3. pain in a nerve root _____

4. excision of a ganglion _____

5. seizure of sleep _____

6. pertaining to one side _____

7. inflammation of the meninges _____

8. paralysis of four (extremities) _____

9. movement that is excessive _____

10. weakness or debility of muscles _____

11. disease of the cerebrum _____

12. pertaining to within the sheath _____

13. hernia(tion) or swelling of the brain _____

14. treatment (using) movement _____

15. suture of the spinal cord _____

Check your answers in Appendix A. Review any material that you did not answer correctly.

Correct Answers _____ X 6.67 = _____ % Score

Learning Activity 15-2

Building Medical Words

Use *encephal/o* (brain) to build words that mean:

1. disease of the brain _____
2. herniation of the brain _____
3. radiography of the brain _____

Use *cerebr/o* (cerebrum) to build words that mean:

4. disease of the cerebrum _____
5. inflammation of the cerebrum _____

Use *crani/o* (cranium [skull]) to build words that mean:

6. herniation (through the) cranium _____
7. instrument for measuring the skull _____

Use *neur/o* (nerve) to build words that mean:

8. pain in a nerve _____
9. specialist in the study of the nervous system _____
10. crushing a nerve _____

Use *myel/o* (bone marrow; spinal cord) to build words that mean:

11. herniation of the spinal cord _____
12. paralysis of the spinal cord _____

Use *psych/o* (mind) to build words that mean:

13. pertaining to the mind _____
14. abnormal condition of the mind _____

Use the suffix *-kinesia* (movement) to build words that mean:

15. movement that is slow _____
16. painful or difficult movement _____

Use the suffix *-plegia* (paralysis) to build words that mean:

17. paralysis of one half (of the body) _____
18. paralysis of four (limbs) _____

Use the suffix *-phasia* (speech) to build words that mean:

19. difficult speech _____

20. lacking or without speech _____

Build surgical terms that mean:

21. destruction of a nerve _____

22. incision of the skull _____

23. surgical repair of the skull _____

24. suture of a nerve _____

25. incision of the brain _____

✓ *Check your answers in Appendix A. Review material that you did not answer correctly.*

Correct Answers _____ X 4 = _____ % Score

Diseases and Conditions

Match the terms with the definitions in the numbered list.

Alzheimer	clonic	Guillain-Barré	paraplegia
ataxia	concussion	hemiparesis	Parkinson
autism	convulsion	ischemic	poliomyelitis
bipolar	dementia	multiple sclerosis	radiculopathy
bulimia	epilepsies	myelomeningocele	shingles

1. weakness in one-half of the body _____

2. cognitive deficit, including memory impairment _____

3. disease associated with formation of small plaques in the cerebral cortex _____

4. eating disorder characterized by binging and purging _____

5. phase of a grand mal seizure characterized by uncontrolled jerking of the body _____

6. autoimmune syndrome that causes acute inflammation of peripheral nerves _____

7. defective muscle coordination _____

8. mental disorder that causes unusual shifts in mood, emotion, and energy _____

9. chronic or recurring seizure disorders _____

10. stroke caused by narrowing of the carotid arteries _____

11. disease caused by the same organism that causes chickenpox in children _____

12. disease of the nerve root associated with the spinal cord _____

13. paralysis of the lower portion of the trunk and both legs _____

14. disease that causes inflammation of the gray matter of the spinal cord _____

15. sudden, violent contraction of one or more voluntary muscles _____

16. most severe form of spina bifida, where the spinal cord and meninges protrude through the spine _____

17. mental disorder characterized by extreme withdrawal and abnormal absorption in fantasy _____

18. disease characterized by head nodding, bradykinesia, tremors, and shuffling gait _____

19. disease characterized by demyelination in the spinal cord and brain _____

20. loss of consciousness caused by trauma to the head _____

✓ *Check your answers in Appendix A. Review any material that you did not answer correctly.*

Correct Answers _____ X 5 = _____ % Score

Learning Activity 15-4

Procedures, Pharmacology, and Abbreviations

Match the terms with the definitions in the numbered list.

antipsychotics	*general anesthetics*	*plasmapheresis*
cryosurgery	*hypnotics*	*psychostimulants*
CSF analysis	*lumbar puncture*	*TIA*
echoencephalography	*myelography*	*tractotomy*
electromyography	*NCV*	*trephination*

1. tests the speed at which impulses travel through a nerve _____

2. treat attention deficit-hyperactivity disorder and narcolepsy _____

3. treat psychosis, paranoia, and schizophrenia by altering chemicals in the brain, including the limbic system, which controls emotions _____

4. act upon the brain to produce complete loss of feeling with loss of consciousness _____

5. ultrasound technique used to study the intracranial structures of the brain _____

6. technique that uses extreme cold to destroy tissue _____

7. radiological examination of the spinal canal, nerve roots, and spinal cord _____

8. stroke with symptoms that resolve in about 24 hours _____

9. laboratory analysis used to diagnose infections, tumors, and intracranial hemorrhage _____

10. recording of electrical signals when a muscle is at rest and during contraction to assess nerve damage _____

11. procedure to extract spinal fluid for diagnostic purposes, introduce anesthetic agents, or remove fluid _____

12. extracorporal procedure to remove autoantibodies in autoimmune diseases _____

13. transection of a nerve tract in the brainstem or spinal cord _____

14. agents that depress central nervous system functions, promote sedation and sleep, and relieve agitation, anxiousness, and restlessness _____

15. incision of a circular opening into the skull to reveal brain tissue and decrease intracranial pressure _____

✓ *Check your answers in Appendix A. Review any material that you did not answer correctly.*

Correct Answers _____ X 6.67 = _____ % Score

DOCUMENTING HEALTH-CARE ACTIVITIES

This section provides practical application activities in the form of exercises to help develop skills in documenting patient care. First, read the medical report. Then complete the activities and exercises that follow.

Documenting Health-Care Activity 15-1

Discharge Summary: Subarachnoid Hemorrhage

General Hospital

1511 Ninth Avenue ■ ■ **Sun City, USA 12345** ■ ■ **(555) 802–1887**

DISCHARGE SUMMARY

ADMISSION DATE: July 5, 20xx   **DISCHARGE DATE:** July 16, 20xx

ADMITTING DIAGNOSIS: Severe headaches associated with nausea and vomiting

DISCHARGE DIAGNOSIS: Subarachnoid hemorrhage

HISTORY OF PRESENT ILLNESS: Patient is a 61-year-old woman who presents at this time complaining of an "extreme severe headache while swimming." She also complains of associated neck pain, occipital pain, nausea, and vomiting.

A CT scan was obtained that showed blood in the cisterna subarachnoidalis consistent with subarachnoid hemorrhage. The patient also had mild acute hydrocephalus. Neurologically, the patient was found to be within normal limits. A cerebral MRI was performed, and no aneurysm was noted.

HOSPITAL COURSE: The patient was hospitalized on 7/5/xx. On 7/7/xx, she had sudden worsening of her headache, associated with nausea and vomiting. Also, she was noted to have meningismus on examination. A lumbar puncture was performed to R/O possible rebleed. At the time of the lumbar puncture, CSF in four tubes was read as consistent with recurrent subarachnoid hemorrhage. A repeat MRI was performed without evidence of an aneurysm.

PROCEDURE: On 7/9/xx, the patient underwent repeat MRI, which again showed no aneurysm. The patient was deemed stable for discharge on 7/10/xx.

ACTIVITY: The patient was instructed to avoid any type of activity that could result in raised pressure in the head. The patient was advised that she should undergo no activity more vigorous than walking.

Michael R. Saadi, MD
Michael R. Saadi, MD

MRS:dp

D: 7–16–20xx
T: 7–16–20xx

Terminology

The terms listed in the table that follows are taken from *Discharge Summary: Subarachnoid Hemorrhage*. Use a medical dictionary such as *Taber's Cyclopedic Medical Dictionary*, the appendices of this book, or other resources to define each term. Then review the pronunciation for each term and practice by reading the medical record aloud.

Term	Definition
aneurysm ĂN-ū-rĭzm	
cerebral MRI sĕ-RĒ-brăl	
cisterna subarachnoidalis sĭs-TĔR-nă sŭb-ă-răk-NOYD-ă-lĭs	
CSF	
hydrocephalus hī-drō-SĔF-ă-lŭs	
lumbar puncture LŬM-băr PŬNK-chūr	
meningismus mĕn-ĭn-JĬS-mŭs	
occipital ŏk-SĬP-ĭ-tăl	
R/O	
subarachnoid sŭb-ă-RĂK-noyd	

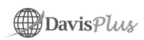 **Davis***Plus*   Visit the *Medical Terminology Systems* online resource center at Davis*Plus* to practice pronunciation and reinforce the meanings of the terms in this medical report.

Critical Thinking

Review *Discharge Summary: Subarachnoid Hemorrhage* to answer the questions.

1. In what part of the head did the patient feel pain?

_____

_____

_____

_____

2. What imaging tests were performed, and what was the finding in each test?

_____

_____

_____

_____

3. What was the result of the lumbar puncture?

_____

_____

_____

_____

4. What was the result of the repeat MRI?

_____

_____

_____

5. Regarding activity, what limitations were placed on the patient?

_____

_____

_____

_____

Consultation Report: Acute-Onset Paraplegia

Physician Center

2422 Rodeo Drive ■ ■ Sun City, USA 12345 ■ ■ (555)788–2427

CONSULTATION

Jacobs, Elaine

August 15, 20xx

CHIEF COMPLAINT: Low back pain and lower extremity weakness

HISTORY OF PRESENT ILLNESS: This is a 41-year-old, right-handed white female with a history of low back pain for the past 15–20 years after falling at work. She has had four subsequent lumbar surgeries, with the most recent on 7/20/xx. She was admitted to the hospital for pain management. The patient had a subarachnoid catheter placement for pain control and management on 7/28/xx, at the T10–11 level. This was followed by trials of clonidine for hypertension and methadone for pain control, with bladder retention noted after clonidine administration. Upon catheter removal, the patient noted the subacute onset of paresis, paresthesias, and pain in the legs approximately 2 1/2–3 hours later. We were consulted neurologically for assessment of the lower extremity weakness.

IMPRESSION: Patient has symptoms of acute-onset paraplegia. Differential diagnoses include a subarachnoid hemorrhage, epidural abscess, and transverse myelitis.

PLAN: Patient will be placed on IV steroids with compression stockings for lymphedema should physical therapy be cleared by cardiology for manipulation of that region. Documentation of spinal fluid will be obtained under fluoroscopy. Her glucose and blood pressures must be carefully monitored.

Jake S. Domer, MD
Jake S. Domer, MD

JSD:st

Terminology

The terms listed in the table that follows are taken from *Consultation Report: Acute-Onset Paraplegia.* Use a medical dictionary such as *Taber's Cyclopedic Medical Dictionary,* the appendices of this book, or other resources to define each term. Then review the pronunciation for each term and practice by reading the medical record aloud.

Term	Definition
abscess ĂB-sĕs	
acute ă-KŪT	
epidural ĕp-ĭ-DOO-răl	
infarct ĬN-fărkt	
lumbar LŬM-băr	
myelitis mī-ĕ-LĪ-tĭs	
paraplegia păr-ă-PLĒ-jē-ă	
paresthesia păr-ĕs-THĒ-zē-ă	
subarachnoid sŭb-ă-RĂK-noyd	
T10–11	

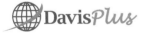

Visit the *Medical Terminology Systems* online resource center at Davis*Plus* to practice pronunciation and reinforce the meanings of the terms in this medical report.

Critical Thinking

Review *Consultation Report: Acute-Onset Paraplegia* to answer the questions.

1. What was the original cause of the patient's current problems, and what treatments were provided?

_____

_____

_____

_____

2. Why was the patient admitted to the hospital?

_____

_____

_____

_____

3. What medications did the patient receive, and why was each given?

_____

_____

_____

_____

4. What was the cause of bladder retention?

_____

_____

_____

_____

5. What occurred after the catheter was removed?

_____

_____

_____

_____

6. What three disorders were listed in the differential diagnosis?

_____

_____

_____

_____

Documenting Health-Care Activity 15-3

Constructing Chart Notes

To construct chart notes, replace the italicized and boldfaced terms in each of the two case studies with one of the listed medical terms.

bradykinesia	neuralgia	Parkinson disease
bradyphasia	neuropathy	sciatica
dysphagia	osteophyte	tremor
herniation		

Mr. K., a 58-year-old male, works at a local newspaper. For most of his life, he has been tying and lifting bundles of papers and placing them in trucks for delivery throughout the city. He complains of (1) *nerve pain* of the lower back and, when standing, (2) *pain that radiates down the nerve* of his right leg, causing his foot to "tingle." The results of an MRI show a (3) *protrusion* of the disc at the L3–L4, compressing the nerve. The MRI also reveals a small (4) *bone spur* impinging on the same nerve. A nerve conduction velocity will be ordered to assess (5) *nerve disease*.

1. _____
2. _____
3. _____
4. _____
5. _____

Mr. M. is an 82-year-old man who was brought to our office by his daughter. She expresses concern because her father frequently has a "far-away stare," and his left hand has developed a noticeable (6) *shake.* His (7) *slow speech* and "word slurring" make it difficult for her to understand and respond to him, causing him further frustration. The daughter notes that her father has (8) *slow movement* and (9) *difficulty in swallowing,* often gagging on his food. The results of a complete medical history, examination, and full neurological workup indicate that this gentleman is suffering from (10) *shaking palsy*. The plan is to begin treatment with Levodopa.

6. _____
7. _____
8. _____
9. _____
10. _____

✓ *Check your answers in Appendix A. Review any material that you did not answer correctly.*

Correct Answers _____ X 10 = _____ % Score

Special Senses

Chapter Outline

Objectives

Upon completion of this chapter, you will be able to:

• Locate and describe the structures of the eye and ear.

• Pronounce, spell, and build words related to the special senses.

• Describe diseases, conditions, and procedures related to the special senses.

• Explain pharmacology related to the treatment of eye and ear disorders.

• Demonstrate your knowledge of this chapter by completing the learning and documenting health-care activities.

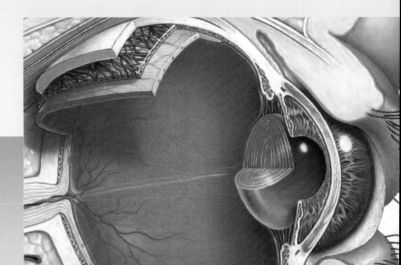

Anatomy and Physiology

General sensations perceived by the body include touch, pressure, pain, and temperature. These sensations are not identified with any specific site of the body. Specific sensations include smell, taste, vision, hearing, and equilibrium (balance). Each specific sensation is connected to a specific organ or structure in the body. This chapter presents information on the sense of vision provided by the eye and the senses of hearing and equilibrium provided by the ear.

Anatomy and Physiology Key Terms

This section introduces important terms associated with the special senses, along with their definitions and pronunciations. Word analyses for selected terms are also provided. Pronounce the term, and place a check mark in the box after you do so.

Term	Definition
accommodation ă-kŏm-ō-DĀ-shŭn ☐	Adjustment of the eye for various distances so that images focus on the retina of the eye
acuity ă-KŪ-ĭ-tē ☐	Clearness or sharpness of a sensory function
adnexa ăd-NĔK-să ☐	Tissues or structures in the body adjacent to or near a related structure *The adnexa of the eye include the extraocular muscles, orbits, eyelids, conjunctiva, and lacrimal apparatus.*
humor	Any fluid or semifluid of the body
labyrinth LĂB-ĭ-rĭnth ☐	Series of intricate communicating passages *The labyrinth of the ear includes the cochlea, semicircular canals, and vestibule.*
opaque ō-PĀK ☐	Substance or surface that neither transmits nor allows the passage of light
perilymph PĔR-ĭ-lĭmf ☐	Fluid that very closely resembles spinal fluid but is found in the cochlea
photopigment fō-tō-PĬG-mĕnt ☐	Light-sensitive pigment in the retinal cones and rods that absorbs light and initiates the visual process; also called *visual pigment*
refractive rĕ-FRĂK-tĭv ☐	Ability to bend light rays as they pass from one medium to another
stereopsis stĕr-ē-ŎP-sĭs ☐	Depth perception provided by visual information derived from two eyes located in slightly different positions so that each produces its own unique view of an object

Pronunciation Help	Long Sound	ā — rate	ē — rebirth	ī — isle	ō — over	ū — unite
	Short Sound	ă — apple	ĕ — ever	ĭ — it	ŏ — not	ŭ — cut

Eye

The eye is a globe-shaped organ composed of three distinct tunics, or layers: the fibrous tunic, the vascular tunic, and the sensory tunic. (See Fig. 16-1.)

Fibrous Tunic

The outermost layer of the eyeball, the **fibrous tunic,** serves as a protective coat for the more sensitive structures beneath. It includes the (1) **sclera,** (2) **cornea,** and (3) **conjunctiva.** The sclera, or "white of the eye," provides strength, shape, and structure to the eye. As the sclera passes in front of the eye, it bulges forward to become the cornea. Rather than being **opaque,** the cornea is transparent, allowing light to enter the interior of the eye. The cornea is one of the few body structures that does not contain capillaries and must rely on eye fluids for nourishment. The conjunctiva covers the outer surface of the eye and lines the eyelids.

Vascular Tunic

The middle layer of the eyeball, the **vascular tunic,** is also known as the **uvea. The uvea** consists of the choroid, iris, and ciliary body. The (4) **choroid** provides the blood supply for the entire eye. It contains pigmented cells that prevent extraneous light from entering the inside of the eye. An opening in the choroid allows the optic nerve to enter the inside of the eyeball. The anterior portion of the choroid contains two modified structures, the (5) **iris** and the (6**) ciliary body.** The iris is a colored, contractile membrane with a perforated center called the (7) **pupil.** The iris regulates the amount of light passing through the pupil to the interior of the eye. As environmental light increases, the pupil constricts; as light decreases, the pupil dilates. The ciliary body is a circular muscle that produces aqueous **humor.** The ciliary body is attached to a capsular bag that holds the (8) **lens** between the (9) **suspensory ligaments.** As the ciliary muscle contracts and relaxes, it

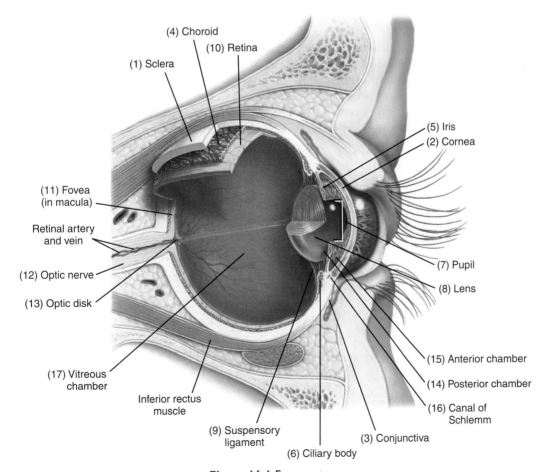

Figure 16-1 Eye structures.

alters the shape of the lens, making it thicker or thinner. These changes in shape allow the eye to focus on an image, a process called **accommodation (Acc)**.

Sensory Tunic

The innermost **sensory tunic** is the delicate, double-layered (10) **retina.** It consists of a thin, outer **pigmented layer** lying over the choroid and a thick, inner **nervous layer,** or visual portion. The retina is responsible for the reception and transmission of visual impulses to the brain. It has two types of visual receptors: rods and cones. **Rods** function in dim light and produce black-and-white vision. **Cones** function in bright light and produce color vision. In the central portion of the retina is a highly sensitive structure called the **macula.** In the center of the macula is the (11) **fovea.** When the eye focuses on an object, light rays from that object are directed to the fovea. Because the fovea is composed of only cones that lie very close to each other, it provides the greatest **acuity** for color vision.

Rods and cones contain a chemical called **photopigment,** or **visual pigment.** As light strikes the photopigment, a chemical change occurs that stimulates rods and cones. The chemical changes produce impulses that are transmitted through the (12) **optic nerve** to the brain, where they are interpreted as vision. The optic nerve and blood vessels of the eye enter at the (13) **optic disc.** Its center is referred to as the **blind spot** because the area has neither rods nor cones for vision.

One of two major fluids **(humors)** of the eye is **aqueous humor.** It is found in the (14) **posterior chamber** and (15) **anterior chamber** of the anterior portion of the eye and provides nourishment for the lens and the cornea. The ciliary body continually produces aqueous humor, which drains from the eye through a small opening called the (16) **canal of Schlemm.** If aqueous humor fails to drain from the eye at the rate at which it is produced, a condition called **glaucoma** results. The second major humor of the eye is **vitreous humor,** a jellylike substance that fills the interior of eye, the (17) **vitreous chamber.** The vitreous humor, lens, and aqueous humor are the **refractive** structures of the eye, focusing light rays sharply on the retina. If any one of these structures does not function properly, vision is impaired.

Adnexa

The **adnexa** of the eye include all supporting structures of the eye globe. Six extraocular muscles control the movement of the eye: the superior, inferior, lateral, and medial rectus muscles and the superior and inferior oblique muscles. These muscles coordinate the eyes so that they move in a synchronized manner. In normal vision, each eye views an image from a somewhat different vantage point, thus transmitting a slightly different image to the brain. The result is binocular perception of depth or three-dimensional space, a phenomenon known as **stereopsis**.

Two movable folds of skin constitute the eyelids, each with eyelashes that are highly sensitive to touch, thus providing a warning that triggers a blink reflex when dust or other irritants are near the eye. (See Fig. 16-2.) The (1) **conjunctiva** lines the inner surface of the eyelids and

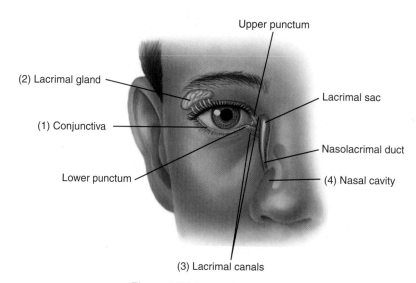

Figure 16-2 Lacrimal apparatus.

the sclera. It lubricates the eye by producing mucus and tears, although a smaller volume than the tears associated with the **lacrimal apparatus.** Lying superior and to the outer edge of each eye are the (2) **lacrimal glands,** which produce tears that bathe and lubricate the eyes. The tears collect at the inner edges of the eyes, the **canthi** (singular, **canthus**), and pass through pinpoint openings, the (3) **lacrimal canals,** to the mucous membranes that line the inside of the (4) **nasal cavity.**

Ear

The ear is the sense receptor organ for two senses: hearing and equilibrium. Hearing is a function of the cochlea. Equilibrium is a function of the semicircular canals and vestibule.

Hearing

The ear consists of three major sections: the outer ear, or **external ear;** the middle ear, or **tympanic cavity;** and the inner ear, or **labyrinth**. (See Fig. 16-3.) The external ear conducts sound waves through air; the middle ear, through bone; and the inner ear, through fluid. This series of transmissions ultimately generates impulses that are sent to the brain and interpreted as sound.

An (1) **auricle** (or *pinna*) collects waves traveling through air and channels them to the (2) **external auditory canal,** also called the **ear canal.** The ear canal is a slender tube lined with glands that produce a waxy secretion called **cerumen.** Its stickiness traps tiny foreign particles and prevents them from entering the deeper areas of the canal. The (3) **tympanic membrane** (also called the **tympanum** or **eardrum**) is a flat, membranous structure drawn over the end of the ear canal. Sound waves entering the ear canal strike against the tympanic membrane, causing it to vibrate. These vibrations cause movement of the three smallest bones of the body, collectively called the **ossicles.** These tiny articulating bones, the (4) **malleus** (or **hammer**), the

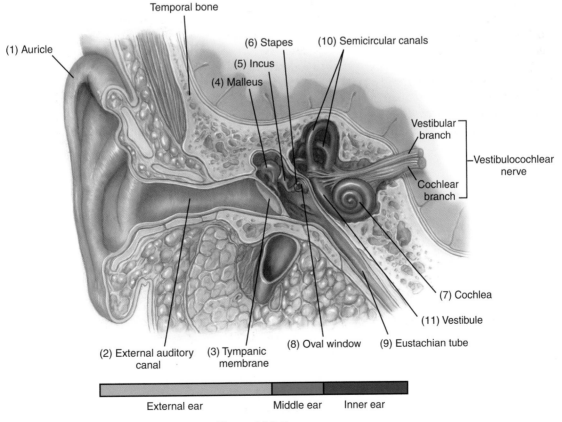

Figure 16-3 Ear structures.

(5) **incus** (or **anvil**), and the (6) **stapes** (or **stirrups**), are located within the tympanic cavity and form a connection between the tympanic membrane and the (7) **cochlea,** the first structure of the inner ear. The cochlea is a snail-shaped structure filled with a fluid called **perilymph**. Its inner surfaces are lined with a highly sensitive hearing structure called the **organ of Corti,** which contains tiny nerve endings called **hair cells.** A membrane-covered opening on the external surface of the cochlea called the (8) **oval window** provides a place for attachment of the stapes. The movement of the ossicles in the middle ear causes the stapes to exert a gentle pumping action against the oval window. The pumping action forces the perilymph to disturb the hair cells, generating impulses that are transmitted to the brain by way of the auditory nerve, where they are interpreted as sound. The (9) **eustachian tube** connects the middle ear to the pharynx. It equalizes pressure on the outer and inner surfaces of the eardrum. When there is an inequality of pressure on either side of the membrane, a deliberate swallow will commonly restore equality.

Equilibrium

The inner ear consists of a system of fluid-filled tubes and sacs and the nerves that connect these structures to the brain. Because of its mazelike design, it is referred to as the **labyrinth.** The labyrinth, which rests inside the skull bones, includes not only the cochlear system (the organ devoted to hearing) but also the vestibular system, which is devoted to the control of equilibrium (balance) and eye movements. The vestibular system contains the (10) **semicircular canals** and the (11) **vestibule.** The vestibule joins the cochlea and the semicircular canals. Many complex structures located in this maze are responsible for maintaining balance.

Anatomy Review: Eye

To review the anatomy of the eye, label the illustration using the listed terms.

anterior chamber	*cornea*	*optic disc*	*retina*
canal of Schlemm	*fovea*	*optic nerve*	*sclera*
choroid	*iris*	*posterior chamber*	*suspensory ligaments*
ciliary body	*lens*	*pupil*	*vitreous chamber*
conjunctiva			

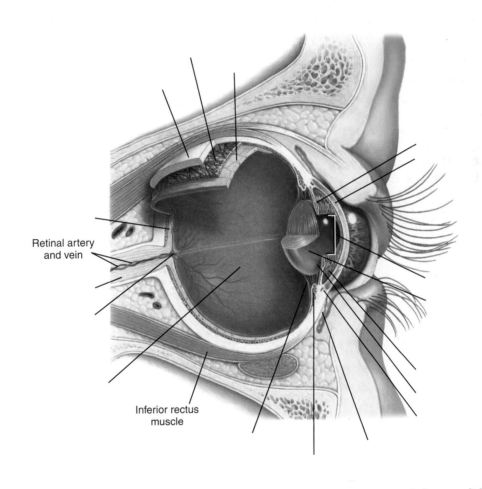

Retinal artery
and vein

Inferior rectus
muscle

 Check your answers by referring to Figure 16-1 on page 563. Review material that you did not answer correctly.

Anatomy Review: Ear

To review the anatomy of the ear, label the illustration using the listed terms.

auricle

cochlea

eustachian tube

external auditory canal

incus

malleus

oval window

semicircular canals

stapes

tympanic membrane

vestibule

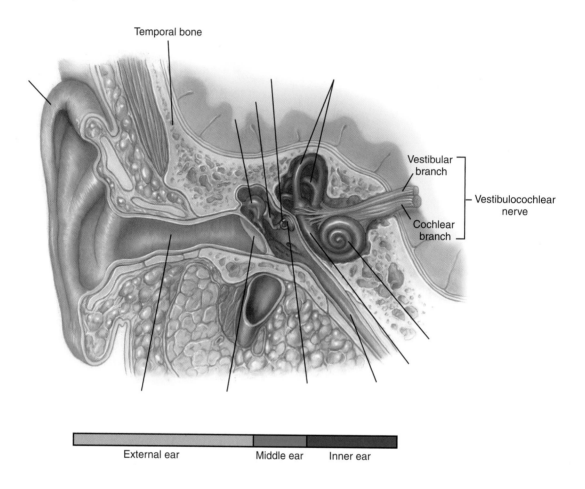

 Check your answers by referring to Figure 16–3 on page 565. Review material that you did not answer correctly.

Medical Word Elements

This section introduces combining forms, suffixes, and prefixes related to the special senses. Word analyses are also provided. From the information provided, complete the meaning of the medical words in the right-hand column. The first one is completed for you.

Element	Meaning	Word Analysis
Combining Forms		
Eye		
ambly/o	dull, dim	**ambly/**opia (ăm-blē-Ō-pē-ă): *dimness of vision* *-opia:* vision *In amblyopia, visual stimulation through the optic nerve of one eye (lazy eye) is impaired, thus resulting in poor or dim vision.*
aque/o	water	**aque/**ous (Ā-kwē-ŭs): _____ *-ous:* pertaining to
blephar/o	eyelid	**blephar/o/**ptosis (blĕf-ă-rō-TŌ-sĭs): _____ *-ptosis:* prolapse, downward displacement
choroid/o	choroid	**choroid/o/**pathy (kō-roy-DŎP-ă-thē): _____ *-pathy:* disease
conjunctiv/o	conjunctiva	**conjunctiv/**al (kŏn-jŭnk-TĪ-văl): _____ *-al:* pertaining to
core/o	pupil	**core/o/**meter (kō-rē-ŎM-ĕ-tĕr): _____ *-meter:* instrument for measuring
pupill/o		**pupill/o/**graphy (pū-pĭ-LŎG-ră-fē): _____ *-graphy:* process of recording
corne/o	cornea	**corne/**al (KOR-nē-ăl): _____ *-al:* pertaining to
cycl/o	ciliary body of the eye; circular; cycle	**cycl/o/**plegia (sī-klō-PLĒ-jē-ă): _____ *-plegia:* paralysis
dacry/o	tear; lacrimal apparatus (duct, sac, or gland)	**dacry/**oma (dăk-rē-Ō-mă): _____ *-oma:* tumor
lacrim/o		**lacrim/o/**tomy (lăk-rĭ-MŎT-ō-mē): _____ *-tomy:* incision
dacryocyst/o	lacrimal sac	**dacryocyst/o/**ptosis (dăk-rē-ō-sĭs-tŏp-TŌ-sĭs): _____ *-ptosis:* prolapse, downward displacement

(continued)

Medical Word Elements—cont'd

Element	Meaning	Word Analysis
glauc/o	gray	**glauc/**oma (glaw-KŌ-mă): _____ -*oma:* tumor *If not treated, glaucoma results in increased intraocular pressure (IOP) that destroys the retina and optic nerve.*
goni/o	angle	**goni/o/**scopy (gŏ-nē-ŎS-kŏ-pē): _____ -*scopy:* visual examination *Gonioscopy helps differentiate the two forms of glaucoma (open- and closed-angle).*
irid/o	iris	**irid/o/**plegia (ĭr-ĭd-ō-PLĒ-jē-ă): _____ -*plegia:* paralysis
kerat/o	horny tissue; hard; cornea	**kerat/o/**tomy (kĕr-ă-TŎT-ō-mē): _____ -*tomy:* incision
ocul/o	eye	**ocul/o/**myc/osis (ŏk-ū-lō-mī-KŌ-sĭs): _____ *myc:* fungus -*osis:* abnormal condition; increase (used primarily with blood cells)
ophthalm/o		**opthalm/o/**logist (ŏf-thăl-MŎL-ō-jĭst): _____ -*logist:* specialist in the study of *Ophthalmologists are physicians who specialize in the medical and surgical management of diseases and disorders of the eyes.*
opt/o	eye, vision	**opt/o/**metry (ŏp-TŎM-ĕ-trē): _____ -*metry:* act of measuring *Optometry is the science of diagnosing, managing, and treating nonsurgical conditions and diseases of the eye and visual system.*
optic/o		**optic/**al (ŎP-tĭ-kăl): _____ -*al:* pertaining to
phac/o	lens	**phac/o/**cele (FĀK-ō-sēl): _____ -*cele:* hernia, swelling *The usual cause of phacocele is blunt trauma to the eye.*
phot/o	light	**phot/o/**phobia (fō-tō-FŌ-bē-ă): _____ -*phobia:* fear *Intolerance to light is associated with people with light-colored eyes and those who suffer from migraines or glaucoma. Some medications also cause a marked intolerance to light.*
presby/o	old age	**presby/**opia (prĕz-bē-Ō-pē-ă): _____ -*opia:* vision *Presbyopia is the loss of accommodation caused by weakening of the ciliary muscles as a result of the aging process.*

Medical Word Elements—cont'd

Element	Meaning	Word Analysis
retin/o	retina	**retin**/osis (rĕt-ĭ-NŌ-sĭs): _____ *-osis:* abnormal condition; increase (used primarily with blood cells) *Retinosis includes any degenerative process of the retina not associated with inflammation.*
scler/o	hardening; sclera (white of eye)	**scler/o**/malacia (sklĕ-rō-mă-LĀ-shē-ă): _____ *-malacia:* softening
scot/o	darkness	**scot/o**/oma (skō-TŌ-mă): _____ *-oma:* tumor *Scotoma is an area of diminished vision in the visual field.*
vitr/o	vitreous body (of the eye)	**vitr**/ectomy (vĭ-TRĔK-tō-mē): _____ *-ectomy:* excision, removal *The removal of the vitreous body allows surgical procedures that would otherwise be impossible, including repair of macular holes and tears in the retina.*
Ear		
audi/o	hearing	**audi/o**/meter (aw-dē-ŎM-ĕ-tĕr): _____ *-meter:* instrument for measuring
labyrinth/o	labyrinth (inner ear)	**labyrinth/o**/tomy (lăb-ĭ-rĭn-THŎT-ō-mē): _____ *-tomy:* incision
mastoid/o	mastoid process	**mastoid**/ectomy (măs-toyd-ĔK-tō-mē): _____ *-ectomy:* excision, removal
ot/o	ear	**ot/o**/py/o/rrhea (ō-tō-pī-ō-RĒ-ă): _____ *py/o:* pus *-rrhea:* discharge, flow
salping/o	tubes (usually fallopian or eustachian [auditory] tubes)	**salping/o**/pharyng/eal: (săl-pĭng-gō-fă-RĬN-jē-ăl): _____ *-al:* pertaining to *pharyng:* pharynx
staped/o	stapes	**staped**/ectomy (stā-pĕ-DĔK-tō-mē): _____ *-ectomy:* excision, removal *Stapedectomy is performed to improve hearing, especially in cases of otosclerosis.*

(continued)

Medical Word Elements—cont'd

Element	Meaning	Word Analysis
tympan/o	tympanic membrane (eardrum)	**tympan/o**/stomy (tĭm-pă-NŎS-tō-mē): _____ *-stomy:* forming an opening (mouth) *Tympanostomy is usually performed to insert small pressure-equalizing (PE) tubes through the tympanum.*
myring/o		**myring/o**/myc/osis (mĭr-ĭn-gō-mī-KŌ-sĭs): _____ *myc:* fungus *-osis:* abnormal condition; increase (used primarily with blood cells)
Suffixes		
-acusia	hearing	an/**acusia** (ăn-ă-KŪ-sē-ă): _____ *an-:* without, not
-cusis		presby/**cusis** (prĕz-bĭ-KŪ-sĭs): _____ *presby:* old age *Presbycusis generally occurs in both ears and primarily affects perception of high-pitched tones.*
-opia	vision	dipl/**opia** (dĭp-LŌ-pē-ă): _____ *dipl-:* double, twofold
-opsia		heter/**opsia** (hĕt-ĕr-ŎP-sē-ă): _____ *heter-:* different
-tropia	turning	eso/**tropia** (ĕs-ō-TRŌ-pē-ă): _____ *eso-:* inward *Esotropia is also called* convergent strabismus *or* crossed eyes.
Prefixes		
exo-	outside, outward	**exo**/tropia (ĕks-ō-TRŌ-pē-ă): _____ *-tropia:* turning *Exotropia is also called* divergent strabismus.
hyper-	excessive, above normal	**hyper**/opia (hī-pĕr-Ō-pē-ă): _____ *-opia:* vision

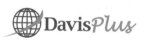 Visit the *Medical Terminology Systems* online resource center at Davis*Plus* for an audio exercise of the terms in this table. Other activities are also available to reinforce content.

⊙ *It is time to review medical word elements by completing Learning Activities 16-1 and 16-2.*

Disease Focus

Common signs and symptoms of eye disorders include a decrease in visual acuity, headaches, and pain in the eye or adnexa. However, many disorders of the eye are serious but asymptomatic; therefore, regular eye checkups are necessary. For diagnosis, treatment, and management of visual disorders, the medical services of a specialist may be warranted. **Ophthalmology** is the medical specialty concerned with disorders of the eye. The physician who treats these disorders is called an **ophthalmologist.** Optometrists work with ophthalmologists in a medical practice or practice independently. **Optometrists** are not medical doctors but are doctors of optometry (O.D.). They diagnose vision problems and eye diseases, prescribe eyeglasses and contact lenses, and prescribe drugs to treat eye disorders. Although they cannot perform surgery, they commonly provide preoperative and postoperative care.

Common signs and symptoms of ear disorders include hearing impairment, ringing in the ears, pain or drainage from the ears, loss of balance, dizziness, and nausea. For diagnosis, treatment, and management of hearing disorders, the medical services of a specialist may be warranted. **Otolaryngology** is the medical specialty concerned with disorders of the ear, nose, and throat (ENT). The physician who treats these disorders is called an **otolaryngologist.** Many otolaryngologists employ audiologists. The **audiologist** specializes in nonmedical management of the auditory and balance systems. Using various testing strategies (such as hearing tests, otoacoustic emission measurements, and electrophysiologic tests), the audiologist aims to determine whether a person can hear within the normal range and, if not, which portions of hearing (high, middle, or low frequencies) are affected and to what degree. If there is a hearing loss or vestibular abnormality, an audiologist may recommend a hearing aid, cochlear implant, or surgery or provide an appropriate medical referral.

Eye Disorders

Common eye disorders include glaucoma and macular degeneration.

Glaucoma

Glaucoma is characterized by increased intraocular pressure (IOP) caused by failure of aqueous humor to drain from the eye through a tiny duct called the **canal of Schlemm.** (See Fig. 16-4, page 574.) The increased pressure on the optic nerve destroys it, and vision is permanently lost.

Although there are various forms of glaucoma, all of them eventually lead to blindness unless the physician detects and treats the condition in its early stages. Glaucoma may occur as a primary or congenital disease or secondary to other causes, such as injury, infection, surgery, or prolonged topical corticosteroid use. Primary glaucoma can be chronic or acute. The **chronic form** is also called **open-angle, simple,** or **wide-angle glaucoma.** The **acute form** is called **angle-closure** or **narrow-angle glaucoma.** Chronic glaucoma may produce no symptoms except gradual loss of peripheral vision over a period of years. Headaches, blurred vision, and dull pain in the eye may also be present. During an ophthalmoscopic examination, cupping of the optic discs is visible. Acute glaucoma causes extreme ocular pain, blurred vision, redness of the eye, and dilation of the pupil. Nausea and vomiting may also occur. If untreated, acute glaucoma causes complete and permanent blindness within 2 to 5 days.

The more common and chronic form of glaucoma is open-angle glaucoma, which is slow to develop and is usually painless. By the time the patient seeks medical attention, it may be too late to restore vision. The rarer form of glaucoma is closed-angle glaucoma. Because of pain and the rapid decrease in vision, the patient generally seeks medical attention before visual field (VF) is lost or blindness has occurred. Treatment for glaucoma includes medications that cause the pupils to constrict **(miotics),** which permits aqueous humor to escape from the eye, thereby relieving pressure. If miotics are ineffective, surgery may be necessary.

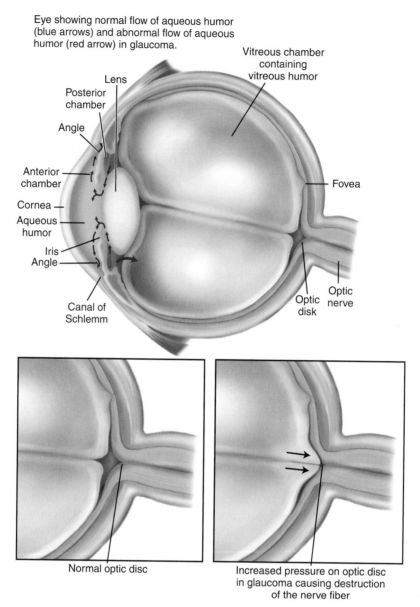

Eye showing normal flow of aqueous humor (blue arrows) and abnormal flow of aqueous humor (red arrow) in glaucoma.

Vitreous chamber containing vitreous humor

Lens

Posterior chamber

Angle

Anterior chamber

Cornea

Aqueous humor

Iris

Angle

Canal of Schlemm

Fovea

Optic disk

Optic nerve

Normal optic disc

Increased pressure on optic disc in glaucoma causing destruction of the nerve fiber

Figure 16-4 Glaucoma.

Macular Degeneration

Macular degeneration is a deterioration of the macula, the most sensitive portion of the retina. The macula is responsible for central, or "straight-ahead," vision required for reading, driving, detail work, and recognizing faces. (See Fig. 16-5.) Although deterioration of the macula is associated with toxic effects of some drugs, the most common type is **age-related macular degeneration (ARMD, AMD).** ARMD is a leading cause of vision loss in the United States. The disease is unpredictable and progresses differently in each individual.

So far, two forms of ARMD have been identified: wet and dry. The less common but more severe form is **wet, or neovascular, ARMD.** It affects about 10% of those afflicted with the disease. Small blood vessels form under the macula. Blood and other fluids leak from these vessels and destroy the vision cells, leading to severe loss of central vision and permanent visual impairment. If identified in its early stages, treatment using a laser beam destroys the newly forming vessels. Unfortunately, the treatment may not be permanent.

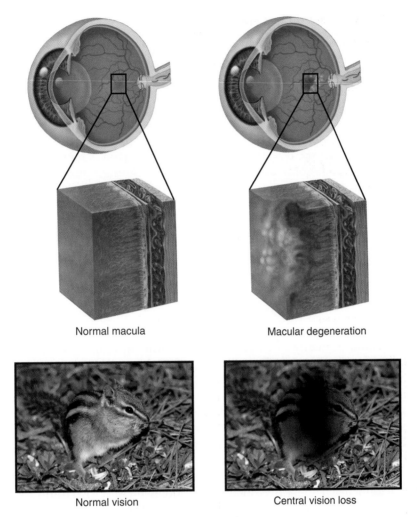

Normal macula

Macular degeneration

Normal vision

Central vision loss

Figure 16-5 Macular degeneration.

The more common form of macular degeneration is **dry ARMD.** Patients with dry ARMD are encouraged to see their ophthalmologist frequently and perform a simple at-home test that identifies visual changes that may indicate the development of the more serious neovascular ARMD.

Ear Disorders

Common ear disorders include otitis media and otosclerosis.

Otitis Media

Otitis media (OM) is an inflammation of the middle ear. This infection may be caused by a virus or bacterium. However, the most common culprit is *Streptococcus pneumoniae.* Otitis media is found most commonly in infants and young children, especially in the presence of an upper respiratory infection (URI). Symptoms may include earache and draining of pus from the ear **(otopyorrhea).** In its most severe form, otitis media may lead to infection of the mastoid process **(mastoiditis)** or inflammation of brain tissue near the middle ear **(otoencephalitis).** Recurrent episodes of otitis media may cause scarring of the tympanic membrane, leading to hearing loss. Treatment consists of bedrest, medications to relieve pain **(analgesics),** and antibiotics. Occasionally, an incision of the eardrum **(myringotomy, tympanotomy)** may be necessary to relieve pressure and promote drainage.

Otosclerosis

Otosclerosis is a disorder characterized by an abnormal stiffness **(ankylosis)** and immobilization of bones of the middle ear that causes hearing loss. The ossicle most commonly affected is the stapes, the bone that attaches to the oval window of the cochlea. The formation of a spongy growth at the footplate of the stapes decreases its ability to move the oval window, resulting in hearing loss. Occasionally, the patient perceives a ringing sound **(tinnitus)** within the ear and experiences dizziness and a progressive loss of hearing, especially of low tones. Development of otosclerosis is typically tied to genetic factors; if one or both parents have the disorder, the child is at high risk for developing the disease. Surgical correction involves removing part of the stapes **(stapedectomy** or, more commonly, **stapedotomy)** and implanting a prosthetic device that allows sound waves to pass to the inner ear. The procedure requires only a local anesthetic and usually lasts only 45 minutes. Hearing is immediately restored.

Oncology

Oncological disorders can occur in almost any structure of the eye or ear as a primary malignancy or spread from other areas of the body to the eye or ear via metastasis.

Eye

Two major **neoplastic diseases** account for more than 90% of all primary intraocular diseases: **retinoblastoma,** found primarily in children, and **melanoma,** found primarily in adults. Most retinoblastomas tend to be familial. The cell involved is the retinal neuron. Vision is impaired, and in about 30% of patients, the disease is found in both eyes **(bilateral).**

Melanoma may occur in the orbit, the bony cavity of the eyeball, the iris, or the ciliary body, but it arises most commonly in the pigmented cells of the choroid. The disease is usually asymptomatic until there is a hemorrhage into the anterior chamber. An ophthalmologist should examine any discrete, fleshy mass on the iris. If malignancy occurs in the choroid, it usually appears as a brown or gray mushroom-shaped lesion.

Treatment for retinoblastoma usually involves the removal of the affected eye(s) **(enucleation),** followed by radiation. Melanoma in which the lesion is on the iris requires iridectomy. For melanoma of the choroid, enucleation is necessary. Many eye tumors are noninvasive and are not necessarily life threatening.

Ear

Malignant and nonmalignant tumors can arise in the external ear, the canal, or the middle ear. Malignant tumors of the ear include basal cell carcinoma and squamous cell tumors.

The most common ear malignancy is **basal cell carcinoma,** which usually occurs on the top of the pinna as the result of sun exposure. It is found more commonly in elderly patients or those with fair skin. Small, craterlike ulcers form as the disease progresses. Basal cell carcinoma does not readily metastasize. However, failure to treat it in a timely manner may result in the need for extensive surgery to remove the tumor.

Squamous cell carcinoma, on the other hand, is much more invasive. However, it is a very rare type of ear tumor. In appearance, it closely resembles basal cell carcinoma, and biopsy is required to make a definitive diagnosis. Squamous cell carcinoma grows more slowly than basal cell carcinoma; however, because of its tendency to metastasize to the surrounding nodes and the nodes of the neck, it must be removed. Surgery combined with radiation therapy is the most effective treatment for squamous cell carcinoma.

Diseases and Conditions

This section introduces diseases and conditions of the eye and ear, along with their meanings and pronunciations. Word analyses for selected terms are also provided.

Term	Definition
Eye	
achromatopsia ă-krō-mă-TŎP-sē-ă *a-:* without, not *chromat:* color *-opsia:* vision	Severe congenital deficiency in color perception; also called *complete color blindness*
ametropia ă-mě-TRŌ-pē-ă *a-:* without, not *metr:* uterus (womb) measure *-opia:* vision	Failure of light rays to focus sharply on the retina as a result of a defect in the lens, cornea, or shape of the eyeball; also called *error of refraction* (See Fig. 16-6.)
astigmatism (Ast) ă-STĬG-mă-tĭzm	Distorted vision resulting from a defective curvature of the cornea or lens causing light rays to diffuse over a large area of the retina rather than being sharply focused *Correction for astigmatism requires the use of lenses that alter the way light enters the eyes.*

hyperopia
  hī-pěr-Ō-pē-ă
  hyper-: excessive, above normal
  -opia: vision
	Visual defect in which the eyeball is too short, and the image falls behind the retina; also called *farsightedness*
	Correction of hyperopia requires the use of biconvex lenses.

myopia mī-Ō-pē-ă	Visual defect in which the eyeball is too long, and the image falls in front of the retina; also called *nearsightedness* *Correction of myopia requires the use of biconcave lenses.*

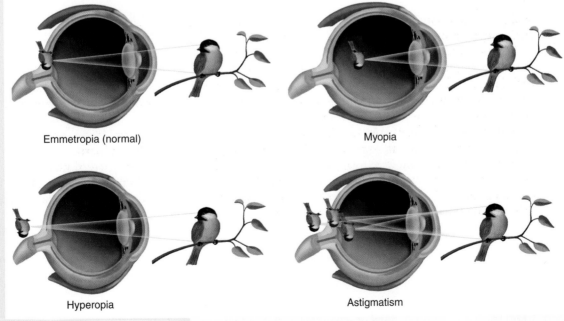

Emmetropia (normal)   Myopia

Hyperopia   Astigmatism

Figure 16-6 Ametropia.

(continued)

Diseases and Conditions—cont'd

Term	Definition
cataract KĂT-ă-răkt	Opacity that forms on the lens and impairs vision, caused by proteins that slowly build up over time *Most cataracts are age related. Surgical treatment to remove the clouded lens and replace it with an artificial intraocular lens (IOL) is one of the safest and most effective surgeries performed in medicine.*
chalazion kă-LĂ-zē-ŏn	Small, hard tumor developing on the eyelid, somewhat similar to a sebaceous cyst; also called *meibomian cyst*
conjunctivitis kŏn-jŭnk-tĭ-VĪ-tĭs *conjunctiv:* conjunctiva *-itis:* inflammation	Inflammation of the conjunctiva and inner eyelids with vascular congestion; also called *pinkeye* *Causes of conjunctiva include irritants, allergy, and viral, bacterial, or fungal infections. The viral form of conjunctivitis is highly contagious. Avoiding contact with others and careful hand washing help control the spread.*
drusen DROO-zĕn	Small yellowish deposits composed of retinal pigment cells that develop under the retina and are associated with an increased risk of developing age-related macular degeneration
ectropion ĕk-TRŌ-pē-ŏn	Eversion, or outward turning, of the edge of the lower eyelid, causing it to pull away from the eye, generally associated with aging and weakness of the small muscles around the eyelid
entropion ĕn-TRŌ-pē-ŏn	Inversion, or inward turning, of the edge of the lower eyelid, commonly causing friction as the eyelashes and outer eyelid rub against the surface of the eye
epiphora ĕ-PĬF-ō-ră	Abnormal overflow of tears *Epiphora is sometimes caused by obstruction of the tear ducts.*
hordeolum hor-DĒ-ō-lŭm	Localized, circumscribed, inflammatory swelling of one of the several sebaceous glands of the eyelid; also called *stye* *Hordeola are commonly caused by a bacterial infection.*
metamorphopsia mĕt-ă-mor-FŎP-sē-ă *meta-:* change; beyond *morph:* form, shape, structure *-opsia:* vision	Visual distortion of objects *Metamorphopsia is commonly associated with errors of refraction, retinal disease, choroiditis, detachment of the retina, and tumors of the retina or choroid.*
nyctalopia nĭk-tă-LŌ-pē-ă *nyctal:* night *-opia:* vision	Impaired vision in dim light; also called *night blindness* *Common causes of nyctalopia include cataracts, vitamin A deficiency, certain medications, and hereditary causes.*
nystagmus nĭs-TĂG-mŭs	Type of involuntary eye movements that appear jerky and may reduce vision or be associated with other, more serious conditions that limit vision
papilledema păp-ĭl-ĕ-DĒ-mă	Swelling and hyperemia of the optic disc, usually associated with increased intracranial pressure; also called *choked disc*

Diseases and Conditions—cont'd

Term	Definition
photophobia fō-tō-FŌ-bē-ă *phot/o:* light *-phobia:* fear	Unusual intolerance of and sensitivity to light *Photophobia commonly occurs in such diseases as meningitis, inflammation of the eyes, measles, and rubella.*
retinopathy rĕt-ĭn-ŎP-ă-thē *retin/o:* retina *-pathy:* disease	Any disorder of retinal blood vessels
strabismus stră-BĬZ-mŭs	Misalignment of the eyes so that they do not focus on the same object at the same time, sending two different images to the brain; also called *heterotropia* or *tropia* (See Fig. 16-7.) *The two most common forms of strabismus are esotropia (ST) and exotropia (XT).*

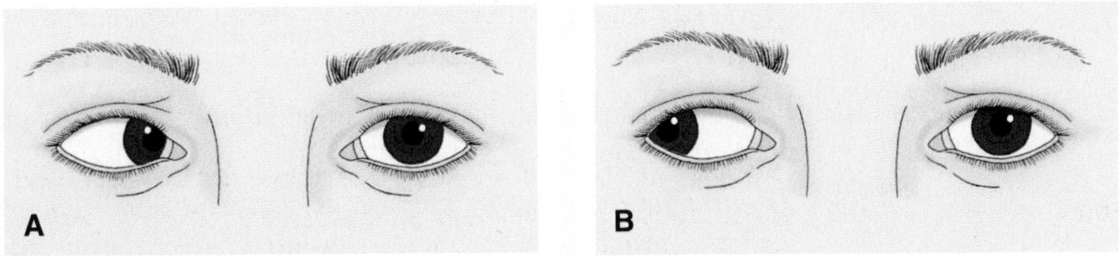

Figure 16-7 Types of strabismus. (A) Esotropia (affected eye turning inward). (B) Exotropia (affected eye turning outward).

Term	Definition
trachoma tră-KŌ-mă	Chronic, contagious form of conjunctivitis that typically leads to blindness

Ear

Term	Definition
anacusis ăn-ă-KŪ-sĭs *an-:* without, not *-acusis:* hearing	Complete deafness; also called *anacusia* *Anacusis may be unilateral or bilateral. Anacusis should not be confused with hearing loss. Hearing loss refers to impairment in hearing, and the individual may be able to respond to auditory stimuli, including speech.*
conduction impairment kŏn-DŬK-shŭn	Blocking of sound waves as they pass through the external and middle ear (conduction pathway)
labyrinthitis lăb-ĭ-rĭn-THĪ-tĭs *labyrinth:* labyrinth (inner ear) *-itis:* inflammation	Inflammation of the inner ear that usually results from an acute viral disease, such as mumps, measles, or influenza *Labyrinthitis may lead to sudden incapacitating vertigo, nausea, and various degrees of hearing loss.*
Ménière disease mĕn-ē-ĀR	Increased fluid pressure of the endolymphatic system that leads to progressive loss of hearing; also called *endolymphatic/labyrinthine hydrops* *Ménière disease is characterized by vertigo, sensorineural hearing loss, and tinnitus.*

(continued)

Diseases and Conditions—cont'd

Term	Definition
noise-induced hearing loss (NIHL)	Condition caused by the destruction of hair cells, the organs responsible for hearing, as a result of sounds that are "too long, too loud, or too close"
	Target shooting, leaf blowing, motorcycle engines, rock concerts, woodworking, and other such environmental noises all produce sounds that may, over time, cause NIHL.
otitis externa ō-TĪ-tĭs ĕks-TĔR-nă *ot:* ear *-itis:* inflammation	Infection of the external auditory canal
	Common causes of otitis externa include exposure to water when swimming (swimmer's ear), bacterial or fungal infections, seborrhea, eczema, and such chronic conditions as allergies.
presbyacusis prĕz-bē-ă-KŪ-sĭs *presby:* old age *-acusis:* hearing	Impairment of hearing resulting from old age; also called *presbyacusia*
	In presbyacusis, patients are generally able to hear low tones but lose the ability to hear higher tones. This condition usually affects speech perception, especially in the presence of background noise, as in a restaurant or a large crowd. This type of hearing loss is irreversible.
tinnitus tĭn-Ī-tŭs	Perception of ringing, hissing, or other sounds in the ears or head when no external sound is present
	Tinnitus may be caused by a blow to the head, ingestion of large doses of aspirin, anemia, noise exposure, stress, impacted wax, hypertension, and certain types of medications and tumors.
vertigo VĔR-tĭ-gō	Sensation of a spinning motion of oneself or of the surroundings
	Vertigo usually results from damage to inner ear structures associated with balance and equilibrium.

 It is time to review pathology, diseases, and conditions by completing Learning Activity 16-3.

Diagnostic, Surgical, and Therapeutic Procedures

This section introduces diagnostic, surgical, and therapeutic procedures used to diagnose and treat eye and ear disorders. Descriptions are provided, along with pronunciations and word analyses for selected terms.

Procedure	Description
Diagnostic	
Clinical	
audiometry aw-dē-ŎM-ĕ-trē *audi/o:* hearing *-metry:* act of measuring	Measurement of hearing acuity at differing sound-wave frequencies and volumes to detect the various types of hearing impairment *Each ear is assessed independently. The patient signals an ability to hear a sound by raising a hand or finger.*
caloric stimulation test	Test that uses different water temperatures to assess the vestibular portion of the nerve of the inner ear (acoustic nerve) to determine whether nerve damage is the cause of vertigo *In the caloric stimulation test, cold and warm water are separately introduced into each ear while electrodes placed around the eye record nystagmus. Eyes move in a predictable pattern when the water is introduced, except with acoustic nerve damage.*
electronystagmography (ENG) ē-lĕk-trō-nĭs-tăg-MŎG-ră-fē	Method of assessing and recording eye movements by measuring the electrical activity of the extraocular muscles *In ENG, electrodes are placed above, below, and to the side of each eye. A ground electrode is placed on the forehead. The electrodes record eye movement relative to the position of the ground electrode.*
gonioscopy gō-nē-ŎS-kō-pē *goni/o:* angle *-scopy:* visual examination	Examination of the angle of the anterior chamber of the eye to determine ocular motility and rotation and diagnose and manage glaucoma
ophthalmodynamometry ŏf-thăl-mō-dī-nă-MŎM-ĕ-trē	Measurement of the blood pressure of the retinal vessels *Ophthalmodynamometry is a screening test used to determine reduction of blood flow in the carotid artery.*
ophthalmoscopy ŏf-thăl-MŎS-kō-pē *ophthalm/o:* eye *-scopy:* visual examination	Visual examination of the interior of the eye using a handheld instrument called an *ophthalmoscope*, which has various adjustable lenses for magnification and a light source to illuminate the interior of the eye *Ophthalmoscopy helps detect eye disorders and other disorders that cause changes in the eye.*

(continued)

Diagnostic, Surgical, and Therapeutic Procedures—cont'd

Procedure	Description
otoscopy ō-TŎS-kō-pē *ot/o:* ear *-scopy:* visual examination	Visual examination of the external auditory canal and the tympanic membrane using an otoscope
pneumatic nū-MĂT-ĭk	Otoscopic procedure that assesses the ability of the tympanic membrane to move in response to a change in air pressure *In pneumatic otoscopy, a tight seal is created in the ear canal, and then a very slight positive pressure and then a negative pressure is applied by squeezing and releasing a rubber bulb attached to the pneumatic otoscope. The fluctuation in air pressure causes movement of a normal tympanic membrane.*
retinoscopy rĕt-ĭn-ŎS-kō-pē *retin/o:* retina *-scopy:* visual examination	Evaluation of refractive errors of the eye by projecting a light into the eyes and determining the movement of reflected light rays *Retinoscopy is especially important in determining errors of refraction in babies and small children who cannot be refracted by traditional methods.*
slit-lamp examination (SLE)	Stereoscopic magnified view of the anterior eye structures in detail, which includes the cornea, lens, iris, sclera, and vitreous humor *The application of fluorescein dye during a slit-lamp examination makes it easier to detect and remove foreign bodies and treat infection, corneal ulcers, and abrasions.*
tonometry tōn-ŎM-ĕ-trē *ton/o:* tension *-metry:* act of measuring	Evaluation of intraocular pressure by measuring the resistance of the eyeball to indentation by an applied force *Tonometry is a standard eye test to detect glaucoma and part of most routine ophthalmic examinations. The applanation method of tonometry uses a sensor to depress the cornea and is the most accurate method of tonometry. (See Fig. 16-8.)*

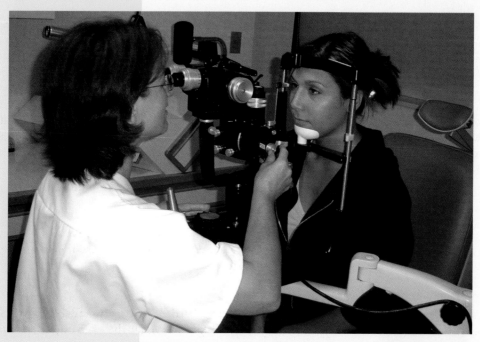

Figure 16-8 Applanation tonometry (courtesy of Richard H. Koop, MD).

Diagnostic, Surgical, and Therapeutic Procedures—cont'd

Procedure	Description
tuning fork tests	Hearing tests using a vibrating tuning fork to determine type of hearing loss
	Conductive hearing loss involves impairment of middle ear structures (malleus, incus, and stapes). Sensorineural hearing loss involves impairment of the inner ear, auditory nerve, or brain.
Rinne RĬN-nē	Tuning fork test that evaluates unilateral hearing loss by comparing sound though bone conduction (BC) versus air conduction (AC); also called *air and bone conduction hearing test*
	In the Rinne test, the physician places a vibrating fork against the mastoid bone (bone conduction) and in front of the auditory meatus (air conduction). In a normal test, air conduction provides longer and louder sound perception than does bone conduction.
Weber	Tuning fork test that determines whether hearing loss occurs in the middle ear (conductive hearing loss) or in the auditory nerves or hair cells of the inner ear (sensorineural); also called *conductive and sensorineural hearing loss test*
	In the Weber test, a vibrating tuning fork placed on the center of the forehead directs sound to each ear simultaneously. If sound perception is equal in both ears, hearing is normal.
visual acuity (VA) test ă-KŪ-ĭ-tē	Part of an eye examination that determines the smallest letters that can be read on a standardized chart at a distance of 20 feet and commonly expressed as a fraction
	The top number refers to the distance from the chart, and the bottom number indicates the distance at which a person with normal eyesight can read the same line. For example, 20/40 indicates that the patient correctly read letters at 20 feet that can be read by a person with normal vision at 40 feet.
Imaging	
dacryocystography dăk-rē-ō-sĭs-TŎG-ră-fē *dacryocyst/o:* lacrimal sac *-graphy:* process of recording	Radiographic imaging procedure of the nasolacrimal (tear) glands and ducts *Dacryocystography is performed for excessive tearing (epiphora) to determine the cause of hypersecretion of the lacrimal gland or obstruction in the lacrimal passages.*
fluorescein angiography floo-RĔS-ēn ăn-jē-ŎG-ră-fē *angio:* vessel (usually blood or lymph) *-graphy:* process of recording	Evaluation of blood vessels and their leakage in and beneath the retina after injection of fluorescein dye, which circulates while photographs of the vessels within the eye are obtained *Fluorescein angiography facilitates the in vivo study of retinal blood flow circulation and is particularly useful in the management of diabetic retinopathy and macular degeneration, two leading causes of blindness.*
Surgical	
blepharoplasty BLĔF-ă-rō-plăs-tē *blephar/o:* eyelid *-plasty:* surgical repair	Cosmetic surgery that removes fatty tissue above and below the eyes that commonly forms as a result of the aging process or excessive exposure to the sun
cochlear implant insertion KŎK-lē-ăr ĬM-plănt *cochle:* cochlea *-ar:* pertaining to	Placement of an artificial hearing device that produces hearing sensations by electrically stimulating nerves inside the inner ear; also called *bionic ear*

(continued)

Diagnostic, Surgical, and Therapeutic Procedures—cont'd

Procedure	Description
cyclodialysis sī-klō-dī-ĂL-ĭ-sĭs *cycl/o:* ciliary body of the eye; circular, cycle *dia:* through, across *-lysis:* separation; destruction; loosening	Formation of an opening between the anterior chamber and the suprachoroidal space for the draining of aqueous humor in glaucoma
enucleation ē-nū-klē-Ā-shŭn	Removal of the eyeball from the orbit *Enucleation is performed to treat cancer of the eye when the tumor is large and fills most of the structure.*
evisceration ē-vĭs-ĕr-Ā-shŭn	Removal of the contents of the eye while leaving the sclera and cornea intact *Evisceration is performed when the blind eye is painful or unsightly. The eye muscles are left intact, and a thin prosthesis called a cover shell is fitted over the sclera and cornea.*
LASIK surgery	Procedure using a specialized laser passed through a temporary flap made in the cornea to reshape underlying corneal tissue *This procedure corrects farsightedness, nearsightedness, and astigmatism. Unfortunately, not all patients are candidates for LASIK surgery. LASIK is the acronym for laser-assisted in situ keratomileusis.*
otoplasty Ō-tō-plăs-tē *ot/o:* ear *-plasty:* surgical repair	Corrective surgery for a deformed or excessively large or small pinna *Otoplasty is also performed to rebuild new ears for those who lost them through burns or other trauma or were born without them.*
phacoemulsification with lens implant fā-kō-ē-mŭl-sĭ-fĭ-KĀ-shŭn	Ultrasonic destruction and removal of a cloudy lens and replacement with a new, clear artificial lens; also called *phaco* (See Fig. 16-9.) *The surgery usually takes less than 15 minutes, and the patient goes home about 2 hours postsurgery.*

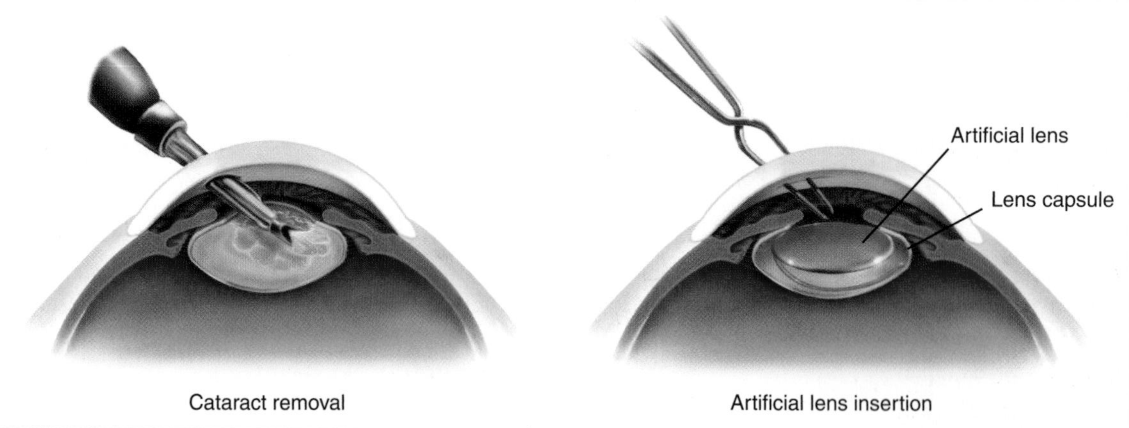

Artificial lens

Lens capsule

Cataract removal

Artificial lens insertion

Figure 16-9 Phacoemulsification for cataract removal.

Diagnostic, Surgical, and Therapeutic Procedures—cont'd

Procedure	Description
pressure-equalizing (PE) tube placement	Insertion of tubes through the tympanic membrane, commonly used to treat chronic otitis media; also called *tympanostomy tubes* or *ventilation tubes* *PE tubes remain in the ear for several months and then fall out on their own or are removed surgically. (See Fig. 16-10.)*

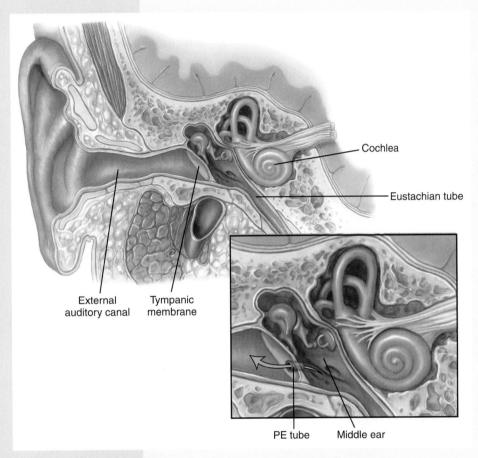

Figure 16-10 Placement of a pressure-equalizing tube.

Procedure	Description
sclerostomy sklĕ-RŎS-tō-mē *scler/o:* hardening; sclera (white of the eye) *-stomy:* forming an opening (mouth)	Surgical formation of an opening in the sclera *Sclerostomy is commonly performed on the anterior chamber in conjunction with surgery for glaucoma for relief of pressure.*
tympanoplasty tĭm-păn-ō-PLĂS-tē *tympan/o:* tympanic membrane (eardrum) *-plasty:* surgical repair	Reconstruction of the eardrum, commonly as a result of perforation; also called *myringoplasty* *Connective tissue located beneath the skin directly behind the ear is used for the tympanic graft.*

(continued)

Diagnostic, Surgical, and Therapeutic Procedures—cont'd

Procedure	Description
Therapeutic	
ear irrigation	Flushing of the ear canal with water or saline to dislodge foreign bodies or impacted cerumen (earwax)
eye refraction test rĕ-FRĂK-shŭn	Visual acuity test to determine the prescription for eyeglasses or contact lenses if required *In an eye refraction test, the patient looks through a device called a phoropter and reads letters or symbols on a wall chart using lenses of differing strengths until vision is corrected to as close to normal as possible.*
retinal photocoagulation rĕ-tin-ŭl fō-tō-kō-ăg-ū-LĀ-shŭn *retin:* retina *-al:* pertaining to	Technique that uses light energy in the form of a laser beam to seal or cauterize retinal tissue; also called *laser photocoagulation* (See Fig. 16-11.) *Retinal photocoagulation is a widely used technique for treating various retinal disorders, including diabetic retinopathy, retinal ischemia, microvascular abnormalities in macular degeneration, adhesions, retinal breaks, and detachment of the retina.*

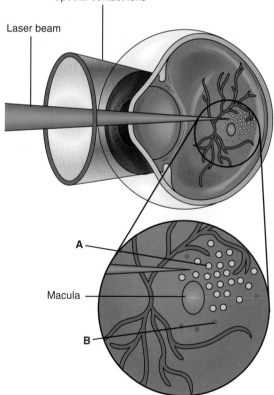

Figure 16-11 Photocoagulation of the retina in diabetic retinopathy. (A) Retinal scars after laser treatment. (B) Untreated blood vessels that continue to bleed and cause visual distortion or blindness.

Pharmacology

Disorders of the eyes and ears are commonly treated with instillation of drops onto the surface of the eye or into the cavity of the ear. The eyes and ears are typically irrigated with liquid solution to remove foreign objects and provide topical application of medications. Pharmacological agents used to treat eye disorders include antibiotics for bacterial eye infections, beta blockers and carbonic anhydrase inhibitors for glaucoma, and ophthalmic decongestants and moisturizers for irritated eyes. Mydriatics and miotics are used not only to treat eye disorders but also to dilate (mydriatics) and contract (miotics) the pupil during eye examinations. Ear medications include antiemetics to relieve the nausea associated with inner ear infections, products to loosen and remove wax buildup in the ear canal, and local anesthetics to relieve the pain associated with ear infections. (See Table 16-1.)

Table 16-1	**Drugs Used to Treat Eye and Ear Disorders**

This table lists common drug classifications used to treat eye and ear disorders, their therapeutic actions, and selected generic and trade names.

Classification	Therapeutic Action	Generic and Trade Names
Eye		
antibiotics, ophthalmic ăn-tĭ-bī-ŎT-ĭks, ŏf-THĂL-mĭk	Inhibit growth of microorganisms that infect the eye *Ophthalmic antibiotics are dispensed as topical ointments and solutions to treat various bacterial eye infections, such as conjunctivitis (pinkeye).*	**tobramycin** TŌ-bră-mī-sĭn *Tobrex* **ciprofloxacin** sĭp-rō-FLŎX-ă-sĭn *Ciloxan*
antiglaucoma agents ăn-tĭ-glaw-KŌ-mă	Increase aqueous humor outflow or decrease its production, resulting in decreased intraocular pressure *Combinations of antiglaucoma drugs that work by different mechanisms are commonly used.*	**timolol** TĪ-mō-lŏl *Betimol* **dorzolamide** dor-ZŌ-lă-mīd *Trusopt* **latanoprost** lă-TĂN-ă-prŏst *Xalatan*
anti-inflammatory, ophthalmics ăn-tĭ-ĭn-FLĂM-ă-tō-rē, ŏf-THĂL-mĭks	Reduce inflammation after corneal injury or ophthalmic surgery or in chronic inflammatory eye conditions	**prednisolone** Prĕd-NĬS-ō-lōn *Pred-Forte* **ketorolac** kē-TOR-ō-lăk *Acular*
artificial tears	Soothe eyes that are dry because of environmental irritants and allergens *Artificial tears generally contain multiple ingredients and are administered topically.*	**cellulose derivatives** SĔL-ū-lōs *Refresh Tears* **glycerin, propylene glycol** GLĬ-sĕr-ĭn, PRŌ-pĭl-ēn GLĪ-cŏl *Moisture Eyes*

(continued)

Table 16-1	Drugs Used to Treat Eye and Ear Disorders—cont'd	

Classification	Therapeutic Action	Generic and Trade Names
mydriatics mĭd-rē-ĂT-ĭks	Disrupt parasympathetic nerve supply to the eye or stimulate the sympathetic nervous system, causing the pupil to dilate *Mydriatics commonly help dilate the pupil to treat inflammatory conditions or in preparation for internal examinations of the eye.*	**atropine sulfate** ĂT-rō-pēn SŬL-fāt
decongestants, ophthalmic dē-kŏn-JĔST-ănts, ŏf-THĂL-mĭk	Constrict the small arterioles of the eye, decreasing redness and relieving conjunctival congestion *Ophthalmic decongestants are over-the-counter products that temporarily relieve the itching and minor irritation commonly associated with allergy.*	**tetrahydrozoline** tĕt-ră-hī-DRŎZ-ō-lēn *Murine, Visine*
Ear		
antiemetics ăn-tĭ-ĕ-MĔT-ĭks	Treat and prevent nausea, vomiting, dizziness, and vertigo by reducing the sensitivity of the inner ear to motion or inhibiting stimuli from reaching the part of the brain that triggers nausea and vomiting *Antiemetics are commonly used to treat vertigo.*	**meclizine** MĔK-lĭ-zēn *Antivert, Bonine*
otic analgesics Ō-tĭk ăn-ăl-JĒ-zĭks	Provide temporary relief from pain and inflammation associated with otic disorders *Otic analgesics may be prescribed for otitis media and otitis externa. Some otic analgesics are also wax emulsifiers.*	**antipyrine and benzocaine** ăn-tĭ-PĪ-rēn, BĔN-zō-kān *Auroguard, Dolotic*
wax emulsifiers ē-MŬL-sĭ-fī-ĕrz	Loosen and help remove impacted cerumen (ear wax) *Excessive wax may be washed out, vacuumed out, or removed using special instruments.*	**carbamide peroxide** KĂR-bă-mīd pĕr-ŎK-sīd *Debrox Drops, Murine Ear Drops*

Abbreviations

This section introduces abbreviations related to the eye and ear, along with their meanings.

Abbreviation	Meaning	Abbreviation	Meaning
Eye			
Acc	accommodation	O.D.	doctor of optometry
ARMD, AMD	age-related macular degeneration	SLE	slit-lamp examination; systemic lupus erythematosus
Ast	astigmatism	ST	esotropia
ENG	electronystagmography	VA	visual acuity
IOL	intraocular lens	VF	visual field
IOP	intraocular pressure	XT	exotropia
LASIK	laser-assisted in situ keratomileusis		
Ear			
AC	air conduction	OM	otitis media
BC	bone conduction	PE	pressure-equalizing (tube); physical examination; pulmonary embolism
ENT	ears, nose, and throat	URI	upper respiratory infection
NIHL	noise-induced hearing loss		

It is time to review procedures, pharmacology, and abbreviations by completing Learning Activity 16–4.

LEARNING ACTIVITIES

The activities that follow provide review of the special senses terms introduced in this chapter. Complete each activity and review your answers to evaluate your understanding of the chapter.

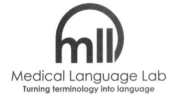

Medical Language Lab
Turning terminology into language

Visit the Medical Language Lab at *medicallanguagelab.com*. Use it to enhance your study and reinforcement of this chapter with the flash-card activity. We recommend that you complete the flash-card activity before starting Learning Activities 16-1 and 16-2.

Learning Activity 16-1
Medical Word Elements

Use the listed elements to build medical words. You may use the elements more than once.

Combining Forms		Suffixes		Prefixes
ambly/o	myring/o	-acusia	-plasty	an-
audi/o	ocul/o	-ar	-ptosis	dipl-
blephar/o	ot/o	-cele	-rrhea	intra-
goni/o	phac/o	-itis	-tomy	
kerat/o	presby/o	-meter		
labyrinth/o	scler/o	-opia		
mastoid/o		-osis		

 1. dimness of vision _____

 2. herniation of the lens _____

 3. double vision _____

 4. downward displacement of the eyelid _____

 5. instrument for measuring the (iridocorneal) angle _____

 6. pertaining to within the eye _____

 7. incision of the cornea _____

 8. discharge from the ear _____

 9. instrument for measuring hearing _____

10. total deafness _____

11. inflammation of the labyrinth of the inner ear _____

12. abnormal condition of hardening of (bones of) the ear _____

13. inflammation of the mastoid _____

14. surgical repair of the eardrum _____

15. (poor) hearing (associated with) old age _____

✓ *Check your answers in Appendix A. Review any material that you did not answer correctly.*

Correct Answers _____ X 6.67 = _____ % Score

Learning Activity 16-2
Building Medical Words

Use *ophthalm/o* (eye) to build words that mean

1. paralysis of the eye _____
2. study of the eye _____

Use *pupill/o* (pupil) to build a word that means

3. examination of the pupil _____

Use *kerat/o* (cornea) to build words that mean

4. softening of the cornea _____
5. instrument for measuring the cornea _____

Use *scler/o* (sclera) to build words that mean

6. inflammation of the sclera _____
7. softening of the sclera _____

Use *irid/o* (iris) to build words that mean

8. paralysis of the iris _____
9. herniation of the iris _____

Use *retin/o* (retina) to build words that mean

10. disease of the retina _____
11. inflammation of the retina _____

Use *blephar/o* (eyelid) to build words that mean

12. paralysis of the eyelid _____
13. prolapse of the eyelid _____

Use *ot/o* (ear) to build a word that means

14. flow of pus from the ear _____

Use *audi/o* (hearing) to build a word that means

15. instrument for measuring hearing _____

Use *myring/o* (tympanic membrane [eardrum]) to build a word that means

16. instrument for cutting the eardrum _____

Use the suffix *-opia* (vision) to build words that mean

17. dim or dull vision _____

18. excessive (farsighted) vision _____

Use the suffix *-acusis* (hearing) to build words that mean

19. without hearing _____

20. excessive (sensitivity to) hearing _____

Build surgical words that mean

21. removal of the stapes _____

22. incision of the labyrinth _____

23. removal of the mastoid process _____

24. surgical repair of the eardrum _____

25. incision of the cornea _____

Check your answers in Appendix A. Review material that you did not answer correctly.

Correct Answers _____ X 4 = _____ % Score

Learning Activity 16-3

Diseases and Conditions

Match the terms with the definitions in the numbered list.

achromatopsia	*drusen*	*nyctalopia*	*otosclerosis*
amblyopia	*epiphora*	*otitis externa*	*presbyacusis*
anacusis	*exotropia*	*otitis media*	*retinoblastoma*
cataract	*hordeolum*	*otoencephalitis*	*tinnitus*
chalazion	*neovascular*	*otopyorrhea*	*vertigo*

1. opacity that forms on the lens and impairs vision _____
2. severe congenital form of color blindness _____
3. impaired vision in dim light _____
4. impaired hearing resulting from old age _____
5. complete deafness _____
6. infection of the external auditory canal _____
7. ankylosis of the middle ear bones resulting in hearing loss _____
8. middle ear infection commonly found in infants and children _____
9. discharge of pus from the ear _____
10. abnormal overflow of tears _____
11. localized, circumscribed inflammatory swelling of a sebaceous gland of the eyelid; stye _____
12. inflammation of the brain tissue near the middle ear _____
13. wet form of macular degeneration _____
14. feeling of dizziness or spinning _____
15. outward deviation of the eye _____
16. small, yellowish deposits that develop on the retina and are associated with macular degeneration _____
17. tumor of the eyelid similar to a sebaceous cyst _____
18. "lazy-eye" syndrome _____
19. neoplastic disease of the eye found primarily in children _____
20. perception of ringing in the ears with no external stimuli _____

✓ *Check your answers in Appendix A. Review any material that you did not answer correctly.*

Correct Answers _____ X 5 = _____ % Score

Terminology

The terms listed in the table that follows are taken from *Operative Report: Retained Foreign Bodies.* Use a medical dictionary such as *Taber's Cyclopedic Medical Dictionary,* the appendices of this book, or other resources to define each term. Then review the pronunciation for each term and practice by reading the medical record aloud.

Term	Definition
bilateral bī-LĂT-ĕr-ăl	
cerumen sĕ-ROO-mĕn	
perforation pĕr-fō-RĀ-shŭn	
supine sū-PĪN	
tympanostomy tĭm-pă-NŎS-tō-mē	

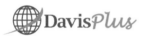 Visit the *Medical Terminology Systems* online resource center at Davis*Plus* to practice pronunciation and reinforce the meanings of the terms in this medical report.

Critical Thinking

Review *Operative Report: Retained Foreign Bodies* to answer the questions.

1. Did the surgery involve one or both ears?

   _____

   _____

   _____

   _____

2. What was the nature of the foreign body in the patient's ears?

   _____

   _____

   _____

   _____

3. What ear structure was involved?

   _____

   _____

   _____

   _____

4. What instrument was used to locate the tubes?

   _____

   _____

   _____

   _____

5. What was the material in which the tubes were embedded?

   _____

   _____

   _____

   _____

6. What occurred when the cerumen and tubes were removed?

_____

_____

_____

_____

7. How was the perforation treated?

_____

_____

_____

_____

Operative Report: Phacoemulsification and Lens Implant

Physicians Day Surgery

1514 Ninth Avenue ■ ■ Sun City, USA 12345 ■ ■ (555) 936–1933

OPERATIVE REPORT

Date: 5/14/xx	Surgeon: Lewis Sloope, MD
Patient: Deetrick, Douglas	Patient ID#: 33422

PREOPERATIVE DIAGNOSIS: Right eye cataract.

POSTOPERATIVE DIAGNOSIS: Right eye cataract.

OPERATION: Phacoemulsification, right eye, with posterior chamber lens implantation.

COMPLICATIONS: None.

PROCEDURE: This 68-year-old male was brought to the operating suite on 8/4/xx as an outpatient. Intravenous anesthesia and retrobulbar block to the right eye were administered. The right eye was prepped in the usual manner. A blepharostat was inserted, and a surgical microscope was positioned. Conjunctival peritomy was performed. Using a keratome, the anterior chamber was entered at the 12 o'clock position. A capsulorrhexis was performed. The cataract was removed by phacoemulsification.

After confirming the 20.5 diopters on the package, the implant was easily inserted into the capsular bag. The wound was observed and shown to be fluid tight. The incision required no sutures. TobraDex ointment was applied, and a sterile patch was taped into place.

Patient was monitored until stable. Postoperative care was reviewed, and patient was released with instructions to return to the office the following day.

Lewis Sloope, MD
Lewis Sloope, MD

rk:bg

D: 5–14–20xx
T: 5–14–20xx

Terminology

The terms listed in the table that follows are taken from *Operative Report: Phacoemulsification and Lens Implant.* Use a medical dictionary such as *Taber's Cyclopedic Medical Dictionary,* the appendices of this book, or other resources to define each term. Then review the pronunciation for each term and practice by reading the medical record aloud.

Term	Definition
blepharostat BLĔF-ă-rō-stăt	
capsulorrhexis kăp-sū-lō-RĔK-sĭs	
cataract KĂT-ă-răkt	
conjunctival kŏn-jŭnk-TĪ-văl	
diopter dī-ŎP-tĕr	
keratome KĔR-ă-tōm	
peritomy pĕr-ĬT-ō-mē	
phacoemulsification fā-kō-ē-mŭl-sĭ-fĭ-KĀ-shŭn	
posterior chamber pŏs-TĒR-ē-or CHĀM-bĕr	
retrobulbar block rĕt-rō-BŬL-băr	
TobraDex TŌ-bră-dĕks	

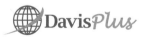

Visit the *Medical Terminology Systems* online resource center at Davis*Plus* to practice pronunciation and reinforce the meanings of the terms in this medical report.

Critical Thinking

Review *Operative Report: Phacoemulsification and Lens Implant* to answer the questions.

1. What technique was used to destroy the cataract?

   _____

   _____

   _____

   _____

2. In what portion of the eye was the implant placed?

   _____

   _____

   _____

   _____

3. What anesthetics were used for surgery?

   _____

   _____

   _____

   _____

4. What was the function of the blepharostat?

   _____

   _____

   _____

   _____

5. What is a keratome?

   _____

   _____

   _____

   _____

6. Where was the implant inserted?

_____

_____

_____

_____

Constructing Chart Notes

To construct chart notes, replace the italicized and boldfaced terms in each of the two case studies with one of the listed medical terms.

antiglaucoma agents	*otalgia*	*pharyngalgia*
asymptomatic	*otorrhea*	*tinnitus*
gonioscopy	*pediatrician*	*tonometry*
hyperopia		

Mrs. B. is an established patient and presents for her annual eye examination. Although she had (1) *no symptoms* in 20xx, the results of the (2) **pressure measurement** of the eyes were above normal. For the last 3 years, she was effectively managed with (3) **medications that decrease intraocular pressure.** The patient now complains of losing "side vision." Results of her eye refraction shows there have been no changes in her (4) **farsightedness.** A (5) **visual examination of the angle** of the anterior chamber of the eyes indicates bilateral open-angle glaucoma that will require surgery. The plan is to schedule Mrs. B. for trabeculo-plasty using a low-level laser.

1. _____
2. _____
3. _____
4. _____
5. _____

Johnny K. was seen at this clinic by Dr. Roberts, a (6) **specialist in children's disorders.** His mother said that for the past 3 days he has complained of an (7) **earache,** (8) a **sore throat,** and (9) **ringing in the ears.** Earlier today, his mother noted an (10) **ear discharge** from the left ear. Upon examination, a perforated eardrum was clearly evident in the left ear. The right eardrum was intact. His tonsillar area showed evidence of strep throat, which was confirmed with a rapid strep test. The patient will begin a regimen of erythromycin with follow-up in 10 days.

6. _____
7. _____
8. _____
9. _____
10. _____

Check your answers in Appendix A. Review any material that you did not answer correctly.

Correct Answers _____ X 10 = _____ % Score

Answer Key

Chapter I—Basic Elements of a Medical Word

Learning Activity I-I
Understanding Medical Word Elements

1. word root *or* root, combining form, suffix, and prefix
2. arthr
3. False—A combining vowel is usually an "o."
4. False—A word root links a suffix that begins with a vowel.
5. True
6. True
7. False—To define a medical word, first define the suffix or the end of the word. Second, define the first part of the word. Third, define the middle of the word.

8. True
9. splen/o
10. hyster/o
11. enter/o
12. neur/o
13. ot/o
14. dermat/o
15. hydr/o

Learning Activity I-2
Identifying Word Roots and Combining Forms

1. nephritis
2. arthrodesis
3. dermatitis
4. dentist
5. gastrectomy
6. chondritis
7. hepatoma
8. muscular

9. gastric
10. osteoma
11. nephr
12. hepat/o
13. arthr
14. oste/o/arthr
15. cholangi/o

Learning Activity I-3
Understanding Pronunciations

1. macron
2. breve
3. long
4. short
5. k

6. n
7. is
8. eye
9. second
10. separate

Learning Activity I-4
Identifying Suffixes and Prefixes

1. -tomy
2. -scope
3. -itis
4. -ic
5. -ectomy

6. an-
7. hyper-
8. intra-
9. para-
10. poly-

Defining Medical Words

Term	Definition
I. gastritis	inflammation of the stomach
2. nephritis	inflammation of the kidney(s)
3. gastrectomy	excision of the stomach
4. osteoma	tumor of bone
5. hepatoma	tumor of the liver
6. hepatitis	inflammation of the liver

Term	Rule	Summary of the Rule
7. arthr/itis	I	Word root (WR) links a suffix that begins with a vowel.
8. scler/osis	I	WR links a suffix that begins with a vowel.
9. arthr/o/centesis	2	Combining form (CF) links a suffix that begins with a consonant.
10. colon/o/scope	2	CF links a suffix that begins with a consonant.
II. chondr/itis	I	WR links a suffix that begins with a vowel.
12. chondr/oma	I	WR links a suffix that begins with a vowel.
13. oste/o/chondr/	3, I	CF links multiple roots to each other. This rule holds true even if the next word root begins with a vowel.
14. muscul/ar	I	WR links a suffix that begins with a vowel.
15. oste/o/arthr/itis	3, I	CF links multiple roots to each other. This rule holds true even if the next word root begins with a vowel. WR links a suffix that begins with a vowel.

Building Medical Words

1. splenectomy
2. appendectomy
3. pancreatectomy
4. cholecystectomy
5. colectomy
6. gastrectomy
7. splenitis
8. hepatitis
9. pancreatitis
10. cholecystitis
11. colitis
12. gastritis
13. hepatomegaly
14. splenomegaly
15. gastromegaly

Chapter 2—Suffixes

Learning Activity 2-1
Building Surgical Words

1. episiotomy
2. colectomy
3. arthrocentesis
4. splenectomy
5. colostomy
6. osteotome
7. tympanotomy
8. tracheostomy
9. mastectomy
10. lithotomy
11. hemorrhoidectomy
12. colostomy
13. colectomy
14. osteotome
15. arthrocentesis
16. lithotomy
17. mastectomy
18. tympanotomy
19. tracheostomy
20. splenectomy

Learning Activity 2-2
Building More Surgical Words

1. arthrodesis
2. rhinoplasty
3. tenoplasty
4. myorrhaphy
5. mastopexy
6. cystorrhaphy
7. osteoclasis
8. lithotripsy
9. enterolysis
10. neurotripsy
11. rhinoplasty
12. arthrodesis
13. myorrhaphy
14. mastopexy
15. cystorrhaphy
16. tenoplasty
17. osteoclasis
18. lithotripsy
19. enterolysis
20. neurotripsy

Learning Activity 2-3
Selecting a Surgical Suffix

1. lithotripsy
2. arthrocentesis
3. splenectomy
4. colostomy
5. dermatome
6. tracheostomy
7. lithotomy
8. mastectomy
9. hemorrhoidectomy
10. tracheotomy
11. mastopexy
12. colectomy
13. gastrorrhaphy
14. hysteropexy
15. rhinoplasty
16. arthrodesis
17. osteoclasis
18. neurolysis
19. myorrhaphy
20. tympanotomy

Learning Activity 2-4
Selecting Diagnostic, Pathological, and Related Suffixes

1. hepatoma
2. neuralgia
3. bronchiectasis
4. dermatosis
5. nephromegaly
6. otorrhea
7. hysterorrhexis
8. blepharospasm
9. cystocele
10. quadriplegia
11. myopathy
12. osteomalacia
13. leukemia
14. osteopenia
15. cardiograph

Learning Activity 2-5
Building Pathological and Related Words

1. bronchiectasis
2. cholelith
3. carcinogenesis *or* carcinogen
4. osteomalacia
5. hepatomegaly
6. neuroma
7. hepatocele
8. neuropathy
9. dermatosis
10. quadriplegia
11. blepharoptosis
12. arteriosclerosis
13. cephalodynia
14. blepharospasm
15. hemophobia

Learning Activity 2-6
Selecting Adjective, Noun, and Diminutive Suffixes

1. gastric *or* gastral
2. bacterial
3. aquatic
4. axillary
5. cardiac *or* cardial
6. spinal *or* spinous
7. membranous
8. internist
9. arteriole
10. sigmoidoscopy
11. alcoholism
12. allergist
13. mania
14. arteriole
15. venule

Forming Plural Words

Singular	Plural	Rule
1. diagnosis	diagnoses	Drop *is* and add *es.*
2. fornix	fornices	Drop *ix* and add *ices.*
3. vertebra	vertebrae	Retain *a* and add *e.*
4. keratosis	keratoses	Drop *is* and add *es.*
5. bronchus	bronchi	Drop *us* and add *i.*
6. spermatozoon	spermatozoa	Drop *on* and add *a.*
7. septum	septa	Drop *um* and add *a.*
8. coccus	cocci	Drop *us* and add *i.*
9. ganglion	ganglia	Drop *on* and add *a.*
10. prognosis	prognoses	Drop *is* and add *es.*
11. thrombus	thrombi	Drop *us* and add *i.*
12. appendix	appendices	Drop *ix* and add *ices.*
13. bacterium	bacteria	Drop *um* and add *a.*
14. testis	testes	Drop *is* and add *es.*
15. nevus	nevi	Drop *us* and add *i.*

Chapter 3—Prefixes

Identifying and Defining Prefixes

Word	Definition of Prefix
1. inter/dental	between
2. hypo/dermic	under, below, deficient
3. epi/dermis	above, upon
4. retro/version	backward, behind

Word	Definition of Prefix
5. sub/lingual	under, below
6. quadri/plegia	four
7. micro/scope	small
8. tri/ceps	three
9. an/esthesia	without, not
10. intra/muscular	in, within
11. supra/pelvic	above, excessive, superior
12. bi/lateral	two
13. peri/odontal	around
14. brady/cardia	slow
15. tachy/pnea	rapid
16. dys/tocia	bad, painful, difficult
17. eu/pnea	good, normal
18. hetero/graft	different
19. post/natal	after, behind
20. circum/renal	around

Learning Activity 3-2

Matching Prefixes of Position, Number and Measurement, and Direction

1. retroversion
2. hypodermic
3. bradypnea
4. subnasal
5. postoperative
6. intercostal
7. epigastric
8. periodontal
9. diarrhea
10. monotherapy
11. suprarenal
12. hemiplegia
13. quadriplegia
14. macrocyte
15. polyphobia

Learning Activity 3-3
Matching Other Prefixes

1. dyspepsia
2. heterograft
3. bradypnea
4. antibacterial
5. bradycardia
6. anticonvulsant
7. amastia
8. anesthesia
9. eupnea
10. tachyphasia
11. tachycardia
12. contraception
13. homograft
14. dystocia
15. homeoplasia

Chapter 4—Body Structure

Learning Activity 4-1
Matching Body Structures and Directional Terms

1. h. ventral cavity that contains digestive, reproductive, and excretory structures
2. k. movement toward the median plane
3. j. part of the spine known as the neck
4. b. tailbone
5. m. away from the surface of the body (internal)
6. f. turning outward
7. l. away from the head; toward the tail or lower part of a structure
8. i. turning inward or inside out
9. n. part of the spine known as the loin
10. a. pertaining to the sole of the foot
11. o. near the back of the body
12. e. lying horizontal with face downward
13. g. nearer to the center (trunk of the body)
14. d. toward the surface of the body (external)
15. c. ventral cavity that contains heart, lungs, and associated structures

Learning Activity 4-2
Basic Word Elements

1. melan/o
2. dist/o
3. cyt/o
4. anter/o
5. leuk/o
6. cyan/o
7. xanth/o
8. dors/o
9. -ar
10. peri-
11. later/o
12. caud/o
13. -ia
14. ultra-
15. ventr/o
16. super-
17. hist/o
18. proxim/o
19. medi/o
20. erythr/o

Building Basic Terms

1. anterior
2. cephalad
3. dorsal
4. ventral
5. cirrhosis

6. erythrocyte
7. melanoma
8. radiologist
9. epigastric
10. hypogastric

Building Medical Words

1. cytologist
2. cytology
3. erythrocyte
4. leukocyte
5. melanocyte

6. ventral
7. proximal
8. medial
9. distal
10. lateral

Diseases and Conditions

1. febrile
2. diagnosis
3. adhesion
4. gangrene
5. hernia
6. peritonitis
7. septicemia
8. suppuration

9. prognosis
10. inflammation
11. rupture
12. symptom
13. edema
14. mycosis
15. perforation

Procedures and Abbreviations

1. percussion
2. curettage
3. CBC
4. ablation
5. endoscopy
6. fluoroscopy
7. Dx
8. electrocautery

9. revision
10. MRI
11. anastomosis
12. nuclear scan
13. palpation
14. I&D
15. computed tomography

Documenting Health-Care Activity 4-1 (Critical Thinking)
Radiological Consultation Letter: Cervical and Lumbar Spine

1. What was the presenting problem?

The patient had neck and lower back pain of more than 2 years' duration.

2. What were the three views of the radiologic examination of June 14, 20xx?

Anterior posterior (AP), lateral, and odontoid

3. Was there evidence of recent bony disease or injury?

There was no evidence of recent bony disease or injury.

4. Which cervical vertebrae form the atlantoaxial joint?

The first cervical vertebra (atlas) and the second cervical vertebra (axis)

5. Was the odontoid fractured?

No, the odontoid was intact.

6. What did the AP and lateral films of the lumbar spine demonstrate?

Apparent minimal spina bifida occulta of the first sacral segment

Documenting Health-Care Activity 4-2 (Critical Thinking)
Radiology Report: Injury of Left Wrist, Elbow, and Humerus

1. Where are the fractures located?

Distal shafts of the radius and ulna

2. What caused the soft tissue deformity?

A fracture caused deformity to the surrounding soft tissue.

3. Did the radiologist take any side views of the left elbow?

The radiologist obtained a single view of the left elbow in the lateral projection.

4. In the AP view of the humerus, what structure was also visualized?

A portion of the elbow

5. What findings are causes of concern for the radiologist?

Lucency through the distal humerus on the AP view along its medial aspect and elevation of the anterior and posterior fat pads

Chapter 5—Integumentary System

Learning Activity 5-1
Medical Word Elements

1. melanoma
2. hypodermic
3. dermatoplasty
4. lipocyte
5. pyoderma
6. dermatologist
7. xeroderma
8. anhidrosis
9. homograft
10. ichthyosis
11. scleroderma
12. mycosis
13. seborrhea
14. trichopathy
15. keratosis

Learning Activity 5-2
Building Medical Words

1. adipoma *or* lipoma
2. adipocele *or* lipocele
3. adipoid *or* lipoid
4. adipocyte *or* lipocyte
5. dermatitis
6. dermatomycosis
7. onychoma
8. onychomalacia
9. onychosis
10. onychomycosis
11. onychocryptosis
12. onychopathy
13. trichopathy
14. trichomycosis
15. dermatology
16. dermatologist
17. adipectomy *or* lipectomy
18. onychectomy
19. onychotomy
20. dermatoplasty *or* dermoplasty

Learning Activity 5-4
Matching Burn and Oncology Terms

1. i. redness of skin
2. e. no evidence of primary tumor
3. h. cancerous; may be life-threatening
4. g. burn that heals without scar formation
5. f. determines degree of abnormal cancer cells compared with normal
6. a. develops from keratinizing epidermal cells
7. b. noncancerous
8. j. primary tumor size, small with minimal invasion
9. c. no evidence of metastasis
10. d. extensive damage to underlying connective tissue

Learning Activity 5-5
Diseases and Conditions

1. pediculosis
2. vitiligo
3. tinea
4. scabies
5. impetigo
6. urticaria
7. chloasma
8. ecchymosis
9. petechiae
10. alopecia
11. abscess
12. erythema
13. eschar
14. pruritus
15. verruca

Learning Activity 5-6
Procedures, Pharmacology, and Abbreviations

1. antifungals
2. fulguration
3. corticosteroids
4. dermabrasion
5. parasiticides
6. keratolytics
7. intradermal test
8. patch test
9. ung
10. xenograft

Documenting Health-Care Activity 5-1 (Critical Thinking)

Pathology Report: Skin Lesion

1. In the specimen section, what does "skin on dorsum left wrist" mean?

Skin was obtained from the back, or posterior, surface of the left wrist.

2. What was the inflammatory infiltrate?

Lymphocytic inflammatory infiltrate in the papillary dermis

3. What was the pathologist's diagnosis for the left forearm?

Nodular and infiltrating basal cell carcinoma near the elbow

4. Provide a brief description of Bowen disease, the pathologist's diagnosis for the left wrist.

Bowen disease is a form of intraepidermal carcinoma (squamous cell) characterized by reddish-brown scaly or crusted lesions that resemble a patch of psoriasis or dermatitis.

Documenting Health-Care Activity 5-2 (Critical Thinking)

Patient Referral Letter: Onychomycosis

1. What pertinent disorders were identified in the past medical history?

History of hypertension and breast cancer

2. What pertinent surgery was identified in the past surgical history?

Mastectomy

3. Did the doctor identify any problems in the vascular system or nervous system?

Vascular and neurological systems were intact.

4. What was the significant finding in the laboratory results?

Alkaline phosphatase was elevated.

5. What treatment did the doctor use for the onychomycosis?

Debridement and medication or Sporanox PulsePak

6. What did the doctor recommend regarding the abnormal laboratory finding?

The doctor recommended a repeat of the liver enzymes in approximately 4 weeks.

Documenting Health-Care Activity 5-3

Constructing Chart Notes

1. erythematous
2. pruritic
3. dermatologist
4. metastasize
5. Mohs surgery
6. asymptomatic
7. biopsy
8. oncologist
9. lymphadenectomy
10. chemotherapy

Chapter 6—Digestive System

Medical Word Elements

1. gingivitis
2. colonoscopy
3. gastroplasty
4. hypogastric
5. dyspepsia
6. sialolith
7. stomatopathy
8. perianal
9. jejunorrhaphy
10. pharyngitis
11. esophagoscope
12. anorexia
13. hematemesis
14. dental
15. dysphagia

Building Medical Words

1. esophagodynia *or* esophagalgia
2. esophagospasm
3. esophagostenosis
4. gastritis
5. gastrodynia *or* gastralgia
6. gastropathy
7. jejunectomy
8. duodenal
9. ileitis
10. jejunoileal
11. enteritis
12. enteropathy
13. enterocolitis
14. colitis
15. colorectal
16. coloptosis
17. colopathy
18. proctostenosis *or* rectostenosis
19. rectocele *or* proctocele
20. proctoplegia *or* proctoparalysis
21. cholecystitis
22. cholelithiasis
23. hepatoma
24. hepatomegaly
25. pancreatitis

Building Surgical Words

1. gingivectomy
2. glossectomy
3. esophagoplasty
4. gastrectomy
5. gastrojejunostomy
6. esophagectomy
7. gastroenterocolostomy
8. enteroplasty
9. enteropexy
10. choledochorrhaphy
11. colostomy
12. hepatopexy
13. proctoplasty *or* rectoplasty
14. cholecystectomy
15. choledochoplasty

Learning Activity 6-4
Diseases and Conditions

1. hematemesis
2. dysphagia
3. hemorrhoids
4. halitosis
5. anorexia
6. melena
7. cirrhosis
8. cachexia
9. obstipation
10. borborygmus
11. ascites
12. Crohn disease
13. steatorrhea
14. leukoplakia
15. flatus

Learning Activity 6-5
Procedures, Pharmacology, and Abbreviations

1. MRCP
2. ESWL
3. IBS
4. antispasmodics
5. choledochoplasty
6. lower GI series
7. gastroscopy
8. antiemetics
9. intubation
10. anastomosis
11. stool guaiac
12. endoscopy
13. laxatives
14. antacids
15. stool culture
16. liver function tests
17. bariatric
18. stat.
19. proctosigmoidoscopy
20. upper GI series

Documenting Health-Care Activity 6-1 (Critical Thinking)
Chart Note: GI Evaluation

1. Referring to Figure 6-3, describe the location of the gallbladder in relation to the liver.

Posterior and inferior portion of the right lobe of the liver

2. Why did the patient undergo the cholecystectomy?

To treat cholecystitis and cholelithiasis

3. What were the patient's prior surgeries?

Tonsillectomy, appendectomy, and cholecystectomy

4. How does the patient's most recent postoperative episode of discomfort (pain) differ from the initial pain she described?

The continuous, deep right-sided pain took on a crescendo pattern and then a decrescendo pattern. Initially, it was intermittent and sharp epigastric pain.

Documenting Health-Care Activity 6-2 (Critical Thinking)
Operative Report: Esophagogastroduodenoscopy with Biopsy

1. What caused the hematemesis?

Etiology was unknown. Inflammation of the stomach and duodenum was noted.

2. What procedures were carried out to determine the cause of bleeding?

During x-ray tomography using the videoendoscope, biopsies were taken of the stomach and duodenum. It was also noted that the patient previously had esophageal varices.

3. How much blood did the patient lose during the procedure?

None

4. Were there any ulcerations or erosions found during the exploratory procedure that might account for the bleeding?

No

5. What type of sedation was used during the procedure?

Demerol and Versed administered intravenously

6. What did the doctors find when they examined the stomach and duodenum?

Diffuse, punctate erythema

Documenting Health-Care Activity 6-3
Constructing Chart Notes

1. dysphagia
2. dyspepsia
3. gastric reflux
4. antacids
5. hiatal hernia
6. anorexia
7. nausea
8. sclerae
9. jaundice
10. hepatomegaly

Chapter 7—Respiratory System

Learning Activity 7-1
Medical Word Elements

1. pleurocentesis
2. bronchoscope
3. tonsillectomy
4. bradypnea
5 dysphonia
6. cyanosis
7. hypoxia
8. laryngoplegia
9. septoplasty
10. sinusotomy
11. hypercapnia
12. eupnea
13. bronchiectasis
14. rhinoplasty
15. pneumonia

Learning Activity 7-2

Building Medical Words

1. rhinorrhea
2. rhinitis
3. laryngoscopy
4. laryngitis
5. laryngostenosis
6. bronchiectasis
7. bronchopathy
8. bronchospasm
9. pneumothorax
10. pneumonitis
11. pulmonologist
12. pulmonary *or* pulmonic
13. dyspnea
14. bradypnea
15. tachypnea
16. apnea
17. rhinoplasty
18. thoracocentesis *or* thoracentesis
19. pulmonectomy *or* pneumonectomy
20. tracheostomy

Learning Activity 7-3

Diseases and Conditions

1. atelectasis
2. empyema
3. rhonchus
4. hypoxia
5. exudate
6. anosmia
7. hypoxemia
8. cystic fibrosis
9. influenza
10. emphysema
11. hemoptysis
12. epistaxis
13. pulmonary edema
14. transudate
15. deviated septum
16. coryza
17. tuberculosis
18. pleurisy
19. consolidation
20. pertussis

Learning Activity 7-4

Procedures, Pharmacology, and Abbreviations

1. sputum culture
2. polysomnography
3. CXR
4. antral lavage
5. antihistamine
6. antitussive
7. sweat test
8. oximetry
9. thoracentesis
10. aerosol therapy
11. decongestant
12. Mantoux test
13. ABGs
14. expectorant
15. throat culture
16. pulmonary function tests
17. laryngoscopy
18. septoplasty
19. pneumonectomy
20. rhinoplasty

Documenting Health-Care Activity 7-1 (Critical Thinking)

SOAP Note: Respiratory Evaluation

1. What symptom caused the patient to seek medical help?

Shortness of breath

2. What was the patient's previous history?

Difficult breathing, high blood pressure, chronic obstructive pulmonary disease, and peripheral vascular disease

3. What were the abnormal findings of the physical examination?

Bilateral wheezes and rhonchi heard anteriorly and posteriorly

4. What changes were noted from the previous film?

Interstitial vascular congestion with possible superimposed inflammatory change and some pleural reactive change

5. What are the present assessments?

Acute exacerbation of chronic obstructive pulmonary disease, heart failure, hypertension, and peripheral vascular disease

6. What new diagnosis was made that did not appear in the previous medical history?

Heart failure

Documenting Health-Care Activity 7-2 (Critical Thinking)

SOAP Note: Chronic Interstitial Lung Disease

1. When did the patient notice dyspnea?

With activity

2. Other than the respiratory system, what other body systems are identified in the history of present illness?

Cardiovascular, urinary, and nervous systems

3. What were the findings regarding the neck?

Supple and no evidence of thyromegaly or adenomegaly

4. What was the finding regarding the chest?

Basilar crackles without wheezing or rhonchi

5. What appears to be the likely cause of the chronic interstitial lung disease?

Combination of pulmonary fibrosis and heart failure

6. What did the cardiac examination reveal?

Trace of edema without clubbing or murmur

Documenting Health-Care Activity 7-3

Constructing Chart Notes

1. dyspnea
2. coryza
3. deviated nasal septum
4. septoplasty
5. T&A
6. myalgia
7. cephalodynia
8. sinusitis
9. pharyngitis
10. antitussive

Chapter 8—Cardiovascular System

Learning Activity 8-1

Medical Word Elements

1. cardiomegaly
2. atheroma
3. arteriorrhexis
4. ventricular
5. transseptal
6. phlebectasis
7. aortogram
8. valvuloplasty
9. sclerosis
10. sclerotherapy
11. thrombolysis
12. arrhythmia
13. periarterial
14. cardialgia
15. aneurysmectomy

Learning Activity 8-2

Building Medical Words

1. atheroma
2. atherosclerosis
3. phlebitis
4. phlebothrombosis
5. venous
6. venospasm
7. cardiologist
8. cardiorrhexis
9. cardiotoxic
10. cardiomegaly
11. angiomalacia
12. angioma
13. thrombogenesis
14. thrombosis
15. aortostenosis
16. aortography
17. cardiocentesis
18. arteriorrhaphy
19. embolectomy
20. thrombolysis

Learning Activity 8-3

Diseases and Conditions

1. infarction
2. angina
3. insufficiency
4. tachycardia
5. varices
6. bruit
7. bradycardia
8. palpitation
9. thrombosis
10. aneurysm
11. embolism
12. arrhythmia
13. regurgitation
14. diaphoresis
15. arteriosclerosis
16. hypertension
17. hyperlipidemia
18. coarctation
19. ischemia
20. stenosis

Learning Activity 8-4
Procedures, Pharmacology, and Abbreviations

1. Holter monitor test
2. echocardiography
3. valvotomy
4. nitrates
5. statins
6. diuretics
7. cardiac biomarkers
8. Doppler
9. stress test
10. defibrillation
11. cardioversion
12. ECG
13. ICD
14. stent placement
15. anticoagulants
16. sclerotherapy
17. CABG
18. endarterectomy
19. PTCA
20. open heart

Documenting Health-Care Activity 8-1 (Critical Thinking)
Chart Note: Acute Myocardial Infarction

1. How long had the patient experienced chest pain before she was seen in the hospital?

Approximately 2 hours

2. Did the patient have a previous history of chest pain?

Yes

3. Initially, what medications were administered to stabilize the patient?

Streptokinase and heparin

4. What two laboratory tests will be used to evaluate the patient?

Partial thromboplastin time and cardiac enzymes

5. During the current admission, what part of the heart was damaged?

The lateral front side of the heart (anterior of the heart)

6. Was the location of damage to the heart for this admission the same as that for the initial MI?

No, in the earlier admission, the damage was to the lower part of the heart.

Documenting Health-Care Activity 8-2 (Critical Thinking)
Operative Report: Right Temporal Artery Biopsy

1. Why was the right temporal artery biopsied?

To rule out arteritis

2. In what position was the patient placed?

Supine

3. What was the incision area?

Right preauricular area

4. How was the temporal artery located for administration of Xylocaine?

By palpation

5. How was the dissection carried out?

Down through the subcutaneous tissue and superficial fascia

6. What was the size of the specimen?

A segment of approximately 1.5 cm

Constructing Chart Notes

1. angina pectoris
2. diaphoresis
3. palpitations
4. hypertension
5. edema

6. myocardial infarction
7. ischemia
8. angioplasty
9. catheter
10. stent

Chapter 9—Blood, Lymphatic, and Immune Systems

Learning Activity 9-1
Medical Word Elements

1. lymphangioma
2. sideropenia
3. splenomegaly
4. thrombosis
5. morphology
6. thymectomy
7. hypochromic
8. microcytic

9. lymphadenopathy
10. erythroblast
11. hemolysis
12. nuclear
13. adenoid
14. agranular
15. hemopoiesis

Learning Activity 9-2
Building Medical Words

1. erythrocytosis
2. leukocytosis
3. lymphocytosis
4. reticulocytosis
5. leukopenia *or* leukocytopenia
6. erythropenia *or* erythrocytopenia
7. thrombocytopenia *or* thrombopenia
8. lymphocytopenia
9. hemopoiesis *or* hematopoiesis
10. leukopoiesis *or* leukocytopoiesis

11. thrombocytopoiesis
12. immunologist
13. immunology
14. splenocele
15. splenolysis
16. splenectomy
17. thymectomy
18. lymphadenectomy
19. splenotomy
20. splenopexy

Learning Activity 9-3
Diseases and Conditions

1. hemoglobinopathy
2. lymphedema
3. lymphadenopathy
4. aplastic
5. anaphylaxis
6. opportunistic
7. Hodgkin disease
8. sensitization
9. erythropenia
10. multiple myeloma
11. mononucleosis
12. sepsis
13. myelogenous
14. Kaposi sarcoma
15. sickle cell
16. thrombocytopenia
17. hemolytic
18. thrombocythemia
19. hemophilia
20. graft rejection

Learning Activity 9-4
Procedures, Pharmacology, and Abbreviations

1. biological
2. lymphangiography
3. monospot
4. anticoagulants
5. WBC
6. homologous
7. ANA
8. lymphoscintigraphy
9. plasmapheresis
10. lymphadenectomy
11. autologous
12. antimicrobials
13. RBC
14. thrombolytics
15. transfusion

Documenting Health-Care Activity 9-1 (Critical Thinking)
Discharge Summary: Sickle Cell Crisis

1. What blood product was administered to the patient?

Two units of packed red blood cells

2. Why was this blood product given to the patient?

The patient was anemic as a result of sickle cell anemia.

3. Why was a CT scan performed on the patient?

To determine the cause of abdominal pain

4. What were the three findings of the CT scan?

Ileus in the small bowel, dilated small bowel loops, and abnormal enhancement pattern in the kidney

5. Why should the patient see his regular doctor?

To follow up on the renal abnormality

Documenting Health-Care Activity 9-2 (Critical Thinking)

Discharge Summary: PCP and HIV

1. How do you think the patient acquired the HIV infection?

From her husband, who died of HIV

2. What were the two diagnoses of the husband?

Multifocal leukoencephalopathy and Kaposi sarcoma

3. What four disorders in the medical history are significant for HIV?

Several episodes of diarrhea, sinusitis, thrush, and vaginal candidiasis

4. What was the x-ray finding?

Diffuse lower lobe infiltrates

5. What two procedures are going to be performed to confirm the diagnosis of *Pneumocystis* pneumonia?

Bronchoscopy and alveolar lavage

Documenting Health-Care Activity 9-3

Constructing Chart Notes

1. lymphadenopathy
2. splenomegaly
3. leukocytosis
4. erythropenia
5. hematologist
6. hemophilia
7. ecchymoses
8. arthralgia
9. hemarthrosis
10. hemostasis

Chapter 10—Musculoskeletal System

Learning Activity 10-1

Medical Word Elements

1. atrophy
2. leiomyoma
3. osteitis
4. patellar
5. chondromalacia
6. arthrodesis
7. ankylosis
8. craniotome
9. osteotomy
10. arthritis
11. dactylitis
12. osteoclast
13. cephalalgia
14. chondroma
15. fascioplasty

Learning Activity 10-2

Building Medical Words

1. osteocytes
2. ostealgia *or* osteodynia
3. osteoarthropathy
4. osteogenesis
5. cervical
6. cervicobrachial
7. cervicofacial
8. myeloma
9. myelosarcoma
10. myelocyte
11. myeloid
12. suprasternal
13. sternoid
14. chondroblast
15. arthritis
16. osteoarthritis
17. pelvimeter
18. myospasm
19. myopathy
20. myorrhexis
21. phalangectomy
22. thoracotomy
23. vertebrectomy
24. arthrodesis
25. myoplasty

Learning Activity 10-3

Diseases and Conditions

1. subluxation
2. rickets
3. spondylolisthesis
4. claudication
5. muscular dystrophy
6. talipes
7. sequestrum
8. myasthenia gravis
9. carpal tunnel
10. ganglion cyst
11. hypotonia
12. Ewing
13. greenstick fracture
14. kyphosis
15. osteoporosis
16. scoliosis
17. chondrosarcoma
18. comminuted fracture
19. spondylitis
20. gout
21. bunion
22. pyogenic
23. necrosis
24. ankylosis
25. phantom limb

Learning Activity 10-4
Procedures, Pharmacology, and Abbreviations

1. myelography
2. open reduction
3. discography
4. CTS
5. laminectomy
6. arthrography
7. arthrodesis
8. amputation
9. HNP
10. salicylates
11. arthroscopy
12. sequestrectomy
13. bone scintigraphy
14. relaxants
15. closed reduction

Documenting Health-Care Activity 10-1 (Critical Thinking)
Operative Report: Right Knee Arthroscopy and Medial Meniscectomy

1. Describe the meniscus and identify its location.

The meniscus is the curved, fibrous cartilage in the knees and other joints.

2. What is the probable cause of the tear in the patient's meniscus?

The continuous pressure on the knees from jogging on a hard surface, such as pavement

3. What does normal ACL and PCL refer to in the report?

The anterior and posterior cruciate ligaments appeared to be normal.

4. Explain the McMurray sign test.

Rotation of the tibia on the femur is used to determine injury to meniscal structures. An audible click during manipulation of the tibia with the leg flexed is an indication that the meniscus has been injured.

5. Why was the surgery performed even though the Lachman and McMurray tests were negative (normal)?

The medial compartment of the knee showed an inferior surface posterior and midmedial meniscal tear that was flipped up on top of itself. The surgeon resected the tear, and the remaining meniscus was contoured back to a stable rim.

Documenting Health-Care Activity 10-2 (Critical Thinking)
Radiographic Consultation: Tibial Diaphysis Nuclear Scan

1. Where was the pain located?

Middle one-third of the left tibia

2. What medication was the patient taking for pain, and did it provide relief?

He was taking NSAIDs but found no relief.

3. How was the blood flow to the affected area described by the radiologist?

Focal, increased blood flow and blood pooling

4. How was the radiotracer accumulation described?

The radiotracer accumulation within the left midposterior tibial diaphysis was delayed.

5. What will be the probable outcome with continued excessive repetitive stress?

The rate of resorption will exceed the rate of bone replacement.

6. What will happen if resorption continues to exceed replacement?

A stress fracture will occur.

Constructing Chart Notes

1. comminuted
2. clavicle
3. open fracture
4. femur
5. orthopedist
6. osteopenia
7. kyphosis
8. spondylalgia
9. osteoporosis
10. pathological fractures

Chapter 11—Urinary System

Learning Activity 11-1
Medical Word Elements

1. nephropathy
2. lithogenesis
3. pyeloplasty
4. anuria
5. glomerulosclerosis
6. cystoscopy
7. dialysis
8. hematuria
9. polyuria
10. ureterectasis
11. meatotome
12. azotemia
13. nephrocele
14. lithotripsy
15. cystogram

Learning Activity 11-2
Building Medical Words

1. nephrolith
2. nephropyosis *or* pyonephrosis
3. hydronephrosis *or* nephrohydrosis
4. pyelography
5. pyelopathy
6. ureterectasis *or* ureterectasia
7. ureterolith
8. ureteralgia
9. cystitis
10. cystoscope
11. cystoplegia
12. vesicocele
13. vesicourethral
14. urethrostenosis
15. urethrotome
16. urology
17. uropathy
18. dysuria
19. oliguria
20. pyuria
21. ureteroplasty
22. cystectomy
23. urethrorrhaphy
24. pyelostomy
25. cystopexy

Learning Activity 11-3

Diseases and Conditions

1. urgency
2. fistula
3. dysuria
4. anuria
5. azotemia
6. hydronephrosis
7. urolithiasis
8. interstitial cystitis
9. oliguria
10. pyelonephritis
11. cystocele
12. enuresis
13. polycystic
14. neurogenic bladder
15. pyuria
16. nephrotic syndrome
17. nocturia
18. reflux
19. Wilms tumor
20. nephrolithiasis

Learning Activity 11-4

Procedures, Pharmacology, and Abbreviations

1. IVP
2. electromyography
3. cystoscopy
4. antibiotics
5. C&S
6. diuretics
7. stent placement
8. ESWL
9. peritoneal
10. renal nuclear scan
11. hemodialysis
12. nephrostomy
13. bladder US
14. potassium
15. UA

Documenting Health-Care Activity 11-1 (Critical Thinking)

Operative Report: Ureterocele and Ureterocele Calculus

1. What were the findings from the resectoscopy?

The prostate and bladder appeared normal, but there was a left ureterocele.

2. What were the name and size of the urethral sound used in the procedure?

#26 French Van Buren

3. What is the function of the urethral sound?

To dilate the urethra

4. In what direction was the ureterocele incised?

Longitudinally

5. Was fulguration required? Why or why not?

Fulguration was not required because there was no bleeding.

Documenting Health-Care Activity 11-2 (Critical Thinking)

Operative Report: Extracorporeal Shock-Wave Lithotripsy

1. What previous procedures were performed on the patient?

ESWL and double-J stent placement

2. Why is the current procedure being performed?

To fragment the remaining calculus and remove the double-J stent

3. What imaging technique was used for positioning the patient to ensure that the shock waves would strike the calculus?

Fluoroscopy

4. In what position was the patient placed in the cystoscopy suite?

Dorsal lithotomy

5. How was the double-J stent removed?

It was removed with grasping forceps as the scope was withdrawn.

Documenting Health-Care Activity 11-3

Constructing Chart Notes

1. hematuria
2. pyuria
3. ureterolithiasis
4. pyelectasis
5. lithotripsy
6. oliguria
7. hypertension
8. proteinuria
9. glomerulonephritis
10. prognosis

Chapter 12—Female Reproductive System

Learning Activity 12-1

Medical Word Elements

1. colposcopy
2. prenatal
3. dystocia
4. hysterorrhexis
5. oophoroma
6. cervicitis
7. amniocentesis
8. perineorrhaphy
9. salpingoplasty
10. primigravida
11. pseudocyesis
12. hemosalpinx
13. multipara
14. menarche
15. galactopoiesis

Learning Activity 12-2
Building Medical Words

1. gynecopathy
2. gynecologist
3. cervicovaginitis
4. cervicovesical
5. colposcope
6. colposcopy
7. vaginitis
8. vaginocele
9. hysteromyoma
10. hysteropathy
11. hysterosalpingography
12. metrorrhagia
13. parametritis
14. uterocele
15. uterocervical
16. uterovesical
17. oophoritis
18. oophorosalpingitis
19. salpingocele
20. salpingography
21. oophoropexy *or* ovariopexy
22. hystero-oophorectomy
23. episiorrhaphy *or* perineorrhaphy
24. hysterosalpingo-oophorectomy
25. amniocentesis

Learning Activity 12-3
Diseases and Conditions

1. pyosalpinx
2. primipara
3. gestation
4. sterility
5. retroversion
6. endocervicitis
7. dystocia
8. atresia
9. Down syndrome
10. septicemia
11. dyspareunia
12. metrorrhagia
13. menarche
14. fibroids
15. oligomenorrhea
16. breech
17. eclampsia
18. choriocarcinoma
19. pathogen
20. primigravida

Learning Activity 12-4
Procedures, Pharmacology, and Abbreviations

1. Pap test
2. hysterosalpingography
3. amniocentesis
4. antifungals
5. colpocleisis
6. cordocentesis
7. cerclage
8. tubal ligation
9. OCPs
10. laparoscopy
11. episiotomy
12. PID
13. chorionic villus sampling
14. estrogens
15. oxytocins
16. cryosurgery
17. IUD
18. hysterectomy
19. lumpectomy
20. prostaglandins

Documenting Health-Care Activity 12-1 (Critical Thinking)

SOAP Note: Primary Herpes 1 Infection

1. Did the patient have any discharge? If so, describe it.

Yes, a brownish discharge

2. What type of discomfort did the patient experience around the vulvar area?

She was experiencing severe itching (pruritus), fever, and blisters.

3. Has the patient been taking her oral contraceptive pills regularly?

Yes

4. Where was the viral culture obtained?

Ulcerlike lesion on the right labia

5. Even though her partner used a condom, how do you think the patient became infected with herpes?

She probably got infected from the cold sore when having oral-genital sex.

Documenting Health-Care Activity 12-2 (Critical Thinking)

Postoperative Consultation: Menometrorrhagia

1. How many pregnancies did this woman have? How many viable infants did she deliver?

Two pregnancies and one viable birth

2. What is a therapeutic abortion?

An abortion performed when the pregnancy endangers the mother's mental or physical health or when the fetus has a known condition incompatible with life

3. Why did the physician propose to perform a hysterectomy?

The patient desired definitive treatment for menometrorrhagia and had declined palliative treatment.

4. What is a vaginal hysterectomy?

Surgical removal of the uterus through the vagina

5. Did the surgeon plan to remove one or both ovaries and fallopian tubes?

The surgeon planned to perform a bilateral (pertaining to two sides) salpingo-oophorectomy.

6. Why do you think the physician planned to use the laparoscope to perform the hysterectomy?

To permit visualization of the abdominal cavity as the the vagina

Documenting Health-Care Activity 12-3

Constructing Chart Notes

1. gravida 3, para 3
2. metrorrhagia
3. menorrhagia
4. dysmenorrhea
5. uterine fibroids
6. nullipara
7. menarche
8. menopause
9. mammography
10. needle biopsy

Chapter 13—Male Reproductive System

Learning Activity 13-1
Learning Activity 13-1
Medical Word Elements

1. spermicide
2. varicocele
3. scrotoplasty
4. prostatomegaly
5. anorchism
6. gonadectomy
7. genitourinary
8. epididymectomy
9. epispadias
10. hypogonadism
11. balanitis
12. androgen
13. perineorrhaphy
14. vasectomy
15. vesiculography

Learning Activity 13-2
Building Medical Words

1. orchiditis
2. orchidoptosis
3. balanorrhea
4. balanocele
5. spermatocyte
6. spermatoblast
7. spermatocele
8. prostatalgia *or* prostatodynia
9. prostatorrhea
10. prostatomegaly
11. prostatolith
12. hypospadias
13. hyperspadias
14. vesiculitis
15. vesiculography
16. gonadopathy
17. balanoplasty
18. vasectomy
19. scrotoplasty
20. perineorrhaphy

Learning Activity 13-3
Diseases and Conditions

1. leukorrhea
2. herpes
3. cryptorchidism
4. hypospadias
5. phimosis
6. varicocele
7. epispadias
8. testicular torsion
9. condyloma
10. anorchidism
11. balanitis
12. priapism
13. prostatitis
14. epididymitis
15. sterility
16. hydrocele
17. chlamydia
18. chancre
19. hypogonadism
20. gynecomastia

Learning Activity 13-4

Procedures, Pharmacology, and Abbreviations

1. semen analysis
2. androgens
3. scrotal
4. cryosurgery
5. vasectomy
6. urethroplasty
7. vasovasostomy
8. antiandrogens
9. TURP
10. PSA
11. antivirals
12. orchiopexy
13. circumcision
14. HPV
15. BPH

Documenting Health-Care Activity 13-1 (Critical Thinking)

Consultation Report: Benign Prostatic Hyperplasia

1. What is the reason for the present admission?

Left inguinal hernia repair and right ventral hernia repair

2. What occurred when the physician removed the Foley catheter?

The patient complained of dysuria, frequency, and a feeling of incomplete emptying with weak stream.

3. What did the patient's previous history indicate regarding these symptoms?

He had a history of hesitancy, weak stream, and voiding every 2 to 3 hours.

4. Why was it difficult to assess for bladder distention?

The incision lies over the bladder area.

5. Was there a definitive diagnosis identified in the impression?

The impression indicates questionable urine retention.

6. What procedure will the physician perform if the patient has difficulty voiding?

The doctor will catheterize the patient.

Documenting Health-Care Activity 13-2 (Critical Thinking)

Chart Note: Acute Epididymitis

1. What were the complaints of the patient?

Severe left-sided groin pain, scrotal pain, and urethritis with a clear urethral discharge

2. What procedure did the physician perform regarding the urethral discharge?

The discharge was expressed upon compression of the glans, and swabs were obtained for testing.

3. What information does the chart note provide regarding the left testicle?

Moderate pain and tenderness, which is alleviated with elevation of the testicles

4. How does the chart note describe the left epididymis?

Palpable, with significant induration and tenderness

5. What did the rectal examination reveal?

Mild prostatic hyperplasia and tenderness

Documenting Health-Care Activity 13-3

Constructing Chart Notes

1. leukorrhea
2. dysuria
3. pruritus
4. orchialgia
5. meatus

6. PSA
7. digital rectal examination
8. prostatomegaly
9. asymptomatic
10. benign

Chapter 14—Endocrine System

Learning Activity 14-1

Medical Word Elements

1. thymoma
2. pancreatitis
3. polydipsia
4. glycogenesis
5. endocrine
6. adipsia
7. exocrine
8. hyperglycemia

9. thymolysis
10. thyromegaly
11. adrenalitis
12. hypocalcemia
13. hyperkalemia
14. acromegaly
15. toxicologist

Learning Activity 14-2

Building Medical Words

1. hyperglycemia
2. hypoglycemia
3. glycogenesis
4. pancreatitis
5. pancreatolysis

6. pancreatopathy
7. thyroiditis
8. thyromegaly
9. parathyroidectomy
10. adrenalectomy

Learning Activity 14-3

Diseases and Conditions

1. acromegaly
2. myxedema
3. diuresis
4. hirsutism
5. cretinism
6. thyroid storm
7. Addison disease
8. exophthalmic goiter

9. hyperkalemia
10. pheochromocytoma
11. type 1
12. hyponatremia
13. glycosuria
14. Cushing syndrome
15. type 2

Learning Activity 14-4
Procedures, Pharmacology, and Abbreviations

1. FBS
2. RAIU
3. corticosteroids
4. growth hormone
5. thyroid scan
6. T_4
7. oral antidiabetics
8. GTT
9. antithyroids
10. transsphenoidal
11. T_3
12. TFT
13. exophthalmometry
14. total calcium test
15. insulin

Documenting Health-Care Activity 14-1 (Critical Thinking)
Consultation Note: Hyperparathyroidism

1. What is an adenoma?

Benign tumor of a gland

2. What does the physician suspect caused the patient's hyperparathyroidism?

Possible parathyroid adenoma

3. What type of laboratory findings revealed parathyroid disease?

Elevated calcium level

4. What is hypercalciuria?

Excessive amount of calcium in the urine

5. If the patient smoked 548 packs of cigarettes per year, how many packs did she smoke in an average day?

Approximately 1½ packs per day (365 days per year/548 packs = 1.5)

Documenting Health-Care Activity 14-2 (Critical Thinking)
SOAP Note: Diabetes Mellitus

1. How long has this patient been experiencing voracious eating?

For the past 10 days

2. Was the patient's obesity a result of overeating or a metabolic imbalance?

It was due to overeating

3. Why did the doctor experience difficulty in examining the patient's abdomen?

Because she was obese

4. Was the patient's blood glucose above or below normal on admission?

Above normal

5. What is the reference range for fasting blood glucose?

The reference range for fasting blood glucose is 70 to 110 mg/dL.

Documenting Health-Care Activity 14-3
Constructing Chart Notes

1. polydipsia
2. polyuria
3. polyphagia
4. hyperglycemia
5. glycosuria
6. lethargy
7. constipation
8. bradycardia
9. hypopnea
10. triiodothyronine and thyroxine

Chapter 15—Nervous System

Medical Word Elements

1. ventriculostomy
2. neuroma
3. radiculalgia
4. gangliectomy
5. narcolepsy
6. unilateral
7. meningitis
8. quadriplegia
9. hyperkinesia
10. myasthenia
11. cerebropathy
12. intrathecal
13. encephalocele
14. kinesiotherapy
15. myelorrhaphy

Building Medical Words

1. encephalopathy
2. encephalocele
3. encephalography
4. cerebropathy
5. cerebritis
6. craniocele
7. craniometer
8. neuralgia *or* neurodynia
9. neurologist
10. neurotripsy
11. myelocele
12. myeloplegia
13. psychotic *or* psychic
14. psychosis
15. bradykinesia
16. dyskinesia
17. hemiplegia
18. quadriplegia
19. dysphasia
20. aphasia
21. neurolysis
22. craniotomy
23. cranioplasty
24. neurorrhaphy
25. encephalotomy

Diseases and Conditions

1. hemiparesis
2. dementia
3. Alzheimer
4. bulimia
5. clonic
6. Guillain-Barré
7. ataxia
8. bipolar
9. epilepsies
10. ischemic
11. shingles
12. radiculopathy
13. paraplegia
14. poliomyelitis
15. convulsion
16. myelomeningocele
17. autism
18. Parkinson
19. multiple sclerosis
20. concussion

Learning Activity 15-4
Procedures, Pharmacology, and Abbreviations

1. NCV
2. psychostimulants
3. antipsychotics
4. general anesthetics
5. echoencephalography
6. cryosurgery
7. myelography
8. TIA
9. CSF analysis
10. electromyography
11. lumbar puncture
12. plasmapheresis
13. tractotomy
14. hypnotics
15. trephination

Documenting Health-Care Activity 15-1 (Critical Thinking)
Discharge Summary: Subarachnoid Hemorrhage

1. In what part of the head did the patient feel pain?

The occipital, the back part of the head

2. What imaging tests were performed, and what was the finding in each test?

CT scan showed blood in the cisterna subarachnoidalis and mild acute hydrocephalus. Cerebral angiogram and MRI showed no aneurysm.

3. What was the result of the lumbar puncture?

The results were consistent with recurrent subarachnoid hemorrhage.

4. What was the result of the repeat MRI?

It again showed no evidence of an aneurysm.

5. Regarding activity, what limitations were placed on the patient?

Avoid activity that could raise the pressure in the head, and perform no activity more vigorous than walking.

Documenting Health-Care Activity 15-2 (Critical Thinking)
Consultation Report: Acute-Onset Paraplegia

1. What was the original cause of the patient's current problems, and what treatments were provided?

Fall at work about 15 to 20 years ago and four subsequent lumbar surgeries

2. Why was the patient admitted to the hospital?

Pain management

3. What medications did the patient receive, and why was each given?

Clonidine for hypertension and methadone for pain

4. What was the cause of bladder retention?

Administration of clonidine

5. What occurred after the catheter was removed?

Subacute onset of paresis, paresthesias, and pain in the legs, approximately 2½ to 3 hours later

6. What three disorders were listed in the differential diagnosis?

Subarachnoid hemorrhage, epidural abscess, and transverse myelitis

Constructing Chart Notes

1. neuralgia
2. sciatica
3. herniation
4. osteophyte
5. neuropathy

6. tremor
7. bradyphasia
8. bradykinesia
9. dysphagia
10. Parkinson disease

Chapter 16—Special Senses

Medical Word Elements

1. amblyopia
2. phacocele
3. diplopia
4. blepharoptosis
5. goniometer
6. intraocular
7. keratotomy
8. otorrhea

9. audiometer
10. anacusia
11. labyrinthitis
12. otosclerosis
13. mastoiditis
14. myringoplasty
15. presbyacusia

Building Medical Words

1. ophthalmoplegia *or* ophthalmoparalysis
2. ophthalmology
3. pupilloscopy
4. keratomalacia
5. keratometer
6. scleritis
7. scleromalacia
8. iridoplegia *or* iridoparalysis
9. iridocele
10. retinopathy
11. retinitis
12. blepharoplegia
13. blepharoptosis

14. otopyorrhea
15. audiometer
16. myringotome
17. amblyopia
18. hyperopia
19. anacusis
20. hyperacusis
21. stapedectomy
22. labyrinthotomy
23. mastoidectomy
24. myringoplasty *or* tympanoplasty
25. keratotomy

Diseases and Conditions

1. cataract
2. achromatopsia
3. nyctalopia
4. presbycusis
5. anacusis
6. otitis externa
7. otosclerosis
8. otitis media
9. otopyorrhea
10. epiphora
11. hordeolum
12. otoencephalitis
13. neovascular
14. vertigo
15. exotropia
16. drusen
17. chalazion
18. amblyopia
19. retinoblastoma
20. tinnitus

Procedures, Pharmacology, and Abbreviations

1. caloric stimulation
2. ophthalmoscopy
3. cochlear implant
4. fluorescein angiography
5. otoplasty
6. mydriatics
7. tonometry
8. visual acuity
9. evisceration
10. antiemetics
11. wax emulsifiers
12. enucleation
13. ST
14. ophthalmic decongestants
15. XT
16. gonioscopy
17. otoscopy
18. audiometry
19. PE
20. otic analgesics

Operative Report: Retained Foreign Bodies

1. Did the surgery involve one or both ears?

It was bilateral, involving both ears.

2. What was the nature of the foreign body in the patient's ears?

Retained tympanostomy tubes

3. What ear structure was involved?

Eardrum, or tympanum

4. What instrument was used to locate the tubes?

Operating microscope

5. What was the material in which the tubes were embedded?

Earwax, or cerumen

6. What occurred when the cerumen and tubes were removed?

It resulted in a large perforation.

7. How was the perforation treated?

The edges were freshened sharply with a pick, and a paper patch was applied.

Documenting Health-Care Activity 16-2 (Critical Thinking)

Operative Report: Phacoemulsification and Lens Implant

1. What technique was used to destroy the cataract?

Phacoemulsification, an ultrasound technique

2. In what portion of the eye was the implant placed?

Posterior chamber

3. What anesthetics were used for surgery?

Intravenous and retrobulbar block

4. What was the function of the blepharostat?

To separate the eyelids during surgery

5. What is a keratome?

A knife used to incise the cornea

6. Where was the implant inserted?

In the capsular bag

Documenting Health-Care Activity 16-3

Constructing Chart Notes

1. asymptomatic
2. tonometry
3. antiglaucoma agents
4. hyperopia
5. gonioscopy
6. pediatrician
7. otalgia
8. pharyngalgia
9. tinnitus
10. otorrhea

Common Abbreviations and Symbols

Common Abbreviations

This table lists common abbreviations used in health care and related fields,* along with their meanings.

Abbreviation	Meaning	Abbreviation	Meaning
A		AOM	acute otitis media
AAA	abdominal aortic aneurysm	AP	anteroposterior
A&P	auscultation and percussion	APC	antigen-presenting cell
A, B, AB, O	blood types in ABO blood group	APTT	activated partial thromboplastin time
AB, Ab, ab	antibody; abortion	ARDS	acute respiratory distress syndrome
ABC	aspiration biopsy cytology	ARF	acute renal failure
ABG	arterial blood gas(es)	ARMD, AMD	age-related macular degeneration
AC	air conduction	AS	aortic stenosis
Acc	accommodation	ASD	atrial septal defect
ACE	angiotensin-converting enzyme (inhibitor)	ASHD	arteriosclerotic heart disease
AChR	acetylcholine receptor	AST	angiotensin sensitivity test; aspartate aminotransferase
ACL	anterior cruciate ligament	Ast	astigmatism
ACS	acute coronary syndrome	ATN	acute tubular necrosis
ACTH	adrenocorticotropic hormone	AV	atrioventricular; arteriovenous
AD	Alzheimer disease	**B**	
ADH	antidiuretic hormone (vasopressin)	Ba	barium
ADHD	attention deficit-hyperactivity disorder	baso	basophil (type of white blood cell)
ADT	androgen deprivation therapy	BBB	bundle branch block
ad lib.	as desired	BC	bone conduction
ADLs	activities of daily living	BCC	basal cell carcinoma
AE	above the elbow	BE	barium enema; below the elbow
AED	automatic external defibrillator; automatic external device	BEAM	brain electrical activity mapping
AFB	acid-fast bacillus (TB organism)	BK	below the knee
AFib	atrial fibrillation	BKA	below-knee amputation
AGN	acute glomerulonephritis	BM	bowel movement
AI	artificial insemination	BMD	bone mineral density
AICD	automatic implantable cardioverter defibrillator	BMI	body mass index
AIDS	acquired immunodeficiency syndrome, acquired immune deficiency syndrome	BMR	basal metabolic rate
		BMT	bone marrow transplant
		BNO	bladder neck obstruction
		BP, B/P	blood pressure
		BPH	benign prostatic hyperplasia; benign prostatic hypertrophy
AK	above the knee	BS	blood sugar
ALL	acute lymphocytic leukemia	BSE	breast self-examination
ALS	amyotrophic lateral sclerosis	BUN	blood urea nitrogen
ALT	alanine aminotransferase	Bx, bx	biopsy
AM, a.m.	in the morning or before noon	**C**	
AML	acute myelogenous leukemia	C&S	culture and sensitivity
ANA	antinuclear antibody	c/o	complains of, complaints
ANS	autonomic nervous system	C1, C2, and so on	first cervical vertebra, second cervical vertebra, and so on
		CA	cancer; chronological age; cardiac arrest
		Ca	calcium; cancer
		CABG	coronary artery bypass graft

Abbreviation	Meaning	Abbreviation	Meaning
CAD	coronary artery disease	CTS	carpal tunnel syndrome
CAH	chronic active hepatitis; congenital adrenal hyperplasia	CV	cardiovascular
		CVA	cerebrovascular accident
		CVD	cardiovascular disease
CAT	computed axial tomography	CVS	chorionic villus sampling
Cath	catheterization; catheter	CWP	childbirth without pain
CBC	complete blood count	CXR	chest x-ray, chest radiograph
CC	cardiac catheterization; chief complaint	cysto	cystoscopy

D

Abbreviation	Meaning	Abbreviation	Meaning
CCU	coronary care unit	D	diopter (lens strength)
CDH	congenital dislocation of the hip	D&C	dilation and curettage
		Decub.	decubitus (lying down)
CF	cystic fibrosis	D.O.	Doctor of Osteopathy
CHD	coronary heart disease	D.P.M.	Doctor of Podiatric Medicine
chemo	chemotherapy	Derm	dermatology
CHF	congestive heart failure	DES	diffuse esophageal spasm; drug-eluting stent
Chol	cholesterol		
CIS	carcinoma in situ	DEXA, DXA	dual energy x-ray absorptiometry
CK	creatine kinase (cardiac enzyme); conductive keratoplasty	DI	diabetes insipidus; diagnostic imaging
		DIC	disseminated intravascular coagulation
CLL	chronic lymphocytic leukemia	diff	differential count (white blood cells)
		DJD	degenerative joint disease
cm	centimeter (1/100 of a meter)	DKA	diabetic ketoacidosis
CML	chronic myelogenous leukemia	DM	diabetes mellitus
		DMARDs	disease-modifying antirheumatic drugs
CNS	central nervous system	DNA	deoxyribonucleic acid
CO	coccygeal nerves	DOE	dyspnea on exertion
CO_2	carbon dioxide	DPI	dry powder inhaler
COLD	chronic obstructive lung disease	DPT	diphtheria, pertussis, tetanus
		DRE	digital rectal examination
COPD	chronic obstructive pulmonary disease	DSA	digital subtraction angiography
		DTR	deep tendon reflex
CP	cerebral palsy	DUB	dysfunctional uterine bleeding
CPAP	continuous positive airway pressure	DVT	deep vein thrombosis; deep venous thrombosis
CPD	cephalopelvic disproportion	Dx	diagnosis

E

Abbreviation	Meaning	Abbreviation	Meaning
CPK	creatine phosphokinase (cardiac enzyme released into the bloodstream after a heart attack)	EBR	external beam radiation
		EBRT	external beam radiotherapy
		EBT	external beam therapy
CPR	cardiopulmonary resuscitation	EBV	Epstein-Barr virus
		ECCE	extracapsular cataract extraction
CRF	chronic renal failure	ECG, EKG	electrocardiogram; electrocardiography
CRRT	continuous renal replacement therapy	ECHO	echocardiogram; echocardiography; echoencephalogram; echoencephalography
C-section, CS	cesarean section		
CSF	cerebrospinal fluid	ECRB	extensor carpi radialis brevis (muscle or tendon)
CT	computed tomography		
CTA	computed tomography angiography	ED	erectile dysfunction; emergency department

(continued)

Abbreviation	Meaning	Abbreviation	Meaning
EEG	electroencephalography	HBV	hepatitis B virus
EF	ejection fraction	HCG	human chorionic gonadotropin
EGD	esophagogastroduodenoscopy	HCl	hydrochloric acid
ELT	endovenous laser ablation; endoluminal laser ablation	HCT, Hct	hematocrit
		HCV	hepatitis C virus
Em	emmetropia	HD	hemodialysis; hip disarticulation; hearing distance
EMG	electromyography		
ENG	electronystagmography	HDL	high-density lipoprotein
ENT	ears, nose, and throat	HDN	hemolytic disease of the newborn
EOM	extraocular movement	HDV	hepatitis D virus
eos	eosinophil (type of white blood cell)	HEV	hepatitis E virus
		HF	heart failure
EPS	electrophysiology studies	Hg	mercury
ESR	erythrocyte sedimentation rate	HHV-8	human herpes virus 8
ESRD	end-stage renal disease	HIV	human immunodeficiency virus
ESWL	extracorporeal shock-wave lithotripsy	H_2O	water
		HMD	hyaline membrane disease
ETT	exercise tolerance test	HNP	herniated nucleus pulposus (herniated disk)
EUS	endoscopic ultrasonography		
F		HP	hemipelvectomy
FBS	fasting blood sugar	HPV	human papillomavirus
FECG, FEKG	fetal electrocardiogram	HRT	hormone replacement therapy
FH	family history	HSG	hysterosalpingography
FHR	fetal heart rate	HSV	herpes simplex virus
FHT	fetal heart tone	HSV-2	herpes simplex virus type 2
FS	frozen section	HTN	hypertension
FSH	follicle-stimulating hormone	Hx	history
FTND	full-term normal delivery	**I, J**	
FVC	forced vital capacity	I&D	incision and drainage
Fx	fracture	IBD	irritable bowel disease
G		IBS	irritable bowel syndrome
G	gravida (pregnant)	IC	interstitial cystitis
GB	gallbladder	ICD	implantable cardioverter-defibrillator
GBP	gastric bypass	ICP	intracranial pressure
GBS	gallbladder series (x-ray studies)	ICU	intensive care unit
		ID	intradermal
GC	gonococcus (Neisseria gonorrhoeae)	IDDM	insulin-dependent diabetes mellitus
		Igs	immunoglobulins
GER	gastroesophageal reflux	IM	intramuscular; infectious mononucleosis
GERD	gastroesophageal reflux disease	IMP	impression (synonymous with diagnosis)
		INR	international normalized ratio
GH	growth hormone	IVP	intravenous pyelogram; intravenous pyelography
GI	gastrointestinal		
GTT	glucose tolerance test	IOL	intraocular lens
GU	genitourinary	IOP	intraocular pressure
GVHD	graft-versus-host disease	IPPB	intermittent positive-pressure breathing
GVHR	graft-versus-host reaction	IRDS	infant respiratory distress syndrome
GYN	gynecology	IS	intracostal space
H		IUD	intrauterine device
HAV	hepatitis A virus	IUGR	intrauterine growth rate; intrauterine growth retardation
Hb, Hgb	hemoglobin	IV	intravenous

Abbreviation	Meaning	Abbreviation	Meaning
IVC	intravenous cholangiogram; intravenous cholangiography	mix astig	mixed astigmatism
		mL	milliliter (1/1,000 of a liter)
IVF	in vitro fertilization	mm	millimeter (1/1,000 of a meter)
IVF-ET	in vitro fertilization and embryo transfer	mm Hg	millimeters of mercury
IVP	intravenous pyelogram; intravenous pyelography	MNL	mononuclear leukocytes
		MPI	myocardial perfusion imaging
K		MR	mitral regurgitation
K	potassium (an electrolyte)	MRA	magnetic resonance angiogram; magnetic resonance angiography
KD	knee disarticulation	MRCP	magnetic resonance cholangiopancreatography
KS	Kaposi sarcoma		
KUB	kidney, ureter, bladder	MRI	magnetic resonance imaging
L		MS	musculoskeletal; multiple sclerosis; mental status; mitral stenosis
L1, L2, and so on	first lumbar vertebra, second lumbar vertebra, and so on	MSH	melanocyte-stimulating hormone
LA	left atrium	MUGA	multiple-gated acquisition (scan)
LASIK	laser-assisted in situ keratomileusis	MVP	mitral valve prolapse
		myop	myopia (nearsightedness)
LAT, lat	lateral	**N**	
LBBB	left bundle branch block	Na	sodium (an electrolyte)
LBW	low birth weight	NB	newborn
LD	lactate dehydrogenase; lactic acid dehydrogenase (cardiac enzyme)	NCV	nerve conduction velocity
		NG	nasogastric
		NIDDM	non–insulin-dependent diabetes mellitus
LDL	low-density lipoprotein	NIHL	noise-induced hearing loss
LES	lower esophageal sphincter	NK cell	natural killer cell
LFT	liver function test	NMT	nebulized mist treatment
LH	luteinizing hormone	NPH	neutral protamine Hagedorn (insulin)
LLQ	left lower quadrant	NSAIDs	nonsteroidal antiinflammatory drugs
LMP	last menstrual period	NSR	normal sinus rhythm
LOC	loss of consciousness	**O**	
LP	lumbar puncture	O_2	oxygen
LPR	laryngopharyngeal reflux	OB	obstetrics
LS	lumbosacral spine	OCG	oral cholecystography
LSO	left salpingo-oophorectomy	OCPs	oral contraceptive pills
lt	left	OD	overdose
LUQ	left upper quadrant	O.D.	Doctor of Optometry
LV	left ventricle	OM	otitis media
lymphos	lymphocytes	OP	outpatient; operative procedure
M		ORTH, ortho	orthopedics
M.D., MD	Doctor of Medicine	OSA	obstructive sleep apnea
MDI	metered-dose inhaler	**P**	
MEG	magnetoencephalography	P	phosphorus; pulse
MG	myasthenia gravis	p̄	after
mg	milligram (1/1,000 of a gram)	PA	posteroanterior; pernicious anemia; pulmonary artery
mg/dl, mg/dL	milligram per deciliter		
MI	myocardial infarction	PAC	premature atrial contraction

(continued)

Abbreviation	Meaning	Abbreviation	Meaning
PAD	peripheral artery disease	PTCA	percutaneous transluminal coronary angioplasty
Pap	Papanicolaou (test)	PTH	parathyroid hormone (also called parathormone)
para 1, 2, 3, and so on	unipara, bipara, tripara, and so on (number of viable births)	PTT	partial thromboplastin time
PAT	paroxysmal atrial tachycardia	PUD	peptic ulcer disease
PBI	protein-bound iodine	PVC	premature ventricular contraction
PCL	posterior cruciate ligament	PVD	peripheral vascular disease
PCNL	percutaneous nephrolithotomy	**Q**	
PCO$_2$	partial pressure of carbon dioxide	qEEG	quantitative electroencephalography
PCP	*Pneumocystis* pneumonia; primary care physician	**R**	
PCTA	percutaneous transluminal coronary angioplasty	RA	right atrium; rheumatoid arthritis
PCV	packed cell volume	RAI	radioactive iodine
PE	physical examination; pulmonary embolism; pressure-equalizing (tube)	RAIU	radioactive iodine uptake
		RBC, rbc	red blood cell
		RD	respiratory distress
		RDS	respiratory distress syndrome
PERRLA	pupils equal, round, and reactive to light and accommodation	RF	rheumatoid factor; radio frequency
		RGB	Roux-en-Y gastric bypass
		RHD	rheumatic heart disease
		RK	radial keratotomy
PET	positron emission tomography	RLQ	right lower quadrant
		R/O	rule out
PFT	pulmonary function tests	ROM	range of motion
PGH	pituitary growth hormone	RP	retrograde pyelogram; retrograde pyelography
pH	symbol for degree of acidity or alkalinity	RSO	right salpingo-oophorectomy
PID	pelvic inflammatory disease	rt	right
PIH	pregnancy-induced hypertension	RUQ	right upper quadrant
		RV	residual volume; right ventricle
PKD	polycystic kidney disease	**S**	
PMH	past medical history	S1, S2, and so on	first sacral vertebra, second sacral vertebra, and so on
PMI	point of maximum impulse	SA, S-A	sinoatrial
PMP	previous menstrual period	SaO$_2$	arterial oxygen saturation
PMN	polymorphonuclear	SD	shoulder disarticulation
PMNL, poly	polymorphonuclear leukocyte	segs	segmented neutrophils
PMS	premenstrual syndrome	SICS	small incision cataract surgery
PND	paroxysmal nocturnal dyspnea	SIDS	sudden infant death syndrome
PNS	peripheral nervous system	SLE	systemic lupus erythematosus; slit-lamp examination
PO$_2$	partial pressure of oxygen		
post	posterior	SNS	sympathetic nervous system
PPD	purified protein derivative	SOB	shortness of breath
PPV	pars plana vitrectomy	sono	sonogram
PRL	prolactin	SPECT	single-photon emission computed tomography
PSA	prostate-specific antigen		
PT	prothrombin time, physical therapy	sp. gr.	specific gravity
		ST	esotropia
pt	patient	stat., STAT	immediately

Abbreviation	Meaning	Abbreviation	Meaning
STD	sexually transmitted disease	TVH	total vaginal hysterectomy
STI	sexually transmitted infection	Tx	treatment
Sx	symptom	**U**	
T		U&L, U/L	upper and lower
T&A	tonsillectomy and adenoidectomy	UA	urinalysis
T1, T2, and so on	first thoracic vertebra, second thoracic vertebra, and so on	UC	uterine contractions
		UGI	upper gastrointestinal
T_3	triiodothyronine (thyroid hormone)	UGIS	upper gastrointestinal series
		ung	ointment
T_4	thyroxine (thyroid hormone)	UPP	uvulopalatopharyngoplasty
TAH	total abdominal hysterectomy	URI	upper respiratory infection
		US	ultrasound; ultrasonography
TB	tuberculosis	UTI	urinary tract infection
TFT	thyroid function test	**V**	
THA	total hip arthroplasty	VA	visual acuity
THR	total hip replacement	VC	vital capacity
ther	therapy	VCUG	voiding cystourethrography
TIA	transient ischemic attack	VD	venereal disease
TKA	total knee arthroplasty	VF	visual field
TKR	total knee replacement	VSD	ventricular septal defect
tPA	tissue plasminogen activator	VT	ventricular tachycardia
TPR	temperature, pulse, and respiration	VUR	vesicoureteral reflux
		W	
TRAM	transverse rectus abdominis muscle (flap)	WBC, wbc	white blood cell
		WD	well developed
TRUS	transrectal ultrasound	WN	well nourished
TSE	testicular self-examination	WNL	within normal limits
TSH	thyroid-stimulating hormone	**X, Y, Z**	
TURBT	transurethral resection of bladder tumor	XP, XDP	xeroderma pigmentosum
		XT	exotropia
TURP	transurethral resection of the prostate		

*For a listing of discontinued, or "Do Not Use," abbreviations, see Appendix H, page 684.

Symbols

This table lists common symbols used in health care and related fields, along with their meanings.

Symbol	Meaning	Symbol	Meaning
@	at	Ø	no
aa	of each	#	number; following a number, pounds
'	foot	÷	divided by
"	inch	/	divided by
Δ	change; heat	×	multiplied by; magnification
℞	prescription, treatment, therapy	=	equals
→	to, in the direction of	≈	approximately equal
↑	increase(d), up	°	degree
↓	decrease(d), down	%	percent
+	plus, positive	♀	female
−	minus, negative	♂	male
±	plus or minus; either positive or negative; indefinite		

Glossary of Medical Word Elements

Medical Word Elements

Element	Meaning	Element	Meaning
A		**-arche**	beginning
a-	without, not	arteri/o	artery
-a	noun ending	arteriol/o	arteriole
ab-	from, away from	arthr/o	joint
abdomin/o	abdomen	-ary	pertaining to
abort/o	to miscarry	asbest/o	asbestos
-ac	pertaining to	-asthenia	weakness, debility
acid/o	acid	astr/o	star
acous/o	hearing	-ate	having the form of, possessing
acr/o	extremity	atel/o	incomplete; imperfect
acromi/o	acromion (projection of the scapula)	ather/o	fatty plaque
-acusia	hearing	-ation	process (of)
-acusis	hearing	atri/o	atrium
-ad	toward	audi/o	hearing
ad-	toward	audit/o	hearing
aden/o	gland	aur/o	ear
adenoid/o	adenoids	auricul/o	ear
adip/o	fat	auto-	self, own
adren/o	adrenal glands	ax/o	axis, axon
adrenal/o	adrenal glands	azot/o	nitrogenous compounds
aer/o	air	**B**	
af-	toward	bacteri/o	bacteria (singular, bacterium)
agglutin/o	clumping, gluing	balan/o	glans penis
agora-	marketplace	bas/o	base (alkaline, opposite of acid)
-al	pertaining to	bi-	two
albin/o	white	bil/i	bile, gall
albumin/o	albumin (protein)	bi/o	life
-algesia	pain	-blast	embryonic cell
-algia	pain	blast/o	embryonic cell
allo-	other, differing from the normal	blephar/o	eyelid
alveol/o	alveolus; air sac	brachi/o	arm
ambly/o	dull, dim	brachy-	short
amni/o	amnion (amniotic sac)	brady-	slow
an-	without, not	bronch/o	bronchus (plural, bronchi)
an/o	anus	bronchi/o	bronchus (plural, bronchi)
ana-	against; up; back	bronchiol/o	bronchiole
andr/o	male	bucc/o	cheek
aneurysm/o	aneurysm (widened blood vessel)	**C**	
angi/o	vessel (usually blood or lymph)	calc/o	calcium
angin/o	choking pain	calcane/o	calcaneum (heel bone)
aniso-	unequal, dissimilar	-capnia	carbon dioxide (CO_2)
ankyl/o	stiffness; bent, crooked	carcin/o	cancer
ante-	before, in front of	cardi/o	heart
anter/o	anterior, front	-cardia	heart condition
anthrac/o	coal, coal dust	carp/o	carpus (wrist bones)
anti-	against	cata-	down
aort/o	aorta	caud/o	tail
append/o	appendix	cauter/o	heat, burn
appendic/o	appendix	cec/o	cecum
aque/o	water		
-ar	pertaining to		

Medical Word Elements—cont'd

Element	Meaning	Element	Meaning
-cele	hernia, swelling	crin/o	secrete
-centesis	surgical puncture	-crine	secrete
cephal/o	head	cruci/o	cross
-ceps	head	cry/o	cold
-ception	conceiving	crypt/o	hidden
cerebell/o	cerebellum	culd/o	cul-de-sac
cerebr/o	cerebrum	-cusia	hearing
cervic/o	neck; cervix uteri (neck of uterus)	-cusis	hearing
		cutane/o	skin
chalic/o	limestone	cyan/o	blue
cheil/o	lip	cycl/o	ciliary body of the eye; circular; cycle
chem/o	chemical; drug	-cyesis	pregnancy
chlor/o	green	cyst/o	bladder
chol/e	bile, gall	cyt/o	cell
cholangi/o	bile vessel	-cyte	cell
cholecyst/o	gallbladder		
choledoch/o	bile duct	**D**	
chondr/o	cartilage		
chori/o	chorion	dacry/o	tear; lacrimal apparatus (duct, sac, or gland)
choroid/o	choroid		
chrom/o	color	dacryocyst/o	lacrimal sac
chromat/o	color	dactyl/o	fingers; toes
-cide	killing	de-	cessation
circum-	around	dendr/o	tree
cirrh/o	yellow	dent/o	teeth
-cision	a cutting	derm/o	skin
-clasia	to break; surgical fracture	-derma	skin
-clasis	to break; surgical fracture	dermat/o	skin
-clast	to break; surgical fracture	-desis	binding, fixation (of a bone or joint)
clavicul/o	clavicle (collar bone)	di-	double
-clysis	irrigation, washing	dia-	through, across
coccyg/o	coccyx (tailbone)	dipl-	double
cochle/o	cochlea	dipl/o	double
col/o	colon	dips/o	thirst
colon/o	colon	-dipsia	thirst
colp/o	vagina	dist/o	far, farthest
condyl/o	condyle	dors/o	back (of the body)
coni/o	dust	duct/o	to lead; carry
conjunctiv/o	conjunctiva	-duction	act of leading, bringing, conducting
-continence	to hold back	duoden/o	duodenum (first part of the small intestine)
contra-	against, opposite		
cor/o	pupil	dur/o	dura mater; hard
core/o	pupil	-dynia	pain
corne/o	cornea	dys-	bad; painful; difficult
coron/o	heart		
corp/o	body	**E**	
corpor/o	body		
cortic/o	cortex	-eal	pertaining to
cost/o	ribs	ec-	out, out from
crani/o	cranium (skull)	echo-	repeated sound
		-ectasis	dilation, expansion
		ecto-	outside, outward

(continued)

Medical Word Elements—cont'd

Element	Meaning	Element	Meaning
-ectomy	excision, removal	-gen	forming, producing, origin
-edema	swelling	gen/o	forming, producing, origin
ef-	away from	-genesis	forming, producing, origin
electr/o	electricity	genit/o	genitalia
-ema	state of; condition	gest/o	pregnancy
embol/o	embolus (plug)	gingiv/o	gum(s)
-emesis	vomiting	glauc/o	gray
-emia	blood condition	gli/o	glue; neuroglial tissue
emphys/o	to inflate	-glia	glue; neuroglial tissue
en-	in, within	-globin	protein
encephal/o	brain	glomerul/o	glomerulus
end-	in, within	gloss/o	tongue
endo-	in, within	glott/o	glottis
enter/o	intestine (usually small intestine)	gluc/o	sugar, sweetness
eosin/o	dawn (rose colored)	glucos/o	sugar, sweetness
epi-	above, upon	glyc/o	sugar, sweetness
epididym/o	epididymis	glycos/o	sugar, sweetness
epiglott/o	epiglottis	gnos/o	knowing
episi/o	vulva	-gnosis	knowing
erythem/o	red	gonad/o	gonads, sex glands
erythemat/o	red	goni/o	angle
erythr/o	red	gon/o	seed (ovum or spermatozoon)
eschar/o	scab	-grade	to go
-esis	condition	-graft	transplantation
eso-	inward	-gram	record, writing
esophag/o	esophagus	granul/o	granule
esthes/o	feeling	-graph	instrument for recording
-esthesia	feeling	-graphy	process of recording
eti/o	cause	-gravida	pregnant woman
eu-	good; normal	gyn/o	woman, female
ex-	out, out from	gynec/o	woman, female
exo-	outside, outward		
extra-	outside	**H**	
		hallucin/o	hallucination
F		hedon/o	pleasure
		hem/o	blood
faci/o	face	hemangi/o	blood vessel
fasci/o	band, fascia (fibrous membrane supporting and separating muscles)	hemat/o	blood
		hemi-	one half
femor/o	femur (thigh bone)	hepat/o	liver
-ferent	to carry	hetero-	different
fibr/o	fiber, fibrous tissue	hidr/o	sweat
fibul/o	fibula (smaller bone of the lower leg)	hist/o	tissue
		histi/o	tissue
fluor/o	luminous, fluorescence	home/o	same, alike
		homeo-	same, alike
G		homo-	same
		humer/o	humerus (upper arm bone)
galact/o	milk	hydr/o	water
gangli/o	ganglion (knot or knotlike mass)		
gastr/o	stomach		

Medical Word Elements—cont'd

Element	Meaning	Element	Meaning
hyp-	under, below, deficient	-ive	pertaining to
hyper-	excessive, above normal	-ization	process (of)
hyp/o	under, below, deficient	**J, K**	
hypn/o	sleep		
hypo-	under, below, deficient	jaund/o	yellow
hyster/o	uterus (womb)	jejun/o	jejunum (second part of the small intestine)
I		kal/i	potassium (an electrolyte)
-ia	condition	kary/o	nucleus
-iac	pertaining to	kerat/o	horny tissue; hard; cornea
-iasis	abnormal condition (produced by something specified)	kern/o	kernel (nucleus)
		ket/o	ketone bodies (acids and acetones)
iatr/o	physician; treatment	keton/o	ketone bodies (acids and acetones)
-iatry	physician; treatment	kinesi/o	movement
-ic	pertaining to	-kinesia	movement
-ical	pertaining to	kinet/o	movement
-ice	noun ending	klept/o	to steal
ichthy/o	dry, scaly	kyph/o	humpback
-ician	specialist	**L**	
-icle	small, minute		
-icterus	jaundice	labi/o	lip
idi/o	unknown, peculiar	labyrinth/o	labyrinth (inner ear)
-ile	pertaining to	lacrim/o	tear; lacrimal apparatus (duct, sac, or gland)
ile/o	ileum (third part of the small intestine)	lact/o	milk
		-lalia	speech, babble
ili/o	ilium (lateral, flaring portion of the hip bone)	lamin/o	lamina (part of the vertebral arch)
		lapar/o	abdomen
im-	not	laryng/o	larynx (voice box)
immun/o	immune, immunity, safe	later/o	side, to one side
in-	in, not	lei/o	smooth
-ine	pertaining to	leiomy/o	smooth (visceral) muscle
infer/o	lower, below	-lepsy	seizure
infra-	below, under	lept/o	thin, slender
inguin/o	groin	leuk/o	white
insulin/o	insulin	lex/o	word, phrase
inter-	between	lingu/o	tongue
intra-	in, within	lip/o	fat
-ion	the act of	lipid/o	fat
-ior	pertaining to	-listhesis	slipping
irid/o	iris	-lith	stone, calculus
-is	noun ending	lith/o	stone, calculus
isch/o	to hold back; block	lob/o	lobe
ischi/o	ischium (lower portion of the hip bone)	log/o	study of
		-logist	specialist in the study of
-ism	condition	-logy	study of
iso-	same, equal	lord/o	curve, swayback
-ist	specialist	-lucent	to shine; clear
-isy	state of; condition	lumb/o	loins (lower back)
-itic	pertaining to	lymph/o	lymph
-itis	inflammation		

(continued)

Medical Word Elements—cont'd

Element	Meaning	Element	Meaning
lymphaden/o	lymph gland (node)	myring/o	tympanic membrane (eardrum)
lymphangi/o	lymph vessel	myx/o	mucus
-lysis	separation; destruction; loosening		
M		**N**	
macro-	large	narc/o	stupor; numbness; sleep
mal-	bad	nas/o	nose
-malacia	softening	nat/o	birth
mamm/o	breast	natr/o	sodium (an electrolyte)
-mania	state of mental disorder, frenzy	necr/o	death, necrosis
mast/o	breast	neo-	new
mastoid/o	mastoid process	nephr/o	kidney
maxill/o	maxilla (upper jaw bone)	neur/o	nerve
meat/o	opening, meatus	neutr/o	neutral; neither
medi-	middle	nid/o	nest
medi/o	middle	noct/o	night
mediastin/o	mediastinum	nucle/o	nucleus
medull/o	medulla	nulli-	none
mega-	enlargement	nyctal/o	night
megal/o	enlargement		
-megaly	enlargement	**O**	
melan/o	black	obstetr/o	pregnancy; childbirth
men/o	menses, menstruation	ocul/o	eye
mening/o	meninges (membranes covering the brain and spinal cord)	odont/o	teeth
		-oid	resembling
meningi/o	meninges (membranes covering the brain and spinal cord)	-ole	small, minute
		olig/o	scanty
menstr/o	monthly discharge of blood	-oma	tumor
ment/o	mind	omphal/o	navel (umbilicus)
meso-	middle	onc/o	tumor
meta-	change, beyond	onych/o	nail
metacarp/o	metacarpus (hand bones)	oophor/o	ovary
metatars/o	metatarsus (foot bones)	-opaque	obscure
-meter	instrument for measuring	ophthalm/o	eye
metr/o	uterus (womb); measure	-opia	vision
metri/o	uterus (womb)	-opsia	vision
-metry	act of measuring	-opsy	view of
micr/o	small	opt/o	eye, vision
micro-	small	optic/o	eye, vision
mono-	one	or/o	mouth
morph/o	form, shape, structure	orch/o	testis (plural, testes)
muc/o	mucus	orchi/o	testis (plural, testes)
multi-	many, much	orchid/o	testis (plural, testes)
muscul/o	muscle	-orexia	appetite
mut/a	genetic change	orth/o	straight
my/o	muscle	-ory	pertaining to
myc/o	fungus (plural, fungi)	-ose	pertaining to; sugar
mydr/o	widen, enlarge	-osis	abnormal condition; increase (used primarily with blood cells)
myel/o	bone marrow; spinal cord	-osmia	smell
myos/o	muscle	oste/o	bone

Medical Word Elements—cont'd

Element	Meaning	Element	Meaning
ot/o	ear	-phobia	fear
-ous	pertaining to	-phonia	voice
ovari/o	ovary	-phoresis	carrying, transmission
ox/i	oxygen	-phoria	feeling (mental state)
ox/o	oxygen	phot/o	light
-oxia	oxygen	phren/o	diaphragm; mind
		-phylaxis	protection
P		-physis	growth
pachy-	thick	pil/o	hair
palat/o	palate (roof of the mouth)	pituitar/o	pituitary gland
pan-	all	-plakia	plaque
pancreat/o	pancreas	plas/o	formation, growth
-para	to bear (offspring)	-plasia	formation, growth
para-	near, beside; beyond	-plasm	formation, growth
parathyroid/o	parathyroid glands	-plasty	surgical repair
-paresis	partial paralysis	-plegia	paralysis
patell/o	patella (kneecap)	pleur/o	pleura
path/o	disease	-plexy	stroke
-pathy	disease	-pnea	breathing
pector/o	chest	pneum/o	air; lung
ped/i	foot; child	pneumon/o	air; lung
ped/o	foot; child	pod/o	foot
pedicul/o	lice	-poiesis	formation, production
pelv/i	pelvis	poikil/o	varied, irregular
pelv/o	pelvis	poli/o	gray; gray matter (of the brain or spinal cord)
pen/o	penis		
-penia	decrease, deficiency	poly-	many, much
-pepsia	digestion	polyp/o	small growth
per-	through	-porosis	porous
peri-	around	post-	after, behind
perine/o	perineum (area between the scrotum [or vulva in the female] and anus)	poster/o	back (of the body), behind, posterior
		-potence	power
		-prandial	meal
peritone/o	peritoneum	pre-	before, in front of
-pexy	fixation (of an organ)	presby/o	old age
phac/o	lens	primi-	first
phag/o	swallowing, eating	pro-	before, in front of
-phage	swallowing, eating	proct/o	anus, rectum
-phagia	swallowing, eating	prostat/o	prostate gland
phalang/o	phalanges (bones of the fingers and toes)	proxim/o	near, nearest
		pseudo-	false
pharmaceutic/o	drug, medicine	psych/o	mind
pharyng/o	pharynx (throat)	-ptosis	prolapse, downward displacement
-phasia	speech	ptyal/o	saliva
phe/o	dusky, dark	-ptysis	spitting
-phil	attraction for	pub/o	pubis (anterior part of the pelvic bone)
phil/o	attraction for		
-philia	attraction for	pulmon/o	lung
phim/o	muzzle	pupill/o	pupil
phleb/o	vein	py/o	pus

(continued)

Medical Word Elements—cont'd

Element	Meaning	Element	Meaning
pyel/o	renal pelvis	ser/o	serum
pylor/o	pylorus	sial/o	saliva, salivary gland
pyr/o	fire	sider/o	iron
		sigmoid/o	sigmoid colon
Q, R		silic/o	flint
		sin/o	sinus, cavity
quadri-	four	sinus/o	sinus, cavity
rachi/o	spine	-sis	state of; condition
radi/o	radiation, x-ray; radius (lower arm bone on the thumb side)	-social	society
		somat/o	body
radicul/o	nerve root	somn/o	sleep
rect/o	rectum	son/o	sound
ren/o	kidney	-spadias	slit, fissure
reticul/o	net, mesh	-spasm	involuntary contraction, twitching
retin/o	retina	sperm/i	spermatozoa, sperm cells
retro-	backward, behind	sperm/o	spermatozoa, sperm cells
rhabd/o	rod shaped (striated)	spermat/o	spermatozoa, sperm cells
rhabdomy/o	rod-shaped (striated) muscle	sphygm/o	pulse
rhin/o	nose	-sphyxia	pulse
rhytid/o	wrinkle	spin/o	spine
roentgen/o	x-rays	spir/o	breathe
-rrhage	bursting forth (of)	splen/o	spleen
-rrhagia	bursting forth (of)	spondyl/o	vertebrae (backbone)
-rrhaphy	suture	squam/o	scale
-rrhea	discharge, flow	staped/o	stapes
-rrhexis	rupture	-stasis	standing still
-rrhythm/o	rhythm	steat/o	fat
rube/o	red	sten/o	narrowing, stricture
		-stenosis	narrowing, stricture
S		stern/o	sternum (breastbone)
		steth/o	chest
sacr/o	sacrum	sthen/o	strength
salping/o	tube (usually the fallopian or eustachian [auditory] tube)	stigmat/o	point, mark
		stomat/o	mouth
-salpinx	tube (usually the fallopian or eustachian [auditory] tube)	-stomy	forming an opening (mouth)
		sub-	under, below
sarc/o	flesh (connective tissue)	sudor/o	sweat
-sarcoma	malignant tumor of connective tissue	super-	upper, above
		super/o	upper, above
scapul/o	scapula (shoulder blade)	supra-	above; excessive; superior
-schisis	a splitting	sym-	union, together, joined
schiz/o	split	syn-	union, together, joined
scler/o	hardening; sclera (white of the eye)	synapt/o	synapsis, point of contact
scoli/o	crooked, bent	synov/o	synovial membrane, synovial fluid
-scope	instrument for examining		
scop/o	to view	**T**	
-scopy	visual examination		
scot/o	darkness	tachy-	rapid
seb/o	sebum, sebaceous	tax/o	order, coordination
semi-	one-half	-taxia	order, coordination
semin/o	semen; seed	tele/o	distant
semin/i	semen; seed	ten/o	tendon
sept/o	septum	tend/o	tendon
sequestr/o	separation		

Medical Word Elements—cont'd

Element	Meaning	Element	Meaning
tendin/o	tendon	uln/o	ulna (lower arm bone on the opposite side of the thumb)
-tension	to stretch	ultra-	excess, beyond
test/o	testis (plural, testes)	-um	structure, thing
thalam/o	thalamus	umbilic/o	umbilicus, navel
thalass/o	sea	ungu/o	nail
thec/o	sheath (usually referring to the meninges)	uni-	one
thel/o	nipple	ur/o	urine, urinary tract
therapeut/o	treatment	ureter/o	ureter
-therapy	treatment	urethr/o	urethra
therm/o	heat	-uria	urine
thorac/o	chest	urin/o	urine, urinary tract
-thorax	chest	-us	condition; structure
thromb/o	blood clot	uter/o	uterus (womb)
thym/o	thymus gland	uvul/o	uvula
-thymia	mind; emotion		
thyr/o	thyroid gland	**V, W**	
thyroid/o	thyroid gland		
tibi/o	tibia (larger bone of the lower leg)	-verse	to turn
		vagin/o	vagina
-tic	pertaining to	valv/o	valve
-tocia	childbirth, labor	valvul/o	valve
tom/o	to cut	varic/o	dilated vein
-tome	instrument to cut	vas/o	vessel; vas deferens; duct
-tomy	incision	vascul/o	vessel (usually blood or lymph)
ton/o	tension		
tonsill/o	tonsils	ven/o	vein
tox/o	poison	ventr/o	belly, belly side
-toxic	pertaining to poison	ventricul/o	ventricle (of the heart or brain)
toxic/o	poison		
trabecul/o	trabecula (supporting bundles of fibers)	-version	turning
		vertebr/o	vertebrae (backbone)
trache/o	trachea (windpipe)	vesic/o	bladder
trans-	across, through	vesicul/o	seminal vesicle
tri-	three	vest/o	clothes
trich/o	hair	viscer/o	internal organs
trigon/o	trigone (triangular region at the base of the bladder)	vitr/o	vitreous body (of the eye)
		vitre/o	glassy
-tripsy	crushing	vol/o	volume
-trophy	development, nourishment	voyeur/o	to see
-tropia	turning	vulv/o	vulva
-tropin	stimulate		
tubercul/o	a little swelling	**X, Y, Z**	
tympan/o	tympanic membrane (eardrum)		
		xanth/o	yellow
U		xen/o	foreign, strange
		xer/o	dry
-ula	small, minute	xiph/o	sword
-ule	small, minute	-y	condition; process

English Terms

Meaning	Element	Meaning	Element
A		backward, behind	retro-
		bacteria (singular, bacterium)	bacteri/o
abdomen	abdomin/o, lapar/o	bad	mal-
abnormal condition (produced by something specified)	-iasis	bad; painful; difficult	dys-
		band, fascia (fibrous membrane supporting and separating muscles)	fasci/o
abnormal condition; increase (used primarily with blood cells)	-osis	base (alkaline, opposite of acid)	bas/o
above, upon	epi-	before, in front of	ante-, pre-, pro-
above; excessive; superior	supra-	beginning	-arche
acid	acid/o	belly, belly side	ventr/o
acromion (projection of the scapula)	acromi/o	below, under	infra-
		between	inter-
across, through	trans-	bile duct	choledoch/o
act of leading, bringing, conducting	-duction	bile vessel	cholangi/o
		bile, gall	bil/i, chol/e
act of measuring	-metry	binding, fixation (of a bone or joint)	-desis
adenoids	adenoid/o		
adrenal glands	adren/o, adrenal/o	birth	nat/o
after, behind	post-	black	melan/o
against	anti-	bladder	cyst/o, vesic/o
against, opposite	contra-	blood	hem/o, hemat/o
against; up; back	ana-	blood clot	thromb/o
air	aer/o	blood condition	-emia
air; lung	pneum/o, pneumon/o	blood vessel	hemangi/o
albumin (protein)	albumin/o	blue	cyan/o
all	pan-	body	corp/o, corpor/o, somat/o
alveolus; air sac	alveol/o		
amnion (amniotic sac)	amni/o	bone	oste/o
aneurysm (widened blood vessel)	aneurysm/o	bone marrow; spinal cord	myel/o
		brain	encephal/o
angle	goni/o	breast	mamm/o, mast/o
anterior, front	anter/o	breathe	spir/o
anus	an/o	breathing	-pnea
anus, rectum	proct/o	bronchiole	bronchiol/o
aorta	aort/o	bronchus (plural, bronchi)	bronch/o, bronchi/o
appendix	append/o, appendic/o	bursting forth (of)	-rrhage, -rrhagia
appetite	-orexia		
arm	brachi/o	**C**	
around	circum-, peri-		
arteriole	arteriol/o	calcaneum (heel bone)	calcane/o
artery	arteri/o	calcium	calc/o
asbestos	asbest/o	cancer	carcin/o
atrium	atri/o	carbon dioxide (CO$_2$)	-capnia
attraction for	-phil, phil/o, -philia	carpus (wrist bones)	carp/o
away from	ef-	carrying, transmission	-phoresis
axis, axon	ax/o	cartilage	chondr/o
		cause	eti/o
B		cecum	cec/o
		cell	cyt/o, -cyte
back (of the body)	dors/o	cerebellum	cerebell/o
back (of the body), behind, posterior	poster/o	cerebrum	cerebr/o

English Terms—cont'd

Meaning	Element	Meaning	Element
cessation	de-	disease	path/o, -pathy
change, beyond	meta-	distant	tele/o
cheek	bucc/o	double	di-, dipl-, dipl/o
chemical; drug	chem/o	down	cata-
chest	pector/o, steth/o, thorac/o, -thorax	drug, medicine	pharmaceutic/o
childbirth, labor	-tocia	dry	xer/o
choking pain	angin/o	dry, scaly	ichthy/o
chorion	chori/o	dull, dim	ambly/o
choroid	choroid/o	duodenum (first part of the small intestine)	duoden/o
ciliary body of the eye; circular; cycle	cycl/o	dura mater; hard	dur/o
clavicle (collar bone)	clavicul/o	dusky, dark	phe/o
clothes	vest/o	dust	coni/o
clumping, gluing	agglutin/o	**E**	
coal, coal dust	anthrac/o	ear	aur/o, auricul/o, ot/o
coccyx (tailbone)	coccyg/o	electricity	electr/o
cochlea	cochle/o	embolus (plug)	embol/o
cold	cry/o	embryonic cell	-blast, blast/o
colon	col/o, colon/o	enlargement	mega-, megal/o, -megaly
color	chrom/o, chromat/o	epididymis	epididym/o
conceiving	-ception	epiglottis	epiglott/o
condition	-esis, -ia, -ism	esophagus	esophag/o
condition; process	-y	excess, beyond	ultra-
condition; structure	-us	excessive, above normal	hyper-
condyle	condyl/o	excision, removal	-ectomy
conjunctiva	conjunctiv/o	extremity	acr/o
cornea	corne/o	eye	ocul/o, ophthalm/o
cortex	cortic/o	eye, vision	opt/o, optic/o
cranium (skull)	crani/o	eyelid	blephar/o
crooked, bent	scoli/o	**F**	
cross	cruci/o	face	faci/o
crushing	-tripsy	false	pseudo-
cul-de-sac	culd/o	far, farthest	dist/o
curve, swayback	lord/o	fat	adip/o, lip/o, lipid/o, steat/o
a cutting	-cision	fatty plaque	ather/o
D		fear	-phobia
darkness	scot/o	feeling	esthes/o, -esthesia
dawn (rose colored)	eosin/o	feeling (mental state)	-phoria
death, necrosis	necr/o	femur (thigh bone)	femor/o
decrease, deficiency	-penia	fiber, fibrous tissue	fibr/o
deficiency, under, below	hyp-, hyp/o	fibula (smaller bone of the lower leg)	fibul/o
development, nourishment	-trophy	fingers; toes	dactyl/o
diaphragm; mind	phren/o	fire	pyr/o
different	hetero-	first	primi-
digestion	-pepsia	fixation (of an organ)	-pexy
dilated vein	varic/o		
dilation, expansion	-ectasis		
discharge, flow	-rrhea		

(continued)

English Terms—cont'd

Meaning	Element	Meaning	Element
flesh (connective tissue)	sarc/o	heat, burn	cauter/o
flint	silic/o	hernia, swelling	-cele
foot	pod/o	hidden	crypt/o
foot; child	ped/i, ped/o	horny tissue; hard; cornea	kerat/o
foreign, strange	xen/o	humerus (upper arm bone)	humer/o
form, shape, structure	morph/o	humpback	kyph/o
formation, growth	plas/o, -plasia, -plasm		
formation, production	-poiesis	**I**	
forming an opening (mouth)	-stomy	ileum (third part of the small intestine)	ile/o
forming, producing, origin	-gen, gen/o, -genesis	ilium (lateral, flaring portion of the hip bone)	ili/o
four	quadri-	immune, immunity, safe	immun/o
from, away from	ab-	in, not	in-
fungus (plural, fungi)	myc/o	in, within	en-, end-, endo-, intra-
G		incision	-tomy
gallbladder	cholecyst/o	incomplete; imperfect	atel/o
ganglion (knot or knotlike mass)	gangli/o	inflammation	-itis
genetic change	mut/a	instrument for examining	-scope
genitalia	genit/o	instrument for measuring	-meter
gland	aden/o	instrument for recording	-graph
glans penis	balan/o	instrument to cut	-tome
glassy	vitre/o	insulin	insulin/o
glomerulus	glomerul/o	internal organs	viscer/o
glottis	glott/o	intestine (usually small intestine)	enter/o
glue; neuroglial tissue	gli/o, -glia	involuntary contraction, twitching	-spasm
gonads, sex glands	gonad/o	inward	eso-
good; normal	eu-	iris	irid/o
granule	granul/o	iron	sider/o
gray	glauc/o	irrigation, washing	-clysis
gray; gray matter (of the brain or spinal cord)	poli/o	ischium (lower portion of the hip bone)	ischi/o
green	chlor/o	**J, K**	
groin	inguin/o	jaundice	-icterus
growth	-physis	jejunum (second part of the small intestine)	jejun/o
gum(s)	gingiv/o	joint	arthr/o
H		kernel (nucleus)	kern/o
hair	pil/o, trich/o	ketone bodies (acids and acetones)	ket/o, keton/o
hallucination	hallucin/o	kidney	nephr/o, ren/o
hardening; sclera (white of the eye)	scler/o	killing	-cide
having the form of, possessing	-ate	knowing	gnos/o, -gnosis
head	cephal/o, -ceps	**L**	
hearing	acous/o, -acusia, -acusis, audi/o, audit/o, -cusia, -cusis	labyrinth (inner ear)	labyrinth/o
heart	cardi/o, coron/o	lacrimal sac	dacryocyst/o
heart condition	-cardia		
heat	therm/o		

English Terms—cont'd

Meaning	Element	Meaning	Element
lamina (part of the vertebral arch)	lamin/o	muscle	muscul/o, my/o, myos/o
large	macro-	muzzle	phim/o
larynx (voice box)	laryng/o		

N

Meaning	Element	Meaning	Element
lens	phac/o	nail	onych/o, ungu/o
lice	pedicul/o	narrowing, stricture	sten/o, -stenosis
life	bi/o	navel (umbilicus)	omphal/o
light	phot/o	near, beside; beyond	para-
limestone	chalic/o	near, nearest	proxim/o
lip	cheil/o, labi/o	neck; cervix uteri (neck of uterus)	cervic/o
liver	hepat/o		
lobe	lob/o	nerve	neur/o
loins (lower back)	lumb/o	nerve root	radicul/o
lower, below	infer/o	nest	nid/o
luminous, fluorescence	fluor/o	net, mesh	reticul/o
lung	pulmon/o	neutral; neither	neutr/o
lymph	lymph/o	new	neo-
lymph gland (node)	lymphaden/o	night	noct/o, nyctal/o
lymph vessel	lymphangi/o	nipple	thel/o
		nitrogenous compounds	azot/o

M

Meaning	Element	Meaning	Element
		none	nulli-
male	andr/o	nose	nas/o, rhin/o
malignant tumor of connective tissue	-sarcoma	not	im-
		noun ending	-a, -ice, -is
many, much	multi-, poly-	nucleus	kary/o, nucle/o
marketplace	agora-		

O

Meaning	Element	Meaning	Element
mastoid process	mastoid/o		
maxilla (upper jaw bone)	maxill/o	obscure	-opaque
meal	-prandial	old age	presby/o
mediastinum	mediastin/o	one	mono-, uni-
medulla	medull/o	one-half	hemi-, semi-
meninges (membranes covering the brain and spinal cord)	mening/o, meningi/o	opening, meatus	meat/o
		order, coordination	tax/o, -taxia
		other, differing from the normal	allo-
menses, menstruation	men/o		
metacarpus (hand bones)	metacarp/o	out, out from	ec-, ex-
metatarsus (foot bones)	metatars/o	outside	extra-
middle	medi-, medi/o, meso-	outside, outward	ecto-, exo-
		ovary	oophor/o, ovari/o
milk	galact/o, lact/o	oxygen	ox/i, ox/o, -oxia
milk	lact/o		

P

Meaning	Element	Meaning	Element
mind	ment/o, psych/o		
mind; emotion	-thymia	pain	-algesia, -algia, -dynia
monthly discharge of blood	menstr/o	palate (roof of the mouth)	palat/o
		pancreas	pancreat/o
mouth	or/o, stomat/o	paralysis	-plegia
movement	kinesi/o, -kinesia, kinet/o	parathyroid glands	parathyroid/o
		partial paralysis	-paresis
mucus	muc/o, myx/o		

(continued)

English Terms—cont'd

Meaning	Element	Meaning	Element
patella (kneecap)	patell/o	red	erythem/o, erythemat/o, erythr/o, rube/o
pelvis	pelv/i, pelv/o		
penis	pen/o		
perineum (area between the scrotum [or vulva in the female] and anus)	perine/o	renal pelvis	pyel/o
		repeated sound	echo-
		resembling	-oid
peritoneum	peritone/o	retina	retin/o
pertaining to	-ac, -al, -ar, -ary, -eal, -iac, -ic, -ical, -ile, -ine, -ior, -itic, -ive, -ory, -ous, -tic	rhythm	-rrhythm/o
		ribs	cost/o
		rod shaped (striated)	rhabd/o
		rod-shaped (striated) muscle	rhabdomy/o
pertaining to poison	-toxic	rupture	-rrhexis
pertaining to sugar	-ose	**S**	
phalanges (bones of the fingers and toes)	phalang/o		
pharynx (throat)	pharyng/o	sacrum	sacr/o
physician; treatment	iatr/o, -iatry	saliva	ptyal/o
pituitary gland	pituitar/o	saliva, salivary gland	sial/o
plaque	-plakia	same	homo-
pleasure	hedon/o	same, alike	home/o, homeo-
pleura	pleur/o	same, equal	iso-
point, mark	stigmat/o	scab	eschar/o
poison	tox/o, toxic/o	scale	squam/o
porous	-porosis	scanty	olig/o
potassium (an electrolyte)	kal/i	scapula (shoulder blade)	scapul/o
power	-potence	sea	thalass/o
pregnancy	-cyesis, gest/o	sebum, sebaceous	seb/o
pregnancy; childbirth	obstetr/o	secrete	crin/o, -crine
pregnant woman	-gravida	seed (ovum or spermatozoon)	gon/o
process (of)	-ation, -ization		
process of recording	-graphy	seizure	-lepsy
prolapse, downward displacement	-ptosis	self, own	auto-
		semen; seed	semin/o, semin/i
prostate gland	prostat/o	seminal vesicle	vesicul/o
protection	-phylaxis	separation	sequestr/o
protein	-globin	separation; destruction; loosening	-lysis
pubis (anterior part of the pelvic bone)	pub/o	septum	sept/o
		serum	ser/o
pulse	sphygm/o, -sphyxia	sheath (usually referring to the meninges)	thec/o
pupil	cor/o, core/o, pupill/o	short	brachy-
pus	py/o	side, to one side	later/o
pylorus	pylor/o	sigmoid colon	sigmoid/o
Q, R		sinus, cavity	sin/o, sinus/o
radiation, x-ray; radius (lower arm bone on the thumb side)	radi/o	skin	cutane/o, derm/o, -derma, dermat/o
		sleep	hypn/o, somn/o
rapid	tachy-	slipping	-listhesis
record, writing	-gram	slit, fissure	-spadias
rectum	rect/o	slow	brady-

English Terms—cont'd

Meaning	Element	Meaning	Element
small	micr/o, micro-	synapsis, point of contact	synapt/o
small growth	polyp/o	synovial membrane,	synov/o
small, minute	-icle, -ole, -ula, -ule	synovial fluid	
smell	-osmia		
smooth	lei/o	**T**	
smooth muscle (visceral)	leiomy/o	tail	caud/o
society	-social	tear; lacrimal apparatus	dacry/o, lacrim/o
sodium (an electrolyte)	natr/o	(duct, sac, or gland)	
softening	-malacia	teeth	dent/o, odont/o
sound	son/o	tendon	ten/o, tend/o,
specialist	-ician, -ist		tendin/o
specialist in the study of	-logist	tension	ton/o
speech	-phasia	testis (plural, testes)	orch/o, orchi/o,
speech, babble	-lalia		orchid/o, test/o
spermatozoa, sperm cells	sperm/i, sperm/o,	thalamus	thalam/o
	spermat/o	the act of	-ion
spine	rachi/o, spin/o	thick	pachy-
spitting	-ptysis	thin, slender	lept/o
spleen	splen/o	thirst	dips/o, -dipsia
split	schiz/o	three	tri-
a splitting	-schisis	through	per-
standing still	-stasis	through, across	dia-
stapes	staped/o	thymus gland	thym/o
star	astr/o	thyroid gland	thyr/o, thyroid/o
state of mental disorder,	-mania	tibia (larger bone of the	tibi/o
frenzy		lower leg)	
state of; condition	-ema, -isy, -sis	tissue	hist/o, histi/o
sternum (breastbone)	stern/o	to bear (offspring)	-para
stiffness; bent, crooked	ankyl/o	to break; surgical fracture	-clasia, -clasis, -clast
stimulate	-tropin	to carry	-ferent
stomach	gastr/o	to cut	tom/o
stone, calculus	-lith, lith/o	to go	-grade
straight	orth/o	to hold back	-continence
strength	sthen/o	to hold back; block	isch/o
stroke	-plexy	to inflate	emphys/o
structure, thing	-um	to lead; carry	duct/o
study of	log/o, -logy	to miscarry	abort/o
stupor; numbness; sleep	narc/o	to one side; side	later/o
sugar, sweetness	gluc/o, glucos/o,	to pull	ill/o
	glyc/o, glycos/o	to see	voyeur/o
surgical puncture	-centesis	to shine; clear	-lucent
surgical repair	-plasty	to steal	klept/o
suture	-rrhaphy	to stretch	-tension
swallowing, eating	phag/o, -phage,	to turn	-verse
	-phagia	to view	scop/o
sweat	hidr/o, sudor/o	toes, fingers	dactyl/o
swelling	-edema	tongue	gloss/o, lingu/o
a little swelling	tubercul/o	tonsils	tonsill/o
sword	xiph/o	toward	-ad, ad-, af-

(continued)

English Terms—cont'd

Meaning	Element	Meaning	Element
trabecula (supporting bundles of fibers)	trabecul/o	uterus (womb); measure	metr/o
trachea (windpipe)	trache/o	uvula	uvul/o
transplantation	-graft	**V**	
treatment	therapeut/o, -therapy	vagina	colp/o, vagin/o
tree	dendr/o	valve	valv/o, valvul/o
trigone (triangular region at the base of the bladder)	trigon/o	varied, irregular	poikil/o
		vein	phleb/o, ven/o
tube (usually the fallopian or eustachian [auditory] tube)	salping/o, -salpinx	ventricle (of the heart or brain)	ventricul/o
		vertebrae (backbone)	spondyl/o, vertebr/o
tumor	-oma, onc/o	vessel (usually blood or lymph)	angi/o, vascul/o
turning	-tropia, -version	vessel; vas deferens; duct	vas/o
two	bi-	view of	-opsy
tympanic membrane (eardrum)	myring/o, tympan/o	vision	-opia, -opsia
		visual examination	-scopy
U		vitreous body (of the eye)	vitr/o
		voice	-phonia
ulna (lower arm bone on the opposite side of the thumb)	uln/o	volume	vol/o
		vomiting	-emesis
		vulva	episi/o, vulv/o
umbilicus, navel	umbilic/o	**W, X, Y, Z**	
under, below	sub-	water	aque/o, hydr/o
under, below, deficient	hyp-, hyp/o, hypo-	weakness, debility	-asthenia
unequal, dissimilar	aniso-	white	albin/o, leuk/o
union, together, joined	sym-, syn-	widen, enlarge	mydr/o
unknown, peculiar	idi/o	without, not	a-, an-
upper, above	super-, super/o	woman, female	gyn/o, gynec/o
ureter	ureter/o	word, phrase	lex/o
urethra	urethr/o	wrinkle	rhytid/o
urine	-uria	x-rays	roentgen/o
urine, urinary tract	ur/o, urin/o	yellow	cirrh/o, jaund/o, xanth/o
uterus (womb)	hyster/o, metri/o, uter/o		

Index of Genetic Disorders

Index of Clinical, Laboratory, and Imaging Procedures

CLINICAL

LABORATORY

A

Antinuclear antibody, Chapter 9, Blood, Lymphatic, and Immune Systems, 289
Arterial blood gas, Chapter 7, Respiratory System, 200

B

Blood chemistry analysis, Chapter 4, Body Structure, 62
Blood culture, Chapter 9, Blood, Lymphatic, and Immune Systems, 289
Blood urea nitrogen, Chapter 11, Urinary System, 374

C, D

Cardiac biomarkers, Chapter 8, Cardiovascular System, 243
Cerebrospinal fluid analysis, Chapter 15, Nervous System, 542
Chorionic villus sampling, Chapter 12, Female Reproductive System, 413
Complete blood count
  Chapter 4, Body Structure, 62
  Chapter 9, Blood, Lymphatic, and Immune Systems, 289
Culture
  Chapter 6, Digestive System, 152
  Chapter 7, Respiratory System, 200
  Chapter 9, Blood, Lymphatic, and Immune Systems, 289
Culture and sensitivity
  Chapter 5, Integumentary System, 105
  Chapter 11, Urinary System, 374

E

Endometrial biopsy, Chapter 12, Female Reproductive System, 414

F

Fasting blood sugar, Chapter 14, Endocrine System, 496

G

Glucose tolerance test, Chapter 14, Endocrine System, 496

H

Hepatitis panel, Chapter 6, Digestive System, 152

I, J, K

Insulin tolerance test, Chapter 14, Endocrine System, 496

L

Lipid panel, Chapter 8, Cardiovascular System, 243
Liver function tests, Chapter 6, Digestive System, 152

M, N, O

Monospot, Chapter 9, Blood, Lymphatic, and Immune Systems, 289

P, Q, R

Pap test, Chapter 12, Female Reproductive System, 414
Papanicolaou test, Chapter 12, Female Reproductive System, 414
Partial thromboplastin time, Chapter 9, Blood, Lymphatic, and Immune Systems, 289
Prostate-specific antigen, Chapter 13, Male Reproductive System, 448, 452
Prothrombin time, Chapter 9, Blood, Lymphatic, and Immune Systems, 289

S

Semen analysis, Chapter 13, Male Reproductive System, 453
Serum bilirubin, Chapter 6, Digestive System, 152
Sputum culture, Chapter 7, Respiratory System, 200
Stool culture, Chapter 6, Digestive System, 152
Stool guaiac, Chapter 6, Digestive System, 152
Sweat test, Chapter 7, Respiratory System, 200

T

Throat culture, Chapter 7, Respiratory System, 200
Thyroid function test, Chapter 14, Endocrine System, 496
Total calcium test, Chapter 14, Endocrine System, 496

U, V, W, X, Y, Z

Urinalysis, Chapter 11, Urinary System, 374

IMAGING

Index of
Pharmacology

Index of Oncological Terms

Index of Discontinued Abbreviations and Eponyms

Discontinued Abbreviations

The Joint Commission (JC) and the Institute for Safe Medication Practices (ISMP) report that the following abbreviations are commonly misinterpreted and have resulted in harmful medical errors. Both organizations have compiled a comprehensive "Do Not Use" list (available on their websites) for health-care providers.

To prevent harmful medical errors from occurring, both organizations recommend discontinuance of those abbreviations. Instead, the abbreviations should be written out. Nevertheless, some of the abbreviations on the "Do Not Use" list are still used by health-care providers. This table lists these abbreviations, along with their meanings.

Abbreviation	Meaning	Abbreviation	Meaning
Medication and Therapy Time Schedule		*Other Related Abbreviations*	
a.c.	before meals	AD	right ear
b.i.d.	twice a day	AS	left ear
hs	half strength	AU	both ears
h.s.	at bedtime	cc	cubic centimeter, same as mL (1/1000 of a liter)
NPO, n.p.o.	nothing by mouth		
p.c.	after meals		*Use mL for milliliters or write out the meaning.*
p.o.	by mouth		
p.r.n.	as required	dc, DC, D/C	discharge; discontinue
qAM	every morning	OD	right eye
q.d.	every day	OS	left eye
q.h.	every hour	OU	both eyes
q.2h.	every 2 hours	subcu, Sub-Q, subQ	subcutaneous (injection)
q.i.d.	four times a day		
q.o.d.	every other day	U	unit
qPM	every evening		
t.i.d.	three times a day		

Discontinued Eponyms

The *International Classification of Diseases*, 10th edition, Clinical Modification (ICD-10-CM) contains the use of eponyms when assigning certain codes for diagnoses and procedures. However, all surgical eponyms have been removed from the *International Classification of Diseases*, 10th edition, Procedure Coding System (ICD-10-PCS). In their place are root terms that describe the objective of the procedure and other parameters to assign proper codes. The ICD-10-PCS procedural codes are more specific and clinically accurate, and they have a more logical structure than the previous coding systems. There are still some diagnostic eponyms in ICD-10-PCS, but most have been replaced with constructed terms that identify the diseases or conditions. This table lists common eponyms, along with ICD-10-PCS constructed words and where each eponym appears in this textbook.

Eponyms	ICD-10-PCS Constructed Word*	Systems, 8th Edition
Addison disease	corticoadrenal insufficiency	Chapter 14, Endocrine System, 489
Alzheimer disease	cerebral degeneration	Chapter 15, Nervous System, 532
Bell palsy	facial nerve palsy	Chapter 15, Nervous System, 536
Bowen disease	carcinoma in situ of skin	Chapter 5, Integumentary System, 97, 99
Colles fracture	fracture of lower end of radius	Chapter 10, Musculoskeletal System, 330
Crohn disease	regional enteritis	Chapter 6, Digestive System, 149
Cushing syndrome	adrenal hyperplasia resulting from excess adrenocorticotropic hormone (ACTH)	Chapter 14, Endocrine System, 489–490
Down syndrome	trisomy 21	Chapter 12, Female Reproductive System, 412
Graves disease	autoimmune hyperthyroidism	Chapter 14, Endocrine System, 488
Guillain-Barré syndrome	infective or idiopathic polyneuritis	Chapter 15, Nervous System, 533
Heberden nodes	generalized osteoarthrosis of hand	Chapter 10, Musculoskeletal System, 330
Hodgkin disease	classical Hodgkin lymphoma	Chapter 9, Blood, Lymphatic, and Immune Systems, 287
Huntington chorea	neurodegenerative genetic disorder	Chapter 15, Nervous System, 533
Kaposi sarcoma	malignant neoplasm of soft tissue	Chapter 9, Blood, Lymphatic, and Immune Systems, 287
Ménière disease	endolymphatic/labyrinthine hydrops	Chapter 16, Special Senses, 579
Parkinson disease	paralysis agitans	Chapter 15, Nervous System, 538
Paget disease	osteitis deformans	Chapter 10, Musculoskeletal System, 334
Reye syndrome	acute noninflammatory encephalopathy and fatty degenerative liver failure	Chapter 15, Nervous System, 538
Wilms tumor	nephroblastoma	Chapter 11, Urinary System, 372
Surgical/Dx Procedures		
Mohs	micrographic surgery	Chapter 5, Integumentary System, 106
Roux-en-Y gastric bypass (RGB)	gastric bypass with gastroenterostomy	Chapter 6, Digestive System, 156
Doppler ultrasonography	ultrasonography using sound pitch	Chapter 8, Cardiovascular System, 243
Rinne tuning fork test	air and bone conduction hearing test	Chapter 16, Special Senses, 583
Weber tuning fork test	conductive and sensorineural hearing loss test	Chapter 16, Special Senses, 583

* The compliance date for implementation of ICD-10-CM/PCS was October 1, 2015, for all entities covered by the Health Insurance Portability and Accountability Act (HIPAA).

Index

W

X

Y

Z

Rules for Singular and Plural Suffixes

This table presents common singular suffixes, the rules for forming plurals, and examples of each.

Rule		Example	
Singular	**Plural**	**Singular**	**Plural**
-*a*	Retain *a* and add *e*.	pleur*a*	pleur*ae*
-*ax*	Drop *x* and add *ces*.	thor*ax*	thora*ces*
-*en*	Drop *en* and add *ina*.	lum*en*	lum*ina*
-*is*	Drop *is* and add *es*.	diagnos*is*	diagnos*es*
-*ix*	Drop *ix* and add *ices*.	append*ix*	append*ices*
-*ex*	Drop *ex* and add *ices*.	ap*ex*	ap*ices*
-*ma*	Retain *ma* and add *ta*.	carcino*ma*	carcino*mata*
-*on*	Drop *on* and add *a*.	gangli*on*	gangli*a*
-*um*	Drop *um* and add *a*.	bacteri*um*	bacteri*a*
-*us*	Drop *us* and add *i*.	bronch*us*	bronch*i*
-*y*	Drop *y* and add *ies*.	deformit*y*	deformit*ies*